BIOCHEMICAL MODULATION of SKIN REACTIONS

Transdermals, Topicals, Cosmetics

Preface

Irritant and allergic contact dermatitis have been a major problem in the topical application to the skin of drugs, cosmetics, or cosmeceuticals. In addition, contact dermatitis is an important occupational health hazard, causing a range of chronic and long-lasting debilitating skin conditions, which the Department of Occupational Safety and Health Agency has rated as the second most common reason for loss of work time. The irritating or sensitizing properties of such occupational toxic agents, cosmetics, and drugs, such as alpha hydroxy acids, clonidine, detergents, diphenhydramine, fragrances, nickel, nicotine, propranolol, p-aminobenzoic acid, phenylaniline, retinoic acid, and many others, have been well documented.

Dermal and especially transdermal delivery of drugs have been hampered by the realization that most drugs, as well as many excipients used in the manufacture of transdermal patches, cause skin irritation or skin sensitization. Since the skin is also an excellent barrier to drug permeation, percutaneous enhancers have been used in most cases to increase drug permeation. Enhancers alter the skin lipid bilayer, thus opening channels for increased permeation of the drug. The alteration of the lipid bilayer causes irritation that is proportional to the degree of lipid bilayer destruction. Thus, irritation and sensitization are the primary limitations in the delivery of drugs to and through the skin. There are more than ten companies primarily involved in the transdermal delivery of drugs, and every large pharmaceutical company has ongoing transdermal delivery programs. Despite this effort and 15 years after the introduction of the nitroglycerin patch, there are only seven transdermal drugs in the marketplace.

Although contact dermatitis is accepted as being a serious problem, until recently the use of protective gloves or hypoallergenic gloves was the only approach recommended to prevent contact dermatitis and the use of steroids to reduce its symptoms. In the last few years, in several academic and industrial laboratories, work has been ongoing to develop biochemical modulators to reduce or abrogate skin reactions, and over 70 patents (see Chapter 14 for patent literature review) have already been issued. At the same time, the science of skin immunology has rapidly evolved where many of the processes underlying irritant and allergic contact dermatitis are beginning to be understood.

This book is an attempt to bring together the knowledge that has been gained the last few years in the field of contact dermatitis, with emphasis on the use of biochemical modulators to abrogate skin reactions. In the initial part of the volume, we have attempted to offer a concise, readable, and in-depth presentation of the basic concepts of topical drug delivery, the structure and function of the skin, the fundamentals and test methods for irritation, sensitization, and phototoxicity, and finally an overview of the mechanisms of allergic and irritant contact dermatitis.

The second part of the volume examines in depth the numerous cellular and molecular factors involved in the development of irritation and sensitization. Separate chapters are presented for Langerhans cells, keratinocytes, T lymphocytes, mast cells, cytokines, and the proinflammatory mediators of the arachidonic acid cascade. The chapters were written by world-renowned authorities in these subjects, who have had a hand in shaping our knowledge in the field.

The third part of the volume presents eight chapters describing different biochemical modulators that can be used to minimize and/or abrogate skin reactions. These chapters would be of greater interest to the pharmaceutical, cosmetic, or occupational health formulation scientists, since they distill the knowledge to specific and practical recommendations.

The final chapter addresses the future prospects and new avenues for study that would allow for exciting new solutions. Dr. Streilein has written a very insightful and challenging chapter, which (although controversial in some ways, as it should be) would allow for out-of-the-box thinking for the researchers in the field.

It is our belief that this volume will fill an unmet need for the audience in the fields of cosmetics, occupational health, dermatology, and especially transdermal drug delivery. It is our hope that the book will also serve as a catalyst for further research in the field and the discovery of better and more potent ways of abrogating irritation and sensitization. This, for example, will allow for many more drugs to be delivered transdermally and the transdermal route of drug administration to enter the mainstream of drug delivery.

Last, we would like to thank the chapter authors for their guidance and encouragement, as well as for their cooperation in adhering to the strict manuscript specifications.

Agis F. Kydonieus

John J. Wille

Editors

Agis F. Kydonieus is President of Samos Phamaceuticals, LLC, Princeton, NJ, a company involved in consulting and development of biomaterials, medical devices, skin care, and drug delivery products. Previously he served as Vice President of Corporate R&D at Convatec, a Bristol-Myers Squibb Company, and President of Hercon Laboratories, a transdermal delivery company. The holder of 30 U.S. patents, he is the author or co-author of over 100 publications and the editor of ten books. Dr. Kydonieus is a co-founder of the Controlled Release Society and Krikos and a member of numerous scientific societies. He received his B.S.Ch.E. summa cum laude (1959) and doctoral degree (1964) in chemical engineering from the University of Florida, Gainesville.

John J. Wille is currently President and Chief Operating Officer of *Hy-Gene, Incorporated*, Ventura, CA, a skin and wound care company. He received a B.A. in zoology from Cornell University, Ithaca, NY, and a doctoral degree in cell biology/genetics from Indiana University, Bloomington, with advanced postgraduate training in biophysics and theoretical biology at the Argonne National Laboratory and the University of Chicago. He has served as professor of cell and molecular biology at the University of Cincinnati, Louisiana State University, and the Mayo Medical School. He was head of cell biology at the Southern Research Institute and later was director of skin and biomaterials research, Bristol-Myers Squibb-Convatec in Skillman, NJ. Dr. Wille is one of the world authorities on the mammalian cell cycle and human keratinocyte cell biology, and is a leading authority on skin and wound care technologies. He has published more than 200 papers, books, and abstracts and holds more than 15 U.S. and foreign patents.

Contributors

Alfred Amkraut, Ph.D.
3358 Kenneth Drive
Palo Alto, CA

Saqib J. Bashir, B.Sc., M.B., Ch.B.
Dept. of Dermatology
University of California
School of Medicine
San Francisco, CA

Nancy Berna, M.S.
Dept. of Histology-Embryology
Facultes Universitaires Notre-Dame de la Paix
Namur, Belgium

Bret Berner, Ph.D.
Cygnus, Inc.
Redwood City, CA

Alain Coquette, Ph.D.
Dept. of Biology
SGS Biopharma SA
Wavre, Belgium

Michel Cormier, Ph.D.
Alza Corporation
Palo Alto, CA

Ralf W. Denfeld, M.D.
Dept. of Dermatology
Albert-Ludwigs University
Freiburg, Germany

Charles A. Dinarello, M.D.
Division of Infectious Diseases
Dept. of Medicine
University of Colorado Health Science Center
Denver, CO

Thomas J. Franz, M.D.
Connetics Corporation
Palo Alto, CA

Anthony A. Gaspari, M.D.
Dept. of Dermatology and Cancer Center
University of Rochester School of Medicine
  and Dentistry
Rochester, NY

Gary S. Hahn, M.D.
Immunology and Allergy Division
Dept. of Pediatrics
University of California, San Diego
and Cosmederm Technologies
La Jolla, CA

B. Homey, M.D.
Dept. of Dermatology
Heinrich-Heine University
Duesseldorf, Germany

Kouichi Ikai, M.D.
Dept. of Dermatology
Kyoto University Graduate School of Medicine
Kyoto, Japan

Richard S. Kalish, M.D., Ph.D.
Dept. of Dermatology
State University of New York at Stony Brook
Stony Brook, NY

Agis F. Kydonieus, Ph.D.
Samos Pharmaceuticals, LLC
Kendall Park, NJ

Paul A. Lehman, M.S.
Dermatopharmacology Laboratory
University of Arkansas for Medical Sciences
Little Rock, AR

P. Lehmann, M.D.
Dept. of Dermatology
Heinrich-Heine University
Duesseldorf, Germany

Howard I. Maibach, M.D.
Dept. of Dermatology
University of California
School of Medicine
San Francisco, CA

Sharmila Masli, Ph.D.
Schepens Eye Research Institute and
Department of Dermatology
Harvard Medical School
Boston, MA

James Matriano, Ph.D.
Alza Corporation
Palo Alto, CA

Bozena B. Michniak, Ph.D.
Dept. of Basic Pharmaceutical Sciences
College of Pharmacy
University of South Carolina
Columbia, SC

Marcia R. Monteiro, M.D.
Division of Diagnostic and Experimental
  Dermatopathology
Dept. of Pathology, Anatomy, and Cell Biology
Jefferson Medical College
Philadelphia, PA

George F. Murphy, M.D.
Division of Diagnostic and Experimental
  Dermatopathology
Dept. of Pathology, Anatomy, and Cell Biology
Jefferson Medical College
Philadelphia, PA

Norbert J. Neumann, M.D.
Dept. of Dermatology
Heinrich-Heine University
Duesseldorf, Germany

Mark R. Pittelkow, M.D.
Dept. of Dermatology, Biochemistry, and
  Molecular Biology
Mayo Clinic
Rochester, MN

Yves Poumay, Ph.D.
Dept. of Histology-Embryology
Facultes Universitaires Notre-Dame de la Paix
Namur, Belgium

Jan C. Simon, M.D.
Dept. of Dermatology
Albert-Ludwigs University
Freiburg, Germany

J. Wayne Streilein, M.D.
Schepens Eye Research Institute and
Department of Dermatology
Harvard Medical School
Boston, MA

Stephen E. Ullrich, Ph.D.
Dept. of Immunology
M.D. Anderson Cancer Center
University of Texas
Houston, TX

H. W. Vohr, M.D.
Research Toxicology
Bayer AG
Wuppertal, Germany

Paul Wakem, Ph.D.
Dept. of Dermatology
University of Rochester School of Medicine
  and Dentistry
Rochester, NY

Philip W. Wertz, Ph.D.
Dows Institute
University of Iowa
Iowa City, IA

John J. Wille, Ph.D.
Bioderm Technologies, Inc.
Trenton, NJ

Donald R. Wilson, M.S.
Cygnus, Inc.
Redwood City, CA

Table of Contents

SECTION III: BIOCHEMICAL MODULATORS AND MODES OF ACTION

Section I

Introduction and General Considerations

1 Fundamental Concepts in Transdermal Delivery of Drugs

Agis F. Kydonieus, John J. Wille, and George F. Murphy

CONTENTS

I. INTRODUCTION

Controlled release may be defined as a technique or method in which active chemicals are made available to a specified target at a rate and duration designed to accomplish an intended effect. Transdermal drug delivery can, therefore, be defined as the controlled release of drugs through intact skin, to obtain therapeutic levels systemically and to affect specified targets for the control of, for example, hypertension, pain, and addictive behavior. Dermal drug delivery is similar to transdermal delivery except that the specified target is the skin itself.

In this chapter, we will discuss the transdermal delivery of drugs, as it has the capability to produce several products with billion dollar potential. Most concepts, however, are equally applicable to dermal delivery. In addition, the immunologic concepts and approaches to the modulation of sensitization and irritation discussed in this volume are pertinent not only to the topical delivery of drugs, but to cosmetic and other applications whereby chemicals come in contact with intact skin.

II. RATIONALE FOR TRANSDERMAL CONTROLLED RELEASE MEDICATION

During the last 15 years, controlled release technology has received increasing attention in the face of a growing awareness that substances ranging from drugs to agricultural chemicals are frequently excessively toxic and sometimes ineffective when administered or applied by conventional means. Thus, conventionally administered drugs in the form of pills, capsules, injectables, and ointments are introduced into the body as pulses that usually produce large fluctuations of drug concentrations in the bloodstream and tissues and, consequently, unfavorable patterns of efficacy and toxicity.

The process of molecular diffusion through polymers and synthetic membranes has been used as an effective and reliable means of attaining transdermal controlled release of drugs and pharmacologically active agents. Central to the development of transdermal controlled delivery systems is the synthesis of the principles of molecular transport in polymeric materials and those of pharmacokinetics and pharmacodynamics. In transdermal drug delivery, pharmacokinetics is an important consideration because target tissues are seldom directly accessible, and drugs must be transported from the portal of entry on the body through a variety of biological interfaces to reach the desired receptor site. During this transport process, the drug can undergo severe biochemical degradation and, thereby, produce a delivery pattern at the receptor site that differs markedly from the pattern of drug release into the system.

A. Conventional Delivery vs. Transdermal Controlled Release of Medication

Conventionally, active agents are most often administered to a system by nonspecific, periodic applications. For example, in medical treatment, drugs are introduced at intervals by ingestion of pills or liquids or by injection. The drugs then circulate throughout much of the body, and the concentration of the active agent rises to high levels, systemwide, at least initially.[1] Both by injection and orally, the initially high concentrations may be toxic and cause side effects both to the target organ and neighboring structures. As time passes, the concentration diminishes, owing to natural metabolic processes, and a second dose must be administered to prevent the concentration from dropping below the minimum effective level. This situation is, of course, very inconvenient and difficult to monitor, and careful calculations of the amount of residual active agent must be made to avoid overdosing. The close attention required, together with the fact that large amounts of the drug are lost in the vicinity of the target organ, makes this type of delivery inefficient and costly. In addition, side effects owing to drugs misdirected to nontarget tissues are also possible.

The ideal transdermal administration provides a constant blood concentration, one that is effective but not toxic and is maintained for the desired time. Advantages of this system for therapeutic agents are (1) reproducible and prolonged constant delivery rate, (2) convenience of less frequent administrations, and (3) reduced side effects because the dose does not exceed the toxic level.

B. Advantages of Transdermal Drug Delivery

The advantages of transdermal medication indicated above are indeed great. However, transdermal systems can impart other important advantages to active agents that could be sufficient to elevate many products to commercial success. Table 1 lists a number of these advantages, the most important of which are discussed below.

1. Clinical Improvements

Transdermal delivery can increase the therapeutic value of many drugs by obviating specific problems associated with the drug. Such problems might include gastrointestinal irritation, low absorption, decomposition due to hepatic "first pass" effect, formation of metabolites that cause side effects, and short half-life necessitating frequent dosing. In transdermal medication, the above problems can be eliminated because the drug diffuses over a prolonged period of time directly into the bloodstream. An excellent example is that of nitroglycerin used in angina pectoris patients as a vasodilator. Nitroglycerin has a 90% hepatic "first pass" effect, so it could not be used orally to

TABLE 1
Some Advantages of Transdermal Medication

Bypass of hepatic "first pass" and gastrointestinal incompatibility
Reduction of side effects due to the optimization of the blood concentration–time profile
Provision of predictable and extended duration of activity
Greater patient compliance due to the elimination of multiple dosing schedules
Enhancement of therapeutic efficacy
Reduction of frequency of dosage
Reversibility of drug delivery which would allow for removal of the drug source
Minimization of inter- and intrapatient variation
Self-administration

prevent angina pectoris attacks. Its main use was as a sublingual pill to abort an attack after it occurred. With the advent of transdermal medication, nitroglycerin is now used as a patch to prevent angina pectoris attacks.

The transdermal delivery of the antihypertensive clonidine provides for a reduced side effect profile by lowering the daily dose required and eliminating peaking concentrations. Dry mouth and drowsiness, the two most important side effects of clonidine, are substantially reduced by transdermal therapy.[2,3] Reduction of side effects can also be accomplished for drugs that are substantially metabolized during the first pass through the liver.[4] Estradiol is a physiological hormone secreted by the ovaries, and it is used therapeutically for systemic estrogen replacement for postmenopausal women and prevention of osteoporosis. A once-daily oral bolus of estradiol has been likened to "hitting the liver with a hammer" every 24 hours, so marked are the hepatic proteins that result. These elevations have been postulated to cause certain serious side effects of exogenous estrogens, including hypertension, hyperlipidemia, and hypercoagulability.[5] Since the skin does not metabolize estradiol significantly, only 5% of the amount used in oral dosing is required, thus minimizing the side effects caused by the metabolite estrone.

2. Patient Compliance

Patient compliance is an important driver for better clinical outcomes and improved cost effectiveness. The practical importance of compliance is apparent. If the patient does not comply, the therapeutic goal is not achieved and the cost of drugs prescribed and not taken as well as the cost for emergency care required become enormous. In all cases where the effect of dosage regimen was studied with hypertensives, antiasthmatics, allergics, diabetics, cancer patients, ulcer patients, and the elderly, the conclusion was that once-per-day medication gave the best compliance.[6–12]

Lusher, in his studies with hypertensives, indicated that 60 to 75% of the patients were well-controlled, but one third to one fourth of the patients were noncompliant. He concluded that with the advent of potent antihypertensive drugs, noncompliance has become the most important limiting factor in the management of hypertension.[6]

Vandereychen, in his article on chronic illness behavior and noncompliance with treatment, concluded that improving adherence to treatment regimen may produce as great an impact upon disability and health as the development of ever-new biomedical assessment and treatment techniques, and may result in greater cost effectiveness of health care services.[13]

Transdermal patches can be made to last for up to 7 days. Patches that could last for 14 days or more are possible if the irritation caused by skin occlusion or by the drug and excipients could be eliminated. For example, the nitroglycerine patch for angina pectoris is administered once daily, the fentanyl patch for analgesia every 3 days, and the estradiol patch for hormone replacement and the clonidine patch for hypertension once per week. Although extensive studies of patient compliance with the patches have not been performed, they are very well tolerated and extremely successful

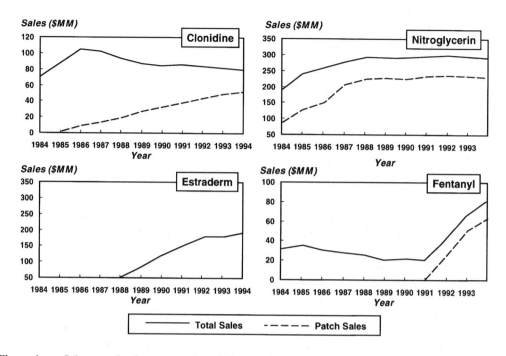

Figure 1   Sales growth of some transdermal therapeutic systems.

in the marketplace. Figure 1 shows the sales in the U.S. of the four transdermal patches mentioned above, as well as the total sales of all dosage forms. The performances of the transdermal patches are impressive. The nitroglycerine patch reached $250 million per year, 5 years after its introduction in 1982. The fentanyl patch rejuvenated a dying market of the oral fentanyl product. The performance of the clonidine and estradiol patches is equally as impressive.

3. Economic and Marketing Considerations

The cost of developing new drug entities, as well as the time it takes to bring such drugs to the marketplace, has been continuously increasing. Thus, in 1975 over $1 billion was spent in pharmaceutical research, and it took an average of 10 years and $60 million to bring a new drug to the marketplace.[14] By contrast, in 1995, almost $15 billion was spent in pharmaceutical research and it took about 12 years and $500 million to take a product from discovery to market.[15]

In transdermal delivery, you may start with a drug that is already approved; therefore, the risks, time to the marketplace, and the research costs are all substantially reduced. These costs will vary from organization to organization, but should not exceed $10 million and 5 years.

In the managed care environment, where cost containment is of primary importance, the development of 7-day transdermal patches of proprietary, as well as generic drugs, should prove cost-effective to health management and purchasing groups and therapeutically significant to the patient. Table 2 summarizes some of the driving reasons for the cost effectiveness of transdermal delivery. Therefore, when transdermal products were introduced into the market, as discussed earlier, they were met with great success.

Transdermal delivery presents marketing advantages to pharmaceutical companies as well. Some of the advantages include product differentiation, higher success rate, patentability and extension of patent coverage, and less time and lower cost to market. Recently, Bristol-Myers Squibb entered into a $40 million agreement ($15 million initial license payment) with the transdermal company Sano for the development of a buspirone patch for anxiety and attention deficit

TABLE 2
Cost Effectiveness of Transdermal Delivery

Finished product price same for oral or transdermal delivery for same course of treatment
Reduced cost due to better clinical outcome produced by improved patient compliance
   Extension of duration of drug activity
   Elimination of multiple dosing schedules
   Reduction of side effects due to optimization of blood concentration time profiles
Patient compliance outcome
   Reduction in emergency care costs
   Reduction in hospitalization costs

disorder. Buspirone is a $400 million/year proprietary Bristol-Myers Squibb drug that is facing a patent expiration issue.[16] It is not surprising, therefore, that a great number of patents (Table 3) are issued each year, trying to protect developments in the field.[17]

TABLE 3
Transdermal Drug Delivery Patents and Patent Applications

	Number of Patents			
	1994	**1995**	**1996**	**1997**
Delivery methods	81	146	143	139
Chemical enhancers	60	57	93	61
Physical enhancers (iontophoresis)	29	32	46	35
Anti-irritants/countersensitizers	11	6	9	8
Grand total	181	241	291	243

Data from the Japanese, European, World, and U.S. patent offices (Reference 17).

Notwithstanding the promise of transdermal drug delivery and the enormous amounts of research, only seven drug entities have been introduced into the U.S. market, due to some severe limitations.

C. LIMITATIONS OF TRANSDERMAL DELIVERY

Though the advantages of transdermal medication are impressive, the merits of each application have to be examined individually, and the positive and negative effects weighed carefully before large expenditures for developmental work are committed.

Only a small percentage of drugs can be delivered transdermally due to three limitations: difficulty of permeation through human skin, skin reactions, and clinical need. However, with the FDA approval of 7-day clonidine and estradiol patches, the clinical need might come in the form of convenience and greater patient compliance due to the elimination of multiple dosing schedules.

1. Skin Permeation

In addition to its use as a physical barrier, the human skin functions as a chemical barrier as well. The outermost layer of the skin, the stratum corneum, is an excellent barrier to almost all chemicals including drugs. The anatomy and biochemistry of skin are presented extensively in many books and review articles and they will not be discussed here.[18,19] It would suffice to say that if the dosage required is more than 10 mg/day, the delivery transdermally will be very difficult, if not impossible. Daily dosages of less than 2 to 3 mg/day are preferred. Thus, very few drugs can permeate this horny layer in sufficient amounts to deliver a therapeutic dose. As far as skin permeability is concerned, the physicochemical properties of the drug, in addition to its potency, will have to be taken into account. Thus drugs with low molecular weight, low melting point, and moderate oil and water solubility will permeate best. Proteins and peptides, even when extremely potent, cannot be delivered transdermally by passive diffusion. Table 4 summarizes the important criteria in selecting drugs that would have good probability of success.[20]

TABLE 4
Important Criteria in the Drug Selection Process

1. Marketing and economic consideration
   - Patent protection, patent infringement issues, drug patent expiration
   - Market potential, present cost of therapy, competition
2. Clinical rationale
   - Extend duration of activity and improve patient compliance
   - Reduce side effects to nontarget tissues
3. Skin acceptability considerations
   - Drug irritation profile
   - Drug sensitization profile
   - Drug metabolization profile
4. Drug administration considerations
   - Adequate skin permeability (melting point, molecular weight, partition coefficient)
   - Oral dosage and bioavailability considerations
   - Drug potency

Fortunately, skin permeation models and adequate experimental data exist that would allow one to make a reasonable prediction of the permeation of a specific drug through skin. One such model based on experimental data from 25 drugs has been presented in graphical form by Kasting and Cooper.[21] From their figure, the maximum, unenhanced flux of any drug can be determined just by knowing its molecular weight and melting point.

Another model based on experimental data developed a global expression for log K_p, the dermal permeability constant, which was only a function of the molecular weight and the log P (octanol/water) partition coefficient of the drug.[22] Magee modified the above expression to use MR (molar refraction) instead of molecular weight.[23]

$$\log K_p = 0.801 \log P - 0.0260\ MR - 2.71$$

He also developed equations with more predictive power for aliphatics and water, steroids, and phenols.[23]

Several other models based on mathematical algorithms have been proposed. For example, Albery and Hadgraft proposed a two-phase model and Berner and Cooper a two-parallel pathway model.[24,25] Guy and Hadgraft proposed a single-compartment model, Higuchi a multicompartment model, and Michaels et al. a brick model.[26–28]

The Berner and Cooper model combines a polar or aqueous pathway and a nonpolar lipophilic pathway. Equations can be derived where the maximum, unenhanced flux can be determined by knowing the molecular weight and melting point of the drug. The octanol/water partition coefficient also affects the flux, but substantially more weakly. Figure 2 presents graphically the solution of the Berner and Cooper equations assuming a log P (octanol/water) of 5.

a. Chemical Enhancers

A chemical enhancer can be defined as a compound that alters the skin barrier function so that a desired drug can permeate at a faster rate. The chemical enhancer by its presence in the stratum

Predictive Model for Skin Permeability

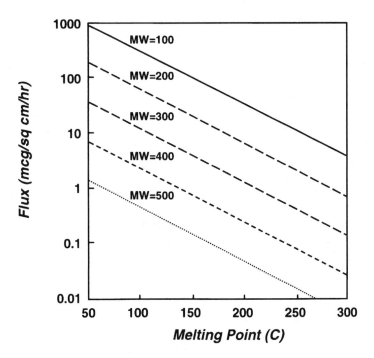

Figure 2   Berner-Cooper predictive model of skin permeability.

corneum could also increase permeation of the desired drug by increasing the concentration of the drug in the skin. Alcohols, amines and amides, amino acetates, sulfoxides, fatty acids, surfactants, urea and unsaturated cyclic ureas, terpenes, liposomes, and many other chemicals have been patented and tested as chemical enhancers.[29] Dozens of chemical enhancers are patented each year (see Table 3) and several books have been written summarizing the work and proposing mechanisms of enhancement.[29–31] However, most of the chemical enhancers cause skin reactions and they are thus limited in actual use. The mechanism of action and the skin reactions caused by some penetration enhancers have been summarized.[32]

b. Physical Enhancing Methods

There are several nonchemical methods that have been used to enhance drug permeation through skin. Iontophoresis, electroporation, and phonophoresis are the most promising methods, and they have been studied extensively. Reviews of all three methods have also been published.[33–35]

Iontophoresis is a process that involves the transport of charged molecules, including proteins and peptides, into the skin by the passage of a direct electric current through an electrolyte solution containing the charged molecules to be delivered, using an appropriate electrode polarity.[33] However, due to the increased transport of water, the flux of noncharged molecules is also enhanced.[36] The Nernst-Planck equation that describes the electrically facilitated transport of molecules through membranes suggests that any required dose of a drug can be delivered by simply increasing the electric current. This would be true if the movement of ionic species through the skin did not cause adverse effects such as uncomfortable and burning sensations, irritation, blister formation, and skin necrosis. These side effects can be minimized if the electric current is held below 0.2 to 0.5 mA/cm^2.[37] It has also been reported that the use of pulsed current reduces irritation potential.[38]

Ledger, as well as Molitor and Fernandez, reviewed the skin effects caused by transdermal iontophoretic delivery of drugs.[39,40]

Electroporation is another process presented recently to enhance skin permeation.[41] Electroporation involves the application of a brief electric field pulse to create aqueous pathways in the lipid bilayers and thus enhance permeation.[42] In contrast to iontophoresis where low current and long-term application of electrical current are required, in electroporation the electric field pulses generate transmembrane potentials of 1 V but last only for 10 µs to 10 ms.[42,43] It is thought that micropores are created with a diameter range of about 10 nm, which can exist for several hours and then disappear under reversible conditions.[44]

In in vivo rat studies with calcein, flux values of 10 to 20 $\mu g/cm^2/h$ were observed with no visible damage to the skin for voltages below 150 V, with erythema and edema being evident at higher voltages.[45] However, the same authors have indicated that it is difficult to ascertain which electrical conditions will be acceptable for clinical use, and many features, including pulse voltage/current/energy, pulse length, pulse frequency, duration of total exposure, and electrode size, site, and design, will be important.[46]

Phonophoresis, the application of ultrasound to increase the permeation of drugs through skin, has also been experimentally investigated. The mechanism for permeation enhancement is not well understood, but it appears to be due to ultrasonic perturbation and decrease in the activation energy of the barrier membrane.[47] In the skin, it has been concluded that phonophoresis affects both the polar and the nonpolar pathways.[48] Although it is known that for increased frequency up to 15 MHz the permeation is progressively enhanced, additional research is required for the development of a practical system, where the intensity, frequency, pulse, duration, permeation rate, and patient tolerance are optimized. As expected, at lower frequencies the treatment is well tolerated, but at higher frequencies, intensities, or duration, erythema, edema, blisters, and other adverse skin reactions are observed.[49–52]

2. Skin Reactions

A serious obstacle to dermal and transdermal delivery of drugs is the possibility of adverse skin reactions collectively known as irritant and contact allergic dermatitis. Irritants and sensitizers are often encountered in the workplace as occupational risks associated with hazardous corrosives, chemical accelerators, and other industrial chemicals. Still others come in daily contact with irritating and sensitizing chemicals in the home setting while working with household cleansers, textiles, jewelry, diaper urine, hair coloring dyes, and cosmetics. A rather severe form of contact dermatitis of the hands is prevalent, and 5 to 10% of all patients seen by dermatologists are diagnosed with hand eczema.[53–56]

In transdermal delivery, as discussed earlier, most drugs cannot be delivered transdermally because they do not permeate through skin in sufficient amounts to produce a therapeutic dose, and when chemical or physical permeation enhancers are used, in most cases, they also increase skin reactions. Drugs themselves cause adverse skin reactions in such a severe way that only seven transdermal products are being marketed in the U.S. after 20 years of research and development by dozens of companies. These include clonidine for the treatment of hypertension, fentanyl for the management of chronic pain, testosterone for replacement therapy, nicotine for smoking cessation, nitroglycerin for the prevention of angina pectoris, scopolamine for the prevention of motion sickness, and estradiol for postmenopausal symptoms and prevention of osteoporosis.

The book *Cutaneous Drug Reactions* is a compilation of skin reactions caused by drugs in general.[57] Delayed-type contact hypersensitivity responses are reported to occur for many topical medicaments surveyed by patch testing, including benzocaine, chlorpheniramine, diphenhydramine, neomycin sulfate, penicillin, promazine, and sulfanilamide.[58] Clinical testing on humans has shown that several antihistamines are sensitizers.[59]

a. Irritation

Generally, an irritant is a substance (e.g., soap) that causes an immediate (minutes to hours) and localized skin inflammatory response manifest as redness (erythema) and swelling (edema) that does not extend beyond the immediate area of original contact, nor does it cause the formation of memory cells.[60]

The main steps by which agents provoke irritant contact dermatitis include a neurological phase, a vascular phase, and a cellular phase. In the neurological phase, transient vasoconstriction occurs typically within 30 s of contact with the irritant. Vasodilation occurs within about 1 to 6 min of contact, followed by margination of neutrophils in the vessels and diapedesis, the outward passage of the corpuscular elements through intact vessel walls. The pathogenesis of irritation is not totally understood and the current understanding of the subject will be discussed in subsequent chapters. It will suffice to state here that almost all skin cells participate in the process either as the source of cytokines, leucotrienes, prostaglandins, and other inflammatory molecules, or as modulators of the process.

Table 5 lists several commercially significant drugs that are irritants.[61]

TABLE 5
Some Common Drugs That Are Topically Irritating

Drug Class	Drug Name
Ace inhibitor	Captopril
	Fostinopril
Antihypertensive	Prazosin
Cold medicine	Dimemorfan
Narcotic antagonist	Naltrexone
Nonsteroidal anti-inflammatory	Ketoproten
	Diclofenac
	Piroxicam
	Flurbiprofen
Several indications	Prostaglandin
Weight control	Mazindol
Antiacne/antiwrinkle	Retinoic acid
	α-Hydroxy acid
Antiseptic	Chlorhexidine
Enhancers	Propylene glycol, oleic acid, alcohol

In addition to drugs, examples of potential skin irritating agents include water, skin cleansers, cosmetics, industrial cleaning agents, alkalis, acids, oils, organic solvents, oxidizing agents, reducing agents, plant matter, animal matter, and combinations thereof.[62]

Current modalities of prevention include use of barrier creams, and protective and/or hypoallergenic gloves.[63,64] It is generally recognized that these approaches offer very limited short-term solutions to a range of chronic and long-lasting debilitating skin conditions that OSHA has rated as the second most common reason for loss of work time.[65] Therapeutic intervention is also limited to hydrocortisone creams, or a high potency topical steroid such as clobetasol.[66] Unfortunately, the very chronicity of eczema and the treatment time course involved in dermal and transdermal drug delivery argue against the chronic use of high potency steroids with their epidermal thinning and skin atrophying effects, loss of dermal mast cells, and general immunosuppressing effects. Hopefully the approaches discussed in Chapters 14 through 22 would allow for the use of a broader spectrum of biochemical modulators to prevent and treat irritation.

b. Sensitization

Allergic reactions of the skin known as sensitization or allergic contact dermatitis (ACD) are immune responses that occur in the skin. They are caused by the penetration of the skin by a foreign substance (e.g., hapten or antigen). ACD is a two-phase process involving an initiation (induction) phase followed by an elicitation phase. The former phase occurs immediately after first-time exposure of the skin to the hapten and is characterized by the formation of immune memory cells, that can subsequently recognize the specific hapten which previously entered the skin. The elicitation phase occurs when the skin is reexposed to the original hapten, and results in an overt but delayed hypersensitivity reaction.[55] Agents that cause ACD are varied and numerous and include, for example, metals (e.g., nickel, chromium, cobalt), fragrances, chemicals, cosmetics, textiles, pesticides, plastics, pollen, and the like.[54]

A major obstacle to the transdermal delivery of drugs is the development of allergic contact dermatitis. For example, transdermal delivery of clonidine causes contact dermatitis reactions in up to 20% of treated patients, as do most beta-blockers, antiasthmatics, and antihistamines that have been tested in humans.[67,68] Table 6 provides a list of commercially important drugs that are sensitizers.[61]

TABLE 6
Some Common Drugs That Are Topically Sensitizing

Class	Drug	1993 Sales ($ millions)
Beta blockers		>1,000
	Nadolol	120
	Timolol	5
	Metaprolol	248
Antihypertensive	Clonidine	>100
Antiasthmatic	Albuterol	>1,000
Antihistamines		1,427
	Clorpheniramine	368
	Diphenhydramine	142
Antianxiety		>1,000
	Alprazolam	624
	Lorazepam	>500
	Fluphenazine	

The sensitization process is not totally understood and the current understanding is discussed in several chapters in this volume. Below we present a hypothetical scheme (Figure 3) which appears to explain why the biochemical modulators discussed in Chapters 15 to 17 are effective.[68]

In this figure, sensitization is depicted to the left, and the challenge reaction (generally applied 10 to 14 days after sensitization of human skin) to the right. Antigen (depicted as cross-hatched triangles) contacts with the epidermal surface during sensitization (Step 1) and is taken up by Langerhans cells (LC; Step 2). These normally freely motile cells traffic via dermal lymphatics (Step 3) and migrate to draining lymph nodes (Step 4). The perivascular dermal connective tissue at this juncture (to the upper left of draining node) may contain low numbers of naive CD4 T cells ($CD4_n$) as well as mononuclear phagocytes and resting, nondegranulating mast cells (latter not shown). In the lymph node, the migrant antigen-containing LC present processed peptide signals to the $CD4_n$ T cells (4), imparting antigen-specific memory ($CD4_\Delta$; Step 5). Upon entering the

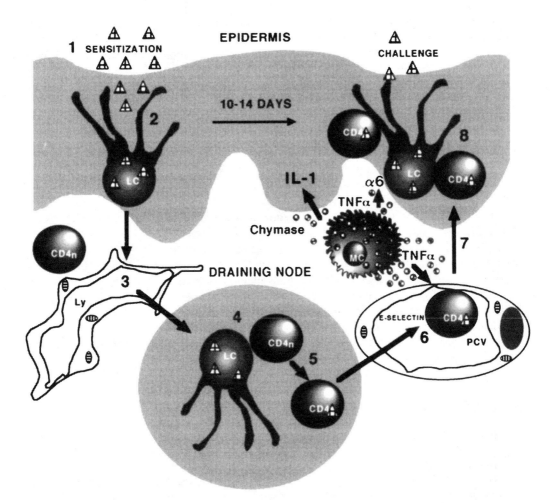

Figure 3   Hypothesis of processes involved in the induction and elicitation of skin immune response.

peripheral circulation, these newly formed $CD4_\Delta T$ cells constitute a small component of the total white blood cell population. During intranodal sensitization, experimental evidence in rodents suggests that another important event also may occur. This involves production of IgE-like, antigen-specific molecules by a second, as yet undefined population of nodal lymphocytes which also receive peptide signals from the antigen-presenting LC. These antibodies circulate and eventually become bound to the membranes of dermal mast cells (MC) situated in the perivascular space of postcapillary venules (PCV).

Upon epicutaneous challenge by the same antigen, several events are now primed to occur. Mast cells may interact with antigen by virtue of cross-linking of surface molecules in an IgE-like fashion. This cross-linking results in mast cell degranulation in the perivascular space of superficial dermal PCVs. TNF-α acutely released from the liberated mast cell granules triggers endothelial activation, with induction of a cascade of leukocyte-endothelial adhesion molecules. One of these, E-selectin, promotes binding of $CD4_\Delta$ to the endothelial surface (Step 6), with subsequent diapedesis into the dermal matrix and ultimately, via adhesive and chemotactic gradients, into the epidermal layer (Step 7). Such endothelial activation and $CD4_\Delta$ recruitment may also be facilitated by cleavage of epidermal interleukin-1 (IL-1) into its active form by the mast cell granule serine proteinase, chymase. Small numbers of pioneer $CD4_\Delta T$ cells now located within the superficial dermis and epidermis interact with processed antigenic peptides (Step 8) presented by LC fixed within the epidermis as an apparent consequence of altered motility. This may result in part from TNF-α–induced upregulation of LC cell surface integrins, such as a6, which promotes binding to basement membrane zone and soluble laminin. $CD4_\Delta T$ cells so stimulated produce and release a repertoire of TH1 cytokines which then drive the inflammatory response, recruiting secondarily responding mononuclear cells. These events correlate clinically and histopathologically with the fully evolved delayed hypersensitivity reaction.

III. SUMMARY

Transdermal delivery offers many advantages which can elevate drugs to significant commercial successes. Such advantages include patient compliance, elimination of side effects, and predictable and extended duration of activity.

There are two limitations which have prevented transdermal delivery from achieving its full potential. These limitations include adequate drug skin permeation to achieve therapeutic effectiveness, and skin reactions caused by the drug and other excipients when they are placed in contact with the skin. The skin permeation problem can be improved by the use of chemical enhancers, as well as physical enhancing methods including iontophoresis, electroporation, and phonophoresis. Unfortunately, when these enhancers are used at levels or intensities adequate to provide a substantial increase in drug permeation, they also potentiate skin reactions, such as skin irritation and sensitization.

Skin reactions are indeed the Achilles' heel of transdermal medication. It is hoped that this volume will provide some answers and impetus for further studies.

REFERENCES

1. Robinson, J. R., Controlled release pharmaceutical systems, in *Chemical Marketing and Economics Reprints*, Long, F. W., O'Neill, W. P., and Steward, R. D., Eds., American Chemical Society, Washington, D.C., 1976, 213.
2. Popli, S., Transdermal clonidine for hypertensive patients, *Clin. Therapy*, 5, 624, 1983.
3. McMahon, F., *Clinical Experience with Clonidine TTS, in Mild Hypertension*, Weber, M. and Mathias, C., Eds., Steinkopff Verlag, Darnstadt, Germany, 1984, 148.
4. Berner, B. and Kydonieus, A., Novel drug delivery systems, in *The Drug Development Process*, Welling, P. G., Ed., Marcel Dekker, New York, 1996.
5. Campbell, S. and Whitehead, M., *The Controversial Climacteric*, MTP Press, Lancaster, England, 1981, 103.
6. Lusher, T. and Vetter, W., *J. Human Hypertension*, 4, 43, 1990.
7. Ruggeri, S. et al., *J. Intern. Med. Res.*, 15, 170, 1987.
8. Bantz, E. et al., *Ann. Allergy*, 59, 341, 1987.
9. Pullan, T. et al., *Clin. Pharmacol. Therap.*, 44, 540, 1988.
10. Gritz, E. et al., *Preventive Med.*, 18, 711, 1989.
11. Bader, J., *J. Clin. Gastroenterol.*, 11, 525, 1989.
12. Stewart, R. et al., *Med. Clin. N. Am.*, 73 (6), 1551, 1989.
13. Vandereychen, J., *Psychother. Psychosom.*, 50, 182, 1988.
14. Katz, M., The birth pangs of a new drug, *Drug Cosmet. Ind.*, 40, 1980.
15. Anon., What Companies are Researching, Medical Adv. News supplement, *What's in the Pipeline*, 3, 1996.
16. *PR Newswire*, file p1103083.305, November 3, 1997.
17. Kydonieus, A., *Controlled Release Newsletter*, Roseman, T., Ed., 15(1) 12, 1998.
18. Bissett, D. L., Anatomy and biochemistry of skin, in *Transdermal Delivery of Drugs*, Kydonieus, A. and Berner, B., Eds., CRC Press, Boca Raton, FL, 1, 29, 1987.
19. Franz, T., Tojo, K., Shah, K., and Kydonieus, A., Transdermal delivery, in *Treatise on Controlled Drug Delivery*, Kydonieus, A., Ed., Marcel Dekker, New York, 1991, 341.

20. Franz, T., Tojo, K., Shah, K., and Kydonieus, A., Transdermal delivery, in *Treatise on Controlled Drug Delivery*, Kydonieus, A., Ed., Marcel Dekker, New York, 1991, 342.

21. Kasting, G. and Cooper, E., Effect of lipid solubility and molecular size on percutaneous absorption, in *Skin Pharmacokinetics*, Shroot, B. and Schaefer, H., Eds., S. Karger, Basel, 1987, 138.

22. Potts, R. O. and Guy R. H., Predicting skin permeability, *Pharm. Res.*, 9, 663, 1992.

23. Magee, P. S., Some new approaches to understanding and facilitating transdermal drug delivery, in *Percutaneous Penetration Enhancers*, Smith, E. W. and Maibach, H. I., Eds., CRC Press, Boca Raton, FL, 1995, 471.

24. Albery, W. J. and Hadgraft, J., Percutaneous absorption: theoretical description, *J. Pharm. Pharmacol.*, 31, 140, 1979.

25. Berner, B. and Cooper, E., Models of skin permeability, in *Transdermal Delivery of Drugs*, Kydonieus, A. and Berner, B., Eds., CRC Press, Boca Raton, FL, 2, 41, 1997.

26. Guy, R. H. and Hadgraft, J., Prediction of drug disposition kinetics in skin and plasma following topical administration, *J. Pharm. Sci.*, 73, 883, 1985.

27. Higuchi, W. I., Simultaneous transport and metabolism of β-estradiol in hairless mouse skin, *Therapeut. Res.*, 10, 149, 1989.

28. Michaels, A. S., Chandrasekaran, S. K., and Shaw, J. E., Drug permeation through human skin, *AICHE J.*, 21, 985, 1975.

29. Smith, E. W. and Maibach, H. I., *Percutaneous Penetration Enhancers*, CRC Press, Boca Raton, FL, 1995.

30. Hsieh, D. S., *Drug Permeation Enhancement*, Marcel Dekker, New York, 1994.

31. Bronaugh, R. L. and Maibach, H. I., *Percutaneous Absorption*, Marcel Dekker, New York, 1985.

32. Bodde, H. E., Verhoeven, J., and Van Driel, L. M. J., The skin compliance of transdermal drug delivery systems, in *Crit. Rev. Therapeut. Drug Carrier Systems*, 6, 94, 1989.

33. Banga, A. K. and Chien, Y. W., Iontophoretic delivery of drugs: fundamentals, developments and biomedical applications, *J. Control. Rel.*, 7, 1, 1988.

34. Bommannan, D., Menon, G. K., Okuyama, H., Elias, P. M., and Guy, R. H., Sonophoresis II. Examination of the mechanisms of ultrasound-enhanced transdermal drug delivery, *Pharm. Res.*, 9, 1043, 1992.

35. Prausnitz, M., Bose, V. G., Langer, R., and Weaver, J. C., Electroporation, in *Percutaneous Penetration Enhancers*, Smith, E. W. and Maibach, H. I., Eds., CRC Press, Boca Raton, FL, 1995, 393.

36. Gangarosa, L. P., *Proc. Soc. Exp. Biol. Med.*, 154, 651, 1977.

37. Harris, R., in *Therapeutic Electricity and Ultraviolet Irradiation.*, Light, S., Ed., Wiley, New York, 1967, 168.

38. Okabe, K., Yamaguchi, H., and Kawai, Y., New Iontophoretic transdermal administration of the beta-blocker Metaprolol, *J. Control. Rel.*, 4, 79, 1986.

39. Ledger, P. W., Skin biological issues in electrically enhanced transdermal delivery, *Adv. Drug Deliv. Rev.*, 9, 289, 1992.

40. Molitor, H. and Fernandez, L., Studies on iontophoresis. I. Experimental studies on the causes and prevention of iontophoretic burns, *Am. J. Med. Sci.*, 198, 778, 1939.

41. Prausnitz, M., Bose, V. G., Langer, R., and Weaver, J. C., Electroporation of mammalian skin: a mechanism to enhance transdermal drug delivery, *Proc. Natl. Acad. Sci. U.S.A.*, 90, 10504, 1993.

42. Weaver, J. C., Electroporation: a general phenomenon for manipulating cells and tissues, *J. Cell. Biochem.*, 51, 426, 1993.

43. Orlowski, S. and Mir, L. M., Cell electropermeabilization: a new tool for biochemical and pharmaceutical studies, *Biochim. Biophys. Acta*, 1154, 51, 1993.

44. Barnett, A. and Weaver, J. C., A unified quantitative theory of reversible electrical breakdown and rupture, *Bioelectrochem. Bioenerg.*, 25, 163, 1991.

45. Prausnitz, M., Seddick, D. S., Kon, A. A., Bose, V. G., Frankenburg, S., Klaus, S. N., Langer, R., and Weaver, J. C., Methods for in vivo tissue electroporation using surface electrodes, *Drug Deliv.*, 1, 125, 1993.

46. Prausnitz, M., Bose, V. G., Langer, R., and Weaver, J. C., Electroporation, in *Percutaneous Penetration Enhancers*, Smith, E. W. and Maibach, H. I., Eds., 1995, 403.

47. Julian, N. T. and Zentner, G. M., Mechanism for ultrasonically enhanced transmembrane solute permeation, *J. Control. Rel.*, 12, 77, 1990.

48. Kost, J., Experimental approaches to elucidate the mechanism of ultrasonically enhanced transdermal drug delivery, Abstr. 17th Int. Symp. on Controlled Release of Bioactive Material, Lee, V. H. L., Ed., 1990, 53.
49. Kirsten, E. B., Zinsser, H., and Reid, J. M., Effect of IMC ultrasound on the genetics of mice, *IEEE Trans. Ultrasonic Eng.*, 112, 1963.
50. Cowden, J. W. and Abell, M. R., Some effects of ultrasonic radiation on normal tissues, *Exp. Mol. Pathol.*, 2, 367, 1963.
51. Tachibana, K., Transdermal delivery of insulin to alloxan-diabetic rabbits by ultrasound exposure, *Pharm. Res.*, 9, 952, 1992.
52. McElnay, J. C., Kennedy, T. A., and Harlaud, R., The influence of ultrasound on the percutaneous absorption of fluocinolone acetonide, *Int. J. Pharm.*, 40, 105, 1987.
53. Halkier-Sorensen, L., Occupational skin diseases, *Contact Dermatitis Suppl.*, 1, 35, 1996.
54. Rycroft, R., Menne, T., Frosch, P., and Benezra, C., Eds., *Textbook of Contact Dermatitis*, Springer-Verlag, New York, 540, 1992.
55. Rietschel, R. L. and Fowler, J. E., Jr., Eds., *Fisher's Contact Dermatitis*, 4th ed., Williams & Wilkins, Baltimore, MD, 1995.
56. Menne, T. and Maibach, H. I., Eds., *Hand Eczema*, CRC Press, Boca Raton, FL, 1994.
57. Zurcher, K. and Krebs, A., Eds., *Cutaneous Drug Reactions*, S. Karger, Basel, 1992.
58. Fischer, A. A., Contact dermatitis from topical medicaments, *Semin. Dermatol.*, 1, 49, 1982.
59. Sequeira, J. A., U.S. Patent 4,834,980 assigned to Schering Plough, Transdermal Delivery of Azatadine, 1989.
60. Willis, C. M., Houng, E., Brandon, D. R., and Wilkinson, J. D., Immunopathological and ultrastructural findings in human allergic and irritant contact dermatitis, *Br. J. Dermatol.*, 115, 305, 1986.
61. Personal experience of authors.
62. Van der Walle, H. B., *Hand Eczema*, Menne, T. and Maibach, H. I., Eds., CRC Press, Boca Raton, FL, 1994, 35.
63. Frosch, P. J., Kurte, A., and Pilz, B., *Contact Dermatitis*, 29, 113, 1994.
64. Estlander, T., Joolanki, R., and Kenerva, L., *Hand Eczema*, Menne, T. and Maibach, H. I., Eds., CRC Press, Boca Raton, FL, 1994, 311.
65. Lushniac, B., NIOSH Report, Presented at NIH Workshop on Irritant Contact Dermatitis, Washington, D.C., March 25, 1996.
66. Moller, H., The atopic hand eczema, in *Hand Eczema*, Menne, T. and Maibach, H. I., Eds., CRC Press, Boca Raton, FL, 1994, 46.
67. Maibach, H. I., Clonidine: irritant and contact dermatitis assays, *Contact Dermatitis*, 12, 192, 1985.
68. Wille, J. J., Njieha, F., Amin, P., and Kydonieus, A., Topical delivery of mast cell degranulating agents for treatment of transdermal drug-induced hypersensitivity, *Proc. Int. Symp. Control. Rel. Bioact. Mater.*, 22, 119, 1995.

2 The Skin as a Barrier: Structure and Function

Thomas J. Franz and Paul A. Lehman

CONTENTS

I. INTRODUCTION

The skin, along with the mucosal linings of the digestive, respiratory, and urogenital tracts, comprises the epithelial system of the body, whose function is to encase and isolate internal structures from the external environment. Like all other epithelia, the skin serves as a barrier, to keep water and other vital substances in and foreign material out. However, the skin is the *only* epithelium that must function in a hostile, nonaqueous environment. Whereas the linings of the gastrointestinal or genitourinary tracts, for example, are bathed by interstitial fluid on the inside and another aqueous phase (gastric juices or urine) on the outside, skin is without aqueous contact on the outside under most normal conditions. To survive in this adverse environment and preserve its own integrity from the destructive effects of desiccation and to fulfill its functional obligations to the body as well, skin has developed a specialized structure of *unique physical–chemical composition*, the stratum corneum. "Indeed, the raison d'etre of the epidermis is to make the stratum corneum; this is its specific biologic mission."[1] Since terrestrial life would be impossible without an efficient water barrier, this extraordinary structure develops *in utero* 6 to 8 weeks prior to delivery. Thus, all normal full-term infants arrive with an effective epidermal barrier.[2,3]

The stratum corneum, which is the outermost layer of skin, is a multilayered structure consisting of flattened cells totally devoid of the usual intracellular organelles. It is commonly referred to as a "dead" tissue to reflect the fact that its cells have no nuclei and, therefore, are incapable of mitosis.

However, very critical enzymatic activities persist and profound biochemical changes take place between the inner and outer stratum corneum.

That the "barrier" properties of skin do indeed reside in the stratum corneum was not known until the work of Winsor and Burch.[4] In a series of simple in vitro experiments, the rate of water loss through full-thickness human cadaver skin was measured. Then, following separation of the skin into epidermis and dermis, its two constituent layers, water loss through each was measured individually. It was discovered that all of the barrier function displayed by full-thickness skin persisted in the separated epidermal tissue. Water moved freely across the isolated dermal layer and the rate was roughly equivalent to the rate of loss from bulk water. In a subsequent experiment, they found that destruction of the outermost portion of the epidermis, the stratum corneum, resulted in loss of the water barrier. The stratum corneum was, therefore, clearly established as the rate-limiting barrier of skin. Since that time, numerous studies have documented that the stratum corneum is not only the rate-limiting barrier to water loss from the body, but the barrier to systemic absorption of substances with which man comes into contact in his environment.

Subsequent work of the last few decades has served to better define the biochemical and ultrastructural basis of the barrier layer. One frequent observation made by many investigators over the years has been the tendency for lipid-soluble molecules to permeate skin better than water-soluble molecules. This is now known to be related to the presence of lipid bilayers in the intercellular space of the stratum corneum, a structural feature not seen in other epithelial systems.[5] Concurrently, our concept of the barrier has changed dramatically. Whereas skin was commonly thought of as being a barrier of high resistance to most substances, it is now recognized to be a barrier of *variable* resistance. In some instances it has been the portal of entry for toxic substances resulting in serious adverse systemic reactions and death;[6] and it is now used as a route for delivery of a small number of therapeutic agents to the systemic circulation, i.e., transdermal drug delivery.

Though those interested in dermal and transdermal drug delivery focus primarily on the skin as a barrier to absorption, it cannot be forgotten that the skin is also a barrier to microorganisms, ultraviolet radiation, electrical energy, and mechanical forces as well, and also serves to support the important thermoregulatory needs of the body.

II. ANATOMY AND BIOCHEMISTRY OF SKIN

A. OVERVIEW OF SKIN STRUCTURE

Skin is one of the largest organs of the body, 15,000 to 20,000 cm^2 in area in most adults, varying in thickness from approximately 1.5 to 4 mm, and weighing approximately 2 kg.[7] It consists of two parts: (1) the cellular outermost layer, epidermis; and (2) the inner, relatively acellular, connective tissue layer, dermis (Figure 1). Lying between these two layers is a submicroscopic structure, the basal lamina or basement membrane zone, which serves as the anchoring structure by which the epidermis and dermis are held together. The blood supply to the skin resides exclusively in the dermis, and the nutritional needs of the epidermis are met entirely by diffusion. Below the dermis is a layer of fatty (adipose) tissue called the hypodermis, which some authors discuss as a third integumentary layer. This layer consists of a network of fat cells (adipocytes) arranged in lobules and separated by fibrous (collagen) bundles which connect the dermis to the fascial layer lying below the hypodermis. Although it is important both as a thermal insulator and cushion to mechanical forces, its relevance to transdermal/dermal delivery has never been established and it will not be discussed further.

The epidermis is composed of two parts (Figure 2): the living cells of the Malpighian layer, which in turn can be divided into several strata; and the dead cells of the stratum corneum, commonly referred to as the horny layer, because it also forms specialized structures such as hair, nails, and the horns of animals. The prime function of the viable cells of the epidermis is to move progressively through a process of differentiation, eventually to die (terminal differentiation), and through this

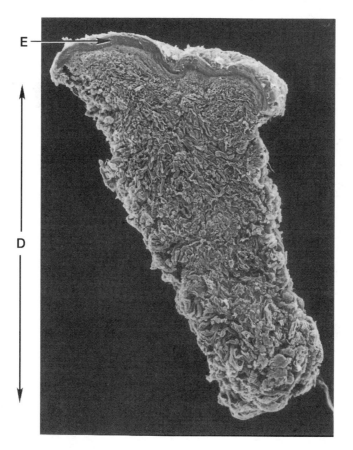

Figure 1 Low magnification (× 80) scanning electron micrograph of skin from the upper back showing relative thinness of epidermis (E) and fibrous nature of dermis (D). (Reprinted with permission from Franz, T. J., Tojo, K., Shah, K. R., and Kydonieus, A., Transdermal delivery, in *Treatise on Controlled Drug Delivery*, Kydonieus, A., Ed., Marcel Dekker, New York, 1991, chap. 8.)

mechanism to generate the barrier layer. As cells undergo differentiation and move from inner to outer epidermis, many extraordinary biochemical and structural changes take place: (1) loss of mitotic activity, (2) synthesis of new organelles (lamellar and keratohyalin granules) and subsequent loss of all cell organelles, (3) total remodeling of cell architecture as cells increase in width, flatten, and lose most of their water content, (4) modification of cell membrane and cell surface antigens and receptors, and (5) synthesis of new lipids, as well as structural and enzymatic proteins.[8]

B. EPIDERMIS

The epidermis is a continually renewing, stratified squamous epithelium covering the entire outer surface of the body. Over most of the body it ranges in thickness from 0.06 to 0.1 mm, though it is much thicker over the palms and soles, due to the increased thickness of the horny layer at those sites. The major cell (80%) of the epidermis is the keratinocyte, so named because of the family of fibrous proteins (keratins) contained within. However, other important cellular elements are present. These include the melanocyte, the source of melanin pigment which gives the skin its color and affords protection from the damaging effects of ultraviolet radiation; the Langerhans cell, which is part of the immune surveillance system and critical to the development of allergic contact dermatitis; and the Merkel cell, which is thought to function as a mechanoreceptor for the sensation of touch.[8]

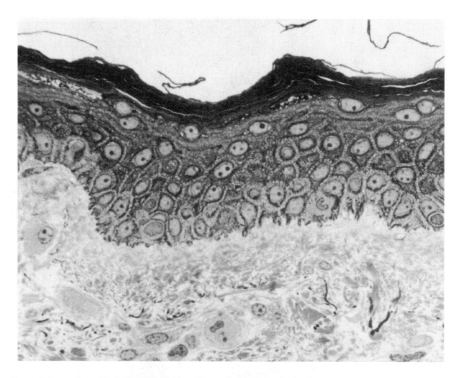

Figure 2   Photomicrograph (× 250) illustrating cellular nature of epidermis and a portion of the relatively acellular, upper dermis. The dark appearing, amorphous layer at the top is the stratum corneum. (Reprinted with permission from Franz, T. J., Tojo, K., Shah, K. R., and Kydonieus, A., Transdermal delivery, in *Treatise on Controlled Drug Delivery*, Kydonieus, A., Ed., Marcel Dekker, New York, 1991, chap. 8.)

Keratinocytes are characterized by the presence of submicroscopic (10 nm) filaments (keratins) and desmosomes, specialized structures occurring at irregular intervals on the cell membrane that serve as points of attachment for adjacent cells. These highly organized intercellular junctions serve to create strong mechanical links between cells. They have one intracellular part, the desmosomal plaque, and one extracellular part, the desmosomal plate. Inside the cell the desmosomal plaque interacts with keratin filaments and serves as an anchoring point for the intracellular keratin cytoskeleton, thus creating a supracellular network of filaments that is essential for mainlining the structural integrity of the epidermis.[9,10]

The adhesive function of the desmosome is thought to be performed by two glycoproteins, desmocollins and desmogleins, both members of the cadherin gene family of Ca^{2+}-dependent cell-to-cell adhesion molecules. The latter proteins are transmembrane glycoproteins, anchored in the desmosomal plaque. Thus, the mechanical properties of individual cells are transferred to the epithelial tissue as a whole via the desmosomes. The structure known as the desmosomal plate results from the interaction between the extracellular, carbohydrate-containing parts of desmogleins from two adjacent cells. Degradation of these parts of the desmogleins would lead to a loss of the cohesive capacity of desmosomes and impairment of the forces holding neighboring cells together. This is thought to occur normally when cells at the outermost layer of the stratum corneum are eventually shed, the process of desquamation.

Keratinocytes are unusually rich in keratin proteins, which comprise up to two thirds of the total dry weight of the cell. The keratins represent a family of alpha-helical, water-insoluble proteins ranging in size from 40 to 70 kDa, which make up the major part of the cytoskeleton of all epithelial cells. Although more than 30 different human keratins have been identified, the particular types expressed depend on the tissue and stage of differentiation, as well as the health of the tissue.[11,12]

Keratins can be divided into two subfamilies: acidic keratins having an isoelectric point < 5.5, and basic keratins having an isoelectric point >6.5. They are rich in serine, glutamic acid, and glycine but have a low cystine content. Four major keratins are found in normal epidermis: acidic 50 and 56.5 kDa, and basic 58 and 65 to 67 kDa. In order for the keratins to form filaments they are coexpressed as pairs, one acidic and one basic. In the epidermis the biochemical composition of the keratin filaments varies with the state of differentiation. The 50/58.5 (acidic/basic)-kDa keratins are synthesized in the basal layer, and the 56.5/65 (acidic/basic)-kDa keratins are synthesized in supra basal cells.

The mitotically active keratinocytes reside in the basal layer or stratum germinativum (Figure 3). As daughter cells move outward through the other strata of the epidermis, they begin to flatten and assume a polyhedral shape. When viewed by light microscopy, the cells appear to have spines due to the dehydration caused by routine histological preparation. As the cells shrink from dehydration, they pull away from each other except where firmly attached by desmosomes, thus, giving rise to the name spinous layer (stratum spinosum).

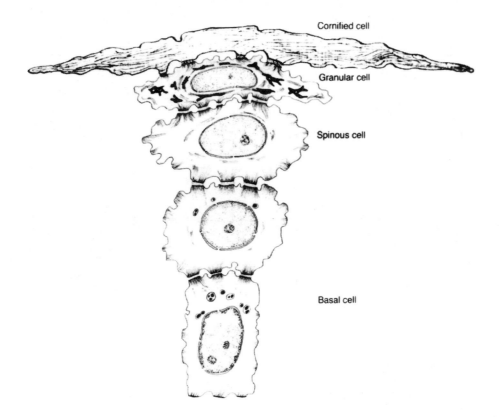

Cornified cell

Granular cell

Spinous cell

Basal cell

Figure 3   Schematic illustration of epidermal differentiation showing transformation of mitotically active, vertically oriented basal cell to "dead," horizontally oriented corneocyte. (Reprinted with permission from Moschella, S. L. and Hurley, H. J., Eds., *Dermatology*, 3rd ed., W. B. Saunders, Philadelphia, 1993, chap 1.)

In the spinous layer keratin filaments become more prominent and a shift toward the synthesis of higher molecular weight keratins begins. Also in this layer a new organelle appears, the lamellar granule (membrane coating granule, Odland body). These 0.2- to 0.3-μm-diameter organelles contain large amounts of lipid and are distinguished by their organization into alternating lamellae (Figure 4). It is the extrusion of these lipids into the intercellular space of the next stratum, the granular layer, that initiates formation of the barrier.[13,14]

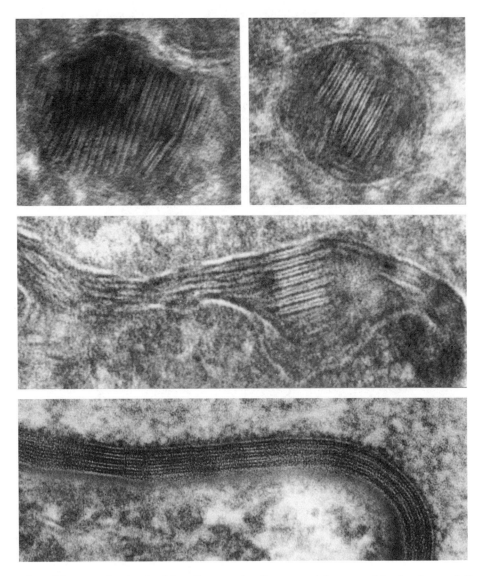

Figure 4   Electron micrograph of lamellar granules from neonatal mouse skin showing evolution of intracellular lipid discs to broad intercellular lamellae. Top panels: "stacked discs" appearance of lipids in lamellar granules of granular cells. Middle panel: extruded lamellar granule contents in intercellular space at interface of granular and horny layers. Fusion of discs is beginning to occur. Bottom panel: only broad lamellar sheets are seen in the outer portion of the stratum corneum. (Courtesy of Dr. Kathi Madison.)

Major changes in cellular architecture occur in the granular layer, named for the basophilic granules (keratohyalin granules) that are so prominently seen under both light and electron microscopy. The cells of this layer continue to flatten and become much wider than the underlying cells. Also in this layer new proteins begin to appear, the major new protein being a high molecular weight, histidine-rich precursor (pro-filaggrin) which is contained in the keratohyalin granule. It will be converted to filaggrin and serve as the matrix in which the keratin filaments are enmeshed in the stratum corneum.[15]

Another protein, cystine-rich involucrin, first appears. It, along with other proteins such as loricin, cystatin-α (keratolinin), and small proline-rich proteins, will become a major component of the thickened cell envelope of the stratum corneum. Ultrastructural studies suggest involucrin is an elongated rod-shaped protein, with more than 100 potential glutamyl donor sites for participation in isopeptide bond formation, which could serve in the formation of the initial scaffolding of the cell envelope.[16]

Lamellar granules become more numerous in the granular layer where they migrate to the cell membrane and release their contents into the intercellular space, the first step in the formation of a barrier which is unique to skin. Studies have shown that large molecular weight substances such as lanthanum and horseradish peroxide, which can diffuse freely from the dermis through the intercellular space of the basal and spinous layers, do not penetrate the granular layer.[17,18]

C. STRATUM CORNEUM

The stratum corneum is the end product of epidermal differentiation and consists of 15 to 25 cell layers over most of the body surface (Figure 5), though it is much thicker over the palms and soles.[19] The transition from granular layer to horny layer must occur abruptly, as intermediate cell types are seldom seen. The nucleus and all cell organelles (microsomes, mitochondria, etc.) of the cells within the granular layer are broken down, a thick (15 nm) band of cross-linked proteins is deposited on the inner surface of the cell membrane to form the cell envelope, and the entire cell is filled with keratin filaments and associated matrix proteins (filaggrin).

The corneocyte is the largest cell in the epidermis, approximately 0.5 μm in thickness and 30 to 40 μm in width. It contains no organelles but is filled with protein, 80% of which is high molecular keratin (>60,000 Da). The intercellular space is filled with lipids organized into multiple bilayers, and these lipids are of unusual composition. Approximately 14% of the stratum corneum, by weight, is lipids. In addition, the stratum corneum has a very low water content, though it can take up to five times its weight in water when placed in an aqueous environment.[20]

Formation of the stratum corneum is also accompanied by the deposition of a 15-nm-thick band of protein on the inner surface of the plasma membrane, the cornified cell envelope, a structure unique to keratinocytes and a hallmark of terminal differentiation.[21] The cornified envelope is a rigid protein scaffold formed through the action of transglutaminases which covalently cross-links protein precursors via the formation of isopeptide bonds between γ-carboxyl groups of peptide-bound glutamine and ε-amino groups of peptide-bound lysine.[22,23] These isodipeptide cross-links, along with disulfide bonds, render the envelope insoluble and very resistant to chemical attack, contributing to the overall barrier properties of the stratum corneum.

Formation of the cornified envelope is accompanied by loss of the normal cell membrane and covalent attachment of an unusual ω-hydroxyceramide to its cell envelope.[24] Phospholipids, which normally make up a large component of cell membranes, are degraded, leaving the barrier layer with little or no phospholipid content. Thus, corneocytes are left with a compound cell envelope consisting of a highly insoluble, cross-linked protein inner surface and a hydroxyceramide mono-layer outer surface. The lipid coating may function as an anchor for the intercellular lipid bilayers and serve to influence their organization as well.[25,26]

The corneocytes are joined together by modified desmosomes and overlap with each other at their edges to form a mechanically strong layer. All the mechanical strength of the epidermis derives from the stratum corneum and it can be prepared in pure form as an intact "membrane" suitable for permeability studies.[27]

A particularly intriguing feature of stratum corneum architecture is its orderly arrangement into columns or stacks,[28] a feature not seen in routine histologic preparations of the skin in which defatting solvents have been used. However, when frozen sections of unfixed skin are swollen (hydrated) with dilute acid or alkali, the cells of the horny layer are neatly aligned (Figure 6). This is most evident in regions where the epidermis is thin (and in animal skin) and the turnover rate is low. It is not seen in areas such as the palms and soles, where the stratum corneum is unusually thick and the turnover rate high. This orderly arrangement of corneocytes may have some relationship to barrier function, as the diffusion coefficient of water in palmar and plantar skin is much higher than elsewhere.[29]

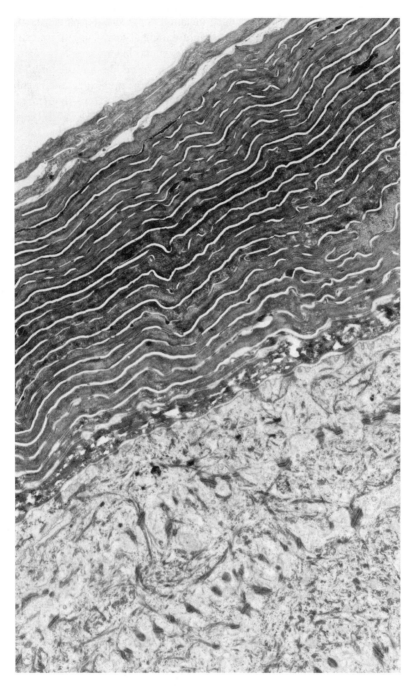

Figure 5   Electron micrograph (× 9,600) through full thickness of stratum corneum and upper layers of living epidermis. The thinness of corneocytes and multilayered nature of the barrier layer are apparent. Absence of structure in the intercellular space is the result of lipid solvents used to prepare the specimen. (Reprinted with permission from Franz, T. J., Tojo, K., Shah, K. R., and Kydonieus, A., Transdermal delivery, in *Treatise on Controlled Drug Delivery*, Kydonieus, A., Ed., Marcel Dekker, New York, 1991, chap. 8.)

D. DESQUAMATION AND TURNOVER TIME

The turnover time of the stratum corneum, the time for a newly formed cell to move from inside to outside and be sloughed, has been found to be approximately 14 days, using two separate

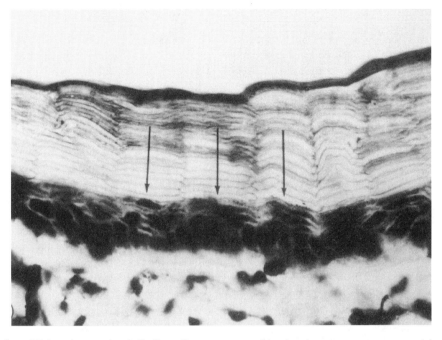

Figure 6   Light micrograph of alkali-swollen mouse ear skin showing corneocytes arranged in vertical columns. (Reprinted with permission from Menton, D. N., *Am. J. Anat.*, 145, 1, 1976.)

techniques. Impregnation of the stratum corneum with the fluorescent dye tetrachlorsalicylanilide, which stains the entire thickness of the stratum corneum, revealed that it took approximately 10 to 15 days for the surface of the skin to lose its fluorescence in regions such as the abdomen, back, and forearm.[30] Using a separate approach in which the cells of the viable epidermis were labeled with ^{14}C-glycine revealed that it took 13 to 14 days for the first labeled cells, i.e., those coming from the granular layer, to reach the skin surface.[31] It should be noted, however, that there is a significant regional variation in stratum corneum renewal.

The process by which corneocytes are shed from the outer surface of the skin is referred to as desquamation. Since stratum corneum thickness is normally relatively constant over each region of the body, the rate of desquamation must be controlled to match the rate of corneocyte formation from below, and something must occur in the outermost portion of the barrier to reduce intercorneocyte binding forces. Though there is incomplete understanding of this homeostatic mechanism, an essential role in the process of desquamation is played by desmosomes, which serve to bond corneocytes together, and serine proteases, which are responsible for their digestion.[32,33] An in vitro model has been developed which shows that the dissociation of corneocytes from plantar stratum corneum is preceded by the degradation of the intercellular portion of desmosomes, loss of desmoglein-1-like (DG-1) protein, and the appearance of lower molecular weight components with DG-1-like immunoreactivity.[34]

Intercellular lipids may also play a role in desquamation. Often assumed to be important cohesive elements in the barrier layer, lipid differences between inner and outer stratum corneum do exist, which lends support to this belief.[35] In addition, it has been shown that there is a loss of the lipid bilayers in the outermost stratum corneum.[36] Recent evidence also suggests that one lipid in particular, cholesterol sulfate, may play a special role in the process by acting as a serine protease inhibitor.[37] This lipid normally exists at low concentration in the outer SC but: (1) has been found to be increased in one condition, recessive X-linked ichthyosis, characterized by a thickened (failure of desquamation) and scaly barrier; and (2) can produce changes in the skin of mice somewhat similar to ichthyosis following direct topical application. Calcium ions may also play a role in regulating desquamation through their inhibitory effect on proteolytic enzymes.[38]

E. Dermis

The dermis is largely an integrated fibroelastic, acellular structure consisting of interwoven fibrous, filamentous, and amorphous connective tissue.[8] It is the largest component of skin and it is from this layer that the skin derives its mechanical strength. The dermis is divided into two parts: the upper, papillary dermis and the lower, reticular dermis. The papillary dermis is the thinner of the two and is distinguished from the reticular dermis by having fiber bundles of much smaller diameter. Its interface with the epidermis is irregular and thrown into folds. The most elevated portions of the papillary dermis are referred to as dermal papillae, and each contains a capillary loop arising from the underlying arteriole plexus. As skin ages there is loss of dermal papillae and a reduction in the number of capillary loops.

Collagen is the major fibrous protein of the dermis, accounting for more than 70% of its dry weight. Bundles of collagen fibers are woven into a network within the dermis, which accounts for the great tensile strength of skin. Interwoven among the collagen fabric is a network of elastic fibers which give skin its resilience, i.e., the ability to restore normal structure following deformation by external forces. It makes up only 1 to 2% of the dry weight of the dermis. Other nonfibrous components of the dermis are the glycosaminoglycans (the amorphous ground substance) and the finely filamentous glycoproteins, both of which contribute to the water-binding properties of dermis.

From the standpoint of percutaneous absorption, perhaps the most important element of the dermis is its vasculature, which serves as the "sink" for absorption. The blood supply to the skin comes from cutaneous branches of musculoskeletal arteries, which ascend from the underlying musculature, penetrate the subcutaneous fat, and enter the dermis. In the deeper regions of the dermis, branches spread horizontally to form a deep vascular plexus running parallel to the surface of the skin. In addition, the parent vessel ascends to the papillary dermis and divides into smaller arterioles which form a superficial plexus. Arising from the superficial plexus are smaller arterioles that give rise to capillary loops running at right angles to the surface of the skin and traversing the dermal papillae to within a few microns of the basement membrane (Figure 7).

The vascular surface available for the exchange of substances between skin and blood has been estimated to be 1 to 2 cm^2 per cm^2 of skin surface.[39] The average blood flow to the skin may vary from 0.5 to 100 ml/min/100 g, although normal resting flow is in the range of 3 to 10 ml/min/100 g.[40] The higher rates of blood flow are only seen under conditions of elevated ambient temperature and exercise, i.e., when there is a heat load to dissipate.

The general model for percutaneous absorption depicts a compound's movement from skin surface to systemic circulation proceeding stepwise as follows: vehicle $\rightarrow$ stratum corneum $\rightarrow$ viable epidermis $\rightarrow$ dermis $\rightarrow$ dermal blood vessels. However, lymphatic vessels are also present in the dermis and can serve as a route of entry into the systemic circulation. In addition, there is some evidence that the dermal vasculature is not 100% effective at extracting all diffusing molecules and that some may permeate directly into deeper tissues, such as muscle or joints.[41]

Blood flow through the skin may influence the rate of percutaneous absorption.[42] This may be important for compounds with very high rates of barrier penetration, as well as in situations in which the barrier is damaged by disease or is altered through the use of penetration enhancers.

F. Skin Appendages

The skin contains a number of appendages whose ducts perforate the stratum corneum and may act as shunts for diffusion. These include the eccrine and apocrine sweat glands, hair follicles, and sebaceous glands. The duct of the sebaceous gland does not itself penetrate the stratum corneum but, over most of the body, empties into the duct of the hair follicle approximately 0.5 mm below the surface of the skin.

The role of skin appendages as pathways for percutaneous absorption has long been debated. Since the openings of appendageal ducts account for only 1% or less of the surface area of the skin, it is frequently argued that their overall contribution to absorption must be relatively small.[43] However, for compounds whose penetration through the unbroken stratum corneum is extremely limited, this

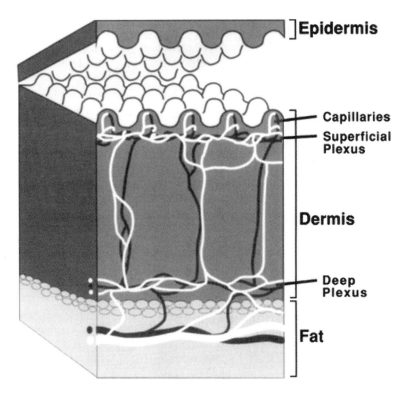

Figure 7 Schematic illustration of cutaneous vasculature showing both a superficial and deep plexus. Capillary loops arise from the superficial plexus and serve as the nutritional source for the living epidermis and the sink for percutaneous absorption. (Reprinted with permission from Franz, T. J., Tojo, K., Shah, K. R., and Kydonieus, A., Transdermal delivery, in *Treatise on Controlled Drug Delivery*, Kydonieus, A., Ed., Marcel Dekker, New York, 1991, chap. 8.)

may represent a significant pathway, perhaps the only pathway for absorption. There is clear evidence that permeation through hair follicles is an important route during iontophoresis.[44,45]

Data obtained from a number of animal and human "model" systems which have no hair follicles also give evidence of a significant contribution of the follicular pathway to percutaneous absorption. Permeation of a number of compounds through rat skin experimentally altered by wounding to eliminate the hair follicles shows two- to fivefold less penetration through the altered skin.[46,47] Likewise, the permeability of newborn rat skin, which lacks hair follicles during the first 5 days after birth, has been shown to increase as the hair follicles emerge.[47,48]

Similar evidence exists for human skin. Epidermal sheets obtained from human scar tissue, histologically confirmed to be free of hair follicles and sebaceous glands, were 1.6- to 3-fold less permeable to a number of steroid compounds than normal, nonscarred skin.[49] These data are also consistent with limited in vivo observations on regional variation in percutaneous absorption in humans. The head, which has a much higher density of follicles than other body sites, is also more permeable to hydrocortisone, parathion, and malathion than other body sites with the exception of the genital area. The increase may be as high as four- to fivefold.[50]

III. ROLE OF LIPIDS IN BARRIER FUNCTION

A. LIPID COMPOSITION

One major element underlying the impermeability of skin is the hydrophobic nature of the stratum corneum. Recent data derived from morphologic, histochemical, and biochemical studies provide strong evidence that the stratum corneum can be viewed as a "heterogeneous two compartment system of protein-enriched cells embedded in lipid-laden intercellular domains."[5] The term "bricks and mortar" is now widely used to describe this organizational model, and the lipids (mortar) are thought to be the major element underlying barrier function, particularly to water and other hydrophilic materials.

Major changes in the lipid composition of the epidermis occur as cells differentiate and move from the basal layer to the horny layer (Figure 8). There is a shift from polar lipids to neutral lipids and almost complete loss of phospholipids. With respect to barrier function, the most important changes occur just beneath the horny layer, in the granular layer, and lead to the deposition of lipids in the intercellular space. These lipids, derived from lamellar granules which have fused with the cell membrane to discharge their contents, first appear as broad discs (Figure 4). As this material moves up into the stratum corneum, modifications occur leading to the formation of broad multi-laminate sheets, not unlike those normally seen in cell membranes. Synchronous with this change in morphology are major biochemical changes in lipid composition which can best be characterized as movement from a polar lipid profile to a very nonpolar lipid profile. Nature's intent seems clear. The prime function of the horny layer is to serve as a barrier to water loss, and this will be accomplished through the generation of a domain of very high hydrophobicity. The resulting biochemical and morphologic structures created are unique to skin.

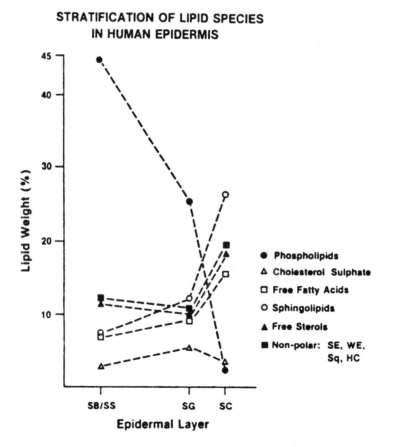

**STRATIFICATION OF LIPID SPECIES
IN HUMAN EPIDERMIS**

● Phospholipids
△ Cholesterol Sulphate
□ Free Fatty Acids
○ Sphingolipids
▲ Free Sterols
■ Non-polar: SE, WE,
            Sq, HC

Figure 8   The composition of lipid species within the epidermis changes as cells differentiate and move from the basal and spinous layers (SB/SS) to the granular layer (SG) and stratum corneum (SC). SE = sterol esters, WE = wax esters, Sq = squalene, HC = hydrocarbons. (Reprinted with permission from Lampe, M. A., Williams, M. L., and Elias, P. M., *J. Lipd Res.*, 24, 131, 1983.)

Changes in the lipid content of human skin with differentiation are known from the work of Lampe et al.[51] A complete analysis of the lipids obtained from abdominal skin was made at three levels within the epidermis. Total lipids were extracted from each layer, fractionated, and quantified using thin-layer chromatography (Table 1). It was found that generation of a fully formed stratum corneum is accompanied by an enrichment of neutral lipids and sphingolipids (ceramides) and virtual elimination of the most polar lipids, phospholipids. Whereas the neutral lipids and ceramides make up less than 60% of the combined basal and spinous layers, they account for more than 95% of the horny layer. Virtually identical results have been obtained with the epidermis of pig skin using a similar experimental design.[52] Thus, it can be assumed that the same phenomena are operative in the skin of most mammals.

TABLE 1
Variations in Lipid Composition During Human Epidermal Differentiation and Cornification[a]

Fraction	Strata Basale/Spinosum (n = 5)			Stratum Granulosum (n = 7)			Stratum Corneum					
							Whole (n = 4)			Outer (n = 8)		
Polar lipids*	44.5	±	3.4	25.3	±	2.6	4.9	±	1.6	2.3	±	0.5
Cholesterol sulfate**	2.4	±	0.5	5.5	±	1.3	1.5	±	0.2	3.4	±	0.5
Neutral lipids	51.0	±	4.5	56.5	±	2.8	77.7	±	5.6	68.4	±	2.1
Free sterols	11.2	±	1.7	11.5	±	1.1	14.0	±	1.1	18.8	±	2.1
Free fatty acids***	7.0	±	2.1	9.2	±	1.5	19.3	±	3.7	15.6	±	3.0
Triglycerides	12.4	±	2.9	24.7	±	4.0	25.2	±	4.6	11.2	±	1.5
Sterol/wax esters[b]	5.3	±	1.3	4.7	±	0.7	5.4	±	0.9	12.4	±	1.9
Squalene	4.9	±	1.1	4.6	±	1.0	4.8	±	2.0	5.6	±	2.1
n-Alkanes	3.9	±	0.3	3.8	±	0.8	6.1	±	2.6	5.4	±	0.8
Sphingolipids	7.3	±	1.0	11.7	±	2.7	18.1	±	2.8	26.6	±	2.3
Glucosylceramides I	2.0	±	0.3	4.0	±	0.3	Trace			Trace		
Glucosylceramides II	1.5	±	0.3	1.8	±	0.2	Trace			Trace		
Ceramides I	1.7	±	0.1	5.1	±	0.4	13.8	±	0.4	19.4	±	0.5
Ceramides II	2.1	±	0.3	3.7	±	0.1	4.3	±	0.4	7.2	±	0.5
Total	99.1			101.1			99.3			100.7		

[a] Weight % ± SEM.

[b] Sterol/wax esters present in approximately equal quantities, as determined by acid hydrolysis.

Significant differences: *, SS/SB vs. SG ($P < 0.01$); SG vs. WSC or SS/SB ($P < 0.001$). **, SG vs. WSC ($P < 0.02$); WSC vs. OSC ($P < 0.01$). ***, SG vs. WSC ($P < 0.05$). ****, SS/SB vs. SG ($P < 0.05$); WSC vs. OSC ($P < 0.05$).

From Lampe, M. A., Williams, M. L., and Elias, P. M., *J. Lipid Res.*, 24, 131, 1983. With permission.

B. Regional Variation

Regional variation in stratum corneum lipid content was evaluated at four sites known to have different permeability properties.[53] Total lipid content varied among the four sites, with face skin, the most permeable site, having the greatest lipid content, and plantar skin, the least permeable site, having the lowest lipid content (Table 2). Neutral lipids comprised the largest percentage of stratum corneum lipids at all four sites, varying from 60 to 78%, and sphingolipids the next largest percentage, 18 to 35%. In trying to correlate these observations with known regional differences in percutaneous absorption, an inverse relationship between the total amount of neutral lipid present and skin permeability is noted.[43] Neutral lipids are highest in the abdomen, where water permeability

TABLE 2
Regional Variations in Lipid Weight Percent and Distribution of Major Lipid Species

	Site										
	Abdomen (n = 4)			**Leg (n = 4)**			**Face (n = 3)**			**Plantar (n = 3)**		
Lipid weight %	6.5	±	0.5	4.3	±	0.8	7.2	±	0.4	2.0	±	0.6
Major species												
Polar lipids	4.9	±	1.6	5.2	±	1.1	3.3	±	0.3	3.2	±	0.89
Cholesterol sulfate[a]	1.5	±	0.2	6.0	±	0.9	2.7	±	0.3	3.4	±	1.2
Neutral lipids	77.7	±	5.6	65.7	±	1.8	66.4	±	1.4	60.4	±	0.9
Sphingolipids[b]	18.2	±	2.8	25.9	±	1.3	26.5	±	0.9	34.8	±	2.1

[a] Significant differences: abdomen vs. leg, $P < 0.01$; leg vs. face, $P < 0.02$; abdomen vs. face, $P < 0.02$; face vs. plantar, $P < 0.01$; abdomen vs. plantar, $P < 0.01$; plantar vs. leg, $P < 0.02$. Cholesterol sulfatte: leg > plantar > face > abdomen.

[b] Significant differences: abdomen vs. leg $P < 0.05$; abdomen vs. face, $P < 0.05$. Spingolipids: planter > face > leg > abdomen.

From Lampe, M. A., et al., *J. Lipid Res.*, 24, 120, 1983. With permission.

is lowest, and lowest in plantar skin, where water permeability is highest. Also noted is the fact that sphingolipids show a direct correlation to water permeability, having just the opposite distribution as the neutral lipids at the same two sites.

A comparison of oral epithelium with skin also points up the important relationship between lipids and barrier properties. Oral epithelium is similar to skin in that it differentiates to form a stratum corneum containing intercellular lipid lamellae, yet is an order of magnitude more permeable to water than skin.[54] In the pig, oral epithelium was found to have approximately 15% less total lipid content per square centimeter surface area than skin, not enough difference to account for the tenfold permeability difference. More important, it contained a lower percentage of ceramides (21% vs. 39%), particularly the linoleate-rich acylceramide unique to keratinizing epithelia and thought to be critical to barrier function. Linoleic acid deficiency has long been known to be associated with formation of an abnormal barrier having increased water permeability.[55] Oral epithelium was also found to contain one tenth the level of covalently bound cell envelope hydroxyceramide as skin, and still retained significant levels of phospholipids, 13% vs. 0% in skin. Thus, qualitative changes is lipid composition can clearly affect barrier function.

IV. INFLAMMATORY AND IMMUNOLOGIC PROCESSES

Positioned as an interface between man and environment, the skin is subject to a diverse collection of both chemical and physical insults and, as a result, is a frequent site of inflammatory reactions. The topical application of medicaments for cosmetic and therapeutic purposes only adds to the problem. Cutaneous inflammation (dermatitis) is mediated by a complex array of both cells and soluble factors, with the final expression of these events being the four classical signs of inflammation: heat, swelling (edema), redness (erythema), and pain. The visible appearance of cutaneous inflammation can vary depending on the stage of the reaction, acute or chronic, and the potency of the offending agent.

The early or acute phase of the reaction is characterized by erythema, edema, and burning or itching (pruritus). This may progress to vesiculation (blister), oozing, crusting, and scaling, depending on the severity of the reaction. If contact with the inciting agent continues, the acute weeping stage may be supplanted by a chronic phase characterized by thickened (lichenified), dry or scaly skin, continued pruritus, and frequently, excoriations. Even after the reaction subsides the site will appear darker (hyperpigmented) than the surrounding skin for some time owing to cellular damage with subsequent loss of melanin pigment into the surrounding tissue. Occasionally, severe dermatitic reactions lead to destruction of melanocytes resulting in hypopigmentation or permanent depigmentation, a particularly distressing problem for darkly pigmented races.

A. ALLERGIC CONTACT DERMATITIS

Cutaneous reactions can be divided into two types, those that have an underlying immunologic or allergic basis (allergic contact dermatitis) and those without an immunologic basis (contact irritant dermatitis). Allergic contact dermatitis is a form of delayed of cell-mediated hypersensitivity.[56] The immune system of the body is divided into two parts. One part, humoral immunity, serves as a defense against bacterial invasion and is derived from the production of circulating antibodies (immunoglobulins) by B lymphocytes. The second part of the immune system, cell-mediated immunity, serves primarily as a defense against intracellular organisms (viruses, fungi, yeast, mycobacteria, intracellular parasites, and undigestible foreign substances) and is derived from the function of T lymphocytes.[57] Allergic contact dermatitis is associated with cell-mediated immunity and, since the "invading" chemical is not a pathogenic microorganism, it can be viewed as a misdirected form of immunity.

Allergic contact dermatitis is a specific acquired hypersensitivity of the delayed type. Through repeated exposures to a particular chemical, a person becomes sensitized or allergic to it, i.e., develops an immunologic mechanism of memory to recognize and react to that specific chemical, now called an allergen or antigen. Not all chemicals are capable of stimulating an allergic reaction, nor is it usual for any one chemical to sensitize all individuals. Most contact allergens sensitize only a small percentage of those exposed. For example, the antihypertensive drug, clonidine, when applied as a transdermal patch evokes allergic reaction in only one of five patients who use it.[58] However, some chemicals are known to be strong sensitizers. The antigens of poison ivy and poison oak will sensitize more than 70% of individuals exposed to them. In the past, the topical use of many drugs has had to be discontinued because of the occurrence of allergic contact dermatitis. The sulfonamides, penicillins, and antihistamines are examples of drug classes that commonly induce sensitization following repeated application to the skin.[59]

The first step in the development of allergic contact dermatitis is the binding of the antigen to the cell membrane of an antigen-presenting cell. T lymphocytes are incapable of interacting directly with antigens even though they possess the appropriate surface receptor for that antigen. In the skin, the prime antigen-presenting cell is the Langerhans cell, which comprises about 3 to 4% of epidermal cells. Due to the presence of multiple dendritic processes, the area of coverage of an individual cell is greatly increased and the small number of cells present form a continuous network for surveillance. As drugs and chemicals diffuse through the skin, some molecules interact with the Langerhans cell membrane and are internalized for "processing" and subsequent presentation to T lymphocytes in the regional lymph nodes. This results in the production of daughter cells genetically programmed to respond to the specific antigen that activated their parent. When sufficient numbers of cells have been formed, they reenter the circulation and return to the skin and other peripheral tissues. This phase of the sensitization process (induction) normally takes 1 to 3 weeks.

When sensitized daughter cells (T lymphocytes) encounter the specific "processed" antigen on the surface of a Langerhans cell or other antigen-presenting cell (macrophage), they become activated, enlarge (blast transformation), and release a number of substances called lymphokines into the surrounding tissue. These substances act as mediators of the inflammatory process and induce migration and activation of other inflammatory cells. Following recontact with the antigen, a cell-mediated response usually takes 12 to 48 h to develop — thus the origin of the term "delayed" hypersensitivity.

An immediate form of hypersensitivity can also occur following topical application of a wide range of agents. Referred to as the "contact urticaria syndrome," it describes a wheal-and-flare response occurring within 30 to 60 min of application and results from histamine and other mediator release from mast cells. Contact urticaria can result from both immunologic (mediated by immunoglobulin-E) and nonimmunologic causes. For example, the penetration enhancer dimethyl sulfoxide directly stimulates histamine release through a nonimmunologic mechanism, as do certain substances released by plants (nettles) and animals (caterpillars, jellyfish).[60]

The clinical appearance of allergic contact dermatitis is dependent upon the duration of the reaction and its location on the body.[61] Acute eruptions are generally characterized by the presence of erythema, papules, and either small blisters (vesicles) or large blisters (bullae). In certain parts of the body (eyelids, penis, scrotum), however, blisters may not develop and only erythema and edema will be noted. Chronic allergic contact dermatitis, however, irrespective of body site, will generally be characterized by thickening (lichenification) of the skin, scaling, and possibly fissuring and erythema. Diagnosis cannot be made on the basis of the clinical signs alone. Diagnostic patch testing should be employed to identify the offending agent.[57]

B. IRRITANT CONTACT DERMATITIS

Contact dermatitis may be produced on an allergic or nonallergic basis. The most common form of contact dermatitis occurs on a nonallergic basis and is referred to as "irritant contact dermatitis." Although frequently thought of as being a single process, it is now considered to be a complex biologic syndrome having a diverse pathophysiology, natural history, and clinical appearance.[62] The clinical picture depends not only on external factors, but on host (internal) factors as well.

The pathogenesis of irritant dermatitis is poorly understood, but it can be thought of as resulting from cell injury or death. The irritant action of caustic or corrosive materials such as strong acids or alkalis is easily understood, since they produce cell death and elicit a reaction after a single application in everyone exposed irrespective of their constitutional susceptibility. These types of reactions can be thought of as chemical "burns" and represent an example of acute irritation. Clinically, the reaction is usually limited to the exposed area, can appear within minutes of exposure, and is characterized by several of the following signs: erythema, edema, pustules, blisters (vesicles/bullae), oozing/crusting, ulceration, and eschar formation. The symptoms of burning, stinging, or pain will accompany the reaction.

Many chemicals, too weak to act as irritants following a single application, can act as irritants when the concentration and duration of exposure are sufficient. Most instances of irritant dermatitis are, in fact, chronic (cumulative irritant contact dermatitis) and develop slowly after a relatively long period of exposure and repeated contact with the offending agent. The clinical picture will differ from that of an acute reaction and is more likely to be characterized by erythema, scaling, dryness, and, perhaps, cracking or fissuring of the skin. The mechanism by which these mild irritants act and the need for repeated application in most instances are not clearly understood. However, frequently used materials such as surfactants and penetration enhancers (dimethyl sulfoxide, decylmethyl sulfoxide, ethanol, propylene glycol, azone) are examples of compounds that will produce irritant reactions in a dose-dependent manner following repeated use.

"Irritant contact dermatitis (ICD) is both clinically and microscopically a highly pleomorphic condition, with an etiology ranging from acute inflammation due to short-term contact with cytotoxic chemicals (primary irritants), through to chronic or accumulative disease arising from repeated exposure to more marginal irritants."[63] Diagnosis is usually made on the basis of exclusion of other possible causes, particularly allergic contact dermatitis. Presently there is no single diagnostic test for irritant contact dermatitis.

REFERENCES

1. Kligman, A. M., The biology of the stratum corneum, in *The Epidermis*, Montagna, W. and Lobitz, W. C., Jr., Eds., Academic Press, New York, 1964, chap 20.
2. Evans, N. and Rutter, N., Transdermal drug delivery to the newborn infant, in *Transdermal Drug Delivery*, Hadgraft, J. and Guy, R. H., Eds., Marcel Dekker, New York, 1989, chap 8.
3. Kalia, Y. N., Nonato, L. B., Lund, C. H., and Guy, R. H., Development of skin barrier function in premature infants, *J. Invest. Dermatol.*, 111, 320, 1998.
4. Winsor, T. and Burch, G. E., Differential roles of layers of human epigastric skin on diffusion rate of water, *Arch. Int. Med.*, 74, 428, 1944.
5. Elias, P. M., Epidermal lipids, barrier function, and desquamation, *J. Invest. Dermatol.*, 80, 44s, 1983.
6. Pines, W. L., The hexachlorophene story, *FDA Papers*, 6, 11, 1972.
7. Rushmer, R. F., Buettner, K. J., Short, J. M., and Odland, G. F., The skin, *Science*, 154, 343, 1966.
8. Holbrook, K. A. and Wolff, K., The structure and development of skin, in *Dermatology in General Medicine*, 4th ed., Fitzpatrick, T. B., Eisen, A. Z., Wolff, K., Freedberg, I. M., and Austen, K. F., Eds., McGraw Hill, New York, 1993, chap 8.
9. Garrod, D. R., Desmosomes and hemidesmosomes, *Curr. Opin. Cell Biol.*, 5, 30, 1993.
10. Buxton, R. S. and Magee, A. I., Structure and interactions of desmosomal and other cadherins, *Semin. Cell Biol.*, 3, 157, 1992.
11. Moll, R. et al., The catalog of human cytokeratins: patterns of expression in normal epithelia, tumors and cultured cells, *Cell*, 31, 11, 1982.
12. O'Guin, W. M. et al., Differentiation-related expression of keratin pairs, in *Cellular and Molecular Biology of Intermediate Filaments*, Goldman, R. D. and Steinert, P. M., Eds., Plenum, New York, 1990, 301.
13. Madison, K. C., Swartzendruber, D. C., Wertz, P. W., and Downing, D. T., Presence of intact intercellular lipid lamellae in the upper layers of the stratum corneum, *J. Invest. Dermatol.*, 88, 714, 1987.
14. Landmann, L., The epidermal permeability barrier, *Anat. Embryol.*, 178, 1, 1988.
15. Dale, B. A., Resing, K. A., and Haydock, P. V., Filaggrins, in *Cellular and Molecular Biology of Intermediate Filaments*, Goldman, R. W. and Steinert, P. M., Eds., Plenum, New York, 1990, 393.
16. Eckert, R. L., Yaffe, M. B., Crish, J. F., Murthy, S., Rorke, E. A., and Welter, J. F., Involucrin-structure and role in envelope assembly, *J. Invest. Dermatol.*, 100, 613, 1993.
17. Squier, C. A., The permeability of keratinized and nonkeratinized oral epithelium to horseradish peroxidase, *J. Ultrastruct. Res.*, 43, 160, 1973.
18. Elias, P. M., McNutt, N. S., and Friend, D. S., Membrane alterations during cornification of mammalian squamous epithelia: a freeze-fracture, tracer, and thin-section study, *Anat. Rec.*, 189, 577, 1977.
19. Holbrook, K. A. and Odland, G. F., Regional differences in the thickness (cell layers) of the human stratum corneum: an ultrastructural analysis, *J. Invest. Dermatol.*, 62, 415, 1974.
20. Scheuplein, R. J. and Morgan, L., "Bound-water" in keratin membranes measured by a microbalance technique, *Nature*, 214, 456, 1969.
21. Matoltsy, A. G. and Balsamo, C. A., A study of cornified epithelium of human skin, *J. Biophys. Biochem. Cytol.*, 1, 339, 1955.
22. Rice, R. H. and Green, H., The cornified envelope of terminally differentiated human epidermal keratinocytes consists of cross-linked protein, *Cell*, 11, 417, 1977.
23. Thacher, S. M. and Rice, R. H., Keratinocyte-specific transglutaminase of cultured human epidermal cells: relation to cross-linked envelope formation and terminal differentiation, *Cell*, 40, 685, 1985.
24. Swartzendruber, D. C., Wertz, P. W., Madison, K. C., and Downing, D. T., Evidence that the corneocyte has a chemically bound lipid envelope, *J. Invest. Dermatol.*, 88, 709, 1987.
25. Wertz, P. W., Madison, K. C., and Downing, D. T., Covalently bound lipids of human stratum corneum, *J. Invest. Dermatol.*, 92, 109, 1989.
26. Swartzendruber, D. C., Wertz, P. W., Kitko, D. J., Madison, K. C., and Downing, D. T., Molecular models of the intercellular lipid lamellae in mammalian stratum corneum, *J. Invest. Dermatol.*, 92, 251, 1989.
27. Kligman, A. M. and Christophers, E., Preparation of isolated sheets of human stratum corneum, *Arch. Dermatol.*, 88, 702, 1963.

28. Menton, D. N., A minimum-surface mechanism to account for the organization of cells into columns in the mammalian epidermis, *Am. J. Anat.*, 145, 1, 1976.

29. Blank, I. H., Further observations on factors which influence the water content of the stratum corneum, *J. Invest. Dermatol.*, 21, 259, 1953.

30. Baker, H. and Kligman, A. M., Techniques for estimating turnover time of human stratum corneum, *Arch. Dermatol.*, 95, 408, 1967.

31. Rothberg, S., Crounse, R. G., and Lee, J. L., Glycine-C^{14} incorporation into the proteins of normal stratum corneum and the abnormal stratum corneum of psoriasis, *J. Invest. Dermatol.*, 37, 497, 1961.

32. Suzuki, Y., Nomura, J., Hori, J., Koyama, J., Takahashi, M., and Horii, I., Detection and characterization of endogenous protease associated with desquamation of stratum corneum, *Arch. Dermatol. Res.*, 285, 372, 1993.

33. Suzuki, Y., Nomura, J., Koyama, J., and Horii, I., The role of proteases in stratum corneum: involvement in stratum corneum desquamation, *Arch. Dermatol. Res.*, 286, 249, 1994.

34. Lundström, A. and Egelrud, T., Evidence that cell shedding from plantar stratum corneum in vitro involves endogenous proteolysis of the desmosomal protein desmoglein 1, *J. Invest. Dermatol.*, 94, 216, 1990.

35. Elias, P. M. and Menon, G. K., Structural and lipid biochemical correlates of the epidermal permeability barrier, in *Advances in Lipid Research*, Vol. 24, Elias, P. M., Ed., Academic Press, San Diego, chap. 1.

36. Rawlings, A. V., Hope, J., Mayo, A. M., Watkinson, A., and Scott, I. R., Skin dryness — what is it? (abst.) *J. Invest. Dermatol.*, 100, 510, 1993.

37. Sato, J., Denda, M., Nakanishi, J., Nomura, J., and Koyama, J., Cholesterol sulfate inhibits proteases that are involved in desquamation of stratum corneum, *J. Invest. Dermatol.*, 111, 189, 1998.

38. Lundstrom, A. and Egelrud, T., Cell shedding from human plantar skin in vitro: evidence that two different types of protein structures are degraded by a chymotrypsin-like enzyme, *Arch. Dermatol. Res.*, 282, 234, 1990.

39. Rothman, S., *Physiology and Biochemistry of Skin*, University of Chicago Press, Chicago, 1954, chap. 4.

40. Ryan, T. J., Cutaneous circulation, in *Biochemistry and Physiology of Skin*, Goldsmith, L. A., Ed., Oxford University Press, New York, 1983, chap. 35.

41. Guy, R. H. and Maibach, H.I., Drug delivery to local subcutaneous structures following topical administration, *J. Pharm. Sci.*, 72, 1375, 1983.

42. Riviere, J. E. and Williams, P. L., Pharmacokinetic implication of changing blood flow in skin, *J. Pharm. Sci.*, 81, 601, 1992.

43. Scheuplein, R. J. and Bronaugh, R. L., Percutaneous absorption, in *Biochemistry and Physiology of Skin*, Goldsmith, L. A., Ed., Oxford University Press, New York, 1983, chap. 58.

44. Burnette, R. R. and Ongpipattanakul, B., Characterization of the pore transport properties and tissue alteration of excised human skin during iontophoresis, *J. Pharm. Sci.*, 77, 132, 1988.

45. Turner, N. G. and Guy, R. H., Visualization and quantitation of iontophoretic pathways using confocal microscopy, *J. Invest. Dermatol.*, Symposium Proceedings 3, 136. 1998.

46. Hueber, F., Besnard, M., Schaefer, H., and Wepierre, J., Percutaneous absorption of estradiol and progesterone in normal and appendage-free skin of the hairless rat: lack of importance of nutritional blood flow, *Skin Pharmacol.*, 7, 245, 1994.

47. Illel, B., Schaefer, H., Wepierre, J., and Doucet, O., Follicles play an important role in percutaneous absorption, *J. Pharm. Sci.*, 80, 424, 1991.

48. Behl, C. R., Bellantone, N. H., and Flynn, G. L., Influence of age on percutaneous absorption of substances, in *Percutaneous Absorption: Mechanism, Methodology, Drug Delivery*, Bronaugh, R. L. and Maibach, H. I., Eds., Marcel Dekker, New York, 1985, chap. 14.

49. Hueber, F., Schaefer, H., and Wepierre, J., Role of transepidermal and transfollicular routes in percutaneous absorption of steroids: in vitro studies on human skin, *Skin Pharmacol.*, 7, 237, 1994.

50. Guy, R. H. and Maibach, H. I., Calculations of body exposure from percutaneous absorption data, in *Percutaneous Absorption: Mechanism, Methodology, Drug Delivery*, Bronaugh, R. L. and Maibach, H. I., Eds., Marcel Dekker, New York, 1985, chap. 35.

51. Lampe, M. A., Williams, M. L., and Elias, P. M., Human epidermal lipids: characterization and modulations during differentiation, *J. Lipid Res.*, 24, 131, 1983.

52. Gray, G. M. and Yardley, H. J., Different populations of pig epidermal cells: isolation and lipid composition, *J. Lipid Res.*, 16, 441, 1975.

53. Lampe, M. A., Burlingame, A. L., Whitney, et al., Human stratum corneum lipids: characterization and regional variations, *J. Lipid Res.*, 24, 120, 1983.

54. Wertz, P. W., Kremer, M., and Squier, C. A., Comparison of lipids from epidermal and palatal stratum corneum, *J. Invest. Dermatol.*, 98, 375, 1992.

55. Hansen, H. S. and Jensen, B., Essential function of linoleic acid esterified in acylglucosylceramide and acylceramide in maintaining the epidermal water permeability barrier: evidence from feeding studies with oleate, linoleate, arachidonate, columbinate and α-linolenate, *Biochim. Biophys. Acta*, 878, 357, 1985.

56. Marzulli, F. N. and Maibach, H. I., Allergic contact dermatitis, in *Dermatotoxicology*, 5th ed., Marzulli, F. N. and Maibach, H. I., Eds., Taylor & Francis, Washington, D.C., 1996, chap. 11.

57. Dahl, M. V., *Clinical Immunodermatology*, 3rd ed., Mosby, New York, 1996.

58. 1998 *Physicians Desk Reference*, p. 711.

59. Fisher, A. A., *Contact Dermatitis*, 3rd ed., Lea & Febiger, Philadelphia, 1986.

60. Amin, S., Lahti, A., and Maibach, H. I., Contact urticaria and the contact urticaria syndrome, in *Dermatotoxicology*, 5th ed., Marzulli, F. N. and Maibach, H. I., Eds., Taylor & Francis, Washington, D.C., 1996, chap 38.

61. Belsito, D. V., Eczematous dermatitis, in *Dermatology in General Medicine*, 4th ed., Fitzpatrick, T. B., Eisen, A. Z., Wolff, K., Freedberg, I. M., and Austen, K. F., Eds., McGraw Hill, New York, 1993, chap. 19.

62. Weltfriend, S., Bason, M., Lammintausta, K., and Maibach, H. I., Irritant dermatitis (Irritation), in *Dermatotoxicology*, 5th ed., Marzulli, F. N. and Maibach, H. I., Eds, Taylor & Francis, Washington, D.C., 1996, chap. 8.

63. Wills, C. M., Histology of irritant contact dermatitis, in *The Irritant Contact Dermatitis Syndrome*, van der Valk, P. G. M. and Maibach, H. I., Eds, CRC Press, Boca Raton, FL, 1996, chap. 31.

3 Epidermal Lipid Metabolism and Barrier Function of Stratum Corneum

Philip W. Wertz and Bozena B. Michniak

CONTENTS

I. INTRODUCTION

As epidermal keratinocytes differentiate, they synthesize lipids, much of which is packaged into small organelles called lamellar granules. Except for linoleic acid, which is an essential fatty acid and must be derived from the diet, the other lipids found in the stratum corneum are synthesized *de novo* in the epidermis from acetate. Most of the energy required for lipid synthesis is produced by anaerobic glycolysis with reduction of the resulting pyruvate to lactate. Late in the differentiation program, the contents of the lamellar granules are exocytosed into the intercellular spaces. Acid hydrolases, also delivered to the intercellular spaces via the lamellar granules, completely break down the remaining phospholipids and convert the glycolipids to ceramides. Ceramides, cholesterol, and fatty acids are the major lipid classes found in the stratum corneum. The lipid processing that accompanies formation of the permeability barrier results in conversion of the initially extruded lamellae into broad multilamellar lipid structures that fill most of the intercellular spaces of the stratum corneum, and it is this intercellular lipid that provides the epidermal permeability barrier. Several lines of evidence suggest that the unusual lipid mixture in the stratum corneum contains gel phase domains in equilibrium with liquid crystalline domains and that the multilayered structures may be highly interdigitated. The purpose of the present chapter is to introduce the major epidermal lipids and their biosynthetic pathways, the hydrolases involved in barrier maturation, and to discuss the possible use of lipid metabolic inhibitors as secondary permeability enhancers.

II. ALTERATION OF EPIDERMAL LIPID COMPOSITION WITH DIFFERENTIATION

Although the structures of many of the lipids present in epidermis and stratum corneum were not known prior to the 1980s, it was recognized as early as 1932 that epidermal lipid composition changes dramatically as a function of differentiation, when Kooymann demonstrated a very low proportion of phospholipid in stratum corneum compared to viable epidermis.[1] Subsequently[2] it was observed that there is a gradual increase in cholesterol and free fatty acid content in going from the basal layer to the stratum corneum, whereas phospholipids accumulated from the basal layer into the granular layer, after which they are catabolized. Gray and co-workers, in the mid to late 1970s, isolated epidermal cell populations enriched in basal cells, granular cells, and stratum corneum and performed the first detailed lipid analyses to account for essentially all of the lipid components.[3–5] It was found that basal cells contain a small amount of cholesterol and high proportions of sphingomyelin, phosphatidylcholine, and phosphatidylethanolamine. The serine and inositol phosphatides are also present, but in relatively low proportions. In the granular cells there is additional cholesterol and phospholipids, and in addition, there are significant proportions of ceramides, glucosylceramides, and free fatty acids. In moving from the granular layer into the stratum corneum, the phospholipids are completely degraded and the glucosylceramides are deglycosylated, leaving ceramides, cholesterol, and fatty acids as the major lipids of the stratum corneum. In addition to alteration of composition, the mass of total lipid per cell increases dramatically with increasing differentiation.

Much of this accumulating lipid is packaged into small organelles known as lamellar granules.[6,7] These organelles are round to ovoid in shape and consist of one, or sometimes several, stacks of lamellar disks surrounded by a unit bounding membrane. The internal disks of the lamellar granules are thought to be flattened lipid vesicles,[7] although it has alternatively been suggested that this internal material could be a membranous sheet folded in an accordion-like manner.[8] In the upper granular layer, the lamellar granules migrate to the apical end of the cell. The bounding membrane of the granule fuses with the plasma membrane, and the granule contents are exocytosed into the intercellular space. The lipids associated with the lamellar granules still include abundant proportions of phospholipids and glycolipids in addition to cholesterol and small proportions of ceramides and fatty acids. Along with lipids, the lamellar granules deliver acid hydrolases to the intercellular space, and these hydrolases complete the conversion of the polar lipids to the mature barrier lipid mixture at the interface between the stratum granulosum and stratum corneum. This lipid processing is associated with the edge-to-edge fusion of the flattened lipid vesicles and the subsequent physical rearrangement from a pair of bilayers to an interdigitated broad–narrow–broad trilaminar unit with an overall periodicity of 13 nm.[9] This lipid remodeling also results in a conversion of liquid crystalline membranes to what is probably a mixture of liquid crystalline and more rigid gel phase domains.[10]

At about the same time that the bounding membrane of the lamellar granule fuses with the plasma membrane, the cornified envelope is forming.[11–13] An unusual hydroxyceramide is derived from the lipid of the bounding membrane of the lamellar granule, and this sphingolipid becomes covalently attached to the outer surface of the cornified envelope.[14,15] This covalently bound lipid layer has the dimensions of a bilayer and appears to provide a monomolecular coating on the outer surface of all of the cornified cells.[15]

The accumulation of lipid and modulation of lipid composition that accompanies keratinization reflects a balance between lipid synthesis and accumulation within the epidermis and the action of catabolic enzymes in the late stages of differentiation. The ultimate mixture of lipids that comprise the covalently bound lipid layer and the intercellular membranes within the stratum corneum is biologically unusual in that phospholipids are absent. These intercellular lipids determine the diffusional resistance and, thereby, the barrier properties of the tissue.

III. MAJOR LIPID BIOSYNTHETIC PATHWAYS

A. FATTY ACIDS SYNTHESIS[16]

Acetate delivered through the circulation is the main carbon source for lipid synthesis in the epidermis. This precursor is converted to acetyl CoA at the expense of one ATP by acetate thiokinase. The first and rate-determining enzymatic step in fatty acid biosynthesis is catalyzed by the biotin-dependent acetyl CoA carboxylase. One ATP is consumed in conversion of acetyl CoA to malonyl CoA. Most of the ATP produced in the epidermis is the result of anaerobic glycolysis with reduction of pyruvate to lactate.[17] The fatty acid synthetase complex, which is cytosolic in location, converts acetyl CoA and malonyl CoA into palmitate (C16:0). Acetate from acetyl CoA and malonate from malonyl CoA are transferred to acyl carrier protein (ACP), and acetate from an acetyl ACP is transferred to carbon 2 of malonyl ACP by a condensing enzyme with the liberation of CO_2 and production of β-ketobutyryl ACP. One NADPH is then used to reduce the β-keto group to a hydroxyl. A double bond is then introduced between carbons 2 and 3 with the removal of water by enoyl ACP hydrase, and in another NADPH-requiring step, the double bond is reduced to yield butyryl ACP. Another malonyl CoA is then condensed with the butyryl group, and this sequence of enzymatic reactions is repeated until a 16-carbon chain has been produced.

The palmityl group is either hydrolyzed from ACP yielding free palmitic acid or transferred to CoA to yield palmityl CoA. The latter can be extended in length through the action of a fatty acid elongase system and double bonds can be introduced through the action of fatty acid desaturases. Both of these enzymes are located in the endoplasmic reticulum. Elongation involves an initial reaction with malonyl CoA followed by a NADPH-dependent reduction. The steps are essentially the same as outlined above for *de novo* synthesis, except that ACP is not involved.

The fatty acids are initially incorporated mainly into triglycerides and phosphoglycerides.[18] After transfer of fatty acids from ACP to CoA, fatty acyl transferases transfer the acyl chains from fatty acyl CoA to glycerol-3-phosphate to produce phosphatidic acid, after which the phosphate is removed, yielding diacylglycerol. Fatty acids found on the 1-position of the glycerol backbone are mostly saturated, and unsaturated fatty acids are found in the 2-position.

The most important metabolic pathway by which polar headgroups become attached to diacylglycerol or ceramide to produce phosphoglycerides or sphingomyelin, respectively, is the Kennedy pathway.[18] In this pathway, choline, for example, is initially phospholylated at the cost of one ATP, followed by condensation with CTP to produce CDP-choline and pyrophosphate. CDP-choline then reacts with 1,2-diacylglycerol yielding phosphatidylcholine. The other phosphatides are produced by an entirely analogous metabolic pathway. Sphingomyelin is produced by transfer of phosphorylcholine from CDP-choline to ceramide.

B. CHOLESTEROL[19]

Basal keratinocytes have plasma membrane-associated low density lipoprotein (LDL) receptors and are, therefore, capable of deriving cholesterol from the circulation. However, as cells move off of the basal lamina and begin to differentiate, the LDL receptors are internalized and degraded.[20] As a result, most of the cholesterol in epidermis must be synthesized *in situ*. The initial steps in conversion of acetate to cholesterol involve the formation of β-hydroxymethylglutaryl CoA (HMG CoA) from 3 acetyl CoAs. Acetyl CoA and acetoacetyl CoA are condensed to produce HMG CoA. The rate-determining step in cholesterol synthesis is then the NADPH-dependent reduction of HMG CoA catalyzed by HMG CoA reductase and yields mevalonate CoA. This reduction requires 2 NADPHs. Free mevalonic acid is then produced by hydrolysis of the CoA thioester, and the resulting mevalonic acid is phosphorylated at the expense of 1 ATP to produce 5-phosphomevalonic acid. A second phosphorylation yields 5-pyrophosphomevalonic acid. A third phosphorylation produces an unstable metabolite which loses CO_2 and one phosphate group to produce 3-isopentenylpyrophosphate, which equilibrates with its isomer, 3,3′-dimethylallyl pyrophosphate. These two isomers are condensed with the release of pyrophosphate and the formation of *trans, trans*-geranyl pyrophosphate. Another isoprenyl pyrophosphate combines with this intermediate, again with loss of pyrophosphate, to yield *trans, trans*-farnesyl pyrophosphate, which equilibrates with its isomer, nerolidol pyrophosphate. These two intermediates undergo an NADPH-dependent reductive condensation to yield squalene. Squalene is acted upon by a mixed function oxidase to yield squalene 2,3-epoxide, which is then converted to lanosterol, a tetracyclic triterpene. Conversion of lanosterol to cholesterol involves the reduction of a double bond in the side chain, a shift of one double bond, and removal of three methyl groups.

HMG CoA reductase activity is regulated by phosphorylation: the dephosphorylated enzyme is active, and the phosphorylated form is inactive.[21] It has been argued that both the level of HMG CoA reductase messenger RNA and the extent of enzyme phosphorylation are regulated by barrier requirements. The evidence and arguments in support of this have been reviewed.[22]

C. Sphingolipids[23]

The rate-determining step in sphingolipid synthesis is catalyzed by serine palmityl transferase, which condenses serine with palmityl CoA in an NADPH-requiring reaction to produce 3-ketodihydrosphingosine with the release of CO_2. This initial product is reduced to dihydrosphingosine by an NADPH-dependent reductase, and N-acylation then yields a ceramide. The dihydrosphingosine moiety of the ceramide can then be converted to sphingosine by the introduction of a trans double bond between carbons 4 and 5, or phytosphingosine may be produced by hydroxylating carbon 4. It appears that hydroxylation of fatty acids on the α position as well as additional hydroxylation on the aliphatic chain of the long-chain base component, as found in the more polar ceramides, occurs after the initial formation of a ceramide in vitamin C-dependent reactions.[24]

As noted previously, ceramides can be converted to sphingomyelins by attachment of a phosphorylcholine to the primary hydroxyl group of the long-chain base. They can also be glucosylated to produce glucosylceramides by transfer of a β-glucopyranosyl residue from CDP-glucose to the primary hydroxyl group of the base. The glycosylation is mediated by a membrane-associated enzyme, ceramide glucosyltransferase.

IV. DEGRADATIVE ENZYMES

Late in the keratinization process, the phospholipids are catabolized and the glycosylceramides are deglycosylated. Fatty acids are cleaved from the 1-position of the phosphoglycerides by a phospholipase A1, while the fatty acids at the 2-position are liberated through the action of phospholipase A2.[25,26] The phosphodiester linkages between the glycerol and the phosphorus of the phosphoglycerides and between the sphingosine and the phosphorus in sphingomyelin are cleaved by phospholipase C.[27] Removal of the glucosyl moiety from the glucosylceramides is mediated by a β-glucocerebrosidase.[28,29] In general, these hydrolases have acidic pH optima, and at least some of these enzymes have been shown to be associated with lamellar granules.[30,31] Accordingly, the activity levels of several of these hydrolytic enzymes is greatest in the upper granular layer where the lamellar granule contents are extruded. The pH in this region of the epidermis may be lowered by the production of lactic acid through anaerobic glycolysis.[31,32] The lipid processing mediated by the acid hydrolases in the late stages of differentiation is thought to be necessary for conversion of the lamellar granule disks into the multilamellar structures of the stratum corneum.[29]

V. STRATUM CORNEUM LIPIDS

Representative structures of the major stratum corneum lipids and their relative proportions are presented in Figure 1.

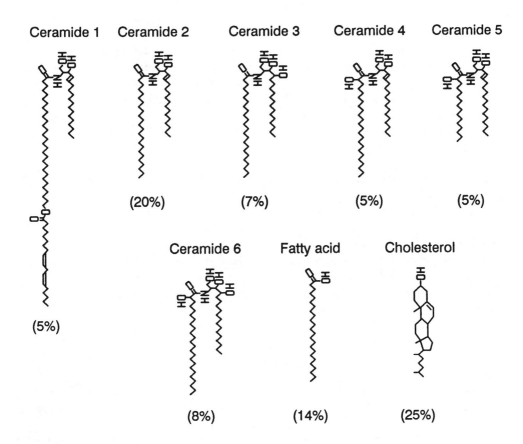

Figure 1   Representative structures and proportions (weight percent) of the major stratum corneum lipids.

The free fatty acids make up between 10 and 15% of the stratum corneum lipid mass and consist of saturated straight chained species.[33] They contain from 14 through 28 carbons with the 22- and 24-carbon species being the most abundant. Free fatty acids and cholesterol sulfate, a quantitatively minor stratum corneum component, are the only ionizable lipids in the stratum corneum and may be required for forming and maintaining a lamellar phase.[34]

Cholesterol represents 25% of the total stratum corneum lipid, and cholesterol sulfate, noted above, accounts for about 5%. Small amounts of cholesterol fatty acid esters are also present.[35] The cholesterol esters are neither bilayer-forming lipids themselves, nor are they well accommodated by bilayers formed from other lipids. Therefore, the cholesterol esters may phase separate into nonlamellar liquid phase domains within the stratum corneum. This may provide a mechanism for isolating unsaturated fatty acids and preventing their fluidizing effect on the intercellular membrane domains.

The ceramides comprise 50% of the total lipid mass in the stratum corneum and are structurally heterogenous.[36] Six chromatographically separable fractions of ceramides have been isolated from porcine epidermis. Each fraction has been characterized by a combination of chemical, chromatographic, and spectroscopic techniques, and representative structures are included in Figure 1. Ceramide 1 is structurally quite unusual. It consists of 30- through 34-carbon ω-hydroxyacids amide-linked to sphingosine and dihydrosphingosine bases and bears ester-linked linoleic acid on the ω-hydroxyl group. It has been proposed that ceramide 1 may serve as a molecular rivet in linking together the intercellular lamellae.[36] More recently a specific model has been proposed in which ceramide 1 plays a key role in formation of the observed

13-nm broad–narrow–broad lamellar arrangement,[10,37] and X-ray diffraction data support this suggestion.[37,38] Ceramide 2 consists of a mixture of sphingosine and dihydrosphingosine bases with amide-linked normal fatty acids. The fatty acid moiety consists of straight-chained saturated fatty acids and are mostly 24, 26, and 28 carbons in length. Ceramide 3 contains the same normal, saturated fatty acids, but now the long-chain base component is a phytosphingosine. Both ceramides 4 and 5 consist of mixtures of sphingosines and dihydrosphingosines with amide-linked α–hydroxyacids. Ceramide 4 contains long 24- through 28-carbon hydroxyacids, whereas ceramide 5 contains almost entirely the 16-carbon entity, α–hydroxypalmitic acid. Ceramide 4 with its longer fatty acid chains is chromatographically more mobile. Finally, ceramide 6 contains α-hydroxyacids amide-linked to phytosphingosines.

Except for the linoleate moiety of ceramide 1, for which a specialized function has been suggested, all of the aliphatic chains in the ceramides as well as the fatty acids are straight, and all of the polar head groups are minimal. All of the ceramides and fatty acids are rod or cylindrical shaped. This makes them ideal for the formation of highly ordered gel phase membrane domains, which are less fluid and less permeable than the more usual liquid crystalline membrane domains found in most biological membranes. Evidence from a number of sources, including calorimetric and infrared spectroscopic measurements,[39] X-ray diffraction studies,[40] and fluorescence spectroscopy,[41] supports the presence of gel phase domains within stratum corneum.

Cholesterol, which is not cylindrical in shape, has the ability to either stiffen or fluidize membranes, depending on the proportion of cholesterol and the nature of the other lipids present. It has been suggested that in the epidermal stratum corneum, cholesterol may provide a degree of fluidity to what could otherwise be very rigid membranes.[10] Overall, it is thought that the stratum corneum membrane system is a highly interdigitated system consisting of microscopic gel phase domains in equilibrium with liquid crystalline domains.

In situations where the barrier function of the skin has been compromised, the topical application of lipids can result in delayed recovery of barrier function, accelerated recovery, or there may be no effect.[42,43] Application of any one or combination of the major classes of barrier lipids (ceramides, cholesterol, fatty acids) results in delayed barrier recovery. An equimolar mixture of ceramides, cholesterol, and free fatty acids allows normal barrier recovery, whereas, if any one of the three components is increased about threefold to achieve a 3:1:1 molar ratio, barrier recovery is accelerated. Optimum lipid mixtures for the acceleration of barrier recovery include, in addition to ceramides and cholesterol, both nonessential and essential fatty acids.[43]

VI. SECONDARY PENETRATION ENHANCERS

A. The Concept

The suggestion that inhibitors of lipid metabolism can be used to locally and reversibly diminish barrier function for the purpose of drug delivery has been advanced by Tsai et al.[44] On the basis that mainly ceramides, cholesterol, and fatty acids in the intercellular spaces determine the barrier function of the skin and a demonstration that barrier function varies inversely with stratum corneum lipid content, it has been proposed that inhibitors of key enzymes involved in the biosynthesis of the major lipid types could provide a means of reducing barrier function. In addition to diminishing the concentration of lipid in the stratum corneum, the selective inhibition of one of the major lipid biosynthetic pathways would lead to an alteration of the proportions of stratum corneum lipids, and it has been shown that the lipid composition is also important for barrier function.

A less thoroughly but closely related area is the potential use of inhibitors of hydrolases to prevent the lipid processing associated with final formation and maturation of the barrier.[45]

Yet another potential variant on the secondary enhancer theme is the potential to reduce barrier function by means of locally induced essential fatty acid deficiency.[46]

B. The Evidence

Almost all of the evidence in support of the suggestion that inhibitors of lipid biosynthesis could be used topically to diminish barrier function comes from experiments on recovery of barrier function in hairless mouse skin following barrier disruption.[44,47–49] One exception is a study in which transepidermal water loss was shown to increase following four to six daily applications of lovastatin, an HMG CoA reductase inhibitor, to hairless mouse skin.[50] In the other supportive studies, barrier function was first disrupted by either removal of stratum corneum lipids by wiping the skin with acetone-soaked cotton balls, by tape stripping, or by the induction of dietary essential fatty acid deficiency. Regardless of the method of barrier disruption as judged by transepidermal water loss, recovery of barrier function can be delayed by the topical application of inhibitors of the rate-limiting enzymes of the major stratum corneum lipids. Barrier recovery can be delayed by topical lovastatin or fluvastatin, both of which inhibit HMG CoA reductase, the rate-limiting enzyme in the synthesis of cholesterol.[47] Cholesterol sulfate, a cholesterol biosynthesis inhibitor of uncertain mechanism, also is effective in delaying barrier recovery.[44] Likewise, 5-(tetradecyloxy)-2-furancarboxylic acid, an inhibitor of fatty acid synthesis, and β-chloroalanine, an inhibitor of serine palmitoyl transferase, are also effective in delaying barrier recovery.[48] In one study, it was demonstrated that inhibition of barrier recovery by inhibitors of fatty acid or cholesterol synthesis did result in increased uptake of lidocaine or caffeine, and the effects of combinations of inhibitors of both metabolic pathways appeared to produce an additive effect.[44] However, it was also shown that at least part of the effect of the inhibitors was thermodynamic rather than metabolic. The octanol/water partition coefficients of the drugs were altered by the inclusion of inhibitors in the common vehicle.

There is only one example of delayed barrier recovery by application of an inhibitor of a hydrolase. Bromoconduritol-β-epoxide, an inhibitor of β-glucocerebrosidase, delays recovery of barrier function following disruption with acetone.[45] It also prevents the conversion of the initially extruded lamellar granule contents into the multilamellar arrays that are normally present in the intercellular spaces of the stratum corneum. It has also been demonstrated that topical application of bromoconduritol-β-epoxide to intact mouse skin progressively and reversibly impaired barrier function.[51]

It is well established that essential fatty acid deficiency results in impairment of the barrier function of the skin manifest as elevated transepidermal water loss.[52] At a biochemical level the increase in transepidermal water loss that accompanies the development of essential fatty acid deficiency correlates with substitution of oleic acid for linoleic acid in the acylceramide.[53] In one set of experiments, it was shown that topically applied methyl oleate could penetrate into the viable epidermis of neonatal mice and enter into lipid metabolism with considerable replacement of linoleate in the acylglucosylceramide that is the immediate precursor.[46] Although barrier function was not assessed in this study, the observed biochemical alterations strongly suggested that one could locally induce essential fatty acid deficiency and thereby compromise barrier function. With topical oleate, there would also be a traditional enhancer effect.

C. Future Prospects

The concept that barrier function can be manipulated by metabolic means is relatively new but promising and draws a great deal of support from experiments employing hairless or neonatal mouse skin. The greatest impediment to the use of topically applied metabolic inhibitors as secondary enhancers may be delivery of sufficient concentrations of inhibitors to the sites of lipid synthesis in human skin, where barrier function is superior. The exploitation of lipid synthesis inhibitors or catabolic inhibitors may require their use in combination with more conventional enhancers or with physical means of enhancement. A problem with the use of oleate to locally induce essential fatty acid deficiency is that this fatty acid is too irritating for repeated or long-term use, although it may be acceptable in situations where only occasional use is required. Overall, there are many questions to be answered before secondary enhancers can be applied to practical problems, but this area has the potential to provide great benefit.

REFERENCES

1. Kooyman, D. J., Lipids in the skin. Some changes in the lipids of the epidermis during the process of keratinization, *Arch. Dermatol. Syph.*, 25, 444, 1932.
2. Long, V. J. W., Variations in lipid composition at different depths in the cow snout epidermis, *J. Invest. Dermatol.*, 55, 269, 1970.
3. Gray, G. M. and Yardley, H. J., Different populations of pig epidermal cells: isolation and lipid composition, *J. Lipid Res.*, 16, 441, 1975.
4. Gray, G. M. and Yardley, H. J., Lipid compositions of cells isolated from pig, human and rat epidermis, *J. Lipid Res.*, 16, 434, 1975.
5. Gray, G. M. and White, R. J., Glycosphingolipids and ceramides in human and pig epidermis, *J. Invest. Dermatol.*, 70, 336, 1978.
6. Elias, P. M. and Friend, D. S., The permeability barrier in mammalian epidermis. *J. Cell Biol.*, 65, 180, 1975.
7. Landmann, L., The epidermal permeability barrier, *Anat. Embryol.*, 178, 1, 1988.
8. Menon, G.K., Feingold, K.R., and Elias, P.M., Lamellar body secretory response to barrier disruption, *J. Invest. Dermatol.*, 98, 279, 1992
9. Madison, K. C., Swartzendruber, D. C., Wertz, P. W., and Downing, D.T., Presence of intact intercellular lamellae in the upper layers of the stratum corneum, *J. Invest. Dermatol.*, 88, 714, 1987.
10. Wertz, P. W. and van den Bergh, B. A. I., The physical, chemical and functional properties of lipids in the skin and other biological barriers, *Chem. Phys. Lipids*, 91, 85, 1998.
11. Rice, R. H. and Green, H., Presence in human epidermal cells of a soluble protein precursor of the cross-linked envelope: activation of the cross-linking by calcium ions, *Cell*, 18, 681, 1979.
12. Rice, R. H. and Green, H., The cornified envelope of terminally differentiated human epidermal keratinocytes consists of cross-linked protein, *Cell*, 11, 417, 1977.
13. Mehrel, T., Hohl, D., Rothnagel, J. A., Longley, M. A., Bundman, D., Cheng, C., Lichti, U., Bisher, M. E., Steven, A. C., Steinert, P. M., Yuspa, S. H., and Roop, D. R., Identification of a major keratinocyte cell envelope protein, loricrin, *Cell*, 61, 1103, 1990.
14. Wertz, P. W. and Downing, D. T., Covalently bound ω−hydroxyacylsphingosine in the stratum corneum, *Biochim. Biophys. Acta*, 917, 108, 1987.
15. Swartzendruber, D. C., Wertz, P. W., Madison, K. C., and Downing, D. T., Evidence that the corneocyte has a chemically bound lipid envelope, *J. Invest. Dermatol.*, 88, 709, 1987.
16. Slabas, A. R., Brown, A., Sinden, B. S., Swinhoe, R., Simon, J. W., Ashton, A. R., Whitfield, P. R., and Elborough, K. M., Pivotal reactions in fatty acid synthesis, *Prog. Lipid Res.*, 33, 39, 1994.
17. Freinkel, R. K., Carbohydrate metabolism of epidermis, in *Physiology, Biochemistry and Molecular Biology of the Skin*, 2nd ed., Goldsmith, L. A., Ed., Oxford University Press, New York, 1993, 452.
18. Kennedy, E. P., The metabolism and function of complex lipids, *Harvey Lect.*, 57, 143, 1962.
19. Russell, D. W., Cholesterol biosynthesis and metabolism, *Cardiovasc. Drugs Ther.*, 6, 103, 1992.
20. Pas, M. F., Lombardi, P., Havekes, L. M., Boonstra, J., and Ponec, M., Regulation of low-density lipoprotein receptor expression during keratinocyte differentiation, *J. Invest. Dermatol.*, 97, 334, 1991.
21. Beg, Z. H., Shonik, J. A., and Brewer, Jr., H. B., 3-Hydroxy-3-methylglutaryl coenzyme A reductase: regulation of enzymatic activity by phosphorylation and dephosphorylation, *Proc. Natl. Acad. Sci. U.S.A.*, 75, 3678, 1978.
22. Feingold, K. R., The regulation and role of lipid synthesis, *Adv. Lipid Res.*, 24, 57, 1991.
23. Radin, N. S., Biosynthesis of the sphingoid bases: a provocation, *J. Lipid Res.*, 25, 1536, 1984.
24. Ponec, M., Weerheim, A., Kempenaar, J., Mulder, A., Gooris G. S., Bouwstra, J. A., and Mommaas, A. M., The formation of competent barrier lipids in reconstructed human epidermis requires the presence of vitamin C, *J. Invest. Dermatol.*, 109, 348, 1997.
25. Kaiser, E., Chiba, P., and Zaky, K., Phospholipases in biology and medicine, *Clin. Biochem.*, 23, 349, 1990.
26. Holleran, W. M., Lipid modulators of epidermal proliferation and differentiation, *Adv. Lipid Res.*, 24, 119, 1991.
27. Bergers, M., van de Kerkhof, P. C., Happle, R., and Mier, P. D., Membrane-bound phospholipase C activity in normal and psoriatic epidermis, *Acta Derm.-Venereol.*, 70, 57, 1990.

28. Wertz, P. W. and Downing, D. T., β-Glucosidase activity in porcine epidermis, *Biochim. Biophys. Acta*, 1001, 115, 1989.

29. Holleran, W. M., Ginns, E. I., Menon, G. K., Grundmann, J. U., Fartasch, M., McKinney, C. E., and Elias, P.M., Consequences of beta-glucocerebrosidase deficiency in epidermis. Ultrastructure and permeability barrier alterations in Gaucher disease, *J. Clin. Invest.*, 93, 1756, 1994.

30. Freinkel, R. K. and Traczyk, T. N., Lipid composition and acid hydrolase content of lamellar granules of fetal rat epidermis, *J. Invest. Dermatol.*, 85, 295, 1985.

31. Menon, G. K., Ghadially, R., Williams, M. L., and Elias, P.M., Lamellar bodies as delivery systems of hydrolytic enzymes: implications for normal and abnormal desquamation, *Br. J. Dermatol.*, 126, 337, 1992.

32. Chang, F., Wertz, P. W., and Squier, C.A., Localization of β–glucosidase activity within keratinizing epithelia, *Comp. Biochem. Physiol.*, 105A, 251, 1993.

33. Wertz, P. W. and Downing, D. T., Stratum corneum: biological and biochemical considerations, in *Transdermal Drug Delivery*, Hadgraft, J. and Guy, R. H., Eds., Marcel Dekker, New York, 1988, 1.

34. Wertz, P. W., Abraham, W., Landmann, L., and Downing, D. T., Preparation of liposomes from stratum corneum lipids, *J. Invest. Dermatol.*, 87, 582, 1986.

35. Wertz, P. W., Swartzendruber, D. C., Madison, K. C., and Downing, D.T., Composition and morphology of epidermal cyst lipids, *J. Invest. Dermatol.*, 89, 419, 1987.

36. Wertz P. W. and Downing, D. T., Ceramides of pig epidermis: structure determination, *J. Lipid Res.*, 24, 759, 1983.

37. Bouwstra, J. A., Gooris, G. S., Dubbelaar, F. E., Weerheim, A. M., Ijzerman, A. P., and Ponec, M., Role of ceramide 1 in the molecular organization of the stratum corneum lipids, *J. Lipid Res.*, 39, 186, 1998.

38. Bouwstra, J. A., Gooris, G. S., Salomons-de Vries, M. A., van den Spek, J. A., and Bras, W., Structure of human stratum corneum: a wide-angle X-ray diffraction study, *Int. J. Pharm.*, 84, 205, 1992.

39. Ongpipattanakul, B., Franceur, M. L., and Potts, R. O., Polymorphism in stratum corneum lipids, *Biochim. Biophys. Acta*, 1190, 115, 1994.

40. Bowstra, J. A., Gooris, G. S., van der Spek, J. A., Lavrijsen, S., and Bras, W., *Biochim. Biophys. Acta*, 1212, 183, 1994.

41. Abraham, W., Wertz, P. W., Potts, R. O., and Garrison, M. D., Investigation of phase transition in oral mucosa by fluorescence spectroscopy, *Proc. Int. Symp. Controlled Release Bioact. Mater.*, 21, 557, 1994.

42. Man, M. Q. M., Feingold, K. R., Thornfeldt, C. R., and Elias, P. M., *J. Invest. Dermatol.*, 106, 1096, 1996.

43. Zettersten, E. M., Ghadially, R., Feingold, K. R., Crumrine, D., and Elias, P. M., *J. Amer. Acad. Dermatol.*, 37, 403, 1997.

44. Tsai, J. C., Guy, R. H., Thornfeldt, C. R., Gao, W. N., Feingold, K. R., and Elias, P. M., Metabolic approaches to enhance transdermal drug delivery. 1. Effect of lipid synthesis inhibitors, *J. Pharm. Sci.*, 85, 643, 1996.

45. Holleran, W.M., Takagi, Y., Menon, G. K., Jackson, S. M., Lee, J. M., Feingold, K. R., and Elias, P. M., Permeability barrier requirements regulate epidermal beta-glucocerebrosidase, *Lipid Res.*, 35, 905, 1994.

46. Feingold, K. R., Man, M. Q., Menon, G. K., Cho, S. S., Brown, B. E., and Elias, P. M., Cholesterol synthesis is required for cutaneous barrier function in mice, *J. Clin. Invest.*, 86, 1738, 1990.

47. Holleran, W. M., Man, M. Q., Gao, W. N., Menon, G. K., Elias, P. M., and Feingold, K. R., Sphingolipids are required for mammalian epidermal barrier function. Inhibition of sphingolipid synthesis delays barrier recovery after acute perturbation, *J. Clin. Invest.*, 88, 1338, 1991.

48. Holleran, W. M., Feingold, K. R., Man, M. Q., Gao, W. N., Lee, J. M., and Elias, P. M., Regulation of epidermal sphingolipid synthesis by permeability barrier function, *J. Lipid Res.*, 32, 1151, 1991.

49. Mao-Qiang, M., Elias, P. M., and Feingold, K. R., Fatty acids are required for epidermal permeability barrier function, *J. Clin. Invest.*, 92, 791, 1993.

50. Feingold, K. R., Man, M. Q., Proksch, E., Menon, G.K., Brown, B. E., and Elias, P.M., The lovastatin-treated rodent: a new model of barrier disruption and epidermal hyperplasia, *J. Invest. Dermatol.*, 96, 201, 1991.

51. Holleran, W. M., Takagi, Y., Menon, G. K., Legler, G., Feingold, K. R., and Elias, P. M., Processing of epidermal glucosylceramides is required for optimal mammalian cutaneous barrier function, *J. Clin. Invest.*, 91, 1656, 1993.

52. Holman, R. T., Essential fatty acid deficiency, *Prog. Chem. Fats Other Lipids*, 9, 275, 1968.

53. Melton, J. L., Wertz, P. W., Swartzendruber, D. C., and Downing, D. T., Effects of essential fatty acid deficiency on O-acylsphingolipids and transepidermal water loss in young pigs, *Biochim. Biophys. Acta*, 921, 191, 1987.

4 Methods for Testing the Irritation and Sensitization Potential of Drugs and Enhancers

Saqib J. Bashir and Howard I. Maibach

CONTENTS

0-8493-2117-4/00/$0.00+$.50
© 2000 by CRC Press LLC

I. METHODS FOR TESTING IRRITATION POTENTIAL

A. INTRODUCTION

Skin forms the interface between humans and their environment. Among its many functions, it is an important barrier that may be disrupted by irritation. For this reason, we must document the potential toxicity of any substance to human skin.

Accurate prediction of the irritation potential of industrial, pharmaceutical, and cosmetic materials is therefore necessary to advise suitable health and safety precautions. Presently, animal models fulfill licensing criteria for regulatory bodies. However, a search for alternative methods is stimulated by difficulties in relating animal data to human settings, and also by humane motives.

Many aspects of irritation have been described, ranging from the visible erythema and edema to molecular mediators such as interleukins and prostaglandins. Therefore, a variety of in vivo and in vitro approaches to experimental assay are possible. However, no model assays inflammation in its entirety. Each model is limited by our ability to interpret and extrapolate features of inflammation to the desired context. Therefore, predicting human responses based on data from nonhuman models requires particular care.

Various human experimental models have also been proposed, providing irritant data for the relevant species. However, these studies are also limited by pitfalls in interpretation and, of course, by the fear of applying new substances to human skin before their irritant potential has been evaluated.

B. ANIMAL MODELS

1. Draize Rabbit Models

The Draize model[1a] and its modifications are commonly used to assay skin irritation using albino rabbits. Various governmental agencies have adopted these methods as standard test procedure. The procedure adopted in the U.S. Federal Hazardous Substance Act (FHSA) is described in Tables 1 and 2.[1-3] Table 3 compares this method with some other modifications of the Draize model.

Draize utilized the above scoring system to calculate the Primary Irritation Index (PII). This is calculated by averaging the erythema scores and also averaging the edema scores of all sites (abraded and nonabraded). These two averages are then added together to give the PII value. A value of <2 was considered nonirritating; 2 to 5 mildly irritating; and >5, severely irritating. A value of 5 defines an irritant by Consumer Product Safety Commission (CPSC) standards. Subsequent laboratory and clinical experience has demonstrated the value judgments (i.e., non-, mild, severely irritating) proposed in 1944 require clinical judgment and perspective — and should not be viewed in an absolute sense. Many materials irritating to the rabbit may be well tolerated by human skin.

Although the Draize scoring system does not include vesiculation, ulceration, and severe eschar formation, all of the Draize-type tests are used to evaluate corrosion as well as irritation. When severe and potentially irreversible reactions occur, the test sites are further observed on days 7 and 14, or later if necessary.

Modifications to the Draize assay have attempted to improve its prediction of human experience. The model is criticized for inadequately differentiating between mild and moderate irritants. However, it serves well in hazard identification, often over-predicting the severity of human skin reactions.[3] Therefore, Draize assays continue to be recommended by regulatory bodies.

2. Cumulative Irritation Assays

Several assays study the effects of cumulative exposure to a potential irritant. Justice et al. administered seven applications of surfactant solutions at 10-min intervals to the clipped dorsum

TABLE 1
Draize-FHSA Model

Number of animals	6 albino rabbits (clipped)
Test sites	2×1 in.^{2} sites on dorsum;
	one site intact, the other abraded,
	e.g., with hypodermic needle
Test materials	Applied undiluted to both test sites
	Liquids: 0.5 ml
	Solids/semisolids: 0.5 g
Occlusion	1 in.^{2} surgical gauze over each test site
	Rubberized cloth over entire trunk
Occlusion period	24 h
Assessment	24 and 72 h
	Visual scoring system

TABLE 2
Draize-FHSA Scoring System[2]

	Score
Erythema and eschar formation	
No erythema	0
Very slight erythema (barely perceptible)	1
Well-defined erythema	2
Moderate to severe erythema	3
Severe erythema (beet redness) to slight eschar formation (injuries in depth)	4
Edema formation	
No edema	0
Very slight edema (barely perceptible)	1
Slight edema (edges of area well defined by definite raising)	2
Moderate edema (raised > 1 mm)	3
Severe edema (raised > 1 mm and extending beyond the area of exposure)	4

TABLE 3
Examples of Modified Draize Irritation Method

	Draize	FHSA	DOT	FIFRA	OECD
No. of animals	3	6	6	6	6
Abrasion/intact	Both	Both	Intact	2 of each	Intact
Dose liquids	0.5 ml undiluted	0.5 ml undiluted	0.5 ml	0.5 ml undiluted	0.5 ml
Dose solids in solvent	0.5 g	0.5 g moistened	0.5 g moistened	0.5 g	0.5 g
Exposure period (h)	24	24	4	4	4
Examination (h)	24, 72	24, 72	4, 48	0.5, 1, 24, 48, 72	0.5, 1, 24, 48, 72
Removal of test materials	Not specified	Not specified	Skin washed	Skin wiped	Skin washed
Excluded from testing	—	—	—	Toxic materials pH ≤ 2 or ≥ 11.5	Toxic materials pH ≤ 2 or ≥ 11.5

Note: FHSA: Federal Hazardous Substance Act;
   DOT: Department of Transportation;
   FIFRA: Federal Insecticide, Fungicide and Rodenticide Act;
   OECD: Organization for Economic Cooperation and Development.

From Esther and Maibach, 1989.

of albino mice.[4] The test site was occluded with a rubber dam to prevent evaporation, and the skin was examined microscopically for epidermal erosion.

Frosch et al. described the guinea pig repeat irritation test (RIT) to evaluate protective creams against the chemical irritants sodium lauryl sulfate (SLS), sodium hydroxide (NaOH), and toluene.[5] The irritants were applied daily for 2 weeks to shaved back skin of young guinea pigs. Barrier creams were applied to the test animals 2 h prior to and immediately after exposure to the irritant. Control animals were treated with the irritant only. Erythema was measured visually and by bioengineering methods: laser Doppler flowmetry and transepidermal water loss. One barrier cream was effective against SLS and toluene, while the other cream tested was not. In a follow-up study, another allegedly protective cream failed to inhibit irritation caused by SLS and toluene and exaggerated irritation to NaOH, contrary to its recommended use.[6] The RIT is proposed as an animal model to test the efficacy of barrier creams, and further proposed as a human version, described below.

Repeat application patch tests have been developed to rank the irritant potential of products. Putative irritants are applied to the same site for 3 to 21 days, under occlusion. The degree of occlusion influences percutaneous penetration, which may in turn influence the sensitivity of the test. Patches used vary from Draize-type gauze dressings to metal chambers. Therefore, a reference irritant material is often included in the test to facilitate interpretation of the results. Various animal species have also been used, such as the guinea pig and the rabbit.[7,8] Wahlberg measured skin fold thickness with Harpenden calipers to assess the edema-producing capacity of chemicals in guinea pigs.[8] This model demonstrated clear dose–response relationships and discriminating power, except for acids and alkalis, where no change in skin fold thickness was found.

Open application assays are also used for repeat irritation testing. Marzulli and Maibach described a cumulative irritation assay in rabbits, which utilizes open applications and control reference compounds.[9] The test substances are applied 16 times over a 3-week period and the results are measured with a visual score for erythema and skin thickness measurements. These two parameters correlated highly. A significant correlation was also demonstrated between the scores of 60 test substances in the rabbit and in man, suggesting that the rabbit assay is a powerful predictive model.

Anderson et al. utilized an open application procedure in guinea pigs to rank weak irritants.[10] A baseline response to SLS solution was obtained after 3 applications per day for 3 days to a 1-cm² test area. This baseline is used to compare other irritants, of which trichloroethane was the most irritant, similar to 2% SLS. Histology demonstrated a mononuclear dermal inflammatory response.

3. Immersion Assay

The guinea pig immersion assay was developed to assess the irritant potential of aqueous surfactant-based solutions, but might be extended to other occupational settings, such as aqueous cutting fluids. Restrained guinea pigs are immersed in the test solution, while maintaining their heads above water. The possibility of systemic absorption of a lethal dose restricts the study to products of limited toxic potential. Therefore, the test concentration is usually limited to 10%.

Ten guinea pigs are placed immersed in a 40°C solution for 4 h daily, for 3 days. A comparison group is immersed in a reference solution. Next, 24 h after the final immersion, the animals' flanks are shaved and evaluated for erythema, edema, and fissures.[11–15] Gupta et al.[15] concomitantly tested the dermatotoxic effects of detergents in guinea pigs and humans, utilizing the immersion test and the patch test, respectively. Epidermal erosion and a 40 to 60% increase in the histamine content of the guinea pig skin were found, in addition to a positive patch test reaction in seven of out eight subjects.

4. Mouse Ear Model

Uttley and Van Abbe applied undiluted shampoos to one ear of mice daily for 4 days, visually quantifying the degree of inflammation as vessel dilatation, erythema, and edema.[16] Patrick and

Maibach measured ear thickness to quantify the inflammatory response to surfactant-based products and other chemicals.[17] This allowed quantification of dose–response relationships and comparison of chemicals. Inoue et al. used this model to compare the mechanism of mustard oil-induced skin inflammation to the mechanism of capsaicin-induced inflammation.[18] Mice were pretreated with various receptor antagonists, such as 5-HT$_2$, H$_1$, and tachykinin antagonists, demonstrating that the tachykinin NK1 receptor was an important mediator of inflammation induced by mustard oil. The mouse models provide simplicity and objective measurements. Relevance for man requires elucidation.

5. Other Methods

Several other assays of skin irritation have been suggested. Humphrey quantified the amount of Evans blue dye recovered from rat skin following exposure to skin irritants.[19] Trush et al. utilized myleoperoxidase in polymorphonuclear leukocytes as a biomarker for cutaneous inflammation.[20]

C. HUMAN MODELS

Human models for skin imitation testing are species relevant, thereby eliminating the precarious extrapolation of animal and in vitro data to the human setting. As the required test area is small, several products or concentrations can be tested simultaneously and compared. Inclusion of a reference irritant substance facilitates interpretation of the irritant potential of the test substances. Prior animal studies can be utilized to exclude particularly toxic substances or concentrations before human exposure.

1. Single Application Patch Testing

The National Academy of Sciences (NAS) outlined a single application patch test procedure determining skin irritation in humans.[21] Occlusive patches may be applied to the intrascapular region of the back or the dorsal surface of the forearms, utilizing a relatively nonocclusive tape for new or volatile materials. More occlusive tapes or chambers generally increase the severity of the responses. A reference material is included in each battery of patches.

The exposure time may vary to suit the study. NAS suggests a 4-h exposure period, although it may be desirable to test new or volatile materials for 30 min to 1 h. Studies greater than 24 h have been performed. Skin responses are evaluated 30 min to 1 h after removal of the patch, using the animal Draize scale (Table 1) or similar. Kligman and Wooding described statistical analysis on test data to calculate the IT50 (time to produce imitation in 50% of the subjects) and the ID50 (dose required to produce irritation in 50% of the subjects after a 24-h exposure).[22]

Robinson et al. suggested a 4-h patch test as an alternative to animal testing.[23] Assessing erythema by visual scoring, they tested a variety of irritants on Caucasians and Asians. A relative ranking of irritancy was obtained, utilizing 20% SLS as a benchmark. Taking this model further, McFadden et al. investigated the threshold of skin irritation in the six different skin types.[24] Again using SLS as a benchmark, they defined the skin irritant threshold as the lowest concentration of SLS that would produce skin irritation under the 4-h occluded patch conditions. They found no significant difference in irritation between the skin types.

2. Cumulative Irritation Testing

Lanman et al.[25] and Phillips et al.[7] described a cumulative irritation assay, which has become known as the "21 day" cumulative irritation assay. The purpose of the test was to screen new formulas prior to marketing. A 1-in. square of Webril is saturated with liquid or 0.5 g of viscous substances and applied to the surface of the pad to be applied to the skin. The patch is applied to the upper back and sealed with occlusive tape. The patch is removed after 24 h, and then reapplied after examination of the test site. This is repeated for 21 days and the IT50 can then be calculated.

Modifications have been made to this method. The chamber scarification test (see below) was developed to predict the effect of repeated applications of a potential irritant to damaged skin, rather than healthy skin. The cumulative patch test described above had failed to predict adverse reactions to skin damaged by acne or shaving, or sensitive areas such as the face.[26]

Wigger-Alberti et al. compared two cumulative models, testing skin reaction to metalworking fluids (MWF).[27] Irritation was assessed by visual scoring, transepidermal water loss, and chromametry. In the first method, MWF were applied with Finn Chambers on the volunteers' midback, removed after 1 day of exposure, and reapplied for a further 2 days. In the second method, cumulative irritant contact dermatitis was induced using a repetitive irritation test for 2 weeks (omitting weekends) for 6 h/day. The 3-day model was preferred because of its shorter duration and better discrimination of irritancy. For low irritancy materials in which discrimination is not defined with visual and palpatory scores, bioengineering methods (i.e., transepidermal water loss) may be helpful.

3. The Chamber Scarification Test

This test was developed to test the irritant potential of products on damaged skin.[28,29] Six to eight l-mm sites on the volar forearm were scratched eight times with a 30-gauge needle, without causing bleeding. Four scratches were parallel and the other four were perpendicular to these. Duhring chambers, containing 0.1 g of test material (ointments, creams, or powders), were then placed over the test sites. For liquids, a fitted, saturated pad (0.1 ml) may be used. Chambers containing fresh materials are reapplied daily for 3 days. The sites are evaluated by visual scoring 30 min after removal of the final set of chambers. A scarification index may be calculated if both normal and scarified skin is tested, to reflect the relative degree of irritation between compromised and intact skin: this is the score of scarified sites divided by the score of intact sites. However, the relationship of this assay to routine use of substances on damaged skin remains to be established. Another compromised skin model, the arm immersion model of compromised skin, is described in the immersion tests section below.

4. The Soap Chamber Test

Frosch and Kligman proposed a model to compare the potential of bar soaps to cause "chapping."[30] Standard patch testing was able to predict erythema, but unable to predict the dryness, flaking, and fissuring seen clinically. In this method, Duhring chambers fitted with Webril pads are used to apply 0.1 ml of an 8% soap solution to the human forearm. The chambers are secured with porous tape, and applied for 24 h on day 1. On days 2 to 5, fresh patches are applied for 6 h. The skin is examined daily before patch application and on day 8, the final study day. No patches are applied after day 5. Applications are discontinued if severe erythema is noted at any point. Reactions are scored on a visual scale of erythema, scaling, and fissures. This test correlates well with skin-washing procedures, but tends to overpredict the irritancy of some substances.[31]

5. Immersion Tests

These tests of soaps and detergents were developed in order to improve irritancy prediction by mimicking consumer use. Kooyman and Snyder describe a method in which soap solutions of up to 3% are prepared in troughs.[32] The temperature was maintained at 105°F while subjects immersed one hand and forearm in each trough, comparing different products (or concentrations). The exposure period ranged from 10 to 15 min, three times each day for 5 days, or until irritation was observed in both arms. The antecubital fossa was the first site to demonstrate irritation, followed by the hands.[4,32] Therefore, antecubital wash tests (see below) and hand immersion assays were developed.[3]

Clarys et al. used a 30-min/4-day immersion protocol to investigate the effects of temperature and also anionic character on the degree of irritation caused by detergents.[33] The irritation was quantified by assessment of the stratum cornum barrier function (transepidermal water loss), skin redness (a* color parameter), and skin dryness (capacitance method). Although both detergents tested significantly affected the integrity of the skin, higher anionic content and temperature, respectively, increased the irritant response.

Allenby et al. describe the arm immersion model of compromised skin, which is designed to test the irritant or allergic potential of substances on damaged skin.[34] Such skin may demonstrate an increased response, which may be negligible or undetectable in normal skin. The test subject immersed one forearm in a solution of 0.5 % sodium dodecyl sulfate for 10 min, twice daily until the degree of erythema reached 1 to 1+ on a visual scale. This degree of damage corresponded to a morning's wet domestic work. Patch tests of various irritants were applied to the dorsal and volar aspects of both the pretreated and untreated forearms, and also to the back. Each irritant produced a greater degree of reaction on the compromised skin.

6. Wash Tests

Hannuksela and Hannuksela compared the irritant effects of a detergent in use testing and patch testing.[35] In this study of atopic and nonatopic medical students, each subject washed the outer aspect of the one forearm with liquid detergent for 1 min, twice daily for 1 week. Concurrently, a 48-h chamber patch test of 5 concentrations of the same detergent was performed on the upper back. The irritant response was quantified by bioengineering techniques: transepidermal water loss, electrical capacitance, and skin blood flow. In the wash test, atopics and nonatopics developed irritant contact dermatitis equally, whereas atopics reacted more readily to the detergent in chamber tests. The disadvantage of the chamber test is that, under occlusion, the detergent can cause stronger irritation than it would in normal use.[36] Although the wash test simulates normal use of the product being tested, its drawback is a lack of standard guidelines for performing the test. Charbonnier et al. included squamometry in their analysis of a hand washing model of subclinical irritant dermatitis with SLS solutions.[37] Squamometry demonstrated a significant difference between 0.1 and 0.75% SLS solutions, whereas visual, subjective, capacitance, transepidermal water loss, and chromametry methods were unable to make the distinction. The authors suggest squamometry as an adjunct to the other bioengineering methods.

Frosch describes an antecubital washing test to evaluate toilet soaps, utilizing two washing procedures per day.[31] Simple visual scoring of the reaction (erythema and edema) allows products to be compared. This comparison can be in terms of average score, or number of washes required to produce an effect.

7. Assessing Protective Barriers

Zhai et al. proposed a model to evaluate skin protective materials. Ten subjects were exposed to the irritants SLS and ammonium hydroxide (in urea) and to *Rhus* allergen.[38] The occluded test sites were on each forearm, with one control site on each. The irritant response was assessed visually, using a 10-point scale, which included vesiculation and maceration unlike standard Draize scales. The scores were statistically analyzed for nonparametric data. Of the barrier creams studied, paraffin wax in cetyl alcohol was found to be the most effective in preventing irritation.

Wigger-Alberti and Elsner investigated the potential of petroleum jelly to prevent epidermal barrier disruption induced by various irritants in a repetitive irritation test and assessed its potential as a standard reference product.[39] White petroleum jelly was applied to the backs of 20 human subjects who were exposed to SLS, NaOH, toluene, and lactic acid. Irritation was assessed by transepidermal water loss and colorimetry, in addition to visual scoring. It was concluded that petroleum jelly was an effective barrier cream against SLS, NaOH, and lactic acid, and moderately effective against toluene.

Frosch et al. adapted the guinea pig RIT described above for use in humans.[40] Two barrier creams were evaluated for their ability to prevent irritation to SLS. In this repetitive model, the irritant was applied to the ventral forearm, using a glass cup, for 30 min daily for 2 weeks. One arm of each subject was pretreated with a barrier cream. As in the animal model, erythema was assessed by visual scoring, laser Doppler flow, and transepidermal water loss. Skin color was also measured by colorimetry (La* value). One barrier cream decreased skin irritation to SLS, the most differentiating parameter being transepidermal water loss and the least differentiating being colorimetry.

8. Bioengineering Methods in Model Development

Many of the models described above did not employ the modern bioengineering techniques available, and therefore data based on these models may be imprecise. Despite the investigation's skill, subjective assessment of erythema, edema, and other visual parameters may lead to confounding by inter- and intra-observer variation. Although the eye may be more sensitive than current spectroscopy and chromametric techniques, the reproducibility and increased statistical power of such data may provide greater benefit. A combination of techniques, such as transepidermal water loss, capacitance, ultrasound, laser Doppler flowmetry, spectroscopy, and chromametric analysis, in addition to skilled observation, may increase the precision of the test. Andersen and Maibach compared various bioengineering techniques, finding that clinically indistinguishable reactions induced significantly different changes in barrier function and vascular status.[41] An outline of many of these techniques is provided by Patil et al.[3]

II. METHODS FOR TESTING THE SENSITIZATION POTENTIAL OF DRUGS AND ENHANCERS

A. Introduction

Prediction of skin sensitization is important to both the consumer and to industry. The consumer is protected by a wealth of data allowing commercial or pharmaceutical substances to be licensed for use. Industry, applying predictive data, can confidently launch products in the marketplace, knowing that they are unlikely to cause significant skin allergy.

Currently, predictive methods consist of a variety of guinea pig assays and some human assays. These can be used to test substances under laboratory conditions, which aim to reflect "in use" conditions. Attempts to replace these varied methods, with their varying strengths and weaknesses, have led to the local lymph node assay and also mathematical modeling of a substance's likelihood of causing allergy, based on its physicochemical properties, discussed in Chapter 5.

B. Guinea Pig Models

The guinea pig assay depends on the expertise of the planner and interpreter. Properly executed and interpreted, the assays provide hazard identification and, with assays such as the OET, risk assessment: the dose that will induce (threshold inducing concentration — TIC) and elicit (threshold eliciting concentration — TEC) allergic contact dermatitis. Conversely, in less sophisticated milieus, sensitivity and specificity may be compromised. Anderson provides a rich background, not only of methodology but also of reliability.[41]

Several guinea pig models exist to predict sensitization. Common features include exposure to a test substance to induce sensitization, a rest period of several days, and reexposure to the same substance at a virgin skin site (challenge exposure). This can be followed by a series of rechallenges over a period of several weeks, to confirm allergy. Alternatively, the sensitized guinea pig can be exposed to putative cross-allergens.

Many variations exist around this core process. Some tests favor intradermal injections to induce allergy, others favor epicutaneous administration. Some tests combine both. Similarly, the challenge exposure may be by these methods. The duration of the initiation also varies from model to model, as does the method of skin irritation. Each model, therefore, should be selected with care, paying particular regard to how that model fits with the purpose of the test, and the nature of the test substance.

Irritation Testing

Initially, a group of four to six animals is used to identify a suitable concentration of the test substance for the induction treatment, which should at most be moderately irritant. The highest nonirritant concentration is used for the challenge dose.

Controls

The control animals are usually treated exactly as the test group, except the test substance is omitted during the induction phase of the experiment. They are then challenged in exactly the same manner as the test animals, and the reactions compared.

Evaluation

Visual scoring of the erythema and edema can be used to evaluate the skin reaction to the test substance. The frequency, intensity, and duration of reactions elicited in test and control animals allows determination of whether sensitization has occurred or not. Several models below attempt to quantify the reaction by measuring the size of the reaction and performing statistical analysis on this data.

Classification

A potential contact sensitizer is considered to be a substance which produces allergic contact dermatitis in 15% of the test animals in a nonadjuvant assay and 8% in an adjuvant assay.[48] A negative result occurs when no allergic reaction is elicited in any of the animals. If less than 15% of the animals demonstrate a reaction, the result is defined as questionable, and rechallenging or study repetition is necessary.

1. Guinea Pig Maximization Test[42,43]

In this assay, 20 test and 10 to 20 control guinea pigs are used. The induction process is in two phases: intradermal injections on day 0 and a 48-h occlusive patch on day 7 (boosting). This is followed by a challenge test on day 21.

Method

Day 0: Paired intradermal injections (0.1 ml each) into the clipped and shaved shoulder region; adjacent injections of:
  - Complete Freund's Adjuvant (FCA)
  - Test article in a vehicle (water, paraffin oil, propylene glycol)
  - Mixture of dissolved or suspended test article with FCA (1:1)
Day 7: Topical occlusive patch applied for 48 h over shoulder (clipped on day 6)
  - Concentration applied should be moderately irritating
  - If substance is nonirritating, then pretreat region with 10% SLS on day 6 freshly after clipping
Day 21: Challenge test is performed on a 4-cm² area on the left flank
  - Shave test region
  - Apply nonirritating concentrations (e.g., via Finn chamber)
  - Apply occluded vehicle for control
Day 28: Rechallenge/cross test at contralateral flank weekly

Challenge reactions are examined at 24 and 48 h after removal of the patch and scored according to a standard rating scale. Control animals are treated similarly to the test animals, except no test substance is applied. Kligman and Basketter recommend in their critique of the test that one control group should receive only FCA, as this substance lowers the irritant threshold of the skin.[44] Without this control, irritant reactions may be interpreted erroneously as allergic reactions, when the skin is challenged with the "nonirritating" concentration identified in preliminary irritation studies. Further, the control group should be exposed to an irritant stimulus comparable in intensity to that of the test substance (e.g., SLS). The purpose of this is to control for excited skin syndrome, which may cause a false positive result. Rechallenge reactions should also be performed to rule out false positive reactions. Truly allergic reactions last for several weeks, whereas nonspecific irritation diminishes after 2 to 3 weeks. Rechallenging is performed weekly, on the contralateral flank.

2. Split Adjuvant Technique

In this assay, involving 2 groups of 10 to 20 guinea pigs each, the test substance is administered separately from the FCA.[45-47]

Method

Day 0: Induction: window dressing fixed on shaved suprascapular region
- Expose 2 cm^2 induction site to "dry ice" for 5 s
- Apply topically 0.2 ml semisolid or 0.1 ml liquid test sample
- Occlude under filter paper for 48 h
Day 2: Induction: open dressing, reapply test substance, and re-occlude
Day 4: Induction: prior to induction application, inject 2 × 0.1 ml FCA into test site
- Apply test substance as before; re-occlude
Day 7: Reapply and re-occlude as before
Day 9: Remove entire dressing
Day 22: Challenge test over normal-appearing skin on midback
- Apply 0.5 ml of semisolid or 0.2 ml of liquid to a clipped area and occlude for 24 h. Challenge readings are taken on days 23, 24, and 25

Control animals are treated similarly except no test substance is added.

This test differs from the guinea pig maximization test, as it uses exclusively topical application of the test substance to elicit sensitization, although FCA is still injected intradermally to enhance sensitivity. Also, dry ice is used to irritate the test site.

In a modified version of this test, the test site is excoriated with sandpaper or tape, and is left open rather than occluded. The aim is to achieve a test close to "in use" conditions (see Reference 48).

3. Optimization Test

Maurer models a test of 20 guinea pigs per test substance and 20 per control group.[49] This test induces sensitization by intradermal injection. The test sites are depilated both mechanically and chemically. The challenge is by intradermal injection and by topical occlusion. Injection solutions are made up in physiological saline solution (0.1%). The reactions were assessed by visual scoring and also quantitatively by measuring skin fold thickness × greatest diameter of erythema to give a "reaction volume."

Method

Week 1: Induction
- 0.1 ml-injections are made into the right flank (0.05 ml) and back (0.1 ml) three times per week (on day 0, two injections to each site)

Week 2: Induction: test compound, suspended in FCA, is injected into the nuchal skin three
  times per week
Week 3: Induction: as for week 2
Week 4: Rest
Week 5: Rest
Week 6: Challenge 1: intradermal injection into contralateral flank
  • Same solution used as week 1 induction (0.05 ml of 0.1% solution)
  • Reactions measured at 24 h
Week 7: Challenge 2: epidermal occlusive challenge
  • Results read at 24, 48, and 72 h

Control animals are treated similarly to test animals, except the test substance is omitted
during induction.

The reaction volume is used to calculate the skin irritant threshold (mean reaction volume + 1
SD). If the challenge reaction volume postinjection is greater than the threshold, the reaction is
considered to be allergic. Visual scoring is used to evaluate the occlusion challenge. The exact
Fisher test is used to determine statistical significance.

4. Freund's Complete Adjuvant Test

For the control and treatment groups, 10 to 20 guinea pigs each are required.[48,50] This test was
devised to test weaker allergens as well as strong to moderate allergens. The test substance is mixed
with FCA in a 1:1 ratio, at a concentration of less than 5%. The induction phase involves intradermal
application, and the challenge phase is an open application of the test substance. The challenge
dose is the minimal irritating dose and the 1:3 nonirritating dilutions. This allows a threshold level
to be estimated.

Method

Day 0: Induction by suprascapular intradermal injection of 0.1 ml test substance into shaved
  test site
Day 4: Repeat above
Day 8: Repeat above
Day 21: Challenge on clipped flank skin
  • Apply up to 6 concentrations (minimal irritating and subsequent dilutions) in vehicle
  • Results interpreted at 24, 48, 72 h and visually scored
  • Rechallenge/cross test at 10- to 14-day intervals on contralateral flank

Control animals are treated similarly, except the test article is omitted during induction.

5. Open Epicutaneous Test (OET)

In this assay, the test substance is applied epicutaneously to a shaved flank, using constant volumes
per square centimeter to standard areas.[48,50] For each test concentration group, 6 guinea pigs are
used, while end-use products are tested on 20 animals. Ten guinea pigs are used in the control group.

The induction period requires daily application over 5 consecutive days per week in the 4-week
study, or daily in the 3-week study, until a total of 20 applications have been made.

Method

Week 1: Induction application over 5 or 7 consecutive days.
  • Apply 0.1 ml of neat test article, or progressive (1:3) dilutions to same 8-cm^2 site

Week 2: Induction as above
Week 3: Induction as above for a total of 20 applications
Week 4: Induction as above over the induction period

Day 21/29: Challenge application of test substance/dilutions at 2-cm^2 test site
- Results interpreted at 24, 48, and 72 h postchallenge
- Rechallenge/cross test at 10- to 14-day intervals on contralateral flank

Control animals are treated similarly, except the test article is omitted during induction.

Klecak suggests that a combination of the open epicutaneous test and the Freund's complete adjuvant test is useful in defining conditions under which borderline substances may be allergenic.[50]

6. Modified Draize Test

The aim of the modifications to the Draize test (see Reference 51) was to increase its sensitivity to weaker allergens. The test consists of two parts, involving ten guinea pigs in the treatment group and in the control group. Skin reactions are assessed for erythema and edema, which is graded, and longitudinal and lateral diameters of reaction are measured to determine reaction size.

The control animals are treated with FCA only during the induction. During the challenge and rechallenge, they are treated as the test animals.

Method

Part 1:
Day 0: Induction intradermal injections of 0.1 ml each onto four sites into clipped skin
- Test sites are over inguinal and axillary lymph nodes
- Test dose is 2.5 times the challenge dose
- Reactions measured and scored at 24 h
Day 14: Challenge test
- 0.1 ml of test substance at nonirritant or slightly irritant concentration injected intradermally to one clipped flank
- 0.1 ml of test substance applied epicutaneously onto 8-cm^2 clipped area of contralateral flank
- Results measured and scored at 24 h
Day 21: Confirmation rechallenge
Day 28: Confirmation rechallenge

Part 2: If the challenge tests are negative in part 1, a second set of intradermal injections is administered on day 35. The challenge procedure is as above; however, rechallenge is performed intradermally at weekly intervals. New control animals are necessary for part 2 of the test.

7. Buehler Test

This test involves three groups of guinea pigs: the test group; the vehicle control, which is treated in the same way as the test group except for the omission of the test substance; and the negative control, which is challenged only (see References 48 and 52).

The induction phase consists of 1 or 3 weekly occlusive applications of the test substance to an 8-cm^2 clipped area of skin over the left shoulder. A 4-cm^2 occlusive patch/chamber containing the highest possible (moderately irritating) concentration is applied for 6 h, during which time the animals are placed in restrainers. The induction lasts between 3 and 9 weeks.

The challenge procedure occurs 14 days after the final induction, when 0.2 to 0.5 ml of the test substance is applied under an occlusive patch on naïve back skin for 6 h. Nonirritating concentrations are used. The guinea pigs are restrained as for induction. Ten control guinea pigs are also challenged. Grading of observed skin reactions occurs at 24 and 48 postchallenge. Rechallenges/cross-tests follow at intervals of 1 to 2 weeks, at virgin sites on the back. If indicated, additional control animals may be used.

Assessment is by a calculation of an incidence index, which is the number of responding animals out of the test group, and a severity index, which is a sum of the reaction grades divided by the number of animals used.

Other models include the modified guinea pig maximization test, the single injection adjuvant test, the tierexperimentaller nachweis (TINA) test, the cumulative contact enhancement test, the epicutaneous maximization test, the ear/flank test, the footpad test, and the guinea pig test adapted to cosmetic ingredients. These are reviewed by Klecak[48] and extensively discussed by Anderson and Maibach.[41]

8. The Local Lymph Node Assay

The murine local lymph node assay (LLNA) measures the activity of injected [^{3}H]-(methyl)thymidine in the lymph nodes draining a topical test site test.[54] This is thought to reflect the clonal expansion of T lymphocytes in these nodes during induction of sensitization.

The test substance is applied topically to the dorsum of both ears, in a vehicle, determined by the solubility of the test material. After 5 days, [^{3}H]-(methyl)thymidine is injected intravenously into test and control mice, which are sacrificed 5 h later. The auricular lymph nodes are then excised and the [^{3}H]-(methyl)thymidine count is measured by β-scintillation spectroscopy. A count three times greater than the control group is consistent with sensitization.

This method has the advantage of objectivity — counting radioactivity. As it is a relatively new assay, we are just learning to deal with its imprecision in terms of specificity and sensitivity. Note that it assays for hazard identification and not risk assessment.

C. Human Tests

Currently, the modified maximization technique[55] and the modified Draize procedure[56,57] are the methods of choice.[58] A large pool of subjects is necessary to ensure statistical validity.

In these studies, the test material is applied to the skin under an occlusive patch. This induction sensitization is repeated seven to ten times over a 3-week induction period. This is followed by a rest period of 10 to 14 days. The challenge is performed on virgin skin, under occlusion using a nonirritating dose. Enhancing techniques may be employed, such as repetition of the chemical insult,[59] using a high concentration of test material[56,57] treating the skin with sodium lauryl sulfate (SLS),[60] skin stripping,[61] or freezing.[62] Freund's adjuvant was among the earliest techniques employed to enhance sensitization.

III. CONCLUSION

Irritation and sensitization tests in dermatology are essential to the production and licensing of many industrial and pharmaceutical products. The obvious variety in laboratory tests obviates the need for a single, scientific, standardized approach to testing. Clearly, any successful model must be validated against current experimental standards. This standardization may be provided in the future by the logical methodology of QSAR models, discussed in the next chapter.

REFERENCES

1. Code of Federal Regulations, Office of the Federal Registrar, National Archive of Records. General Services Administration, 1985, title 16, parts 1500.40-1500.42.

1a. Draize, J.H., Woodard, G., and Calvery, H.O., Methods for study of irritation and toxicity of substances applied topically to the skin and mucous membranes, *J. Pharmacol. Exp. Ther.*, 82, 377, 1944.

2. Patrick, E. and Maibach, H.I., Comparison of the time course, dose response and mediators of chemically induced skin irritation in three species, in *Current Topics in Contact Dermatitis*, Frosch, P.J. et al., Eds., Springer-Verlag, New York, 1989, 399.

3. Patil, S.M., Patrick, E., and Maibach, H.I., Animal, human and in vitro test methods for predicting skin irritation, in *Dermatotoxicology Methods: The Laboratory Worker's Vade Mecum*, Marzulli, F. N. and Maibach, H.I., Eds., Taylor & Francis, Washington, D.C., 1998, 89.

4. Justice, J.D., Travers, J.J., and Vinson, L.J., The correlation between animal tests and human tests in assessing product mildness, *Proc. Scientific Section of the Toilet Goods Assoc.*, 35, 12, 1961.

5. Frosch, P.J., Schulze-Dirks, A., Hoffmann, M., Axthelm, I., and Kurte, A., Efficacy of skin barrier creams (I). The repetitive irritation test (RIT) in the guinea pig, *Contact Dermatitis*, 28 (2), 94, 1993.

6. Frosch, P.J., Schulze-Dirks, A., and Hoffmann, M., Axthelm. I. Efficacy of skin barrier creams (II). Ineffectiveness of a popular "skin protector" against various irritants in the repetitive irritation test in the guinea pig, *Contact Dermatitis*, 29(2), 74, 1993.

7. Phillips, L., Steinberg, M., Maibach, H.I., and Akers, W.A., A comparison of rabbit and human skin responses to certain irritants, *Toxicol. Appl. Pharmacol.*, 21, 369, 1972.

8. Wahlberg, J.E., Measurement of skin fold thickness in the guinea pig. Assessment of edema-inducing capacity of cutting fluids acids, alkalis, formalin and dimethyl sulfoxide, *Contact Dermatitis*, 28, 141, 1993.

9. Marzulli, F.N. and Maibach, H.I., The rabbit as a model for evaluating skin irritants: a comparison of results obtained on animals and man using repeated skin exposure, *Food Cosmet. Toxicol.*, 13, 533, 1975.

10. Anderson, C., Sundberg, K., and Groth, O., Animal model for assessment of skin irritancy, *Contact Dermatitis*, 15, 143, 1986.

11. Opdyke, D.L. and Burnett, C.M., Practical problems in the evaluation of the safety of cosmetics, *Proc. Scientific Section, Toilet Goods Assoc.*, 44, 3, 1965.

12. Calandra, J., Comments on the guinea pig immersion test, *CTFA Cosmet. J.*, 3 (3), 47, 1971.

13. Opdyke, D.L., The guinea pig immersion test — a 20 year appraisal, *CTFA Cosmet. J.*, 3 (3), 46, 1971.

14. MacMillan, F.S.K., Ram, R.R., and Elvers, W.B., A comparison of the skin irritation produced by cosmetic ingredients and formulations in the rabbit, guinea pug, beagle dog to that observed in the human, in *Animal Models in Dermatology*, Maibach, H.I., Ed., Churchill Livingstone, Edinburgh, 1975, 12.

15. Gupta, B.N., Mathur, A.K., Srivastava, A.K., Singh, S., Singh, A., and Chandra, S.V., Dermal exposure to detergents, *Vet. Hum. Toxicol.*, 34 (5), 405, 1992.

16. Uttley, M. and Van Abbe, N.J., Primary irritation of the skin: mouse ear test and human patch test procedures, *J. Soc. Cosmet. Chem.*, 24, 217, 1973.

17. Patrick, E. and Maibach, H.I., A novel predictive assay in mice, *Toxicologist*, 7, 84, 1987.

18. Inoue, H., Asaka, T., Nagata, N., and Koshihara, Y., Mechanism of mustard oil-induced skin inflammation in mice, *Eur. J. Pharmacol.*, 333(2-3), 231, 1997.

19. Humphrey, D.M., Measurement of cutaneous microvascular exudates using Evans blue, *Biotech. Histochem.*, 68(6), 342, 1993.

20. Trush, M.A., Egner, P.A., and Kensler, T.W., Myeloperoxidase as a biomarker of skin irritation and inflammation, *Food Chem. Toxicol.*, 32(2), 143, 1994.

21. National Academy of Sciences, Committee for the Revision of NAS Pub. 1138, *Principles and Procedures for Evaluating the Toxicity of Household Substances*, National Academy of Sciences, Washington, D.C., 1977, 23.

22. Kligman, A.M. and Wooding, W.M., A method for the measurement and evaluation of irritants on human skin, *J. Invest. Dermatol.*, 49, 78, 1967.

23. Robinson, M.K., Perkins, M.A., and Basketter, D.A., Application of a 4-h human patch test method for comparative and investigative assessment of skin irritation, *Contact Dermatitis*, 38(4), 194, 1998.

24. McFadden, J.P., Wakelin, S.H., and Basketter, D.A., Acute irritation thresholds in subjects with type I—type VI skin, *Contact Dermatitis*, 38(3), 147, 1998.

25. Lanmnan, B.M., Elvers, W.B., and Howard, C.S., The role of human patch testing in a product development program, in *Proc. Joint Conf. Cosmetic Sci.*, Toilet Goods Association, Washington, D.C., 1968, 135.

26. Battista, C.W. and Rieger, M.M. Some problems of predictive testing, *J. Soc. Cosmet. Chem.*, 22, 349, 1971.

27. Wigger-Alberti, W., Hinnen, U., and Elsner, P., Predictive testing of metalworking fluids: a comparison of 2 cumulative human irritation models and correlation with epidemiological data, *Contact Dermatitis*, 36 (1), 14, 1997.

28. Frosch, P.J. and Kligman, A.M., The chamber scarification test for irritancy, *Contact Dermatitis,* 2, 314, 1976.

29. Frosch, P.J. and Kligman, A.M., The chamber scarification test for testing the irritancy of topically applied substances, in *Cutaneous Toxicity*, Drill, V.A. and Lazar, P., Eds., Academic Press, New York, 1977, 150.

30. Frosch, P.J. and Kligman, A.M., The soap chamber test. A new method for assessing the irritancy of soaps, *J. Am. Acad. Dermatol.*, 1(1), 35, 1979.

31. Frosch, P.J., The irritancy of soap and detergent bars, in *Principles of Cosmetics for the Dermatologist*, Frost, P. and Howitz, S.N., Eds., C. V. Mosby, St. Louis, 1982, 5.

32. Kooyman, D.J. and Snydern, F.H., The test for mildness of soaps, *Arch.. Dermatol Syphilol.*, 46, 846, 1942.

33. Clarys, P., Manou, I., and Barel, A.O., Influence of temperature on irritation in the hand/forearm immersion test, *Contact Dermatitis*, 36(5), 240, 1997.

34. Allenby, C.F., Basketter, D.A., Dickens, A., Barnes, E.G., and Brough, H.C., An arm immersion model of compromised skin (I). Influence on irritation reactions, *Contact Dermatitis*, 28(2), 84, 1993.

35. Hannuksela, A. and Hannuksela, M., Irritant effects of a detergent in wash, chamber and repeated open application tests, *Contact Dermatitis*, 34(2), 134, 1996.

36. Van der Valk, P.G. and Maibach, H.I., Post-application occlusion substantially increases the irritant response of the skin to repeated short-term sodium lauryl sulfate (SLS) exposure, *Contact Dermatitis*, 21(5), 335, 1989.

37. Charbonnier, V., Morrison, B.M., Jr., Paye, M., and Maibach, H.I., Open application assay in investigation of subclinical dermatitis induced by sodium lauryl sulfate (SLS) in man: advantage of squamometry, *Skin Res. Technol.*, 4, 244, 1998.

38. Zhai, H., Willard, P., and Maibach, H.I., Evaluating skin-protective materials against contact irritants and allergens. An in vivo screening human model, *Contact Dermatitis*, 38(3), 155, 1998.

39. Wigger-Alberti, W. and Elsner, P., Petrolatum prevents irritation in a human cumulative exposure model in vivo, *Dermatology*, 194(3), 247, 1997.

40. Frosch, P.J., Schulze-Dirks, A., Hoffmann, M., Axthelm, I., and Kurte, A., Efficacy of skin barrier creams (I). The repetitive irritation test (RIT) in the guinea pig, *Contact Dermatitis*, 28(2), 94, 1993.

41. Andersen, P.H. and Maibach, H.I., Skin irritation in man: a comparative bioengineering study using improved reflectance spectroscopy, *Contact Dermatitis*, 33(5), 315, 1995.

42. Magnusson, B. and Kligman, A.M., The identification of contact allergens by animal assay, the guinea pig maximization test, *J. Invest. Derm.*, 52(3), 268, 1969.

43. Magnusson, B. and Kligman, A.M., *Allergic Contact Dermatitis in the Guinea Pig*, Thomas, Springfield, 1970.

44. Kligman, A.M. and Basketter, D.A., A critical commentary and updating of the guinea pig maximization test, *Contact Dermatitis*, 32(3), 129, 1995.

45. Maguire, H.C., Jr., The bioassay of contact allergens in the guinea pig, *J. Soc. Cosmet. Chem.*, 24, 121, 1973.

46. Maguire, H.C., Jr., Estimation of the allergenicty of prospective human contact sensitizers in the guinea pig, in *Animal Models in Dermatology*, Maibach, H.I., Ed., Churchill Livingstone, New York, 1975, 67.

47. Maguire, H.C., Jr., and Cipriano, D., Allergic contact dermatitis in laboratory animals, in *Cutaneous Toxicicty*, Drill and Lazar, Eds., Raven Press, New York, 1984, 55.

48. Klecak, G., Allergic contact dermatitis in animals, in *Dermatotoxicology Methods: The Laboratory Worker's Vade Mecum*, Marzulli, F.N. and Maibach, H.I., Eds., Taylor & Francis, Washington, D.C., 1998, chap. 11.

49. Maurer, T., The optimization test, *Curr. Probl. Dermatol.*, 14, 114, 1985.

50. Klecak, G., The Freund's complete adjuvant test and the open epicutaneous test. A complimentary test procedure for realistic assessment of allergenic potential, *Current Probl. Dermatol.*, 14, 152, 1985.

51. Johnson, A.W. and Goodwin, B.F.J., The Draize test and modifications, in *Contact Allergy. Predictive Tests in Guinea Pigs*, Anderson, K.E. and Maibach, H.I., Eds., *Current Problems in Dermatology*, Karger, Basel, 14, 31, 1985.

52. Buehler, E.V., A rationale for the selection of occlusion and elicit delayed contact hypersensitivity in the guinea pig. A prospective test, *Current Probl. Dermatol.*, 14, 39, 1985.

53. Anderson, K.E. and Maibach, H.I., Eds., *Contact Allergy. Predictive Tests in Guinea Pigs, Current Problems in Dermatology*, Vol. 14, S. Karger, Basel, 1985.

54. Kimber, I., The local lymph node assay, in *Dermatotoxicology Methods: The Laboratory Worker's Vade Mecum*, Marzulli, F.N. and Maibach, H.I., Eds., Taylor & Francis, Washington, D.C., 1998, Chap. 12.

55. Kligman, E. and Epstein, W.L., Updating the maximization test for identifying contact allergens, *Contact Dermatitis*, 1, 231, 1975.

56. Marzulli, F.N. and Maibach, H.I., Antimicrobials: experimental contact sensitization in man, *J. Soc. Cosmet. Chem.*, 20, 67, 1973.

57. Marzulli, F.N. and Maibach, H.I., The use of graded concentrations in studying skin sensitizers: experimental contact sensitization in man, *Food Cosmet. Toxicol.*, 12, 219, 1974.

58. Marzulli, F.N. and Maibach, H.I., Test methods for allergic contact dermatitis in humans, in *Dermatotoxicology Methods: The Laboratory Worker's Vade Mecum*, Marzulli, F.N. and Maibach, H.I., Eds., Taylor & Francis, Washington, D.C., 1998, Chap. 13.

59. Shelanski, H.A., Experience with and considerations of the human patch test method, *J. Soc. Cosmet. Chem.*, 2, 324, 1951.

60. Kligman, A.M., The SLS provocative patch test in allergic contact sensitization, *J. Invest. Dermatol.*, 46, 571, 1966.

61. Spier, H.W. and Sixt, I., Untersuchungen uber die Abhangigkeit des Ausfalles der exzem Lappshen-praben von der Hornschichtdicke, *Hautarzt*, 6, 152, 1955.

62. Epstein, W.L., Kligman, A., and Senecal, I.P., Role of regional lymph nodes in contact sensitization, *Arch. Dermatol.*, 88, 789, 1963.

63. Freund, J., Effect of paraffin oil and mycobacteria on antibody formation and sensitization; review, *Am. J. Clin. Path.*, 6, 227, 1951.

5 Quantitative Structure Analysis Relationships in the Prediction of Skin Sensitization Potential

Saqib J. Bashir and Howard I. Maibach

CONTENTS

I. INTRODUCTION

Prediction of skin sensitization is important both to the consumer and to industry. The consumer is protected by a wealth of data allowing commercial or pharmaceutical substances to be licensed for use. Industry, applying predictive data, can confidently launch products in the marketplace, knowing that they are unlikely to cause significant skin allergy.

Currently, predictive methods consist of a variety of guinea pig assays and some human assays. These can be used to test substances under laboratory conditions, which aim to reflect "in use" conditions. Attempts to replace these varied methods, with their varying strengths and weaknesses, have led to the mathematical modeling of a substance's likelihood of causing allergy, based on its physicochemical properties.

II. QUANTITATIVE STRUCTURE–ACTIVITY RELATIONSHIPS (QSAR)

The premise behind QSAR is that physicochemical data available on previously identified sensitizers can be used to predict the likelihood of the test substance being a sensitizer. As many sensitizers have been reported, their properties can be catalogued to form a vast database, upon which correlations between their structures and sensitizing ability can be drawn. The larger this database, the more likely statistically significant mathematical relationships can be identified between structural elements (independent variables) and biological activity (dependent variables). The structures that are significantly associated with allergy in the database may also be associated with allergy in vivo. If QSAR models can accurately predict sensitization, then expensive, time-consuming animal and human studies can be avoided. Potential new compounds can be analyzed for sensitivity prior to development, allowing manufacturers to modify products at a conceptual stage.

A. CLASSIFICATION MODEL

This model has been developed to discriminate between allergens and nonallergens,[1-4] utilizing a database of structures that had been reported to cause allergic contact dermatitis over a 20-year period. These structures were analyzed for size, polarity, and protein reactive functions such as amino and alcohol groups, aldehydes, and esters. Similar data were obtained for structures which are nonallergenic, thereby creating a pool of characteristics responsible for sensitization and the degree of reactivity.

Importantly, this model is based on both features that contribute to allergenicity: a combination of the *diffusion ability* of the compound across the stratum corneum, and *protein reactivity* of the compound. The former is reflected by transport/binding descriptors and the latter by a count of dichotomous descriptors (1/0) of toxophores (haptens and prohaptens). These descriptors are demonstrated in Table 1.

TABLE 1
QSAR Descriptors

Determinant	Descriptor	Definition		Variable
Protein reactivity	IX	Reactive aliphatic/aromatic halides		Dichotomous
	IUNIQ	Strong nucleophiles/reactive electrophiles		Dichotomous
	ICOOR	Simple aliphatic esters		Dichotomous
	ICONJ	Conjugated olefins: activated by SH/NH$_2$ Michael addition		Dichotomous
	IArOH	Easily metabolized phenols	} of quinone	Dichotomous
	IArNH	Easily metabolized anilenes	} precursors	Dichotomous
	IOH	Oxidizable primary alcohols		Dichotomous
Transport/binding	MR	Polarizable molecular volume		Continuous
	PL	Lipophilic contribution of log *P*		Continuous
	HBA	Hydrogen bond acceptor groups (count of electron pairs on N and O)		Ordinal
	HBD	Hydrogen bond donor groups (count of N-H and O-H)		Ordinal

Each descriptor has a coefficient value, which is used in an algorithm. This expresses the *Y*-estimate, which scores allergens and nonallergens above and below 0.5, respectively. Values in the range 0.4 to 0.6 are considered indeterminate. Hostýnek et al.[1] modeled six randomly selected chemicals not previously investigated for allergenicity, validating the results in vivo. Full concordance was found between the model analysis and the murine local lymph node assay.

Enslein et al.[7] tested the model on 74 known allergenic and nonallergenic compounds. Of these, 12 compounds fell in the indeterminate range, 57 were correctly predicted, and 5 were incorrectly predicted. These 5 compounds were reported as allergens in literature, but falsely identified as negative by the QSAR model. No false positives were predicted, suggesting that the model more accurately identifies nonallergens (100% specificity, 90% sensitivity).

B. THE RANK MODEL

In contrast to the classification model above, this model attempts to rank the allergic response to a substance as nonallergenic, weak, moderate, and strong, on a scale of 1 to 4, respectively. The descriptors are identical in both the rank and discriminatory models, although the coefficient values assigned to each descriptor vary. Rank 1 (non) is clearly distinct from rank 4 (strong) in this model; however, there is considerable overlap between the intermediate ranks.

Testing this model on the same 74 compounds above, Enslein et al.[7] demonstrated model sensitivity of 95%, allowing an error of ±1 rank in prediction. This error margin was considered equivalent to experimental assays.[8] The model specificity was 60%.

Combining the two models provided an overall concordance of 93%, one model being able to identify some of the "false negatives" predicted in the other.

C. THE DEREK SYSTEM

The QSAR knowledge-based computer system DEREK was developed under the collaboration of a multinational group of expert toxicologists. In addition to skin sensitization prediction, it is also used to predict genotoxicity.

Test structures can be input into the computer graphically, and analysis is carried out by screening each structure against the structural alerts in the DEREK database. Toxophores are identified, and the computer provides information on the toxic effect and also lists literature references. User interpretation is required to assess the risk posed if several toxophores are identified, and also if no toxophores are identified. The latter does not simply reflect safety of the the compound, but also reflects the depth of the database.

The database consists of separate rule sets, which can be chosen according to the user's needs. The standard rule set, developed originally by Sanderson and Earnshaw,[9] contains 52 rules, with end points such as carcinogenicity, neurotoxicity, and some adverse reproductive effects. This has been expanded on by the developmental rule set, which resulted from collaborative work: utilizing a Unilever database from approximately 300 guinea pig maximization tests, 40 structural alerts to skin sensitizers were derived. Substances were grouped according to their most likely mechanism of reaction with skin proteins. Where no mechanism could be identified, structural alerts were created for groups of chemicals with similar functional groups. However, this system does not account for stratum corneum penetration, unlike the classification and rank models described above. Therefore, structural alerts may be identified in a particular query, when in practice the test substance's skin permeability is too low to cause sensitization.

A further FDA rule set pertains to structural alerts for toxophores considered of interest to the U.S. Food and Drug Administration.

The DEREK model has been tested on a dataset of 37 chemicals, of which 25 were skin sensitizers and 12 nonsensitizers. Of the sensitizers, DEREK correctly identified 24 containing structural alerts for skin sensitization. Of the 12 nonsensitizers, 2 were incorrectly identified as skin sensitizers, perhaps a result of the inability of the system to consider perctaneous penetration. (see Ridings et al.[10] for review).

III. CONCLUSION

The predictive power of QSAR depends directly on the quality of the database and our understanding of the mechanisms of skin sensitization. As knowledge in both spheres expands, so shall the power of predictive modeling. Clinical reports of allergy must be reliable to ensure that compounds entered into the database are true allergens. Diagnostic patch tests with adequate controls are required to make the diagnosis of allergic contact dermatitis to a particular allergen.

The above studies demonstrate that QSAR is rapidly developing into a useful technique in the sphere of contact allergy. Accurate predictive mathematical modeling may allow us to forego the lengthy, cumbersome, and labor-intensive experimental techniques for skin sensitization. Prospective studies of novel compounds are necessary to judge the usefulness of this technique in the real life setting.

REFERENCES

1. Hostýnek., J.J., Lauerma, A.I., Magee, P.S., Bloom, E., and Maibach, H.I., A local lymph-node assay validation study of a structure-activity relationship model for contact allergens, *Arch. Dermatol. Res.*, 287(6), 567, 1995 (published erratum appears in *Arch. Dermatol. Res.*, 287(8), 767, 1995).

2. Hostýnek., J.J., Magee, P.S., and Maibach, H.I., QSAR predictive of contact allergy: scope and limitations, *Prevention of Contact Dermatitis*, Vol. 25, Elsner, P., Lachapelle, J.M., and Wahlberg, J.E., Eds., Karger, Basel, 1996, 18.

3. Hostýnek, J.J., Structure-activity relationships in contact sensitization, in *Dermatotoxicology Methods: The Laboratory Worker's Vade Mecum*, Marzulli, F.N. and Maibach, H.I., Eds., Taylor & Francis, Washington, D.C., 1998, Chap. 10.

4. Magee, P.S., Hostýnek, J.J., and Maibach, H.I., A classification model for contact dermatitis, *Quant. Struct.-Act. Relat.*, 13, 22, 1994.

5. Magee, P.S., Hostýnek, J.J., and Maibach, H.I., Modeling allergic contact dermatitis, in *In Vitro Skin Toxicology: Irritation, Phototoxicity, Sensitization*, Rougier, A., Goldberg, A.M., and Maibach, H.I., Eds., Mary Ann Liebert, New York, 1994, 281.

6. Magee, P.S., Hostýnek, J.J., and Maibach, H.I., Toward a predictive model for allergic contact dermatitis, in *Animal Test Alternatives: Refinement-Reduction-Replacement,* Salem, H., Ed., Marcel Dekker, New York, 1994, 159.

7. Enslein, K., Gombar, V.K., Blake, B.W., Maibach, H.I., Hostýnek, J.J., Sigman, C.C., and Bagheri, D., A quantitative structure-toxicity relationships model for the dermal sensitization guinea pig maximization assay, *Food Chem. Toxicol.*, 35(10-11), 1091, 1997.

8. Gad, S.C., A scheme for the prediction and ranking of relative potencies of dermal sensitizers based on data from several systems, *J. Appl. Toxicol.*, 8, 361, 1988.

9. Sanderson, D.M. and Earnshaw, C.G., Computer prediction of possible toxic action from chemical structure; the DEREK system, *Hum. Exp. Toxicol.*, 10, 261, 1991.

10. Ridings, J.E., Barratt, M.D., Cary, R., et al., Computer prediction of possible toxic action from chemical structure: an update on the DEREK system, *Toxicology,* 106, 267, 1996.

6 Methods for Testing the Phototoxicity and Photosensitization of Drugs

N. J. Neumann, B. Homey, H. W. Vohr, and P. Lehmann

CONTENTS

I. INTRODUCTION

The increasing use of toiletries and cosmetics, as well as the topical or systemic application of newly developed pharmaceutical products, increases the potential risk for consumers to be exposed to unknown photosensitizers. For the investigation and prediction of phototoxic or photosensitizing properties of chemicals, a large number of in vitro and in vivo tests are available. In this work, the relevant tests are summarized, and special emphasis is placed on recently released or modified test procedures.

An outstanding example of an epidemic appearance of chemical-induced photoallergy was the release of tetrachlorsalicylanilide (TCSA), which was used as a disinfectant in soaps and other toiletries in England from 1960 to 1993. Furthermore, musk ambrette, a synthetic fragrance and preservative, used worldwide in cosmetic products, has proven to be an important photosensitizer. Following the results of a Scandinavian multicenter study, musk ambrette caused the highest rate of photosensitization out of all the substances tested.[1]

In 1985, restrictive guidelines of the International Fragrance Association concerning the use of musk ambrette in cosmetics led to a remarkable decrease of the musk ambrette-induced photosensitizations. Recently released photopatch test trays incorporate musk ambrette only as a "historical photoallergen."[2]

The Austrian, Swiss, and German photopatch test study group (DAPT) reported that nonsteroidal anti-inflammatory drugs (NSAIDs), disinfectants, sunscreens, phenothiazines, and fragrances are the most relevant photosensitizers (Tables 1 and 2).

Besides these synthetic photosensitizers, there also exist exogenous or endogenous natural phototoxic agents in plants such as the Leguminosae, Moraceae, Rutaceae, and Umbiliferae. Furthermore, porphyrins are important photosensitizers, which accumulate in several tissues and cells bearing distinct enzymatic defects, leading to clinically relevant phototoxic skin reactions after UV light exposure.[3,4]

Many photosensitizers are able to cause both phototoxic and photoallergic reactions, and unfortunately, often an exact clinical or histopathological discrimination is impossible.[5,6]

TABLE 1
Ranking List of Phototoxic Reactions (1985–1990)

Substances	Frequencies (%)
1. Tiaprofenic acid	30.41
2. Promethazine	21.33
3. Carprofen	8.50
4. Chlorpromazine	8.00
5. Fragrance mix	5.54
6. Wood tar	5.16
7. Hexachlorophene	4.36
8. Balsam of Peru	3.38
9. Fenticlor	3.29
10. Triclosan	2.93
11. 4-Isopropyldibenzoylmethane	2.58
12. 6-Methylcumarine	2.17
13. Tetrachlorsalicylanilide	1.98
14. Compositae mix	1.97
15. Tolbutamid	1.86
16. Cyclamate	1.72
17. Saccharin	1.61
18. Colophony	1.60
19. Bithionol	1.60
20. 3-(4-Methylbenzyliden)–camphor	1.60
21. Monobromsalicylchloranilide	1.53
22. Buclosamide	1.52
23. Furosemide	1.47
24. Sulfanilamide	1.33
25. Hydrochlorothiazide	1.27
26. Moschus mix	1.26
27. Thiourea	1.11
28. Tribromsalicylanilide	1.10
29. Moschus ambrette	1.08
30. Chinidinsulfate	1.07
31. Para-aminobenzoic acid	0.80
32. 2-Hydroxy-4-methoxybenzophenone	0.62

TABLE 2
Ranking List of Photoallergic Reactions (1985–1990)

Substances	Frequencies (%)
1. Tiaprofenic acid	3.15
2. Fenticlor	1.60
3. Carprofen	1.34
4. 4-Isopropyldibenzoylmethane	0.89
5. 2-Hydroxy-4-methoxybenzophenone	0.71
6. Promethazine	0.71
7. Tetrachlorsalicylanilide	0.54
8. Moschus ambrette	0.54
9. Fragrance mix	0.37
10. Moschus mix	0.36
11. Chlorpromazine	0.36
12. Bithionol	0.27
13. Triclosan	0.27
14. 6-Methylcumarin	0.18
15. Hexachlorophene	0.18
16. Compositae mix	0.10
17. Cyclamate	0.09
18. Chinidinsulfate	0.09
19. Buclosamide	0.09
20. Para-aminobenzoic acid	0.09
21. Wood tar	0.09
22. Monobromsalicylchloranilide	0.00
23. Tribromsalicylanilide	0.00
24. Sulfanilamide	0.00
25. Hydrochlorothiazide	0.00
26. Furosemide	0.00
27. 3-(4-Methylbenzyliden)–camphor	0.00
28. Saccharin	0.00
29. Colophony	0.00
30. Balsam of Peru	0.00
31. Tolbutamide	0.00
32. Thiourea	0.00

II. DIAGNOSTIC PROCEDURES

The diagnosis of photoreactions is based on medical history, clinical, and histological findings, and especially on photodiagnostic test procedures.[7–13]

Earlier, Stephan Epstein emphasized the eminent role of photopatch testing for the identification of photosensitizers.[14–16] Nevertheless, until the early 1980s the photopatch test procedure was not standardized and varied between different countries and dermatological centers with respect to test tray substance concentrations and vehicles, as well as to the readings, and the classification of test reactions.[17]

A. PHOTOPATCH TEST

The first standard procedure for photopatch testing was defined by the Scandinavian Photodermatitis Research Group (SPDRG) in 1982.[18] Guided by the SPDRG, 45 dermatological centers from Austria, Germany, and Switzerland founded the Austrian, German, and Swiss Photopatch Test

TABLE 3
Photopatch Test

Application of test substances in Finn-Chambers
24 h occlusive to the back
Irradiation 10 J/cm² UVA (320–400 nm)
Controls: Unirradiated patch test
                         UVA-irradiated skin without patch test

TABLE 4A
Photopatch Test Gradings

0	No reaction
1+	Erythema
2+	Erythema and infiltrate
3+	Erythema and papulovesicles
4+	Erythema, bullae, or erosions

TABLE 4B
Classification of Test Reaction

Contact reaction
Every positive reaction in the control area without 1+
  immediately after removal of the test tray

Phototoxic reaction
1+ or 2+, immediate or delayed, as decrescendo reaction

Photoallergic reaction
3+ or 4+, delayed, as crescendo reaction as well as the
  reaction 0, 1+, 2+, 3+

Group (Deutschsprachige Arbeitsgemeinschaft Photopatch-Test: DAPT) in 1984.[19] Their standardized test procedure is summarized in Tables 3, 4A, and 4B. The substances investigated by the DAPT from 1985 to 1996 are listed in Tables 5A and 5B (Figure 1).

After evaluation of the first test period, some substances were dismissed from the test tray since, topically applied, they caused no relevant photoallergic reactions (e.g., furosemide) or had photosensitized some patients via test procedure (e.g., tiaprofenic acid). Additionally, a new set of sunscreens was integrated in the test tray. In the second test period (1990 to 1996), photopatch test data from 1261 patients were evaluated. Out of nearly 1500 positive test reactions, 28.7% were excluded as plain contact reactions and 71.3% were classified as photo-induced, among which 8.06% were indentified as photoallergic reactions.

In comparision to the results of the first test phase, the second photopatch test period revealed a notably reduced number of positive reactions per patient (2.6 vs. 1.1) and the percentage of photoallergic reactions increased significantly (from 3.8% up to 8.1%). Thus, the test modifications led to a remarkable improvement of the photopatch test .

Following the results of the DAPT photopatch test study, nonsteroidal anti-inflammatory drugs, disinfectants, phenothiazines, and sunscreens represent the leading photoallergens in central Europe.

TABLE 5A
List of Substances: Photopatch Test (1985–1990)

Substances	Concentrations (%)
1. Tetrachlorsalicylanilide	0.10
2. Monobromsalicylchloranilide	1.00
3. Tribromsalicylanilide	1.00
4. Buclosamide	5.00
5. Fenticlor	1.00
6. Hexachlorophen	1.00
7. Bithionol	1.00
8. Triclosan	2.00
9. Sulfanilamide	5.00
10. Chlorpromazine	0.10
11. Promethazine	1.00
12. Carprofen	5.00
13. Tiaprofenic acid[a]	5.00
14. Quinidine	1.00
15. Moschus ambrette	5.00
16. Moschus mix[a]	5.00
17. Fragrance mix[a]	8.00
18. 6-Methylcumarine[a]	1.00
19. Para-aminobenzoic acid	5.00
20. Hydrochlorothiazide	1.00
21. Furosemide[a]	1.00
22. 2-Hydroxy-4-methoxybenzophenone	2.00
23. 3-(4-Methylbenzyliden)–camphor	5.00
24. 4-Isopropyldibenzoylmethane	5.00
25. Cyclamate[a]	1.25
26. Saccharin[a]	0.40
27. Wood tar[a]	3.00
28. Colophony[a]	20.00
29. Balsam of Peru	25.00
30. Compositae mix	6.50
31. Tolbutamid[a]	5.00
32. Thiourea[a]	0.10

[a] Substances were discharged from the test tray in 1990, since they only caused a few or no relevant photo reactions or they are supposed to provoke a photoallergy via test procedure.

If the test substance could not penetrate the stratum corneum during the test period, the photopatch test (PPT) revealed, sometimes, a false negative result. In such cases, the photoscratch or the photoprick test could be useful alternative test procedures to detect relevant photosensitizers.

B. Photoscratch and Photoprick Test

The photoscratch and photoprick tests are modifications of the PPT. In contrast to the PPT, the stratum corneum has to be perforated (e.g., by a lancet) in both test procedures before the test substance can be applied. Thus, the supposed photosensitizers come in contact with the epidermis without the penetration process through the stratum corneum.[20]

Systemically applied drugs predominantly revealed false negative photopatch test results, because metabolites are probably the relevant photosensitizers instead of the topically applied test substances themselves. Therefore, systemic photoprovocation might be a helpful test procedure.[11,21,22]

TABLE 5B
List of Substances: Photopatch Test (1991–1996)

Substances	Concentrations (%)
1. Tetrachlorsalicylanilide	0.10
2. Monobromsalicylchloranilide	1.00
3. Tribromsalicylanilide	1.00
4. Buclosamide	5.00
5. Fenticlor	1.00
6. Hexachlorophene	1.00
7. Bithionol	1.00
8. Triclosan	2.00
9. Sulfanilamide	5.00
10. Chlorpromazine	0.10
11. Promethazine	0.10
12. Carprofen	5.00
13. Chinidinsulfate	5.00
14. Moschus ambrette	5.00
15. Hydrochlorothiazide	1.00
16. Balsam of Peru	25.00
17. Compositae mix	6.50
18. Para-aminobenzoic acid	5.00
19. 2-Hydroxy-4-methoxybenzophenone	2.00
20. 3-(4-Methylbenzyliden)–camphor	5.00
21. 4-Isopropyldibenzoylmethane	10.00
22. 4-*tert*-Butyl-4′-methoxydibenzolmethane[a]	10.00
23. 2-Ethylhexyl-*p*-dimethylaminobenzoate[a]	10.00
24. 2-Ethylhexyl-*p*-methoxyzinamate[a]	10.00
25. Phenylbenzimidazolsulfonic acid[a]	10.00
26. p-Methoxy-isoamyl-cinnamate[a]	10.00

[a] Substances newly integrated in the test tray in 1991.

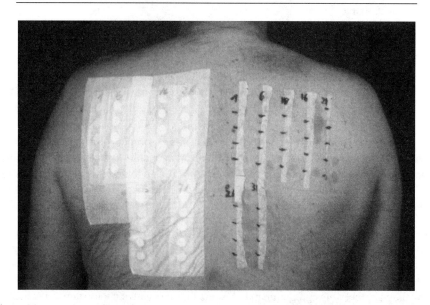

Figure 1   Photopatch test 24 h after application. The control site is still closed and the irradiated test site showed first photoreactions.

C. Photoprovocation Test

After the first irradiation of test areas (preferably located on the back), the supposed photoallergic drug should be applied orally, if possible, at twice the dose normally used. With consideration of the pharmacokinetics, additional skin areas should be exposed subsequently to 10 J/cm^2 UVA treatment (e.g., 1, 2, 3, 5, 8, and 12 h after the drug application). The readings should be performed immediately, and 24, 48, and 72 h after the first irradiation. An example of a positive photoreaction (after systemic quinidine application) is depicted in Figure 2.[11,21,22]

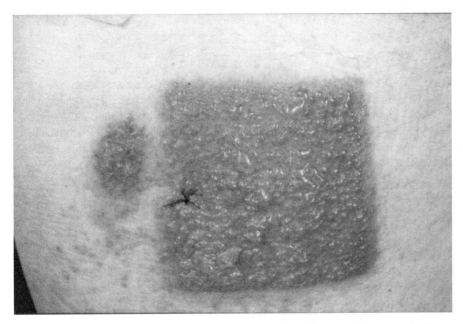

Figure 2   Quinidine-induced photoallergy (positive test reaction after systemic provocation).

III. PREDICTIVE TEST PROCEDURES

Concerning the risk evaluation of contact allergic or contact irritant reactions, the Commission of the European Communities and the Scientific Commitee on Cosmetology recommended several test systems (e.g., Buehler´s test, the optimization test, guinea pig test, mouse ear swelling test, local lymph node assay).[23] Although official guidelines for the risk assessment of the photoreactive potency of newly developed substances are still lacking, the European Community demanded procedures to determine the potential photoallergic and phototoxic risk of skin care products in 1997.* Since UV-absorbing filters (if applied to the skin and irradiated subsequently with UV light) had been accused of causing severe phototoxic and photoallergic reactions, the authorities requested procedures for the safety assessment of sunscreens. Moreover, almost simultaneously they appealed for the abandonment animal testing.

A variety of biological systems were employed to evaluate phototoxicity. In general, phototoxic effects can be investigated by in vitro or in vivo test procedures (Table 6).

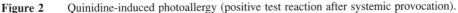

* Commission of the European Communities, Scientific Commitee on Cosmetology, 6th Amendment to the Cosmetics Directive (EC); Guidelines for Safety Assessment of a Cosmetic Product 1997.

TABLE 6
Typical In Vitro Test Systems for
Phototoxicity

Photohemolysis test with erythrocytes
Photo-basophils-histamine-releasing test
Fibroblasts-indol-red uptake test
Candida albicans inhibition test
Paramecium aurelia lethality test
Photo hen's egg test

A. Paramecia

In 1900, initial studies to investigate photosensitizers were performed by Raab, using freshwater ciliate protozoans (paramecia).[24] Raab observed that paramecia exposed simultaneously to a dye called "acridine" and to sunlight died; but paramecia exposed only to "acridine" tolerated the dye without any side effects. Since then this model has been employed by numerous investigators. The paramecia test procedure is inexpensive and relatively easy to perform and, therefore, may serve as a phototoxicity model for large test series.

B. Candida albicans

Another phototoxicity test procedure based on *Candida albicans* was introduced by Daniels in 1965.[25] He exposed *C. albicans* on Sabouraud´s medium to a photosensitizer and UVA as a screening model for phototoxicity. Based on the phototoxic inhibition of growth, the *C. albicans* test is a very simple, inexpensive, and effective method, which was especially useful in testing the phototoxic properties of psoralen.[26,27] However, the well-known phototoxic agents sulfanilamide and dimethylchlortetracycline elicited no phototoxic reactions in the "candida inhibition test system."

C. Red Blood Cells

In 1909, Hasselbach investigated photohemolysis using dyes. Human erythrocytes are cells without a nucleus and cytoplasmic organelles. Thus, erythrocytes provide the opportunity to investigate membrane damage caused by phototoxic chemicals.[28] The experimental conditions are inexpensive and the procedures are easy to perform. Induction of photohemolysis indicates a phototoxic reaction. Erythrocytes received from one individual only and exposure to a phototoxic agent showed a wide range of different results. So, pooled erythrocytes gained from different individuals are necessary for testing. However, well-known potent phototoxic substances (e.g., psoralen) elicited no adequate phototoxic reaction in this test system.

D. White Blood Cells

In 1987, Przybilla et al. demonstrated the phototoxic effects of the nonsteroidal anti-inflammatory drugs (NSAID), e.g., diclofenac, indoprofen, ketoprofen, tiaprofenic acid, in vitro by the photo-basophil-histamine-release test (PBHRT) performed with human leukocytes.[29] Cell suspensions incubated with the test compounds were exposed from 1 to 100 J/cm^2 UVA. The histamine release served as the test parameter after UVA irradiation. Maximum histamine release was observed with tiaprofenic acid, carprofen, and ketoprofen, and no phototoxic effect was detected with indoprofen. These results revealed that most of the NSAIDs can cause phototoxic effects, known from clinical observations as well as other in vitro experiments. Thus, PBHRT might be a promising method for identification of phototoxic chemicals.[29]

Similar in vitro test systems based on leukocytes, fibroblasts, or keratinocytes to test phototoxic agents have been described.[30,31]

E. Cell Cultures

Cultured keratinocytes and fibroblasts obtained from healthy skin samples are useful for phototoxicity testing. Fibroblasts have to be cultured to confluency and keratinocytes until multilayers have been produced. For phototoxicity testing, the highest nontoxic concentration of a test chemical has to be added to cell cultures for an incubation period of 24 h. Afterward, some cells are additionally exposed to UVA. Cells that have been incubated only with the test substance without additionally applied UVA irradiation and cells not incubated with the test substance but irradiated with UVA alone served as controls. Subsequently, after a 24-h incubation period, the morphological changes of the cells are analyzed microscopically, and cell viability is observed — e.g., via neutral red uptake-assay.[32]

F. Dermal Equivalent Model

Two three-dimensional models are suitable for phototoxicty testing: a dermal equivalent (DE) and a skin equivalent (SE) model. The DE model is based on a collagen–glycosaminoglycan–chitosan porous matrix colonized by human fibroblasts. Nontoxic concentrations of test compounds are applied to dermal equivalent test samples and additionally irradiated with UVA (e.g., 3 J/cm^2). Non-UVA-treated dermal equivalent samples serve as controls to exclude non-UVA-induced irritant reactions.

G. Skin Equivalent Model

The DE model combined with an overlay of human keratinocytes, representing a complete differentiated epidermis, is called a skin equivalent (SE) model.

Nontoxic concentrations of test substances are applied to skin equivalents and after 24 h, the 3-(4,5-dimethylthiazol-2-yl)-2,5-diphenyltetrazolium bromide test (MTT) is usually employed to measure the cellular viability in treated (substance application plus UVA irradiation) and untreated (nonirradiated) tissue equivalents. Another useful procedure for the assessment of the inflammatory response is the interleukin-1-alpha release assay. Several studies suggest that both test models could be useful in predicting the phototoxic potential of newly developed chemicals.[33]

H. The Photo Hen's Egg Test (PHET)

In a search for photobiological test systems more advanced than cell cultures which avoid animal models, Neumann et al. established the extra-embryonal vasculature of the incubated hen's egg in combination with UV-irradiation as a screening model for phototoxicity of different chemicals.[30,32,34,35] A similar test was originally introduced by toxicologists as a screening model for mucocutaneous toxicity as an alternative to the Draize test (rabbit's eye test).[36–38]

First, a nontoxic level of the test substance and a nontoxic UVA dose have to be defined. Preliminary studies showed that 5 J/cm^2 UVA does not induce any visible pathological effects on the yolk sac blood vessel system (YS).

The second part of the PHET has a 2×2 factorial test design with the factors being "irradiation" and "substance application," and the determinants "yes" and "no."

During a period of 24 h, the following parameters are evaluated: embryolethality, membrane discoloration, and hemorrhage (Figures 3 to 5).

Fertilized white Leghorn eggs (Shaver Starcross 288A, Lohmann, Cuxhaven, Germany) are incubated in a horizontal position using a commercial incubator at 37.5°C and 65% relative humidity. After 3 days of incubation, all eggs are candled in order to discard those that are defective.

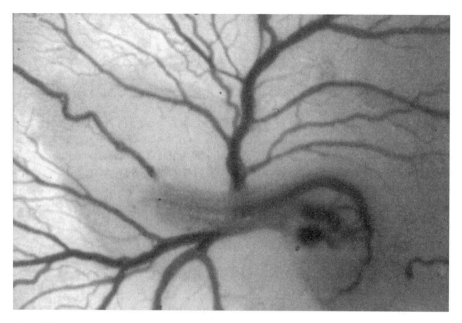

Figure 3   Photo hen's egg test. Normal yolk sac blood vessel system at day 3 of incubation.

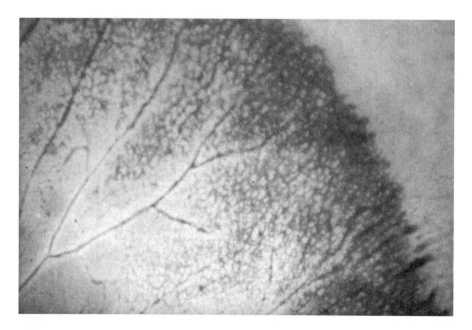

Figure 4   Photo hen's egg test. Severe hemorrhage 24 h after application of 8-MOP followed by 5 J/cm^2 UVA irradiation.

Without damaging the shell membrane, a hole is drilled into the shell, through which 5 ml of egg white is sucked out to lower the embryo and its surrounding YS. Afterward a 1.5 × 2.5-cm window is sawed out of the shell and the eggs are covered with a wax sheet and placed back into the incubator. At day 4 of incubation, only eggs with normally developed embryos and blood vessel systems are used for testing.

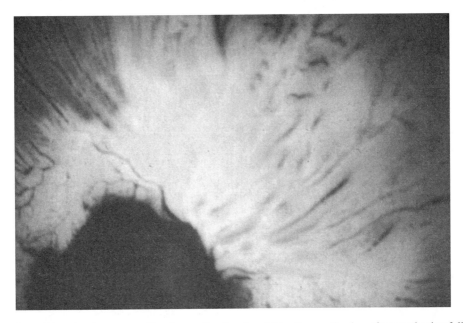

Figure 5 Photo hen's egg test. Membrane discoloration 24 h after application of promethazine followed by 5 J/cm^2 UVA irradition.

Since we are interested in plain phototoxic reactions, in the PHET, the yolk sac blood vessel system of an embryo is exposed to a proven nontoxic concentration of a test substance and to a nontoxic UVA dose simultaneously.

At day 4 of the incubation period, Group 1 (each group consists of 12 eggs) is exposed to a test substance, immediately followed by an irradiation with 5 J/cm^2 UVA (320 to 400 nm, Philips TL 09/40W, Hamburg, Germany). Isotonic sodium chloride solution (NaCl) is normally used as vehicle. Serving as controls, three additional groups are exposed only to NaCl and 5 J/cm^2 UVA or to NaCl or to the test substance alone. Readings are performed 24 h after irradiation. During the observation period, morphological parameters such as membrane discoloration (MD), hemorrhage (HR) [monitored and graded following a four-point scale (Table 7) using a macroscope (M 420, Leitz, Wetzlar, Germany)], and the embryo lethality are assessed.

TABLE 7
Photo Hen´s Egg Test Classification of Membrane Discoloration (MD) and Hemorrhage (HE)

Level 0 (no)	No visible MD / HE
Level 1 (slight)	Just visible MD / HE
Level 2 (moderate)	Visible MD / HE, structures are covered partially
Level 3 (severe)	Visible MD / HE, structures are covered totally

The test parameters MD and HR, as well as embryo lethality, can be summarized in a morphology and lethality index, respectively (Table 8). Employing these indices, the relative phototoxic potential of an assumed photosensitizer compared to other well-known photosensitizers is easily obtained. Based on the PHET results, a list of several photosensitizers is ranked in Table 9. Methoxypsoralen (8-MOP), a classic severe phototoxic substance (with no known photoallergic potential), is the leading phototoxic agent. On the other hand, olaquindox, a well-known photoallergen, revealed no phototoxic effect in the PHET.

TABLE 8
Lethality and Morphology Factors of the Photo Hen´s Egg Test

Relative lethality factor	Lethality rate of the interaction group (L_i) minus the average lethality rate of controls $L_c = (l_{c1} + l_{c2} + l_{c3})/3$
	Relative lethality factor $L = L_i - L_c$
	Relative lethality factor L (%) = $\dfrac{L \times 100}{12}$
Relative morphology factor	Sum of the morphological gradings $(m + h)$ from the interaction group (M^i) minus the sum of the average morphological gradings $(m + h)$ of controls (M_c) $M_c = [(m_{c1} + h_{c1}) + (m_{c2} + h_{c2}) + (m_{c3} + h_{c3})]/3$
	Relative morphology factor $M = M_i - M_c$
	Relative morphology factor M (%) = $\dfrac{M \times 100}{12}$
Test period	24 h after substance application

TABLE 9
Phototoxicity Ranking List Based on Results of the PHET

Substances	Relative Lethality Factor (%)	Relative Morphology Factor (%)
1. 8-MOP	100.00	67.60
2. Promethazine	94.50	54.64
3. Protoporphyrine IX	94.50	64.82
4. Sparfloxacin	58.33	50.90
5. Acridine	58.33	49.54
6. TCSA	44.50	32.42
7. Hematoporphyrine	41.67	58.81
8. Lomefloxacin	30.58	35.67
9. Ciprofloxacin	0.00	62.50
10. Tetracyclin	0.00	2.79
11. Olaquindox	< 0	< 0

In summary, the PHET is an uncomplicated and easy-to-perform test procedure, which represents an inexpensive, valid new screening model for phototoxicity, helping to reduce animal tests.

IV. IN VIVO TEST METHODS

In order to investigate the photoallergenicity of chemicals in the 1960s, erythema tests with an induction and a challenge phase (in vivo test systems) were developed.[39] The erythema tests were later improved with special pretreatments, leading to increased penetration rates, higher immunological reactivity, and a better photosensitivity of the skin. These pretreatments included: mechanical skin irritation (brushing), injection of an adjuvant (e.g., Freund's adjuvant), or application of irritants (e.g., sodium laurylsulfate). Using these improved test systems, even very weak photoallergens were detected. On the other hand, these techniques are very laborious, time consuming (up to 63 days), and expensive.[40,41] Moreover, large numbers of animals are needed, and subjective criteria are used to classify test reactions (erythema scores).

A. MOUSE EAR SWELLING TEST

The first test system based on an objective readout parameter was the MEST, the "mouse ear swelling test."[42–44] A relatively short test period (8 days), a low number of animals, and an objective test parameter (the thickness of the ear) are the major advantages of the MEST. Unfortunately, the ear swelling test is unspecific and does not provide a differentiation between phototoxic and photoallergic reactions. Therefore, the UV-dependent lymph node test has proven to be a more appropriate test procedure.

B. THE UV-DEPENDENT LYMPH NODE ASSAY

Recently, a local lymph node assay (LLNA) was described as a predictive assay for identifying the contact-sensitizing potential of chemicals in mice.[45,46] In comparison with the widely used Buehler's occluded patch test and other guinea pig test data, the LLNA has proven to be a rapid and cost-effective alternative method for the detection of at least moderate-to-strong contact sensitizers.[47–51] In contrast to guinea pig models and the mouse ear swelling test, the LLNA is based upon the detection of a primary immune response as a function of auricular lymph node activation following topical application of chemicals on the dorsal surface of ears. Mainly, in vivo ^{3}[H]-thymidine incorporation is measured as a function of lymph node cell (LNC) proliferation and activation. Recently, we described a modified LLNA based on the detection of increases in lymph node weight and cell counts as a nonradioactive alternative to the original LLNA. Furthermore, additional UVA irradiation allowed the identification of photoreactive compounds.[52]

Although the LLNA was first described to selectively detect allergic skin immune responses, recent studies showed that (photo)irritant test compounds also induce LNC proliferation in vivo.[53–59]

Previous studies showed that optimal sensitization and hapten-induced activation of skin-draining LNC were obtained after sensitizer treatment on 3 consecutive days.[39,42,46] Therefore, five female NMRI mice per group were topically treated on the dorsal surfaces of both ears with 25 µl of photoallergic (e.g., TCSA) or phototoxic (e.g., 8-MOP) standards or vehicle alone on 3 consecutive days. For the induction of photocontact allergy and photoirritancy, mice were irradiated with 10 J/cm^2 UVA immediately after topical treatment. On day 0 and day 3, ear thickness was measured using a spring-loaded micrometer (Oditest; Kroeplin, Schuechtern, Germany), and mean ear swelling was calculated. Furthermore, mice were sacrificed and auricular lymph nodes from each animal were removed and pooled (for each individual mouse) on day 3. LNC proliferation was determined after automatic counting of LNCs per mouse (Coulter Counter ZM, Coulter, Heidelberg, Germany) and calculation of LNC count indices. Lymph node cell count indices (LN index) were defined as the ratio of mean LNC counts from mice treated with the test compound to corresponding results of vehicle-treated control groups. Positive test reactions were defined as either significant ear swelling or significant increase in LNC counts.

The principal findings concerning the differentiation of photoallergic and phototoxic skin reactions are as follows:

1. Photocontact allergens as well as photoirritants induce skin-draining LNC activation.
2. Photoirritants, however, predominantly induce skin inflammation which, in turn, induces draining lymph node proliferation.
3. Induction of photocontact allergy causes only marginal skin inflammation, but a vigorous activation of skin-draining lymph nodes.

Referring to the mechanisms of phototoxic and photoallergic skin reactions, the results of the LLNA show that the development of an integrated model may provide accurate criteria to distinguish between a phototoxic and photoallergic potential of a compound by comparing local draining lymph node activation with skin inflammation.

In this context, validation studies with both LLNA and MEST have resulted in the recognition of these methods by the OECD. These tests have been classified as suitable for screening chemicals for sensitizing activity, as the first stage of an assessment process. Chemicals may be designated as potential photosensitizers if a positive response is recorded in these assays.

In conclusion, the modified LLNA provides a nonradioactive method to differentiate between chemical-induced allergic and irritant skin reactions. Compared with guinea pig tests, this model is objective, measures immunological relevant end points, is markedly less expensive, requires less vivarium space, is of shorter duration (4 days), requires smaller amounts of test substances, and is able to evaluate colored materials.[42,43,45] Furthermore, the monophasic treatment protocol offers the chance to skip the assessment of minimal phototoxic or maximal nonirritant doses of a test compound.

Based on these observations, a differentiation index (DI) was defined, which clearly distinguishes between chemical-induced photoallergic and photoirritant reactions (DI > 1 = [photo]allergy; DI < 1 = photoirritancy).[56]

REFERENCES

1. Thune, A., Jansén, C., Wennersten, G., Rystedt, I., Brodthagen, H., and McFadden, N., The Scandinavian multicenter photopatch study 1980–1985: final report, *Photodermatology*, 5, 261–269, 1988.
2. Rünger, T.M., Lehmann, P., Neumann, N.J., Matthies, C., Schauder, S., Ortel, B., Münzberger, C., and Hölzle, E., Empfehlung einer Photopatch-Test Standardreihe durch die deutschsprachige Arbeitsgruppe "Photopatch-Test," *Hautarzt*, 46, 240–243, 1995.
3. Lehmann, P., Scharfetter, K., Kind, P., and Goerz, G., Erythropoetische Protoporphyrie: Synopsis von 20 Patienten, *Hautarzt*, 42, 570–574, 1991.
4. Neumann, N.J., Fritsch, C., Goerz, G., Ruzicka, T., and Lehmann, P., δ-Aminolevulinic acid in the photo hen's egg test, *Arch. Dermatol. Res.*, 289 (Suppl), A49, 1997.
5. Hölzle, E., Plewig, G., and Lehmann, P., Photodermatoses — diagnostic procedures and their interpretation, *Photodermatol. Photoimmunol. Photomed.*, 4, 109-114, 1987.
6. Neumann, N.J., Hölzle, E., Lehmann, P., Benedikter, S., Tapernoux, B., and Plewig, G., Pattern analysis of photopatch test reactions, *Photodermatol. Photoimmunol. Photomed.*, 10(2), 65-73, 1994.
7. Lehmann, P., Die deutschsprachige Arbeitsgemeinschaft Photopatch-Test (DAPT), *Hautarzt*, 41, 295-297, 1990.
8. Lehmann, P., Photodiagnostische Testverfahren in der Dermatologie, In: Macher, E., Kolde, G., and Bröcker, B., (Eds.), *Jahrbuch der Dermatologie* 1992/1993, Biermann Verlag, Zülpich, 1992, 81-100.
9. Lehmann, P., Principles of photo testing and photopatch testing: a European perspective, *Retinoids Today and Tomorrow*, 31, 36-42, 1991.
10. Lehmann, P., Principles of photo testing and photopatch testing, In: Altmeyer, P., Hoffmann, K., and Stücker, M., (Eds.), *Skin Cancer and UV Radiation*, Springer-Verlag, Berlin, 1997.
11. Lehmann, P., Hölzle, E., and Plewig, G., Photoallergie auf Neotri mit Kreuzreaktion auf Teneretic Nachweis durch systemische Photoprovokation, *Hautarzt*, 39, 38-41, 1988.
12. Lehmann, P., Hölzle, E., von Kries, R., and Plewig, G., Übersicht – Neue Konzepte. Lichtdiagnostische Verfahren bei Patienten mit Verdacht auf Photodermatosen, *Zbl. Hautkr.*, 152, 667-682, 1986.
13. Epstein, S., Photoallergy and primary photosensitivity to sulfanilamide, *J. Invest. Dermatol.*, 2, 43-51, 1939.
14. Epstein, S., "Masked" photopatch tests, *J. Dermatol.*, 41, 369-370, 1963.
15. Epstein, S., The photopatch test. Its technique, manifestations, and significance, *Ann. Allergy*, 22, 1-11, 1964.
16. Epstein, S., Simplified photopatch testing, *Arch. Dermatol.*, 93, 216-220, 1966.
17. Hölzle, E., Plewig, G., Hofmann, C., and Braun-Falco, O., Photopatch testing. Results of a survey on test procedures and experimental findings, *Zbl. Hautkr.*, 151, 361-366, 1985.
18. Jansén, C.T., Wennerstein, G., Rystedt, I., Thune, P., and Brodthagen, H., The Scandinavian standard photopatch test procedure, *Contact Dermatitis*, 8, 155-158, 1982.

19. Hölzle, E., Neumann, N., Hausen, B., Przybilla, B., Schauder, S., Hönigsmann, H., Bircher, A., and Plewig, G., Photopatch testing: the 5-year experience of the German, Austrian, and Swiss Photopatch Test Group, *J. Am. Acad. Dermatol.*, 25, 59-68, 1991.

20. Bourrain, J.L., Paillet, C., Woodward, C., Beani, J.C., and Amblard, P., Diagnosis of photosensitivity to flupenthixol by photoprick testing, *Photodermatol. Photoimmunol. Photomed.*, 4, 159-161, 1997.

21. Schürer, N.Y., Lehmann, P., and Plewig, G., Chinidininduzierte Photoallergie. Eine klinische und experimentelle Studie, *Hautarzt*, 42, 158-161, 1991.

22. Schürer, N.Y., Hölzle, E., Plewig, G., and Lehmann, P., Photosensitivity induced by quinidine sulfate: experimental reproduction of skin lesions, *Photodermatol. Photoimmunol. Photomed.*, 9, 78-82, 1992.

23. OECD (Organisation for Economic Cooperation and Development), Guideline 406 for Testing Chemicals. Adopted 1992.

24. Raab, O., Über die Wirkung fluorescierender Stoffe auf Infusorien, *Z. Biol.*, 39, 524-546, 1900.

25. Daniels, F., A simple microbiological method for demonstrating phototoxic compounds, *J. Invest. Dermatol.*, 44, 259-263, 1965.

26. Gibbs, N.K., An adaption of the *Candida albicans* phototoxicity test to demonstrate photosensitizer action spectra, *Photodermatology*, 4, 312-316, 1987.

27. Knudson, E.A., The Candida phototoxicity test. The sensitivity of different strains of *Candida*, standardization attempts and analysis of the dose-response curves for 5- and 8-methoxypsoralen, *Photodermatology*, 2, 80-85, 1985.

28. Kahn, G. and Fleischaker, B., Evaluation of phototoxicity of salicylanilides and similar compounds by photohemolysis, *J. Invest. Dermatol.*, 56, 91-97, 1971.

29. Przybilla, B., Schwab-Przybilla, U., Ruzicka, T., and Ring, J., Phototoxicity of non-steroidal anti-inflammaotry drugs, demonstrated in vitro by a photo-basophil-histamin-release test, *Photodermatology*, 4, 73-78, 1987.

30. Freeman, R.G., Murtishaw, W., and Knox, J.M., Tissue culture techniques in the study of cell photobiology and phototoxicity, *J. Invest. Dermatol.*, 54, 164-169, 1970.

31. Maurer, T., Phototoxicity testing — in vivo and in vitro, *Food Chem. Toxic.*, 25, 407-414, 1987.

32. Maier, K., Schmitt-Landgraf, R., and Siegmund, B., Development of an in vitro test system with human skin cells for evaluation of phototoxicity, *Toxicol. in Vitro*, 5/6, 457-461, 1991.

33. Johnson, B. E., Walker, E. M., and Hetherington, A. M., In vitro models for cutaneous phototoxicity. In: Marks, R. and Plewig, G. (Eds.), *Skin Models — Models to Study Function and Disfunction of Skin*, 1986.

34. Neumann, N.J., Hölzle, E., Lehmann, P., Rosenbruch, M., Klaucic, A., and Plewig, G., Photo hen's egg test: a model for phototoxicity, *Br. J. Dermatol.*, 136, 326-330, 1997.

35. Neumann, N.J., Klaucic, A., Hölzle, E., Lehmann, P., Evaluation of the phototoxic potential of ciprofloxacin in the phot hen's egg test, *Arch. Dermatol. Res.*, 287, 384, 1995.

36. Draize, H.J., Intracutaneous sensitization test on guinea pigs, In: *Appraisal of the Safety of Chemicals in Food, Drugs and Cosmetics*. Association of Food and Drug Officials of the United States, Austin, TX, 1959.

37. Duffy, P.A., Irritancy testing — a cultured approach, *Toxicol. In Vitro*, 3, 157-158, 1989.

38. Rosenbruch, M., Toxizitätsuntersuchungen am bebrüteten Hühnerei, *Derm. Beruf. Umwelt.*, 38, 5-11, 1990.

39. Vinson, L.J., Borselli, V.F., and Singer, E.F., Realistic methods for determining photosenzitization potential of topical agents, *Am. Perfum. Cosmet.*, 83, 37, 1968.

40. Maurer, T., Experimentelle Modelle des photoallergischen Ekzems, *Allergologie*, 9, 3-7, 1986.

41. Maurer, T., Thomann, P., Weirich, E.G., and Hess, R., The optimization test in the guinea pig, *Agents Actions*, 5, 174, 1975.

42. Gad, S.C., The mouse ear swelling test (MEST) in the 1990s, *Toxicology*, 93, 33, 1994.

43. Gad, S.C., Dunn, B.J., Dobbs, D.W., Reilly, C., and Walsh, R.D., Development and validation of an alternative dermal sensitization test: the mouse ear swelling test (MEST), *Toxicol. Appl. Pharmacol.* 84, 93, 1986.

44. Gerberick, G.F. and Ryan, C.A., A predictive mouse ear swelling model for investigating topical photoallergy, *Food Chem. Toxicol.*, 28 (5), 361, 1990.

45. Kimber, I., Dearman, R.J., Scholes, E.W., and Basketter, D.A., The local lymph node assay: developments and applications, *Toxicology,* 93, 13, 1994.

46. Kimber, I. and Weisenberger, C., A murine local lymph node assay for the identification of contact allergenes. Assay development and results of initial validation study, *Arch. Toxicol.*, 63, 274, 1989.
47. Bühler, E.V., Delayed contact hypersensitivity in the guinea pig, *Arch. Dermatol.*, 91, 171, 1965.
48. Magnusson, B. and Kligman, A.M., The identification of contact allergens by animal assay. The guinea pig maximization test, *J. Invest. Dermatol.*, 52, 268, 1969.
49. Maguire, H.C., The bioassay of contact allergens in the guinea pig, *J. Soc. Cosmet. Chem.*, 24, 51, 1973.
50. Vinson, L.J. and Borselli, V.F., A guinea pig assay of photosensitizing potential of topical germicides, *J. Soc. Cosmet. Chem.*, 17, 123, 1966.
51. Maguire, H.C. and Chase, M.W., Jr., Studies of the sensitization of animals with simple chemical compounds. 13. Sensitization of guinea pigs with picric acid, *J. Exp. Med.*, 135, 357, 1972.
52. Vohr, H.W., Homey, B., Schuppe, H.C., and Kind, P., Detection of photoreactivity demonstrated in a modified local lymph node assay in mice, *Photodermatol. Photoimmunol. Photomed.*, 10, 57-64, 1994.
53. Homey, B., Neubert, T., Arens, A., Schuppe, H.C., Vohr, H.W., Ruzicka, T., and Lehmann, P., Sunscreen and immunosuppression, *J. Invest. Dermatol.*, 109, 395, 1997.
54. Homey, B., Schuppe, H.C., Assmann, T., Vohr, H.W., Lauerma, A.I., Ruzicka, T., and Lehmann, P., A local lymph node assay to analyse immunosuppressive effects of topically applied drugs, *Eur. J. Pharmacol.*, 325, 199, 1997.
55. Homey, B., Vohr, H.W., Schuppe, H.C., and Kind, P., UV-dependent local lymph node reactions: photoallergy and phototoxicity testing, In *Curr. Probl. Dermatol.*, Surber, C., Elsner, P., and Bircher, A.L., (Eds.), 22, 44, 1995.
56. Ikarashi, Y., Tsukamoto, Y., Tsuchiya, T., and Nakamura, A., Influence of irritants on lymph node cell proliferation and the detection of contact sensitivity to metal salts in the murine local lymph node assay, *Contact Dermatitis*, 29, 128, 1993.
57. Schilling, C., Homey, B., Ruzicka, T., Lehmann, P., Schuppe, H.C., and Vohr, H.W., Characterization of the induction phase of contact hypersensitivity in murine epidermal and local draining lymph node cells, *J. EADV*, 7, A37, 1996.
58. Shivji, G.M., Gupta, A.K., and Suder, D.R., Role of cytokines in irritant contact dermatitis, In: *Alternative Methods in Toxicology Series, Volume 10*: *In Vitro Skin Toxicology: Irritation Phototoxicity, Sensitization*. Rougier, A., Goldberg, A.M., and Maibach, H.I., (Eds.), Mary Ann Liebert Publishers, New York, 1994, 13-21.

Section II

Cellular and Humoral Regulation and Pathogenesis

7   Mechanisms of Allergic and Irritant Contact Dermatitis

*Paul Wakem and Anthony A. Gaspari**

CONTENTS

I. INTRODUCTION

Both allergic contact dermatitis (ACD) and irritant contact dermatitis (ICD) are very common and important conditions in clinical and occupational dermatology. With the increased industrialization of our society has come a corresponding increase in our exposure to chemicals, pollutants, and noxious substances, both at home and in the workplace. As our reliance on technology accelerates, exposure to these chemicals will continue to increase as well. Our bodies' first defense against these substances is the skin, and in the majority of individuals, this defense is sufficient and acts without adverse effects. However, as our exposure to chemicals becomes more widespread and frequent, the incidence of pathological responses to this exposure in the population also has increased dramatically. In 1983, the National Center for Health Statistics reported that eczematous dermatitis was one of the most common specific dermatoses encountered in the outpatient setting.[1] Dermatitis resulting from incidental or inadvertent exposure to occupational hazards has been estimated to account for approximately 30% of all occupational disease, with more than 90% of all cases due to ICD or ACD.[2] A Danish study estimated that 2.5% of Danish workers on permanent disability suffered from hyperkeratotic hand eczema at a national cost of $15 million per year.[3] A direct extrapolation to the U.S., based on population alone, would imply an impact of nearly $750 million per year, solely for hand eczema. Thus, contact dermatitis is a disorder of significant economic dimension. This chapter will compare both ICD and ACD and describe the immune mechanisms involved in contact dermatitis.

---

* Grant support from 1RO-1AR/OH46108-01.

II. CATEGORIES OF CONTACT DERMATITIS

There are several categories of contact dermatitis, classified by their etiologies. ICD is a non-immunological, local inflammatory reaction characterized by erythema, edema, or corrosion following a single or repeated exposure of a chemical to an identical cutaneous site,[4] which occurs primarily as a result of chemical toxicity to epidermal cells leading to an inflammatory response in the dermis. A second category, ACD, is a cell-mediated immune type IV hypersensitivity reaction. This type of contact dermatitis requires preexisting genetic susceptibility, an immunocompetent individual (however, some HIV patients can develop ACD),[5–7] and a chemical antigen capable of transepidermal absorption. Photocontact dermatitis, both the toxic and allergic variants, requires that the phototoxin or allergen be activated by exposure to ultraviolet light. The last major category of contact dermatitis is contact urticaria, which involves a wheal and flare response to cutaneous insult and can be subdivided into allergic (immunoglogulin [Ig] E-dependent) and nonallergic (IgE-independent) categories.

ICD can be caused by either acute exposure to particularly toxic substances or chronic exposure to mild irritants. ICD can be induced by acids, which coagulate epidermal proteins; alkali, surfactants, and solvents, which remove surface lipids; and oxidants, which alter epidermal integrity. The severity of dermatitis caused by these irritants depends on the particular compound encountered, its concentration, length of exposure to the irritant, and an individual's susceptibility to a specific compound. Individuals may be predisposed to developing ICD due to: age, with the very young and very old being most susceptible; an individual's genetic factors (i.e., a history of eczema); weather conditions which cause dry and cracked skin such as cold, wind, and low ambient humidity. Other risk factors for ICD include the presence of an active dermatitis or the atopic state of the skin;[8] excessive humidity which increases skin permeability to exogenous substances; skin injury, whether induced by friction, abrasion, or frank laceration, as well as an individual's behavior which increases exposure levels.[9]

In contrast, ACD results from a cell-mediated immune response to a particular chemical hapten. ACD begins with an initial refractory period, followed by an inductive phase lasting from several days to several weeks during which sensitization occurs, and an efferent phase after antigenic reexposure which can precipitate rapid and even severe responses. Susceptibility may wane over time, but tends to persist indefinitely. While the overall sensitization rate of contact allergens is small among exposed individuals, ACD alone contributes to 30% of occupational skin disease.

Predisposition to contact allergy depends on interactions between the patient, the allergen, and the environment.[10] For example, patients with a history of ICD and inflammatory skin lesions have an increased risk of antigen absorption and ACD development, while patients with a history of atopic dermatitis may actually have a decreased risk of developing ACD, but be predisposed to develop ICD. Age, genetic background, and pregnancy can also be contributing factors for ACD, as well as environmental factors, including the application of pressure, friction, exposure to heat, immersion, humidity, temperature, and season.

The development of ACD is affected by the molecular weight and chemical reactivity, as well as the concentration and dose of the allergen, its site of contact, the number of exposures to the chemical, and the frequency of exposure. While it is difficult to predict which substances possess allergenic potential, some chemical families have emerged as more likely allergens than others. For example, aromatics which contain polar or ionic side groups, such as para-aminophenol and hydroquinone, can be potent sensitizers.[11] Some well-known, natural allergens include the resinous secretions of the poison ivy and poison oak plants, which can lead to further incidence of ACD by inducing cross-sensitivity to components found in certain lacquers, varnishes, and oils derived from exotic trees.[12] Synthetic allergens can be grouped into the following categories: rubber products; plastic resins; organic dyes; topical medications, including corticosteroids, germicidals and biocidals; and certain ingredients found in topical medications. Some refined metals such as nickel, cobalt, and chromium may also cause ACD. These allergens may be easily recognized, or more insidious, occurring on such vehicles as cement dust, saw dust, and in soldering rosin. In addition, certain allergens have even been found to penetrate gloves. Hairdressers who have a history of hand dermatitis found that rubber gloves did not provide protection to their hands from chemicals causing their dermatitis, and glyceryl thioglycolate, a notorious contact allergen for hairdressers, penetrated through all but the thickest rubber gloves.[13] All these factors combined generate a substantial role for these compounds in occupational and domestic hazards.

The most common contact allergens in the U.S. are nickel, found in jewelry, metal accouterments on clothing, and in coins; potassium dichromate, found in cement, leather, paper, metallic paint, timber, and household detergent; and paraphenylenediamine, found in hair dyes, printer's ink, radiographic fluid, and fur dyes.

The third category of contact dermatitis is photosensitivity dermatitis which can be classified into phototoxic and photoallergic variants. Lesions resemble those of ICD and ACD, but are localized to sun-exposed areas of the skin including the face (particularly the malar area), the dorsum of the hands, and forearms. Patients may report a stinging or burning sensation of the skin under sunlight, and rapid resolution of symptoms in the shade. Phototoxins and photoallergens require ultraviolet light (UV) of 315 to 400 nm wavelength to generate toxic or sensitizing products. Compounds which can induce photosensitivity include fragrances, lotions containing musk ambrette, suntanning products containing 6-methyl-coumarin, homosalicylate, or para-aminobenzoic acid (PABA), and antibacterials in soaps.[14] Phototoxicity can be induced by psoralens found in the oil of lime skins and in coal tar.[15] Systemic medications such as nalidixic acid, phenothiazines, sulfonamides, sulfonylureas, tetracyclines, and thiazide diuretics can cause photoallergic reactions especially among health care workers who handle medications (pharmacists, pharmaceutical manufacturers, nurses, etc.).[16] Sensitivity to these agents is often determined by photopatch testing.

The final category of contact dermatitis is the wheal and flare response of contact urticaria, which develops rapidly in response to an insult. Immunologic contact urticaria is a type I hypersensitivity reaction mediated by IgE. The response can be local or widespread resulting in rash accompanied by asthma, conjunctivitis, rhinitis, lingual and labial edema, or gastrointestinal complaints,[17] and in extreme cases can result in anaphylactic shock requiring urgent resuscitation. Causative agents for contact uticaria include protein antigens (such as feline saliva proteins), medications, foods, household products, fabrics, and cosmetics. Nonimmunologic contact urticaria can be induced by mild organic acids (acetic, butyric, cinnamic, sorbic), alcohols, balsam of Peru, benzocaine, cobalt chloride, dimethylsulfoxide, formaldehyde, witch hazel, sodium benzoate, ammonium persulfate (used to dye hair platinum-blond), and nicotinic acid esters. Cold, sunlight, water, and perspiration also can be associated with contact urticaria.

Lesions caused by most types of contact dermatitis are very similar in nature.[18] Responses are divided into acute, subacute, and chronic phases. Acute lesions consist of multiple vesicles or bullae, filled with clear fluid, surmounted on erythematous, edematous bases. After vesicle rupture, skin becomes eroded and oozing. Subacute lesions are characterized by more erythema, less edema, and the replacement of vesicles with papules, while chronic lesions display minimal redness and swelling and more pronounced scaling and lichenification.

Progression of contact dermatitis depends on the degree and extent of sensitization. Usually, the dermatitis is localized and resolves within 3 to 4 weeks if reexposure to antigen is avoided. This interval may shorten with appropriate therapy. On rare occasions, the acute stage may progress to a generalized, erythrodermic state in highly sensitive patients who have undergone extensive antigen exposure. This result is believed to be due to clonal expansion of sensitized, hapten-reactive T cells.[19]

III. COMPARISON OF ACD AND ICD

Comparative studies of ACD and ICD suggest that although their clinical definitions seem to be separate and distinct, these two types of contact dermatitis are actually very similar, with considerable overlap in their features (Table 1). In summary, both the histologic and clinical features of ACD and ICD are strikingly similar.

TABLE 1
Comparison of Clinical, Histologic, and Immunologic Features of Irritant and Allergic Contact Dermatitis 1

Feature	Irritant Contact Dermatitis [Ref.]	Allergic Contact Dermatitis [Ref.]
Clinical morphology	Dermatitis can be similar to ACD in mild to moderate reactions [1, 2]	Dermatitis can be similar to ICD; kinetics of resolution may be slower than ICD during patch testing [1, 2]
Histology	Spongiosis, exocytosis, dermal edema, and a mononuclear infiltrate; occasionally, neutrophil-rich infiltrates [3]	Same as ICD; neutrophils usually less prominent [3]
Frequency of hapten-specific T cells in infiltrate	Not known	Estimated to be approximately 1:100-1:1000 [4]
Immunochemistry[a]		
Of T cells	Predominantly CD4+ T cells; some CD8+ T cells; activated state indicated by IL-2 receptor expression [5, 6]	Predominantly CD4+, some CD8+ T cells; activated state indicated by IL-2 receptor expression [5, 6]
Of Langerhans cells Number Morphology	No consistent changes; alterations noted, but are highly dependent on chemical [4, 7]	Decreased, then recovery; alterations noted; particularly with high doses of hapten [4, 8]
Of accessory molecules		
CD36	No effect [9]	Increased [10]
HLA-DR	No effect [9], increased [13]	Increased [11–14]
ICAM-1	Increased [9]	Increased [14, 15]
B7-1	Increased [our unpublished data, 1998]	Increased [16]
Cytokine profiles[b] (mRNA studies)		
TNF-α	Increased [17, 18]	Increased [17, 18]
IFN-γ	Increased [17, 18]	Increased [17–19]
IL-2	Increased [18]	Increased [18]
GM-CSF	Increased [17]	Increased [17]
IL-1α	No change [17][c]	Increased [17][c]
	Increased [20][5]	Dependent on allergen [19, 21][d]
IL-1β	No change [17][c]	Increased [17][c]
	Increased [22, 23][d]	Increased [22, 23][d]
IP-10	No change [17][c]	Increased [17][c]
MIP-2	No change [17][c]	Increased [17][c]
IL-4	Not determined	Increased [24, 25]
IL-6	Not determined	Increased [26][c]
IL-7	Not determined	Not determined
IL-8	Not determined	No change [19]
IL-10	No change [27][c]	Increased [27][c]
IL-12 p35	No change [28][d]	No change [28][d]
IL-12 p40	No change [28][d]	Increased [28][d]
IL-15	Not determined	Not determined
IL-18	Not determined	Not determined
Transgenic mice[6] (in vivo ear swelling assays)		
Overexpression of		
B7-1 by KC	Increased [29]	Increased [29]
B7-2 by KC	No change [30]	No change [30]
ICAM-1 by KC	No change [31]	Not studied [31]

TABLE 1 (CONTINUED)
Comparison of Clinical, Histologic, and Immunologic Features of Irritant and Allergic Contact Dermatitis 1

IL-7 by KC	Increased [32]	Increased [32]
IFN-γ by KC	Not determined	Increased [33]
IL-1-R1 by KC	Not determined	Increased [34]
IL-1-R2 by KC	Not determined	No change [35]
Knockout mice		
ICAM-1	Decreased [36]	Decreased [36]
TNF-α R1	Decreased [37]	Increased [38]
TNF-α R2	No change [37, 39]	Decreased [37, 39]
CD4	Decreased [40]	Decreased [40, 41]
CD28	Decreased [42]	Decreased [42]
IL-1 β	Not determined	Decreased [43]
Immunodeficient mice[d]		
SCID	Decreased [44]	Decreased [44]
Athymic nude	Decreased [44]	Decreased [44]

[a] Immunochemistry of histology sections of skin biopsy samples.

[b] Studies of cytokine mRNA expression from skin biopsy samples at control or irritant- or allergen-challenge skin sites.

[c] Studies only completed in mouse model, with limited number of irritants and allergens. These studies have not been confirmed in humans or using human cells.

[d] Studies completed in human cells.

[e] Data summarized represent in vivo ear swelling studies of irritants or allergens in defined mouse models.

Adapted from Reference 45.

References

1. Rietschel, R. L., Irritant dermatitis. Diagnosis and treatment, in *Exogenous Dermatoses: Environmental Dermatitis*, Menne, T., Maibach, H. I., Eds., CRC Press, Boca Raton, FL, 1991, 375.

2. Fregert, S., Occupational dermatitis in a 10-year period, *Contact Dermatitis*, 1, 96, 1975.

3. Lever, W. F., Schaumberg-Lever, G., *Histopathology of the Skin*, J. B. Lippincott, Philadelphia, 1990, 106.

4. Kalish, R. S., Johnson, K. L., Enrichment and function of urushiol (poison ivy) specific T-lymphocytes in lesions of allergic contact dermatitis to urushiol, *J. Immunol.*, 145, 3706, 1990.

5. McMillan, E. M., Stoneking, L., Burdick, S., Cowan, I., Latafat Husain-Hamzavi, S., Immunophenotype of lymphoid cells in positive patch tests of allergic contact dermatitis, *J. Invest. Dermatol.*, 84, 229, 1985.

6. Brasch, J., Burgard, J., Sterry, W., Common pathogenetic pathways in allergic and irritant contact dermatitis, *J. Invest. Dermatol.*, 98, 166, 1992.

7. Willis, C. M., Stephens, C. J. M., Wilkinson, J. D., Differential effects of structurally unrelated chemical irritants on the density and morphology of epidermal CD1+ cells, *J. Invest. Dermatol.*, 95, 711, 1990.

8. Weinlich, G., Sepp, N., Koch, F., Schuler, G., Romani, N., Evidence that Langerhans cells rapidly disappear from the epidermis in response to contact sensitizers but not to tolerogens/nonsensitizers, *Arch. Dermatol. Res.*, 281, 556, 1989.

9. Willis, C. M., Stephens, C. J. M., Wilkinson, J. D., Selective expression of immune-associated surface antigens by keratinocytes in irritant contact dermatitis, *J. Invest. Dermatol.*, 96, 505, 1991.

10. Simon, M., Jr., Hunyadi, J., Expression of OKM5 antigen on human keratinocytes in positive intracutaneous tests for delayed-type hypersensitivity, *Dermatolagica*, 1745, 1211, 1987.

11. Mackie, R. M., Turbitt, M. L., Quantification of dendritic cells in normal and abnormal human epidermis using monoclonal antibodies directed against Ia and HTA antigens, *J. Invest. Dermatol.*, 81, 216, 1983.

12. Scheynius, A., Fischer, T., Phenotypic differences between allergic and irritant patch test reactions in man, *Contact Dermatitis*, 14, 297, 1986.

continued

TABLE 1 (CONTINUED)
Comparison of Clinical, Histologic, and Immunologic Features of Irritant and Allergic Contact Dermatitis 1

13. Gawkrodger, D. J., Carr, M. M., McVittie, E., Guy, K., Hunter, J. A. A., Keratinocyte expression MHC class II antigens in allergic sensitization and challenge reactions and in irritant contact dermatitis, *J. Invest. Dermatol.*, 88, 11, 1987.

14. Verheyen, A., Mathieu, L., Lambert, J., An immunohistochemical study of contact irritant and contact allergic patch tests. in *Irritant Dermatitis: New Clinical and Experimental Aspects*, Elsner, P., Maibach, H. I., Eds., S. Karger, New York, 1995, 108.

15. Wantzin, G. L., Ralfkiaer, E., Lisby, S., Rothlein, R., The role of intracellular adhesion molecules in inflammatory skin reactions, *Br. J. Dermatol.*, 119, 141, 1988.

16. Simon, J. C., Dietrich, A., Mielke, V., Wuttig, C., Vanscheidt, W., Linsley, P. S., Schopf, E., Sterry, W., Expression of the B7/BB-1 activation antigen and its ligand CD28 in T-cell mediated skin diseases, *J. Invest. Dermatol.*, 103, 539, 1994.

17. Enk, A. H., Katz, S. I., Early molecular events in the induction phase of contact hypersensitivity, *Proc. Natl. Acad. Sci. U.S.A.*, 89(4), 1398, 1992.

18. Hoefakker, S., Caubo, M., van't Erve, E. H. M., Roggeveen, M. J., Boersma, W. J. A., van Joost, T., Notten, W. R. F., Claassen, E., In vivo cytokine profiles in allergic and irritant contact dermatitis, *Contact Dermatitis*, 33, 258, 1995.

19. Howie, S. E. M., Aldridge, R. D., McVittie, E., Forsey, R. J., Sands, C., Hunter, J. A. A., Epidermal keratinocyte production of interferon-γ immunoreactive protein and mRNA is an early event in allergic contact dermatits, *J. Invest. Dermatol.*, 106, 1218, 1996.

20. Corsini, E., Bruccoleri, A., Marinovich, M., Galli, C. L., Endogenous interleukin-1α is associated with skin irritation induced by tributyltin, *Toxicol. Appl. Pharmacol.*, 138, 268, 1996.

21. Pastore, S., Shivji, G. M., Kondo, T., McKenzie, R. C., Segal, L., Somers, D., Sauder, D. N., Efects of contact sensitizers neomycin sulfate, benzoxaine and 2,4-dinitrobenzene-1-sulfonate, sodium salt on viability, membrane integrity and IL-1α mRNA expression of cultured normal human keratinocytes, *Food Chem. Toxicity*, 33, 57, 1995.

22. Brand, C. U., Hunziger, T., Yawalkar, N., Braathen, L. R., IL-1β protein in human skin lymph does not discriminate allergic from irritant contact dermatitis, *Contact Dermatitis*, 35, 152, 1996.

23. Zepter, C., Haffner, A., Soohoo, L. F., De Luca, D., Tang, H., Fisher, P., Chavinson, J., Slmets, C. A., Induction of biologically active IL-1b-converting enzyme and mature IL-1b in human keratinocytes by inflammatory and immunologic stimuli, *J. Immunol.*, 159, 6203, 1997.

24. Asada, H., Linton, J., Katz, S. I., Cytokine gene expression during the elicitation phase of contact sensitivity: regulation by endogenous IL-4, *J. Invest. Dermatol.*, 108, 406, 1997.

25. Rowe, A., Bunker, C. B., Interleukin-4 and the interleukin-4 receptor in allergic contact dermatitis, *Contact Dermatitis*, 38, 36, 1998.

26. Flint, M. S., Dearman, R. J., Kimber, I., Hotchkiss, S. A., Production and in situ localization of cutaneous tumour necrosis factor alpha (TNF-alpha) and interleukin 6 (IL-6) following skin sensitization, *Cytokine*, 10(3), 213, 1998.

27. Enk, A. H., Katz, S. I., Identification and induction of keratinocyte-derived IL-10, *J. Immunol.*, 149, 92, 1992.

28. Muller, G., Saloga, J., Germann, T., Bellinghausen, I., Mohamadzadeh, M., Knop, J., Enk, A. H., Identification and induction of human keratinocyte-derived IL-12, *J. Clin. Invest.*, 94, 1799, 1994.

29. Gaspari, A. A., Burns, R. P., Kondo, S., Nasir, A., Kurup, A., Mlodynia, D., Sauder, D., Barth, R. K., Characterization of the altered cutaneous reactivity of transgenic mice whose keratinocytes overexpress B7-1, *Clin. Immunol. Immunopathol.*, 86(3), 259, 1998.

30. Burns, R., Nasir, A., Ferbel, B., Ramirez, D., Barth, R., Gaspari, A. A., The T-cell costimulatory molecules B7-1 (CD80) and B7-2 (CD86) when expressed on keratinocytes deliver different signals during contact hypersensitivity responses, *J. Invest. Dermatol.*, 110, 477, 1998.

31. Williams, I. R., Kupper, T. S., Epidermal expression of intercellular adhesion molecule 1 is not a primary inducer of cutaneous inflammation in transgenic mice, *Proc. Natl. Acad. Sci., U.S.A.*, 91, 9710, 1994.

32. Uehira, M., Matsuda, H., Hikita, I., Sakata, T., Fujiwara, H., Nishimoto, H., The development of dermatitis infiltrated by gamma delta T cells in IL-7 transgenic mice, *Int. Immunol.*, 5, 1619, 1993.

33. Carroll, J. M., Crompton, T., Seery, J. P., Watt, F. M., Trandgenic mice expressing IFN-γ in the epidermis have eczema, hair hypopigmentation, and hair loss, *J. Invest. Dermatol.*, 108, 412, 1997.

TABLE 1 (CONTINUED)
Comparison of Clinical, Histologic, and Immunologic Features of Irritant and Allergic Contact Dermatitis 1

34. Groves, R. W., Rauschmayr, T., Nakamura, K., Sarkar, S., Williams, I. R., Kupper, T. S., Inflammatory and hyperproliferative skin disease in mice that express elevated levels of the IL-1 receptor (type I) on epidermal keratinocytes. Evidence that IL-1-inducible secondary cytokines produced by keratinocytes in vivo can cause skin disease, *J. Clin. Invest.*, 98, 336, 1996.

35. Rauschmayr, T., Groves, R. W., Kupper, T. S., Keratinocyte expression of the type 2 interleukin 1 receptor mediates local and specific inhibition of interkeukin 1-mediated inflammation, *Proc. Natl. Acad. Sci. U.S.A.*, 94, 5814, 1997.

36. Sligh, J., Jr., Ballantyne, C. M., Rich, S. S., Hawkins, H. K., Smith, C. W., Bradley, A., Beaudet, A. L., Inflammatory and immune responses are impaired in mice deficient in intercellular adhesion molecule 1, *Proc. Natl. Acad. Sci. U.S.A.*, 90, 8529, 1993.

37. Kondo, S., Sauder, D. N., Tumor necrosis factor (TNF) receptor type 1 (p55) is a main mediator for TNF-α-induced skin inflammation, *Eur. J. Immunol.*, 27, 1713, 1997.

38. Kondo, S., Wang, B., Fujisawa, H., Shivji, G. M., Echtenacher, B., Mak, T. W., Sauder, D. N., Effect of gene-targeted mutation in TNF receptor (p55) on contact hypersensitivity and ultraviolet B-induced immunosuppression, *J. Immunol.*, 155, 3801, 1995.

39. Wang, B., Fujisawa, H., Zhuang, L., Kondo, S., Shivji, G. M., Kim, C. S., Mak, T. W., Sauder, D. N., Depressed Langerhans cell migration and reduced contact hypersensitivity response in mice lacking TNF receptor p75, *J. Immunol.*, 159, 6148, 1997.

40. Kondo, S., Beissert, S., Wang, B., Fujisawa, H., Kooshesh, F., Stratigos, A., Granstein, R. D., Mak, T. W., Sauder, D. N., Hyporesponsiveness in contact hypersensitivity and irritant dermatitis in CD4 gene targeted mice, *J. Invest. Dermatol.*, 106, 993, 1996.

41. Fujisawa, H., Kondo, S., Wang, B., Shivji, G. M., Sauder, D. N., The role of CD4 molecules in the induction phase of contact hypersensitivity cytokine profiles in the skin and lymph nodes, *Immunology*, 89, 250, 1996.

42. Kondo, S., Kooshesh, F., Wang, B., Fujisawa, H., Sauder, D. N., Contribution of the CD28 molecule to allergic and irritant-induced skin reactions in CD28 –/– mice, *J. Immunol.*, 157, 4822, 1996.

43. Shornick, L. P., De Togni, P., Mariathasan, S., Goellner, J., Strauss-Schoenberger, J., Karr, R. W., Ferguson, T. A., Chaplin, D. D., Mice deficient in IL-1β manifest impaired contact hypersensitivity to dinitrochlorobenzene, *J. Exp. Med.*, 183, 1427, 1996.

44. Kalish, R. S., T-cells and other leukocytes as mediators of irritant contact dermatitis, *Immunol. Allergy Clin. N. Am.*, 17(3), 407, 1997.

45. Gaspari, A. A., The role of keratinocytes in the pathogenesis of contact dermatitis, *Immunol. Allergy Clin. N. Am.*, 17(3), 377, 1997.

ACD and ICD are usually difficult to distinguish histologically in biopsy specimens.[18] In acute ACD, spongiosis (intercellular edema between epidermal spinous cells) may be mild or moderate, and may be accompanied by a superficial perivascular infiltrate of lymphocytes, histiocytes, and eosinophils. Progressive epidermal edema can lead to keratinocyte (KC) separation and vesicle formation. Parakeratosis may be observed in the stratum corneum along with possible erosions and ulcerations. In subacute ACD, spongiosis is observed in the context of an acanthotic epidermis, with edema in the papillary dermis. Chronic lesions display a scale crust in the stratum corneum, irregular epidermal hyperplasia, and a thickened, fibrotic papillary dermis.

ICD progresses through the same stages and may be variably distinguished by reticular changes, epidermal necrosis, and the presence of neutrophils in addition to the above-mentioned infiltrating cells. These differences are subtle and not reliable; thus, routine histologic study of skin biopsy specimens is not typically helpful in the diagnosis. In circumstances where there is a broader differential diagnosis, histologic study of skin biopsy specimens is useful in diagnosing, for example, erythema multiforme, lichenoid eruption to gold, and psoriasiform changes in hand eczema.

Immunohistochemistry studies examining the cellular nature of the infiltrate also do not distinguish these two types of dermatitis. Although haptens consistently decrease epidermal Langerhans cell (LC) number, some irritants also decrease LC, suggesting that this is not a consistent feature that will distinguish ACD from ICD. Also immunohistochemistry studies of the expression of accessory molecules such as ICAM-1 and B7-1 show no differences between ACD and ICD. However, the accessory molecules CD36 and possibly HLA-DR show an increase in expression during ACD with no comparable increase in expression during ICD, although the expression of HLA-DR has been reported to be increased by the irritant anthralin[20] and to be unaffected by six other irritants,[21] so the expression of HLA-DR may be irritant specific.

Reverse transcription/polymerase chain reaction (RT-PCR) has been used to amplify mRNA expressed by inflammatory or stromal cells in ACD or ICD to study cytokine gene expression. The majority of cytokines described in Table 1 are expressed at increased levels in both ACD and ICD, and two cytokines, interleukin (IL)-8 and IL-12 p35, show no change in expression. However, some subtle differences in cytokine expression during ACD and ICD are evident. The expression of IL-1α, IL-1β, inducible protein (IP)-10, macrophage inhibitory protein (MIP)-2, IL-10, and IL-12 p40 is increased during ACD but unchanged in ICD, although in the case of IL-1α and IL-1β these differences are species specific, while IP-10, MIP-2, and IL-10 expression has only been determined in mouse epidermis and IL-12 p40 only in human epidermis.

Finally, the use of transgenic mice has also led to some useful insights into the similarities between ACD and ICD. The two types of transgenic mice include mice which overexpress a gene and knockout mice, in which a gene is disrupted. In the former case (overexpression), a foreign gene containing a tissue-specific promoter is introduced into genomic DNA, allowing the study of the overexpression of a gene product or a gain of function of an immunologically relevant cytokine or adhesion molecule. The latter type of transgenic mouse is the so-called "knockout mouse," in which a molecularly engineered, disrupted gene is allowed to replace a normal, healthy gene (homologous recombination). Mice are initially chimeric for the disrupted gene, but they are successively bred until they are homozygous for the genetic flaw. These animals are then studied to examine the effects of the loss of a gene product in vivo on a specific biologic phenomenon. As described in Table 1, both types of transgenic mice confirm that ACD and ICD are very similar.

Are there critical differences between ACD and ICD? First, hapten specific Th-lymphocytes can be identified in the skin lesions and draining lymph nodes of experimental animals or humans with ACD, but not in ICD. Second, some of the early studies of cytokine profiles suggest there may be some differences in expression between ACD and ICD. However, these studies have been limited to a mouse model, using only a few haptens or irritants. So it remains to be determined whether these cytokine profile differences are seen using other chemicals and, more important, in human ACD vs. ICD. Other critical features that distinguish ACD and ICD have yet to be determined.

One of the reasons ACD and ICD are so similar is likely related to the limited repertoire of the pathologic responses to skin injury. It is probable that autoreactive T lymphocytes (either conventional CD4+, TCR α/β+ or CD8+, TCR α/β+ or nonconventional T cells such as CD4−CD8−, TCR α/β, or TCR γ/δ) may dominate the infiltrate after skin injury by a hapten, irritant, or other types of skin damage. This hypothesis has yet to be proven, but is worthy of further research.

The above data (Table 1) suggest considerable similarities in ACD and ICD. Since a great deal of information is known about ACD immune mechanisms, but very little information about the immunology of ICD, it is appropriate to review the immunology of ACD. It seems likely that T lymphocytes, LC, and KC perform similar roles in both ACD and ICD.

IV. MECHANISMS OF ACD

A. ACD: AN OVERVIEW

ACD is a prototypical delayed-type hypersensitivity reaction, dependent on epidermal LC presenting haptenated self-proteins to CD4+ T-lymphocytes in regional lymph nodes. Current data support

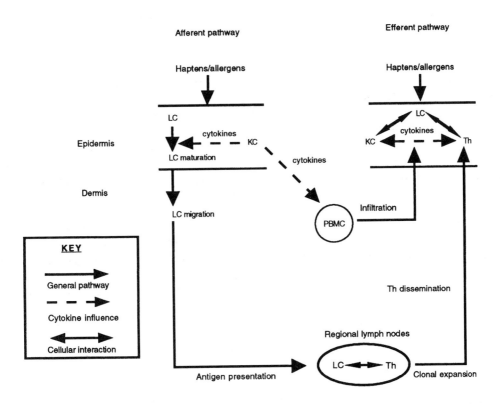

Figure 1   Dual-phase model of ACD. In this model of ACD, LC are important in the afferent (primary or inductive) phase as well as the efferent (secondary or elicitation) phase of ACD. During the afferent phase, hapten-bearing LC migrate from the skin to the paracortical areas of the draining lymph nodes and present antigen to naïve Th cells (primary immune response). In the efferent phase (secondary immune response) hapten-bearing LC migrate from the skin to the paracortical areas of the draining lymph nodes and activate memory Th cells. The activated Th cells then migrate to the site of allergen application.

the dual phase model for ACD (see Figure 1), in which low-molecular-weight hapten penetrates the skin and covalently binds to a host moiety.[22] LC present the hapten–carrier complex to antigen-reactive T cells in regional lymph nodes. Antigen presentation leads to the development of antigen-specific T cell proliferation. This clonally expanded population of T cells resides in the local lymph nodes or may migrate to the skin or other sites to serve as a pool of memory T cells (afferent, inductive, or primary phase).

In the efferent (elicitation or secondary) phase of ACD, a reexposure to antigen results in a similar uptake and processing by LC cells. After processing, LC present the antigen to an expanded pool of memory T cells which are present in the skin, regional lymph nodes, and circulating in the peripheral blood. This second interaction results in a vigorous T cell-mediated response which involves an intricate interplay among epidermal cells, bone marrow-derived cells, lymphokines, and cytokines. The response typically peaks in 24 to 48 h and resolves in 1 to 2 weeks. LC, T cells, and keratinocytes each play important roles in ACD.

B. Role of LC in ACD

LC are dendritic epidermal cells found in stratified squamous epithelia, first discovered in 1868 by Paul Langerhans, who observed LC after staining human skin sections with gold chloride.[23] The cells were originally thought to be of neuronal origin and function, because of their rarity, their dendritic appearance, and because gold chloride had been developed to stain neural tissue. However, in 1963, Breathnach proposed that LC represented effete melanocytes,[24] and in 1976 Potten and Allen theorized that LC may regulate keratinocyte growth.[25] The first accurate hints about LC function began to emerge in 1973.[26] Ultrastructural studies by Silberberg revealed tight apposition among infiltrating lymphocytes and epidermal dendritic LC in ACD, suggesting that LC functioned as antigen-presenting cells. This hypothesis initiated an interest in Langerhans cell research by many investigators,[27–29] and LC have been the subject of intense immunological investigation ever since.

Ultrastructurally, LC are identified by their Birbeck granules, which have been described as either "rod-shaped" or "tennis racket-shaped" organelles with a central "zipper-like" striation.[30] Three-dimensional reconstruction suggests that these organelles are flat, disk, or cup shaped.[31] While their function is unclear, some appear to be continuous with the external compartment of the cell and so are believed to be involved in the endolysosomal uptake and processing of antigen.[32] LC also can be stained with ATPase,[33] which is useful in epidermal but not extra-epidermal sites, plus a variety of specialized monoclonal antibodies.[34]

LC express several cell surface markers including class I MHC in association with β2-microglobulin[35] and class II MHC, which is expressed constitutively (the only epidermal cells to do so) even in the resting state.[36] Class II MHC molecules are noncovalently associated with a 31-kDa molecule (identified in LC), the invariant chain (Ii).[37] Levels of class II MHC have been shown to correlate quantitatively with antigen presentation potential.[38] In fact, it is believed that while LC constitutively express class II MHC, they do not do so at constant levels and the upregulation of class II MHC expression in LC may be caused by KC-derived cytokines. These KC-derived cytokines are critical in the maturation of LC into potent APC.[22,36,39–41]

LC express the lymphocyte markers, CD1a and CD1c, which may be cognate molecules for CD4−CD8− α/β and CD4−CD8− γ/δ T lymphocytes, respectively.[22,42] CD4-bearing LC have been described in normal and in diseased human skin, where the levels appear to be upregulated.[43] These cells have been shown to serve as a target for HIV infection and as a reservoir for HIV replication.[44,45] An intriguing recent finding has been the observation of γ/δ T cell receptor-specific monoclonal antibody immunoreactivity in a subpopulation of normal LC. B cell markers identified on LC are B7-1, B7-2, and the CD40 antigens.[22] In addition, LC have been shown to express several receptors and adhesion molecules[30,46] such as: low- and high-affinity IgE receptor, C3 receptor, integrins (CD11b,c, CD18, CD29, VLA-1 to VLA-6), ICAM-1, LFA-3, CD15, CD45 (a marker for bone marrow-derived cells, also referred to as common leukocyte antigen), and S-100 antigen (a 100-kDa antigen present on a variety of different cell types that is therefore not specific for LC).

LC originate in the bone marrow. Katz and colleagues observed that in adoptive allogeneic bone marrow transplantation experiments into X-irradiated host mice, the host LC were of donor origin, while KC remained of host origin.[47] Furthermore, in human bone marrow grafts involving a female recipient and a male donor, LC were Y chromosome positive.[48] Surface marker studies (particularly class II MHC, CD45, C3bi R, and FcγR) indicate that LC are derived from the monocytes/macrophages lineage.[49] Birbeck granule negative CD1a+ cells have been identified in the peripheral blood. These cells increase in number in burn victims — and in human cord blood, which is believed to be enriched in stem cell precursors.[50] While it is possible that epidermal LC arise from migration of these CD1a+ precursors from the peripheral blood, some LC levels may be maintained by *in situ* epidermal mitosis. Mitosis has been demonstrated by electron microscopy, radioactive thymidine uptake, flow cytometric studies, and human skin transplantation onto nude mice.[51–53] Current evidence suggests that both repopulation and division contribute to LC maintenance.

LC density ranges from 450/mm² in adult human skin to 60/mm² in the sole of the foot, and while these densities are constant, they are not static, but result from an equilibrium of LC circulation, suggesting that LC have a mean epidermal transit time of 3 weeks.[54]

LC are sufficiently networked to create a tight mesh capable of trapping antigen entering almost anywhere on the skin surface. Following the application of allergen, LC undergo a variety of phenotypic and morphological changes, including the uptake of antigen by an increase in the concentration of Birbeck granules, increased rough endoplasmic reticulum prominence, and an increase in the number of coated pits, endosomes, and lysosomes.[55] LC also undergo increased class II MHC expression and loss of ATPase activity.[56,57] Occasionally, LC with swollen mitochondria, cell membrane rupture, hypodense cytoplasm, and decreased arborization of dendrites have been observed, consistent with degenerative changes.[58] The above effects are not seen in the absence of either sensitizing agent or irritant and are dependent on the allergen, its dose, and exposure time. LC can present a variety of haptens, including nickel ions, tetanus toxoid, purified protein derivative of *Mycobacterium*, *Candida albicans* proteins, and even complex antigens such as sheep red blood cells.[59] Some haptens do not require uptake and may bind directly to MHC, such as nickel ion.[60]

LC are essential for the afferent phase of contact sensitization. In the epidermis, LC numbers decrease by more than 50% following antigen application. This decrease is not the result of cell death, but instead due to migration, specifically via dermal lymphatics to the paracortical (T-dependent) zones of draining lymph nodes,[61] as shown by fluorescent sensitizer labeling experiments, radioactive precursor labeling experiments, and in nude mice with an immunocompetent donor graft. In contrast to other classical antigen-presenting cells, which can only activate memory T cells, LC can activate memory and resting "virgin" T cells. After reaching the draining lymph node, LC are thought to present antigen to virgin CD4+ T lymphocytes, a hypothesis supported by several studies. First, LC recovered from lymph nodes 24 h after mice are sensitized with a contact agent can transfer reactivity to previously unsensitized hosts,[62] with as few as ten donor LC able to sensitize a recipient. This suggests the potency and possible role in allograft rejection of LC.[63] Second, graft survival can be prolonged by LC depletion of donor allografts.[64] Finally, ACD cannot be induced in skin sites where epidermal LC are not present, either by using a skin locale where LC numbers are usually low (mouse tail), or by using physical agents to deplete LC (tape stripping of the epidermis, or UV-B irradiation of the skin).[65]

Dermal dendritic cells (DC) may also play a role in ACD, since ACD may occur in some experimental systems using higher doses of hapten in the relative absence of epidermal LC. This suggests that dermal dendritic cells (which may be a dermal subset of LC) can complement the APC functions of epidermal LC. These cell types are being investigated.[66]

Hapten-specific sensitization can be transferred to naive hosts after donation of hapten-modified LC-enriched epidermal cell populations but not with hapten-modified LC-depleted epidermal cells.[67] Hapten-modified LC can break tolerance in a peritoneal exudate model and also can sensitize T cells in vitro.[68] These T cells, when expanded and transferred to a naive host, induce hapten-specific sensitization.[69]

The role LC play in the efferent (elicitation) phase of ACD is less clear. As in the afferent phase, they may uptake and process antigen, migrate to the draining lymph node, and present antigen to an expanded population of memory T cells. Following their migration, LC remain in lymph nodes for several days and then disappear.[70] They are not usually observed in efferent lymphatics. One hypothesis proposed for the downregulation of the CHS response suggests that LC may be actively eliminated (either by hapten-specific IgM, by CTL, or by natural killer activity).[71] In fact, damaged hapten-bearing LC have been frequently observed in ACD.[58] Our work presents an alternative, and possibly concomitant, mechanism for ACD downregulation (discussed below).

The phenotypic, morphological, and functional changes which LC undergo in culture appear to recapitulate the process of LC maturation in vivo. Freshly isolated epidermal cell suspensions contain LC which only weakly stimulate T cells. These same fresh LC (fLC), however, efficiently process intact antigen and present it to MHC class II-restricted T cell clones or hybridomas. In contrast, cultured LC (cLC) are potent antigen-presenting cells which possesses an immunostimulatory capacity 10- to 100-fold greater than fresh LC.[72] However, these cLC poorly process native antigen (that requires processing) and are inefficient at presenting it to T cell clones or hybridomas.[73,74] These cLC are potent at presenting immunogenic peptide fragments that do not require processing, whereas fLC are weak in this regard.

These differences between cLC and fLC can be partially explained by a change in phenotype (see Table 2). Cultured LC, but not fLC, upregulate the expression of a number of cell surface markers which include MHC class I and II, CD23, CD49d, ICAM-1, ICAM-3, LFA-3, CD40, B7-1, and B7-2. In contrast, the expression levels of other cell surface markers, including CD1a, CD1c, CD32, CD11b, CD11c, and E-cadherin are decreased on activated, cultured LC. The fLC preferentially present antigen to sensitized T cells, while cLC preferentially present antigen to naive T cells.[75] Therefore, fLC may reflect LC which present antigen to memory/effector T cells in the efferent phase of CHS, and cLC may parallel LC which present antigen to naive unprimed T cells.

TABLE 2
Phenotype of Resting and Activated LC

Cell Surface Antigen	Resting (Fresh LC)	Activated (Cultured LC)
Class I MHC	++	+++
Class II MHC (Ia)	++	+++
CD1a	++	±
CD1c	+	±
CD4	+	?
FcεRI	+	?
CD23 (FcεRII)	-	+
CD32 (FcγR type II)	+	±
CD11a (LFA-1)	-	-
CD11b (C3bi R)	+	-
CD11c (gp 150/95)	+	-
CD49d (VLA-4)	±	+++
CD54 (ICAM-1)	+ or -	++
ICAM-3	++	+++
CD58 (LFA-3)	+	++
CD40	±	+
E-Cadherin	+	±
B7-1 (CD80)	±	+++
B7-2 (CD86)	±	+++

Note: (−) indicates no expression;

      (±) indicates weak or heterogeneous expression;

      (+ to +++) indicates increasing expression.

Data abstracted from Table References 1–13.

References

1. Gaspari, A. A., Advances in the understanding of contact hypersensitivity, *Am. J. Contact Dermatol.*, 4, 138, 1993.

2. Bos, J. D., Zonneveld, I., Das, P., Grief, S. R., Van der Loos, C. M., Kapsenberg, M. L., The skin immune system (SIS): distribution and immunophenotype of lymphocyte subpopulations in normal human skin, *J. Invest. Dermatol.*, 88, 569, 1987.

3. Bos, J. D., Kapsenberg, M. L., The skin immune sistem (SIS): its cellular constituents and their interactions, *Immunol. Today*, 7, 235, 1986.

4. Teunissen, M. B. M., Dynamic nature and function of epidermal Langerhans cells in vivo and in vitro: a review, with emphasis on human Langerhans cells, *Histochem. J.*, 24, 697, 1992.

5. Gaspari, A. A., Furue, M., Aiba. S., Katz, S. I., Human epidermal Langerhans cells, when cultured, exhibit increased class II MHC expression and become potent immunostimulatory cells, *J. Invest. Dermatol.*, 92, 433, 1989.

TABLE 2 (CONTINUED)
Phenotype of Resting and Activated LC

6. Vedel, J., Vincendeau, P., Bezian, J. H., Taieb, A., Flow cytometry analysis of adhesion molecules on human Langerhans cells, *Clin. Exp. Dermatol.*, 17, 240, 1992.

7. Dezutter-Dambuyant, C., Schmitt, D. A., Dusserre, N., Hanau, D., Kolbe, H. V. J., Kieny, M. P., Gazzolo, L., Mace, K., Pasquali, J. L., Olivier, R., Schmitt, D., Trypsin-resistant gp120 receptors are upregulated on short-term cultured human epidermal Langerhans cells, *Res. Virol.*, 142, 129, 1991.

8. Bieber, T., De la Salle, H., Wollenberg, A., Hakimi, J., Chizzonite, R., Ring, J., Hanau, D., De la Salle, C., Human epidermal Langerhans cells express the high affinity receptor for immunoglobulin E (FcεRI), *J. Exp. Med.*, 175, 1285, 1992.

9. Wang, B., Rieger, A., Kilgus, O., Ochiai, K., Maurer, D., Fodinger, D., Kinet, J., Stingl, G., Epidermal Langerhans cells from normal human skin bind monomeric IgE via FcεRI, *J. Exp. Med.*, 175, 1353, 1992.

10. Bieber, T., Rieger, A., Neuchrist, C., Prinz, J. C., Rieber, E. P., Bolz-Nitulescu, G., Scheiner, O., Kraft, D., Ring, J., Stingl, G., Induction of FcεRII/CD23 on human epidermal Langerhans cells by human recombinant interleukin 4 and γ interferon, *J. Exp. Med.*, 170, 309, 1989.

11. Aiba, S., Nakagawa, S., Ozawa, H., Miyake, K., Yagita, H., Tagami, H., Up-regulation of α4 integrin on activated Langerhans cells: analysis of adhesion molecules on Langerhans cells relating to their migration from skin to draining lymph nodes, *J. Invest. Dermatol.*, 100, 143, 1993.

12. Acevedo, A., Del Pozo, M. A., Arroyo, A. G., Sanchez-Mateos, P., Gonzalez-Amaro, R., Sanchez-Madrid, F., Distribution of ICAM-3-bearing cells in normal human tissues; expression of a novel counter-receptor for LFA-1 in epidermal Langerhans cells, *Am. J. Pathol.*, 143, 774, 1993.

13. Tang, A., Amagai, M., Granger, G., Stanley, J. R., Udey, M. C., Adhesion of epidermal Langerhans cells to keratinocytes mediated by E-cadherin, *Nature*, 361, 82, 1993.

LC cultured in the absence of KC do not undergo any of these changes, but instead die.[76] When LC are cultured with a KC-conditioned supernatant, they survive and undergo the phenotypic, morphological, and functional changes described above, suggesting a role for soluble factors.[77] Further studies identified several soluble keratinocyte-derived cytokines which were responsible for LC survival and maturation. These cytokines included TNF-α (tumor necrosis factor alpha, originally described as a serum factor causing hemorrhagic necrosis of certain tumors; it is toxic to tumor cells in vitro, mediates shock, cachexia, and fever), which facilitated LC survival alone; and GM-CSF (granulocyte macrophage colony-stimulating factor) and IL-1 (interleukin one), which were conducive to both survival and maturation.[39–41] This response of LC to KC-derived cytokines suggests an intimate relationship between KC and LC. Several possibilities can explain the role of this interaction in an allergic response. Contact allergens, which may be irritating or noxious in nature, may cause epidermal keratinocyte injury and result in the release of cytokines.[78] These cytokines may induce LC activation and maturation in either the afferent or efferent phase of a ACD response. Alternatively, direct damage to LC may also lead to LC derived IL-1 release and autocrine or paracrine (LC to LC) LC activation. These findings suggest the importance of KC in ACD.

C. ROLE OF T CELLS IN ACD

Cellular components of the epidermal immune system include LC, KC, and in mice (but not humans) Thy 1+ dendritic epidermal T cells. Epidermotropic lymphocytes were originally identified in studies of cutaneous T cell lymphomas and leukemias. Characterization of the infiltrating cells revealed that CD4[+] T cells made up the majority.[79] Several lines of evidence suggest that these lymphocytes both migrate to the skin in inflammatory states, and normally reside in the skin in small numbers. That such T cells have cutaneous homing capacity was demonstrated in expanded populations of immunized T lymphocytes isolated from lymph nodes draining sensitized skin; the T cells preferentially migrated to the skin.[80] Studies of normal human skin revealed that 98% of identifiable T cells are located in the dermis, largely around postcapillary venules. These T cells are equally divided into CD4[+] and CD8[+] classes. Only 2% of skin T cells were identified in human epidermis; most are CD8[+].[81] It was thus believed that resident T lymphocytes gave rise to infiltrating T cell leukemias and lymphomas.

D. ROLE OF KC IN ACD

Several studies on KC suggested that they function in skin biology simply as an inert barrier providing structural integrity. Any damage to this barrier would result in a nonspecific inflammatory response to generalized tissue damage. Mediators such as free radicals, complement, and arachidonic acid metabolites would be released and cause damage to nearby KC, followed by a wound-healing response.[82] KC were first recognized as being important in the modulation of the immune response in skin in 1981, when it was observed that KC produce epidermal cell thymocyte-activating factor (ETAF),[83,84] later shown to be IL-1α and IL-1β. Since then, KC have been shown to produce a wide variety of different cytokines that have diverse biological effects on epidermotrophic lymphocytes that mediate immune responses in the skin (Table 3). These KC-produced cytokines have the potential to initiate, amplify, and even terminate lymphocyte-mediated inflammation in the skin. While a variety of epidermal cell types, such as LC and melanocytes, can be induced to secrete soluble cytokines, KC are overwhelmingly the predominant cell type in the epidermis, and hence likely to represent a major source of epidermal cytokines.

In addition, KC can participate in cell-mediated immunity by the constitutive expression or upregulation of expression of several important immune accessory molecules.[85–89] The expression of these adherence molecules by KC enhances the migration of epidermotrophic lymphocytes into the epidermis and facilitates KC–lymphocyte interactions in T cell-mediated immunity. Finally, KC can also be induced to express class II MHC in cutaneous graft vs. host disease and ACD.[90–92] All of these findings suggest that KC can function as immunocompetent cells, and may serve as "signal transducers," converting external stimuli into forms recognizable by the host immune system.[78]

1. KC-Derived Cytokines

Some KC-derived cytokines are produced constitutively and their levels can be modified by either cell injury or death. The cytokines produced by KC tend to have pleiotropic effects on a wide variety of cell types, both lymphoid and nonlymphoid, and are thus capable of influencing several limbs of an ACD response. KC also express cytokine receptors on their surface, allowing them to respond to their own cytokines in autocrine fashion, or to soluble factors in their microenvironment. One example is IL-1 receptor, which is normally expressed at low levels, but following IL-1 receptor activation, KC are stimulated to produce IL-6 and GM-CSF.[93] Alternatively, KC cytokines can modulate nearby cell types, causing them to express their own pattern of cytokines, which may, in turn, have an effect on KC in secondary or tertiary interactions. For example, TGF-β, a product of KC, has been shown to alter the influence of other cytokines on LC functional activation.[94] Thus, an intricate cytokine-based signaling network in the epidermis can form the basis of a cascading inflammatory response, such as that found in ACD.

The majority of KC-derived cytokines important in ACD are proinflammatory molecules which stimulate proliferation or differentiation of various cell types including T cells and LC, act as chemoattractants for certain cells, and can amplify those cellular responses which stimulate and

TABLE 3
Cytokine Production By Human and Murine Keratinocytes

Cytokine		Human [Ref.]	Murine [Ref.]	Relevance to ACD
Interleukin-1	IL-1α	+[1]	+[2, 3]	Amplifies T cell responses, activates LC,
	IL-1β	+[1]	+[2, 3]	proinflammatory molecules
Interleukin-6	IL-6	+[4, 5]	?	Actions similar to IL-1 except that it may not activate LC
Interleukin-7	IL-7	+[6]	+[7]	Stimulates T cell proliferation
Interleukin-8	IL-8	+[8]	?	Potent neutrophil chemotactic and activating factor, proinflammatory molecule
Interleukin-10	IL-10	–[9]	+[10]	Suppressive cytokine that may downregulate DTH by decreasing APC function and inhibiting Th1 proliferation
Interleukin-12	IL-12	+[11–13]	?	KC constitutively express α chain of α/β heterodimer; upregulation of biologically active IL-12 by KC can enhance Th1 responses, thereby amplifying DTH
Interleukin-15	IL-15	+[14, 15]	?	Enhances proliferation of stimulated T cells, Th1 responses and killer cells; chemoattractant for T cells
Interleukin-18	IL-18	+[16]	+[17]	IFN-γ-inducing factor which stimulates proliferation and differentiation of Th1 cells
Colony stimulating factors	IL-3	–[18]	+[19, 20]	All cytokines stimulate hematopoiesis in a lineage specific manner; IL-3 acts on mast cells, which play a role in the early phases of CHS; GM-CSF activates LC; the specific role of G-, M-CSF in CHS is less well defined
	G-CSF	+[21]	?	
	M-CSF	+[22]	+[22]	
	GM-CSF	+[23]	+[24, 25]	
Interferons	IFN-α	+[26]	?	Increase in MHC expression,
	IFN-β	+[26]	?	antiproliferation effect, enhances CTL
	IFN-γ	+[27]	?	activity
Tumor necrosis factor	TNF-α	+[28]	+[29]	Induces the expression of adherence molecules by KC; promotes survival of LC but may inhibit migration
Transforming growth factor	TGF-α	+[30, 31]	?	Inhibits T cell proliferation
	TGF-β	?	+[32]	

References

1. Kupper, T. S., Ballard, D. W., Chua, A. O., McGuire, J. S., Flood, P. M., Horowitz, M. C., Langdon, R., Lightfoot, L., Gubler, U., Human keratinocytes contain mRNA indistinquishable from monocyte interleukin 1α and β mRNA, *J. Exp. Med.*, 164, 2095, 1986.

2. Luger, T. A., Stadler, B. M., Katz, S. I., Oppenheim, J. J., Epidermal cell (keratinocyte)-derived thymocyte-activating factor (ETAF), *J. Immunol.*, 127(4), 1493, 1981.

3. Sauder, D. N., Carter, C. S., Katz, S. I., Oppenheim, J. J., Epidermal cell production of thymocyte activating factor (ETAF), *J. Invest. Dermatol.*, 79, 34, 1982.

4. Kupper, T. S., Min, K., Sehgal, P., Mizutani, H., Birchall, N., Ray, A., May, L., Production of IL-6 by keratinocytes. Implications for epidermal inflammation and immunity, *Ann. N.Y. Acad. Sci.*, 557, 454, 1989.

5. Kirnbauer, R., Kock, A., Schwarz, T., Urbanski, T., Krutmann, J., Borth, W., Damm, D., Shipley, G., Ansel, J. C., Luger, T. A., IFN-β2, B cell differentiation factor 2, or hybridoma growth factor (IL-6) is expressed and released by human epidermal cells and epidermoid carcinoma cell lines, *J. Immunol.*, 142, 1922, 1989.

6. Dalloul, A., Laroche, L., Bagot, M., Mossalayi, D., Fourcade, C., Thacker, D. J., Hogge, D. E., Merle-Beral, H., Debre, P., Schmitt, C., Interleukin-7 is a growth factor for Sezary cells, *J. Clin. Invest.*, 90, 1054, 1992.

continued

TABLE 3 (CONTINUED)
Cytokine Production By Human and Murine Keratinocytes

7. Heufler, C., Young, D., Peschel, G., Schuler, G., Murine keratinocytes express interleukin-7, *J. Invest. Dermatol.*, 94, 534,1990.

8. Larsen, C. G., Anderson, A. O., Oppenheim, J. J., Matsushima, K., Production of interleukin-8 by human dermal fibroblasts and keratinocytes in response to interleukin-1 or tumor necrosis factor, *Immunology*, 68(1), 31, 1989.

9. Teunissen, M. B. M., Koomen, C. W., Jansen, J., De Waal Malefyt, R., Schmitt, E., Van Den Wijngaard, R. M. J. G. J., Das, P. K., Bos, J. D., In contrast to their murine counterparts, normal human keratinocytes and human epidermoid cell lines A431 and HaCaT fail to express IL-10 mRNA and protein, *Clin. Exp. Immunol.*, 107, 213, 1997.

10. (T1) Enk, A. H., Katz, S. I., Identification and induction of keratinocyte-derived IL-10, *J. Immunol.*, 149, 92, 1992.

11. (T1) Muller, G., Saloga, J., Germann, T., Bellinghausen, I., Mohamadzadeh, M., Knop, J., Enk, A. H., Identification and induction of human keratinocyte-derived IL-12, *J. Clin. Invest.*, 94, 1799, 1994.

12. Aragane Y., Riemann, H., Bhardwaj, R. S., Schwarz, A., Sawada, Y., Yamada, H., Luger, T. A., Kubin, M., Trinchieri, G., Schwarz, T., IL-12 is expressed and released by human keratinocytes and epidermoid carcinoma cell lines, *J. Immunol.*, 153, 5366, 1994.

13. Yawalker, N., Limat, A., Brand, C. U., Braathen, L. R., Constitutive expression of both subunits of interleukin-12 in human keratinocytes, *J. Invest. Dermatol.*, 106, 80, 1996.

14. Barbulescu, K., Hemmerlein-Kraus, M., Mohamadzadeh, M., Enk, A., Knop, J., Lohmann, S., Identification of human keratinocyte-derived IL-15, *J. Invest. Dermatol.*, 105(3), 480, 1995.

15. Blauvelt, A., Asada, H., Klaus-Kovtun, V., Altman, D. J., Lucey, D. R., Katz, S. I., Interleukin-15 mRNA is expressed by human keratinocytes, Langerhans cells, and blood-derived dendritic cells and is downregulated by ultraviolet B radiation, *J. Invest. Dermatol.*, 106, 1047, 1996.

16. Naik, S. M., Singh, S., Cannon, G., Stipetic, M., Swerlick, R. A., Caughman, S. W., Human interleukin-18 is differentially expressed by cutaneous cells, *J. Invest. Dermatol.*, 110(4), 502, 1998.

17. Stoll, S., Muller, G., Kurimoto, M., Saloga, J., Tanimoto, T., Yamauchi, H., Okamura, H., Knop, J., Enk, A. H., Production of IL-18 (IFN-γ-inducing factor) messenger RNA and functional protein by murine keratinocytes, *J. Immunol.*, 159, 298, 1997.

18. Kondo, S., Ciarletta, A., Turner, K. J., Sauder, D. N., McKenzie, R. C., Failure to detect interleukin (IL)-3 mRNA or protein in human keratinocytes: antibodies to granulocyte macrophage-colony-stimulating factor or IL-6 (but not IL-3) neutralize "IL-3" bioactivity, *J. Invest. Dermatol.*, 104, 335, 1995.

19. Luger, T. A., Kock, A., Kirnbauer, R., Schwarz, T., Ansel, J. C., Keratinocyte-derived interleukin 3, *Ann. N.Y. Acad. Sci.*, 548, 253, 1989.

20. Kupper, T. S., Horowitz, M., Birchall, N., Mizutani, H., Coleman, D., McGuire, J., Flood, P., Dower, S., Lee, F., Hematopoietic, lymphopoietic, and proinflammatory cytokines produced by human and murine keratinocytes, *Ann. N.Y. Acad. Sci.*, 548, 262, 1989.

21. Denburg, J. A., Sauder, D. N., Granulocyte colony stimulating activity derived from human keratinocytes, *Lymphokine Res.*, 5, 261, 1986.

22. Chodakewitz, J. A., Lacy, J., Coleman, D. L., Macrophage colony stimulating factor production by murine and human keratinocytes: enhancement by bacterial lipopolysaccharides, *J. Immunol.*, 144, 2190, 1990.

23. Kapp, A., Danner, M., Luger, T. A., Hauser, C., Schopf, E., Granulocyte-activating mediators (GRAM) II. generation by human epidermal cells-relation to GM-CSF, *Arch. Dermatol. Res.*, 279, 470, 1987.

24. Kupper, T. S., Lee, F., Coleman, D., Chodakewitz, J., Flood, P., Hprowitz, M., Keratinocyte derived T-cell growth factor (KTGF) is identical to granulocyte macrophage colony stimulating factor (GM-CSF), *J. Invest. Dermatol.*, 91, 185, 1988.

25. Gallo, R. L., Staszewski, R., Sauder, D. N., Knisely, T. L., Granstein, R. D., Regulation of GM-CSF and IL-3 production from the murine keratinocyte cell line PAM 212 following exposure to ultraviolet radiation, *J. Invest. Dermatol.*, 97, 203, 1991.

26. Fujisawa, H., Kondo, S., Wang, B., Shivji, G. M., Sauder, D. N., The expression and modulation of IFN-α and IFN-β in human keratinocytes, *J. Interferon Cytokine Res.*, 17, 721, 1997.

27. Howie, S. E. M., Aldridge, R. D., McVittie, E., Forsey, R. J., Sands, C., Hunter, J. A. A., Epidermal keratinocyte production of interferon-γ imunoreactive protein and mRNA is an early event in allergic contact dermatitis, *J. Invest. Dermatol.*, 106, 1218, 1996.

TABLE 3 (CONTINUED)
Cytokine Production By Human and Murine Keratinocytes

28. Kock, A., Schwarz, T., Kirnbauer, R., Urbanski, A., Perry, P., Ansel, J. C., Luger, T. A., Human keratinocytes are a source for tumor necrosis factor alpha: evidence for synthesis and release upon stimulation with endotoxin or ultraviolet light, *J. Exp. Med.*, 172, 1609, 1990.

29. Piguet, P. F., Grau, G. E., Hauser, C., Vassalli, P., Tumor necrosis factor is a critical mediator in hapten induced irritant and contact hypersensitivity reactions, *J. Exp. Med.*, 173, 673, 1991.

30. Coffey, R. J., Derynck, R., Wilcox J. N., Bringman, T. S., Goustin, A. S., Moses, H. L., Pittelkow, Production and auto-induction of transforming growth factor-α in human keratinocytes, *Nature*, 328, 817, 1987.

31. Gottlieb, A. B., Chang, G. K., Posnett, D. N., Fanelli, B., Tam, J. P., Detection of transforming growth factor alpha in normal, malignant and hyperproliferative human keratinocytes, *J. Exp. Med.*, 167(2), 670, 1988.

32. Akhurst, R. J., Fee, F., Balmain, A., Localized production of TGF-β mRNA in tumor promoter-stimulated mouse epidermis, *Nature*, 331, 363, 1988.

prolong delayed-type hypersensitivity (Table 3). While the cytokines IL-1, GM-CSF, and TNF-α affect a number of cell types in a variety of ways, they are believed to potently affect LC survival and maturation in vitro. KC-derived cytokines are critical in the maturation of LC into potent APC.[22,46,49–51,95] In vivo, TNF-α (either directly applied to epidermis, or derived from KC stimulated with either UV-B or a contact irritant) has been shown to induce LC migration.[77,96] T cells have been shown to express receptors for IL-1, IL-6, and GM-CSF, all produced by KC.[97] Allergens may exert their effects on LC morphology, migration, and potent antigen presentation to unprimed T cells in the afferent phase of CHS or memory T cells in the efferent phase of CHS via their ability to induce KC to produce cytokines. Therefore, a particular set of allergens may induce KC to produce a particular array of cytokines.

Both human and murine KC secrete cytokines with IL-3-like activity which acts primarily on dermal mast cells, causing them to proliferate and degranulate.[91,92,98] Recent studies have shown that murine KC produce IL-3, while human KC do not, and the IL-3-like activity secreted by human KC is due instead to GM-CSF and IL-6.[101–103] Mast cell degranulation occurs early in ACD, and hence KC may initiate or amplify this event.

Both IL-1 and TNF-α upregulate the expression of adherence molecules such as ICAM-1 and ELAM-1. These molecules are believed to be important for the binding of lymphocytes to endothelial vessels at the site of inflammation, an important initial step in the transmigration of lymphocytes from the circulation to the skin. The same cytokines induce KC to express ICAM-1, a ligand for the lymphocyte receptor LFA-1.[104–106] Some KC-derived cytokines can exert endocrine effects on bone marrow precursors, priming the immune system for subsequent challenge with either the same or different antigens.[107]

In addition to producing proinflammatory cytokines, KC produce inhibitory cytokines such as IL-10 (murine KC but not human KC) and TGF.[108,109] IL-10 has been shown in vitro to be a potent cytokine synthesis inhibitory factor. That is, it inhibits Th1-mediated activity by suppressing the production of T cell-derived IFN-γ.[110] IL-10 production is enhanced in an ACD response, and may therefore play a role in the termination of the response.[111] TGF similarly plays an immunosuppressive role and may also be involved in damping a CHS response.[112]

KC can constitutively or inducibly produce a wide array of cytokines which affect different target cells and tissues including other KC, lymphocytes, LC, mast cells, blood vessel endothelium, monocytes, macrophages, granulocytes, and bone marrow precursors. While the evidence for these cytokine networks is piecemeal, a testable theoretical framework can be devised which allows for KC to express combinations of cytokine profiles which are active throughout all phases of ACD, ranging from the initiation and amplification to inhibitory effects over the course of a response.

2. KC-Derived Accessory Molecules

During an inflammatory response, KC can be induced to express unique cell surface markers which can include ICAM-1, CD36, B7-1, and class II MHC. ICAM-1 expression can be induced by IFN-γ, a Th1-derived cytokine. Th1 cells, in turn, express LFA-1 and have been shown to adhere to IFN-γ treated KC. This expression has been shown, both in in vitro studies and on human volunteers sensitized to urushiol, to be temporally related to key events in the ACD response.[95,113] Thus, KC-derived cytokines and ICAM-1 can facilitate T cell migration, diapedesis, and chemotaxis.

KC class II MHC expression is observed in a number of dermatologic conditions where there is a lymphocytic infiltrate.[114] The source of MHC is KC derived, and not passive adsorption from the cell surroundings.[115] In humans, IFN-γ is directly responsible for class II MHC expression.[116] The Th1 cells which produce this cytokine have been shown to play an important role in delayed-type hypersensitivity responses both in humans and in animals. Therefore, as Th1 cells infiltrate a cutaneous site in ACD, they induce, by their cytokine profile, local KC to express class II MHC on their surface.

Normally class II MHC expression is observed in antigen-presenting cells of lymphoid origin. The discovery of ectopic class II MHC expression on nonlymphoid cells such as KC, particularly in the disease state, led investigators to speculate on the role class II MHC (Ia) expressing KC may play in pathological processes. In contrast to classical antigen-presenting cells, such as Ia$^+$ LC, Ia$^+$ KC do not present antigen to Th1.[117] The interaction between Ia$^+$ KC and Th1 is not passive and merely ineffectual. Rather, an active signaling event takes place which renders Th1 incubated with haptenated Ia$^+$ KC nonresponsive. The T cells are paralyzed immunologically, in a state known as immunologic tolerance or clonal anergy. The anergic T cells are viable and respond to growth factors, but do not respond to T cell receptor-mediated stimuli. Thus, these T cells are incapable of producing cytokines or proliferating in response to functional antigen presentation, i.e., from Ia$^+$ LC. This tolerance has been shown to be cell-autonomous and nontransferable.[118] That is, tolerized T cells are unable to suppress activated T cells in their environs.

One can infer, however, that anergic T lymphocytes may be able to compete with Ia$^+$ LC for T cell receptor occupancy on the cell surface of Th and by consuming local cytokines and growth factors. Furthermore, when class II MHC is induced on KC during the course of ACD, small numbers of Ia$^+$ LC must compete with large numbers of Ia$^+$ KC (present in 50- to 100-fold excess) to present antigen to T lymphocytes.[119] Coupled with decreasing numbers of epidermal LC following antigen application (see above), this situation favors tolerogenic antigen presentation in the epidermis.[55]

This model of T cell clonotypic anergy supplants an older hypothesis of antigen clearance. It was formerly believed that removal of antigen from the epidermis would lead to resolution of DTH. Allergens have been shown to persist for years, however, at sites of positive patch tests, in persistent light reactions, and in long-standing dichromate sensitivity.[120–122] Clonal anergy can account for ACD resolution, even in the presence of uncleared antigen, and conversely, abnormalities in the clonal anergy mechanism may lead to dermatologic disease.

V. CONCLUSIONS

The clinical spectrum of contact dermatitis ranges from benign to life-threatening, and its impact on society in terms of morbidity and cost is appreciable. The evolution of the concept of the skin from a passive barrier to a dynamic, immunologically active organ has led to a number of advances in understanding the pathophysiology of contact dermatitis. Contact hypersensitivity is a prototypical T cell-mediated allergic response. The key role of antigen presentation by LC to T cells in regional lymphoid tissues is clear. A number of factors in addition to T cell regulatory circuits and LC have been identified. These include the recognition that KC actively participate in all phases of the hypersensitivity response as immunocompetent cells. They do this by expressing adhesion molecules, liberating proinflammatory and inhibitory cytokines, and presenting antigen in tolerogenic form to downregulate immune responsiveness. Superimposed upon these participants is an array of dermal cell types, bone marrow-derived cells, endothelial cells, and components of the nervous system, each of which respond to and produce their own subsets of signaling molecules.

ICD shares clinical, histologic, immunohistochemical, and molecular features with ACD. Hapten-specific Th lymphocytes are thought to be necessary for ACD, but not ICD. However, it is apparent that some of the same inflammatory immune mechanisms are operating for both ACD and ICD. Thus, these apparently simple clinical entities (ACD and ICD), recognized in the literature for centuries, are actually mediated by a sophisticated network of interdigitating components.

Since ACD and ICD responses appear to be so similar, it is imperative that distinquishing differences between the two processes be identified. Areas which should be studied more thoroughly are the effects of ACD and ICD on the expression of cytokines and immune accessory molecules by both DC and KC. As shown in Table 1 these studies are incomplete. For example, the expression of the accessory molecules CD40 and B7-2 have never been studied in DC and KC for upregulation by treatments with either allergens or irritants. Although B7-2 has not been identified on the surface of normal human KC, no studies have determined if B7-2 can be induced on the surface of KC following treatment with allergen or irritant. In addition, several proinflammatory cytokines, important in ACD, have not been tested for their upregulation by either ACD (IL-7, IL-15, and IL-18) or ICD (IL-4, IL-6, IL-8, IL-15, and IL-18), or have only been tested in a mouse system (IP-10, MIP-2, IL-6, and IL-10). Some accessory molecules (HLA-DR) and cytokines (IL-1α) have been reported to have variable effects during either ACD or ICD, which may be dependent on the particular antigen or irritant used. Most studies so far have utilized only a small number of allergens or irritants. It is essential that more allergens and irritants be used to test for differences in accessory molecule and cytokine expression during ACD and ICD. More complete studies of this kind should provide clues of any functional differences between the important dermatological conditions of ACD and ICD.

REFERENCES

1. Adams, R. M., Contact dermatitis due to irritation and allergic sensitization, in *Occup. Skin Dis.*, Adams, R. M., Ed., W. B. Saunders, Philadelphia, 1983, 1.
2. Mathias, E. G., Occupational dermatoses, *J. Am. Acad. Dermatol.*, 19, 1107, 1988.
3. Menné, T., Bachman, E., Permanent disability from skin diseases, *Dermatosen*, 27, 37, 1979.
4. Mathias, C. G. T., Maibach, H. I., Dermatotoxicology monographs I: cutaneous irritation: factors influencing the response to irritants, *Clin. Toxicol.*, 13, 333, 1978.
5. Lane, H. C., Acquired immunodeficiency syndrome, *Dermatol. Clin.*, 8, 771, 1990.
6. Zunich, K. M., Lane, H. C., The immunology of HIV infection, *J. Am. Acad. Dermatol.*, 22, 1202, 1990.
7. Stingl, G., Rappersberger, K., Tschachler, E., Gartner, S., Groh, V., Mann, D. L., Wolff, K., Popovic, M., Langerhans cells in HIV infection, *J. Am. Acad. Dermatol.*, 22, 1210, 1990.
8. Nassif, A., Chan, S. C., Storrs, J., Hanifin, J. M., Abnormal skin irritancy in atopic dermatitis and in atopy without dermatitis, *Arch. Dermatol.*, 130, 1402, 1994.
9. Hall, A. H., Hogan, D. J., Contact dermatitis and urticaria from environmental exposures, *Am. Fam. Phys.*, 48, 773, 1993.
10. Suskind, R. R., Environment and the skin, *Med. Clin. N. Am.*, 74, 307, 1990.
11. Fisher, A. A., *Contact Dermatitis*, Lea & Febiger, Philadelphia, 1986, 892.
12. Dannaker, C., Maibach, H. I., Poison ivy and poison oak dermatitis, in *Plants and the Skin*, Lovell, C. R., Ed., Blackwell, Boston, 1993, 105.
13. Storrs, F. J., Permanent wave contact dermatitis: contact allergy to glycerol monothioglycolate, *J. Am. Acad. Dermatol.*, 11, 74, 1984.
14. Phototesting and photopatch testing, Appendix III, in *Photosensitivity Diseases*, Harbers, L. C., Bickers, D. R., Eds., W. B. Saunders, Philadelphia, 1981, 322.

15. Drug induced photosensitivity (phototoxic and photoallergic drug reactions), in *Photosensitivity Diseases, Principles of Diagnosis and Treatment*, Harber, L. C., Bickers, D. R., Eds., B. C. Decker, Philadelphia, 1989, 160.

16. Epstein, J. H., Photocontact allergy in humans, in *Dermatotoxicology*, Marzulli, F., Maibach, H. I., Eds., Hemisphere, Washington, D.C., 1983, 391.

17. Von Krogh, G., Maibach, H. I., The contact urticaria syndrome and associated disease entities, in *Dermatology*, Moshella, S. L., Hurley, J. H., Eds., W. B. Saunders, Philadelphia, 1985, 323.

18. Lever, W. F., Schaumberg-Lever, G., Noninfectious vesicular and bullous diseases, in *Histopathology of the Skin*, Lever, W. F., Schaumberg-Lever, G., Eds., J. B. Lippincott, Philadelphia, 1990, 92.

19. Hauxthausen, H., Generalized 'ids' (autosensitization) in varicose eczema, *Acta Derm. Venereol.*, 35, 271, 1955.

20. Willis, C. M., Stephens, C. J. M., Wilkinson, J. D., Selective expression of immune-associated surface antigens by keratinocytes in irritant contact dermatitis, *J. Invest. Dermatol.*, 96, 505, 1991.

21. Gawkrodger, D. J., Carr, M. M., McVittie, E., Guy, K., Hunter, J. A. A., Keratinocyte expression of MHC class II antigens in allergic sensitization and challenge reactions and in irritant contact dermatitis, *J. Invest. Dermatol.*, 88, 11, 1987.

22. Gaspari, A. A., Advances in the understanding of contact hypersensitivity, *Am. J. Contact Dermatol.*, 4, 138, 1993.

23. Langerhans, P., Über die Nerven der menschlichen Haut, *Virchows Arch. Pathol. Anat.*, 44, 325, 1868.

24. Breathnach, A. S., A new concept of the relation between the Langerhans cell and the melanocyte, *J. Invest. Dermatol.*, 40, 279, 1963.

25. Potten, C. S., Allen, T. D., A model implicating the Langerhans cell in keratinocyte proliferation control, *Differentiation*, 5, 43, 1976.

26. Silberberg, I., Apposition of mononuclear cells to Langerhans cells in contact allergic reactions, An ultrastructural study, *Acta Derm. Venereol. (Stockh.)*, 53, 1, 1973.

27. Silberberg-Sinakin, I., Bear, R. L., Thorbecke, G. J., Langerhans cells. A review of their nature with emphasis on their immunologic functions, *Progr. Allergy*, 24, 268, 1978.

28. Silberberg-Sinakin, I., Thorbecke, G. J., Bear, R. L., Rosenthal, S. A., Berezowsky, V., Antigen-bearing Langerhans cells in skin, dermal lymphatics and in lymph nodes, *Cell Imunol.*, 25, 137, 1976.

29. Silberberg-Sinakin, I., Gigli, I., Bear, R. L., Thorbecke, G. J., Langerhans cell: role in contact hypersensitivity and relationship to lymphoid dendritic cells and to macrophages, *Immunol. Rev.*, 53, 203, 1980.

30. Birbeck, M. S., Breathnach, A. S., Everall, J. D., An electron microscope study of basal melanocytes and high-level clear cells (Langerhans cells) in vitiligo, *J. Invest. Dermatol.*, 37, 51, 1961.

31. Sagebiel, R. W., Reed, T. H., Serial reconstruction of the characteristic granule of the Langerhans cell, *J. Cell. Biol.*, 36, 595, 1968.

32. Takigawa, M., Iwatsuki, K., Yamada, M., Okamoto, H., Imamura, S., The Langerhans cell granule is an adsorptive endocytic organelle, *J. Invest. Dermatol.*, 85, 12, 1985.

33. Wolff, K., The Langerhans cell, *Cur. Probl. Dermatol.*, 4, 79, 1972.

34. Kashihara, M., Ueda, M., Horiguchi, Y., Furukawa, F., Hanaoka, M., Imamura, S., A monoclonal antibody specific to human Langerhans cells, *J. Invest. Dermatol.*, 87, 602, 1986.

35. Gielen, V., Schmitt, D., Thivolet, J., HLA class I antigen (heavy and light chain) expression by Langerhans cells and keratinocytes of the normal human epidermis: ultrastructural quantitation using immunogold labelling procedure, *Arch. Dermatol. Res.*, 280, 131, 1988.

36. Klareskog, L., Malmnas-Tjernlund, U., Forsum, U., Peterson, P. A., Epidermal Langerhans cells express Ia antigens, *Nature*, 268, 248, 1977.

37. Jones, P. P., Murphy, D. B., Hewgill, D., McDevitt, H. O., Detection of a common polypeptide chain in I-A and I-E sub-region immunoprecipitates, *Mol. Immunol.*, 16, 51, 1978.

38. Matis, L. A., Glimcher, L. H., Paul, W. E., Schwartz, R. H., Magnitude of resonse of histocompatibility-restricted T-cell clones is a function of the product of the concetrations of antigen and Ia molecules, *Proc. Natl. Acad. Sci., U.S.A.*, 80(19), 6019, 1983.

39. Witmer-Pack, M. D., Olivier, W., Valinsky, J., Schuler, G., Steinman, R. M., Granulocyte/macrophage colony-stimulating factor is essential for the viability and function of cultured murine epidermal Langerhans cells, *J. Exp. Med.*, 166, 1484, 1987.

40. Heufler, C., Koch, F., Schuler, G., GM-CSF and IL-1 mediate the maturation of murine epidermal Langerhans cells into potent immunostimulatory dendritic cells, *J. Exp. Med.*, 167, 700, 1988.

41. Koch, F., Heufler, C., Kampgen, E., Schneeweiss, D., Bock, G., Schuler, G., Tumor necrosis factor alpha maintains the viability of murine epidermal Langerhans cells in culture but in contrast to GM-CSF does not induce functional maturation, *J. Exp. Med.*, 171, 159, 1990.

42. Schmitt, D., Dezutter-Dambuyant, C., Brochier, J., Thivolet, J., Subclustering of CD1 monoclonal antibodies based on the reactivity on human Langerhans cells, *Immunol. Lett.*, 12, 231, 1986.

43. Groh, V., Tani, M., Harrer, A., Wolff, K., Stingl, G., Leu3/T4 expression on epidermal Langerhans cells in normal and diseased skin, *J. Invest. Dermatol.*, 86, 115, 1986.

44. Braathen, L. R., Ramirez, G., Kunze, R. O. F., Gelderblom, H., Langerhans cells as primary target cells for HIV infection, *Lancet*, 2, 1094, 1987.

45. Tschachler, E., Groh, V., Popovic, M., Mann, D. L., Konrad, K., Safai, B., Eron, L., Dimarzo Veronese, F., Wolff, K., Stingl, G., Epidermal Langerhans cells—a target for HTLV-III/LAV infection, *J. Invest. Dermatol.*, 88, 233, 1987.

46. Teunissen, M. B. M., Wormmeester, J., Krieg, S. R., Peters, P. J., Bogels, I. M. C., Kapsenberg, M. L., Bos, J. D., Human epidermal Langerhans cells undergo profound morphological and phenotypical changes during in vitro culture, *J. Invest. Dermatol.*, 94, 166, 1990.

47. Katz, S. I., Tamaki, K., Sachs, D. H., Epidermal Langerhans cells are derived from cells originating in bone marrow, *Nature*, 282, 324, 1979.

48. Perrault, C., Pelletier, M., Landry, D., Gyger, M., Study of Langerhans cells after allogenic bone marrow transplantation, *Blood*, 63, 807, 1984.

49. De Fraissinette, A., Schmitt, D., Dezutter-Dambuyant, C., Guyotat, D., Zabot, M. T., Thivolet, J., Culture of putative Langerhans cell bone marrow precursors: characterization of their phenotype, *Exp. Hematol.*, 16, 764, 1988.

50. Gothelf, Y., Sharon, N., Gazit, E., A subset of human cord blood mononuclear cells is similar to Langerhans cells of the skin: a study with peanut agglutinin and monoclonal antibodies, *Hum. Immunol.*, 15, 164, 1986.

51. MacKenzie, I. C., Labelling of murine epidermal Langerhans cells with 3H-thymidine, *Am. J. Anat.*, 144, 127, 1975.

52. Czernielewski, J., Vaigot, P., Prunieras, M., Epidermal Langerhans cells—a cycling cell population, *J. Invest. Dermatol.*, 84, 424, 1985.

53. Miyuachi, S., Hashimoto, K., Mitotic activities of normal epidermal Langerhans cells, *J. Invest. Dermatol.*, 92, 120, 1989.

54. Bos, J. D., Kapsenberg, M. L., The skin immune sistem (SIS): its cellular constituents and their interactions, *Immunol. Today*, 7, 235, 1986.

55. Teunissen, M. B. M., Dynamic nature and function of epidermal Langerhans cells in vivo and in vitro: a review, with emphasis on human Langerhans cells, *Histochem. J.*, 24, 697, 1992.

56. Hanau, D., Babre, M., Schmitt, D. A., Pepoittevin, J . P., Stamph, J. L,. Grosshans, E., Benezra, C., Cazenave, J. P., ATPase and morphologic changes in Langerhans cells induced by epicutaneous application of a sensitizing dose of DNFB, *J. Invest. Dermatol.*, 92, 689, 1989.

57. Kolde, G., Knop, J., Different cellular reaction patterns of epidermal Langerhans cells after application of contact sensitizing, toxic and tolerogenic compounds. A comparative ultrastructural and morphometric time-course analysis, *J. Invest. Dermatol.*, 89, 19, 1987.

58. Picut, C. A., Lee, C. S., Lewis, R. M., Ultrastructural and phenotypic changes in Langerhans cells induced in vitro by contact allergens, *Br. J. Dermatol.*, 116, 773, 1987.

59. Halliday, G. M., Muller, H. K., Langerhans cell presentation of sheep red blood cells induces antibody production, *Immunol. Cell Biol.*, 65, 71, 1987.

60. Kapsenberg, M. L., Van der Pouw-Kraan, T., Stiekema, F. E., Schootemeijer, A., Bos, J. D., Direct and indirect nickel-specific stimulation of T lymphocytes from patients with allergic contact dermatitis to nickel, *Eur. J. Immunol.*, 18, 977, 1988.

61. Weinlich, G., Sepp, N., Koch, F., Schuler, G., Romani, N., Evidence that Langerhans cells rapidly disappear from the epidermis in response to contact sensitizers but not to tolerogens/nonsensitizers, *Arch. Dermatol. Res.*, 281, 556, 1989.

62. Hauser, C., Cultured epidermal Langerhans cells activate effector T cells for contact sensitivity, *J. Invest. Dermatol.*, 95, 436, 1990.

63. Rico, M. J., Streilein, J. W., Comparison of alloimmunogenicity of Langerhans cells and keratinocytes from mouse epidermis, *J. Invest. Dermatol.*, 89, 607, 1987.

64. Thivolet, J., Faure, M., Demidem, A., Mauduit, G., Long-term survival and immunological tolerance of human epidermal allografts produced in culture, *Transplantation*, 42, 274, 1986.

65. Rheins, L. A., Nordlund, J. J., Modulation of the population density of identifiable epidermal Langerhans cells associated with enhancement or suppression of cutaneous immune reactivity, *J. Immunol.*, 136, 867, 1986.

66. Tse, Y., Cooper, K. D., Cutaneous dermal Ia⁺ cells are capable of initiating delayed-type hypersensitivity responses, *J. Invest. Dermatol.*, 94, 267, 1990.

67. Tamaki, K., Fujiwara, H., Katz, S. I., The role of epidermal Langerhans cells in the induction and suppression of contact sensitivity, *J. Invest. Dermatol.*, 76, 275, 1981.

68. Ptak, W., Rozyka, D., Askenase, P. W., Gershon, R. K., Role of antigen-presenting cells in the development and persistence of contact hypersensitivity, *J. Exp. Med.*, 151, 362, 1980.

69. McKinney, E. C., Streilein, J. W., On the extraordinary capacity of allogeneic epidermal Langerhans cells to prime cytotoxic T cells in vivo, *J. Immunol.*, 143, 1560, 1989.

70. Macatonia, S. E., Knight, S. C., Edwards, A. J., Griffiths, S., Fryer, P., Localization of antigen on lymph node dendritic cells after exposure to the contact sensitizer fluorescein isothiocyanate. Functional and morphological studies, *J. Exp. Med.*, 166, 1654, 1987.

71. Asherson, G. L., Colizzi, V., Watkins, M. C., Immunogenic cells in the regional lymph nodes after painting with contact sensitizers picryl chloride and oxazolone: evidence for the presence of IgM antibody on their surface, *Immunology*, 48, 561, 1983.

72. Streilein, J. W., Grammer, S. F., In vitro evidence that Langerhans cells can adopt two functionally distinct forms capable of antigen presentation to T lymphocytes, *J. Immunol.*, 143, 3925, 1989.

73. Aiba, S., Katz, S. I., The ability of cultured Langerhans cells to process and present antigens is MHC-dependent, *J. Immunol.*, 146, 2479, 1991.

74. Gaspari, A. A., Furue, M., Aiba, S., Katz, S. I., Human epidermal Langerhans cells, when cultured, exhibit increased class II MHC expression and become potent immunostimulatory cells, *J. Invest. Dermatol.*, 92, 433, 1989.

75. Dai, R., Grammer, S. F., Streilein, J. W., Fresh and cultured Langerhans cells display differential capacities to activate hapten-specific T cells, *J. Immunol.*, 150, 59, 1993.

76. Vedel, J., Vincendeau, P., Bezian, J. H., Taieb, A., Flow cytometry analysis of adhesion molecules on human Langerhans cells, *Clin. Exp. Dermatol.*, 17, 240, 1992.

77. Fritsch, P., Diem, E., Honigsmann, H., Langerhans cells in cell culture. Survival and identification, *Arch. Derm. Forsch.*, 248, 123, 1973.

78. Barker, J. N. W. N., Mitra, R. S., Griffiths, C. E. M., Dixit, V. M., Nickoloff, B. J., Keratinocytes as initiators of inflammation, *Lancet*, 337, 211, 1991.

79. Edelson, R. L., Cutaneous T cell lymphomas: clues to a skin-thymus interaction, *J. Invest. Dermatol.*, 67, 419, 1976.

80. McWilliams, M., Philips-Guagliata, J. M., Lamm, M. E., Characteristics of mesenteric lymph node cells homing to gut associated lymphoid tissue in syngeneic mice, *J. Immunol.*, 115, 54, 1975.

81. Bos, J. D., Zonneveld, I., Das, P., Grief, S. R., Van der Loos, C. M., Kapsenberg, M. L., The skin immune system (SIS): distribution and immunophenotype of lymphocyte subpopulations in normal human skin, *J. Invest. Dermatol.*, 88, 569, 1987.

82. Nickoloff, B. J., Pathophysiology of cutaneous inflammation, *Arch. Dermatol. Res.*, 284, S10, 1992.

83. Luger, T. A., Stadler, B. M., Katz, S. I., Oppenheim, J. J., Epidermal cell (keratinocyte)-derived thymocyte-activating factor (ETAF), *J. Immunol.*, 127(4), 1493, 1981.

84. Sauder, D. N., Carter, C. S., Katz, S. I., Oppenheim, J. J., Epidermal cell production of thymocyte activating factor (ETAF), *J. Invest. Dermatol.*, 79, 34, 1982.

85. Spinola, S. M., Wild, L. M., Apicella, M. A., Gaspari, A. A., Campagnari, A. A., Experimental human infection with Haemophilus ducreyi, *J. Infect. Dis.*, 169, 1146, 1994.

86. Tamaki, K., Saitoh, A., Gaspari, A. A., Yasaka, N., Furue, M., Migration of Thy-1+ dendritic epidermal cells (Thy-1+DEC); Ly-48 and TNF-α are responsible for the migration of the Thy-1+DEC to the epidermis, *J. Invest. Dermatol.*, 103, 290, 1994.

87. Nasir, A., Ferbel, B., Salminen, W., Barth, R. K., Gaspari, A. A., Exaggerated and persistent cutaneous-delayed type hypersensitivity in transgenic mice whose epidermal keratinocytes constitutively express B7-1 antigen, *J. Clin. Invest.*, 94, 892, 1994.

88. Gaspari, A. A., Epidermal Langerhans cells: potent stimulators of epidermal immunity, *Dendritic Cells*, 4, 1, 1994.

89. Slater, C. A., Sickel, J. Z., Visvesvara, G. S., Pabico, R. C., Gaspari, A. A., Successful treatment of disseminated acanthamoeba infection in an immunocompromised renal transplant patient, *N. Engl. J. Med.*, 331, 85, 1994.

90. Luger, T. A., Stadler, B. M., Katz, S. I., Epidermal cell derived thymocyte activating factor, *J. Immunol.*, 127, 1493, 1981.

91. Kupper, T. S., Ballard, D. W., Chua, A. O., McGuire, J. S., Flood, P., Horowitz, M. C., Langdon, R., Lightfoot, L., Gubler, U., Human keratinocytes contain mRNA indistinguishable from monocyte interleukin 1 alpha and beta mRNA. Keratinocyte epidermal cell derived thymocyte activating factor is identical to interleukin 1, *J. Exp. Med.*, 164, 2095, 1986.

92. Lampert, I. A., Suitters, A. J., Chisholm, P. M., Expression of Ia antigen on epidermal keratinocytes in graft-versus-host disease, *Nature*, 293, 149, 1981.

93. Kupper, T. S., Lee, F., Birchall, N., Clark, S., Dower, S., Interleukin 1 binds to specific high affinity receptors on human keratinocytes and induces granulocyte macrophage colony stimulating factor mRNA and protein: a potential autocrine role for IL-1 in epidermis, *J. Clin. Invest.*, 82, 1787, 1988.

94. Epstein, S. P., Baer, R. L., Thorbecke, G. J., Belsito, D. V., Immunosuppressive effects of transforming growth factor beta: inhibition of the induction of Ia antigen on Langerhans cells by cytokines and of the contact hypersensitivity response, *J. Invest. Dermatol.*, 96, 832, 1991.

95. Barker, J.N.W.N., Role of keratinocytes in allergic contact dermatitis, *Contact Dermatol.*, 26, 145, 1992.

96. Enk, A. H., Katz, S. I., Early molecular events in the induction phase of contact sensitivity, *Proc. Natl. Acad. Sci. U.S.A.*, 89, 1398, 1992.

97. Zola, H., Flego, L., Expression of interleukin-6 receptor on blood lymphocytes without in vitro activation, *Immunology*, 76, 338, 1992.

98. Cumberbatch, M., Kimber, I., Dermal tumour necrosis factor alpha induces dendritic cell migration to draining lymph nodes, and possibly provides one stimulus for Langerhans cell migration, *Immunology*, 75, 257, 1992.

99. Danner, M., Luger, T. A., Human keratinocytes and epidermoid carcinoma cell lines produce a cytokine with interleukin 3-like activity, *J. Invest. Dermatol.*, 88, 353, 1987.

100. Luger, T. A., Wirth, U., Kock, A., Epidermal cells synthesize a cytokine with interleukin 3-like properties, *J. Immunol.*, 134, 915, 1986.

101. Heufler, C., Young, D., Peschel, G., Schuler, G., Murine keratinocytes express interleukin-7, *J. Invest. Dermatol.*, 94, 534,1990.

102. Larsen, C. G., Anderson, A. O., Oppenheim, J. J., Matsushima, K., Production of interleukin-8 by human dermal fibroblasts and keratinocytes in response to interleukin-1 or tumor necrosis factor, *Immunology*, 68(1), 31, 1989.

103. Teunissen, M. B. M., Koomen, C. W., Jansen, J., De Waal Malefyt, R., Schmitt, E., Van Den Wijngaard, R. M. J. G. J., Das, P. K., Bos, J. D., In contrast to their murine counterparts, normal human keratinocytes and human epidermoid cell lines A431 and HaCaT fail to express IL-10 mRNA and protein, *Clin. Exp. Immunol.*, 107, 213, 1997.

104. Pober, J. S., Gimbrone, M. A., Lapierre, L. A., Mendrick, D. L., Fiers, W., Rothlein, R., Springer, T. A., Overlapping patterns of activation of human endothelial cells by interleukin 1, tumor necrosis factor and immune interferon, *J. Immunol.*, 137, 1893, 1986.

105. Dustin, M. L., Singer, K. H., Tuck, D. T., Springer, T. A., Adhesion of T lymphoblasts to epidermal keratinocytes is regulated by interferon-gamma and is mediated by intercellular adhesion molecule 1 (ICAM-1), *J. Exp. Med.*, 167, 1323, 1988.

106. Veijlsgaard, G., Ralfkiaer, E., Avnstorp, C., Czajkowski, M., Marlin, S. D., Rothlein, R., Kinetics and characterisation of intercellular adhesion molecule-1 (ICAM-1) expression on keratinocytes in various inflammatory skin lesions and malignant cutaneous lymphomas, *J. Am. Acad. Dermatol.*, 20, 782, 1989.

107. Kupper, T. S., Lee, F., Coleman, D., Chodakewitz, Z. J., Flood, P., Horowitz, M., Keratinocyte derived T-cell growth factor (KTGF) is identical to granulocyte macrophage colony stimulating factor (GM-CSF). *J. Invest. Dermatol.*, 91, 185, 1988.

108. Enk, A. H., Katz, S. I., Identification and induction of keratinocyte-derived IL-10, *J. Immunol.*, 149, 92, 1992.

109. Epstein, S. P., Baer, R. L., Thorbecke, G. J., Belsito, D. V., Immunosuppressive effects of transforming growth factor beta: inhibition of the induction of Ia antigen on Langerhans cells by cytokines and of the contact hypersensitivity response, *J. Invest. Dermatol.*, 96, 832, 1991.

110. Fiorentino, D. F., Bond, M. W., Mosmann, T. R., Two types of mouse helper T cells. IV. Th2 clones secrete a factor that inhibits cytokine production by Th1 clones, *J. Exp. Med.*, 170, 2081, 1989.

111. Grewe, M., Gyufko, K., Schopf, E., Krutmann, J., Lesional expresion of interferon-gamma in atopic eczema, *Lancet*, 343, 25, 1994.

112. Wrann, M., Bodmer, S., De Martin, R., Siepl, C., Hofer-Warbinek, R., Frei, K., Hofer, E., Fontana, A., T cell supressor factor from human glioblastoma cells is a 12.5 kD protein closely related to transforming growth factor-beta, *EMBO J.*, 6, 1633, 1987.

113. Griffiths, C. E. M., Barker, J. N. W. N., Kunkel, S., Nickoloff, B. J., Modulation of leucocyte adhesion molecules, a T-cell chemotaxin (IL-8) and a regulatory cytokine (TNF-alpha) in allergic contact dermatitis (rhus dermatitis), *Br. J. Dermatol.*, 124, 519, 1991.

114. Aubock, J., Romani, N., Grubauer, G., Fritsch, P., HLA-DR expression on keratinocytes is a common feature of diseased skin, *Br. J. Dermatol.*, 121, 465, 1986.

115. Breathnach, S. M., Katz, S. I., Keratinocytes synthesize Ia antigen in acute cutaneous graft vs host disease, *J. Immunol.*, 131, 2741, 1983.

116. Basham, T. Y., Nickoloff, B. J., Merigan, T. C., Morhenn, V. B., Recombinant gamma interferon induces HLA-DR expression on cultured human keratinocytes, *J. Invest. Dermatol.*, 83, 88, 1984.

117. Gaspari, A. A., Jenkins, M. K., Katz, S. I., Class II MHC-bearing keratinocytes induce antigen-specific unresponsiveness in hapten-specific TH1 clones, *J. Immunol.*, 141, 2216, 1988.

118. Gaspari, A. A., Katz, S. I., Induction of in vivo hyporesponsiveness to contact allergens by hapten-modified Ia+ keratinocytes, *J. Immunol.*, 147, 4155, 1991.

119. Berman, B., Chen, V. L., France, D. S., Dotz, W. I., Petroni, G., Anatomical mapping of epidermal Langerhans cell densities in adults, *Br. J. Dermatol.*, 109, 5536, 1983.

120. Willis, I., Kligman, A. M., The mechanism of the persistent light reactor, *J. Invest. Dermatol.*, 51, 385, 1968.

121. Halbert, A. R., Gebauer, K. A., Wall, L. M., Prognosis of occupational chromate dermatitis, *Contact Dermatitis*, 27, 214, 1992.

122. Pryce, D. W., Irvine, D., English, J. S. C., Rycroft, R. J., Soluble oil dermatitis: a follow-up study, *Contact Dermatitis*, 21, 28, 1989.

8 The Langerhans Cell: Antigen Processing/Antigen Presentation*

Ralf W. Denfeld and Jan C. Simon

CONTENTS

I. INTRODUCTION

Many tissues contain a trace population of antigen-presenting cells (APC) with unusual dendritic shape and strong stimulatory function for T lymphocytes, i.e., the Langerhans cells of the epidermis. These dendritic cells (DC) comprise a system that occupies discrete portions of nonlymphoid and lymphoid organs and is interconnected by defined pathways of movement. The most notable feature common to DC is their ability to capture antigens and initiate T cell-mediated immune responses. The exact mechanisms of DC action are important for understanding how resting T cells are primed and how one might begin to manipulate the immune response at the early sensitization phase of immunity. Three areas of DC function must be considered for the initiation of T cell responses: (1) a sentinel role in which DC capture and present antigen, followed by (2) a migratory function in which DC, now loaded with antigen, move to the T cell-dependent areas of lymphoid organs and bind antigen-specific T cells, and finally (3) their role as "nature's adjuvant" in which T cell growth and effector function are induced.[1-3]

Epidermal Langerhans cells (LC) were originally described in 1868 as nerve cells within human skin located above the basal layer of proliferating keratinocytes.[4,5] After more than a century of speculations about their origin, they were finally recognized to be hematopoietic cells.[6-8] Today it is generally accepted that LC are a constituent of the skin immune system and the principal APC in imperturbed epidermis. Freshly isolated LC are weak T cell stimulators, but excellent at antigen capturing. These characteristics change dramatically following encounter of immunological stimuli, during in vitro culture or in vivo in response to cytokines produced at the site of local tissue damage.

* This work was supported by grants from the Deutsche Forschungsgemeinschaft (Si 397/7-1, 8-1) and the Deutsches Zentrum für Luft- und Raumfahrt (1GC9701/7).

Then, LC rapidly express high levels of major histocompatibility complex (MHC) and costimulatory molecules and lose their endocytic activity. This is thought to reflect the process of differentiation LC undergo en route from the epidermis to the skin-draining lymph nodes in vivo in search of naive T cells. Furthermore, the constitutive expression of MHC molecules and the ability to trap, process, and present antigen ensure that LC are well equipped for the initiation of T cell responses. This potent capacity of LC to act as APC for T cells has been shown for a wide spectrum of antigens, including nominal proteins, superantigens, virus-derived proteins, tumor antigens, and reactive haptens.[1-3] In this review, we shall focus on how antigen is processed and presented by DC, especially by LC.

II. ANTIGEN CAPTURE BY DENDRITIC CELLS

DC play a central role in antigen presentation. In their immature state, they capture antigen at peripheral sites and migrate to secondary lymphoid organs, where they, now fully matured, trigger naive T cells. DC must be able to internalize efficiently any foreign antigen and to regulate coordinately antigen uptake, migration, and T cell stimulatory capacity.[1-3] The endocytic activity of DC isolated ex vivo has been investigated extensively.[9] In particular, it has been shown that fresh DC isolated from nonlymphoid organs are able to capture and process antigen, but rapidly lose this property upon maturation in culture. Work in the early 1990s has established that fresh LC during in vitro culture lose antigen-capturing and -processing ability, MHC class II molecule synthesis, and acidic organelles, and mature into immunostimulatory DC.[10-12] These changes parallel those occuring in vivo when LC migrate from the epidermis to the draining lymph nodes. Similarly, DC can efficiently internalize a diverse array of antigen for processing and loading onto MHC class II molecules. Immature DC are characterized by a high level of endocytic activity, which is lost upon maturation.[9]

The mechanisms of antigen uptake have been studied primarily in human monocyte-derived DC generated in culture with GM-CSF and IL-4 that have the properties of immature DC, i.e., LC, with high endocytic activity but low T cell-stimulatory capacity.[3,13-15] Antigen uptake by these cells occurs via three distinct mechanisms. The first is macropinocytosis, which is a clathrin-independent, but cytoskeleton-dependent type of fluid-phase endocytosis mediated by membrane ruffling and the formation of large (0.2 to 5 μm) vesicles. DC have a very high level of constitutive macropinocytosis which enables a single DC to take up a very large volume of fluid, i.e., half of the cell's volume per hour, although as yet it is unclear how internalized ligands are concentrated in macropinosomes.[14,16] For example, DC can present a soluble antigen taken up via macropinocytosis at 10^{-10} M, being as efficient as antigen-specific B cells that use their membrane immunoglobulins as specific receptors.[13,14] In DC and macrophages, though not epithelial cells, the macrosolutes are concentrated and accumulate in the cytosol for processing and presentation on MHC class I molecules or in lysosomal compartments that contain MHC class II molecules and proteases.[14-18] It is an appealing concept that sentinel DC in the periphery may be able to internalize vast quantities of a variety of antigens by macropinocytosis, which represents a unique pathway in DC for efficient channeling of antigenic peptide to both the MHC class I and class II pathways, and, eventually, prime naive T cells to mount an immune response.

The second mechanism of antigen capture is receptor mediated. Sentinel DC, i.e., LC, express different Fc receptors (FcR), specific for most immunoglobulin isotypes, especially the low-affinity receptors for IgG, FcγRII (CD32), and FcγRIII (CD16),[19] the high-affinity receptor for IgE (FcϵRI),[20-22] and the mannose receptor (MR).[14,23] On DC, FcϵRI functions to augment allergen presentation in an IgE-dependent manner, and FcγRII and III are capable of internalizing IgG-antigen complexes, enabling efficient capture of antigen–antibody complexes by DC.[13,20-22,24] Antigens complexed with antibodies are presented at >100-fold lower concentrations compared to unbound antigen.[16] The FcR expressed by LC and other DC may not be endocytosed for the destruction of opsonized particles in phagolysosomes but rather internalized for antigen processing and presentation. Additionally, the MR is a pattern-recognition molecule containing multiple carbohydrate binding domains that mediate endocytosis of a variety of antigen, i.e., Gram-negative and Gram-positive bacteria, yeasts, parasites, and mycobacteria, which expose mannose or fucose residues.[14,23,25] Especially, in immature DC, i.e., LC within skin, the MR appears to be an important endocytic pathway for receptor-mediated antigen uptake and subsequent delivery to MHC class II compartments. Indeed, mannosylated, and possibly fucosylated proteins are presented with up to 1000-fold higher efficiency than unglycosylated proteins by DC.[14,26,27] In macrophages and immature DC, the MR is present almost entirely within the endocytic apparatus, although it does not colocalize with MHC class II molecules. Following transit to the cell surface, the MR recycles constitutively from the cell surface through the endocytic apparatus, binding ligands externally at neutral pH and dissociating at the more acidic pH within endosomes.[25] Interestingly, in mature DC, the MR, although expressed on the cell surface, displays a greatly reduced endocytic capacity and its proposed role is the capture of carbohydrate antigens.[14,23] Thus, unlike Fc receptors, which are degraded together with bound antigen in endosomal compartments, the MR releases its cargo at endosomal pH and recycles to the cell surface. It therefore allows uptake and accumulation of many ligands in successive rounds by a small number of receptors, providing a sustained capacity for antigen capture.[25] Hence, mannosylation may represent an effective way to target antigen to DC in vivo. Another pathway involves the recently described CD1b pathway of antigen presentation, in which the MR appears to play a critical role in the processing of mycobacterially derived glycolipids in conjunction with CD1b.[28] It was shown that the MR was responsible for the uptake of the mycobacterial lipoglycan lipoarabi-nomannan, which then became internalized and transported to endosomal compartments. MR and CD1b colocalized, suggesting that the MR could deliver the lipoglycans to the endocytic pathway for loading onto CD1b. Thereby, the MR may play a critical role in the processing of carbohydrate antigens. Additional receptors like the MR may be involved in antigen capture by DC.[28] For example, in mice a C-type lectin, DEC-205, is expressed by DC and is likely to have a ligand specificity different from that of the MR.[29] Very recently the human analogue of DEC-205 was cloned.[30] However, a precise role for DEC-205 in antigen processing has not been determined yet.

Finally, DC can take up particles of less than 0.2 μm diameter by micropinocytosis and particles or microbes (0.5 to 6 μm) by phagocytosis. Micropinocytosis encompasses both fluid-phase uptake and, in contrast to macropinocytosis, receptor-mediated endocytosis via clathrin-coated vesicles.[31] Phagocytosis can be mediated probably by macropinocytosis or a receptor-mediated process, utilizing pattern-recognition molecules like the MR or FcR.[23,32–37]

In addition to the efficient antigen capture, LC and other immature DC fulfill other requirements for antigen presentation and T cell stimulation: they synthesize high levels of MHC molecules, possess a very prominent MHC class II compartment, and express abundant levels of adhesion and costimulatory molecules. These features allow DC to perform as the most efficient APC for soluble antigen.

III. ANTIGEN PROCESSING AND PRESENTATION BY LANGERHANS CELLS

The vast majority of either endogenous or foreign protein antigens must be converted into short peptides before they can trigger an immune response. In general, these immunogenic peptides are bound to MHC molecules that are expressed on the surface of APC. The peptide–MHC complexes serve as ligands for antigen-specific receptors on T cells which, once triggered by these peptide–MHC complexes, become activated and differentiate into effector cells. Principally, any cell type that expresses the appropriate MHC products can serve as an APC. In contrast to the expression of MHC class I molecules, which are expressed by almost all nucleated cells, the expression of MHC class II molecules is usually restricted to a subset of professional APC, i.e., DC-like LC, macrophages, and B cells.

A. MHC Class II Antigen Processing and Presentation Pathways

MHC class II molecules are synthesized in the endoplasmatic reticulum (ER) as type I transmembrane glycoproteins, comprising dimerized α- and β-chains of which the C-terminal lumenal domains form the peptide binding groove.[38–40] Transcription of human MHC class II genes, located on chromosome 6, is mainly regulated by the MHC class II transactivator protein, termed CIITA, which also controls the expression of invariant chain (Ii) and HLA-DM, suggesting CIITA to be a critical regulator of antigen presentation.[41,42] In the ER, three such αβ dimers assemble with one Ii trimer, a non-MHC-encoded type II integral membrane glycoprotein, to form nonamers. A lumenal domain of Ii interacts with the putative peptide-binding groove of MHC class II, rendering the groove inaccessible to peptides present in the ER. Once the nonameric complexes are formed, the so-called "calnexin/calreticulin-based quality control system" at the ER-cis-Golgi interface allows egress from the ER and transport to the Golgi complex, suggesting a chaperone function for Ii in the ER. In the Golgi, the α-, β-, and Ii-subunits are terminally glycosylated and transported to the *trans*-Golgi network (TGN), a tubulo-vesicular organelle located at the *trans*-face of the Golgi stacks. From here, most of the nonamers are targeted to the endocytic pathway due to a sorting signal contained in the Ii's cytoplasmatic tail. Reaching the endocytic pathway is required for class II dimers to encounter antigenic peptides.[38–40,43]

All entries into the cell converge at endosomes. In general, the endocytic pathway comprises an extremely pleiomorphic interconnected array of vesicles, larger vacuoles, and tubules that communicate with each other, the plasma membrane (PM), and the TGN. The complex morphology and plasticity of the endocytic pathway, its dispersed intracellular distribution, and the lack of reliable discriminative molecular markers have hampered defining its compartments. However, a number of operational terms have been introduced and have proved to be useful. Early endosomes (EE) are the first structures receiving endocytosed material. They have a less acidic pH than later endocytic compartments and exhibit relatively little proteolytic activity. In the cell periphery, EE are engaged in the sorting of soluble and membrane proteins for transport further down the endocytic pathway, as well as to the PM and the TGN. Centrally, located next to the Golgi area, they are enriched in recycling PM proteins. Internalized material that does not recycle from the EE is subsequently transported to multivesicular late endosomes (LE), which gradually undergo transition into multilaminar lysosomes. In contrast to EE, LE acquire lysosomal membrane proteins (LAMP), which accumulate in lysosomes. They contain a full set of acid hydrolases, have a relatively acidic pH, and like lysosomes are degradative compartments. Thus, EE are involved in receptor/ligand sorting and recycling, LE in accumulating cargo for transport to lysosomes representing the final destination for material internalized by endocytosis.[40]

The majority of the newly synthesized nonameric MHC class II-Ii complexes that have departed from the TGN are thought to arrive at the endocytic pathway via a direct route;[38–40] some may be transported to the cell surface, from where they are cleared by endocytosis due to an internalization signal in the cytoplasmic tail of the Ii and delivered to EE.[44] In a variety of APC, including LC and other tissue DC, the majority of intracellular MHC class II is found in LE and lysosomes, indicating late endocytic structures to be important for MHC class II-mediated antigen presentation.[45–49] Despite their morphological heterogeneity, these structures were collectively designated MHC class II compartments (MIIC). Nevertheless, both EE and MIIC have been implicated as entry sites to which class II–Ii complexes are first delivered. Recently, late EE and/or early MIIC containing abundant Ii were independently identified morphologically and biochemically as the entry site where most of the TGN-derived class II–Ii complexes enter the endocytic tract.[49,50]

Normally, correct trafficking to endosomes requires aminoterminal Ii cytoplasmic sequences, and trafficking within endosomes is dependent on the proteolytic processing of Ii,[43] although, in DC, alternative Ii-independent mechanisms for class II transport and peptide loading have also been suggested.[51] Delayed degradation of Ii within endosomes results in transport of MHC class II–Ii complexes to lysosomes, where they move only slowly to the cell surface, whereas rapid Ii degradation favors endosomal acquisition of peptide and rapid cell surface expression.[52] Ii is degraded by endoproteases found in endosomes or lysosomes, resulting in the disassembly of the nonamers into three αβ dimers bound to a fragment of Ii termed the class II-associated Ii peptide (CLIP), containing a promiscuous peptide sequence that apparently occupies the peptide-binding groove of all nascent MHC class II dimers, thereby inhibiting peptide loading.[43] Although a number of proteases have been implicated in Ii processing, recent studies indicate a special role for cathepsin S. Ii degradation occurs in a stepwise or sequential fashion with two cleavage steps due to cysteine proteases, i.e., cathepsins L and S, and/or aspartyl proteases, i.e., cathepsin D and E, beginning with the luminal carboxy-terminal region, generating a 10-kDa fragment of Ii, termed p10 fragment.[53–55] The p10 fragment of Ii is comprised of the amino-terminal cytoplasmatic domain and terminates in CLIP that remains part of the nonamer. Then cathepsin S efficiently catalyzes the digestion of p10, leading to CLIP formation that causes nonamer dissociation, yielding αβ dimers still bound to CLIP. Selective inhibition of cathepsin S blocks Ii processing beyond the p10 fragment and therefore blocks CLIP generation.[53,56] This results in markedly delayed loading of MHC class II dimers with peptides and delayed appearance of newly synthesized MHC class II dimers on the cell surface. Similar results were recently observed in vivo in unfractionated splenocytes by specific inhibition of cathepsin S after systemic administration of the vinyl-sulfone inhibitor LHVS.[57] Interestingly, cathepsin S is selectively expressed by professional APC and is also unique among cysteine proteases in its stability and activity at neutral as well as acidic pH.[53] Thus cathepsin S is capable of processing Ii into CLIP in a wide variety of endosomes of varying pH, including early endosomes, which reportedly have a relatively high pH and are enriched for MHC class II-Ii complexes.[49,50]

Recent studies point to the capacity of DC to regulate MHC class II trafficking, depending on their state of maturation.[50,58,59] Immature, endocytically active DC, i.e., LC, synthesize large quantities of class II, but transport (or retain) most of it to late endosomal/lysosomal compartments, with little reaching the PM or appearing in late EE/early MIIC. Upon maturation, transport to nonlysosomal late EE/early MIIC begins and, subsequently, when fully matured into potent APC, almost all class II molecules are expressed on the cell surface PM. This process of maturation for antigen presentation was found to take 24 to 48 h, with a more than sixfold increase of the half-life of class II surface molecules.[50,58] Hence, DC like LC are able to delay antigen display by regulating class II transport and compartmentalization representing a property crucial to their role in immunosurveillance. Since this alternative pattern of MHC class II trafficking to lysosomes rather than to the cell surface is reminiscent of trafficking in B cells when Ii processing is inhibited by leupeptin, a cathepsin S inhibitor,[52] one might expect involvement of cathepsin S regulation in immature DC, i.e., LC. Indeed, very recently it was shown that in immature DC, i.e., LC, ineffective Ii proteolysis due to low cathepsin S activity leads to the transport of class II–Ii complexes to lysosomes, while in mature DC, elevated cathepsin S activity results in efficient delivery of class II αβ dimers to the PM. This process is controlled by a novel mechanism involving alterations in the expression and localization of an endogenous cathepsin S inhibitor, namely, cystatin C, implying the ratio of cystatin C to cathepsin S to regulate Ii cleavage and MHC class II trafficking in developing DC, especially LC.[60] Moreover, very recently it was demonstrated that inactivation of cathepsin S strongly reduced IgE/FcεRI-mediated antigen presentation by immature DC, indicating IgE-bound allergens to be channeled via the high affinity FcεRI to MIIC, resulting in MHC class II presentation which is dependent on cathepsin S.[61] In that regard, it is notable that expression of cathepsin S, although induced by IFN-γ, is not driven by the CIITA transcription factor necessary for MHC class II expression, but instead responds to several proinflammatory cytokines, including TNF-α.[62] Taken together, cathepsin S is the most potent catalyst of CLIP formation, thereby modulating antigen presentation in immature DC, i.e., LC, by regulating the trafficking of MHC class II within these cells.

Furthermore, a direct connection between protease activity and antigen presentation was revealed by the finding that the p41 fragment of Ii is a potent inhibitor of cathepsin L (but not cathepsin S).[63,64] Interestingly, the p41 form of Ii is known to be expressed at low level in B cells, whereas in LC it represents almost half of the total Ii,[12] implying an inhibitory role in Ii cleavage. However, a recent report has demonstrated cathepsin L to be necessary for Ii degradation in thymic epithelial cells but not in DC, indicating a critical role for cathepsin L in T cell selection.[65] Nevertheless, the balance between Ii forms and the endosomal protease profile including yet undefined proteases and their physiological inhibitors in antigen presentation remains to be elucidated in more detail.[66]

Following endocytosis and transport through EE, exogenous antigens are proteolytically processed into immunogenic peptides that need to be loaded onto empty MHC class II molecules which, as mentioned earlier, are primarily derived from the biosynthetic route.[38–40] Similarly, endogenous, cytosolically derived peptides can bind to MHC class II molecules following fusion with endocytic compartments[67] or translocation across MIIC membranes by a receptor-mediated process requiring ATP and heat shock proteins.[68] It must be noted, however, that immunogenic peptides need to have a certain "resistance" to endosomal degradation. For example, multiple antigens of the common house dust mite, a major allergen in asthma and atopic dermatitis, have been recently shown to be digestive enzymes.[69] Also, food allergens such as peanuts and shrimp reveal a remarkable resistance to protease destruction.[70] The loading of empty MHC class II dimers with peptides requires MHC class II-CLIP dimers to interact with a nonpolymorphic MHC-encoded dimer, HLA-DM (murine H2-M), which catalyzes the dissociation of CLIP from MHC class II.[71,72] This was confirmed in H2-M–deficient mice that express surface MHC class II molecules entirely occupied by CLIP and are markedly deficient in peptide loading and antigen presentation.[73,74] In addition, it was shown that high levels of HLA-DM could minimize the importance of CLIP formation by promoting dissociation of p10 from class II and stabilizing empty dimers until a suitable peptide is captured.[75] Also, variation in HLA-DM levels was reported to modify rates of peptide loading onto MHC class II dimers.[76] *In situ*, HLA-DM can be detected in early MIIC, but is most abundant in later MIIC,[49,50,72] indicating the compartments for peptide loading onto empty MHC class II dimers. Recently, HLA-DO has been identified as a counterregulator of HLA-DM, inhibiting MHC class II-restricted antigen processing. Both are closely linked, since HLA-DO requires association with HLA-DM for transportation in the endocytic pathway.[77,78] So HLA-DM and HLA-DO also serve to edit the range of bound immunogenic peptides, by allowing for the dissociation of peptides of relatively low affinity.

Once loaded, class II molecules reach the PM where they can interact with antigen-specific T cell receptors, thereby selecting individual T cells for activation. How class II molecules ultimately reach the PM remains unknown but is dependent on the stability of the class II-peptide complexes.[79] Conceivably, this last step in transport may involve multiple budding and fusion events.[80] However, a small amount of multivesicular MIIC can fuse directly with the PM, releasing the internal vesicles (exosomes) into the extracellular media being able to stimulate specific T cells.[81,82] Last, recycling MHC class II molecules have been described which are able to capture a new set of antigenic peptides in an HLA-DM- and Ii-independent pathway.[83]

Taken together, the critical events in peptide processing and selection for class II presentation are posited to be dependent on four main factors: (1) the timing, kinetics, and efficiency of Ii's proteolytic processing to CLIP within the endosomes, which seems to be a function of cathepsin S expression in LC; (2) the level of HLA-DM and HLA-DO; (3) the ability of peptides to persist among the multicatalytic endosomal proteases; and (4) the relative avidity of MHC class II dimers for Ii and peptide which is to be critically dictated by the individual MHC class II haplotype.

B. MHC Class I Antigen Processing and Presentation Pathways

MHC class I molecules are expressed on the cell surface of almost all nucleated mammalian cell types. The fully assembled human MHC class I molecule is composed of two type I transmembrane glycoproteins: a polymorphic heavy chain (HC), comprised of three extracellular globular domains

(α1, α2, α3), noncovalently associated with the soluble invariant light chain, the β2 microglobulin (β2m), via the α3 domain. The polymorphism of the HC is mainly resident in the α1 and α2 domains, forming the peptide binding groove which is capable of retaining the free amino- and carboxy-groups at the ends of the peptide. In humans, the HC of the MHC class I molecules are encoded by the HLA genes on chromosome 6, whereas the β2m gene is on chromosome 15. Following their synthesis and equipped with signal sequences, both the HC and β2m enter the ER.[41,84] There, preceding peptide loading, these newly synthesized subunits carry out a sequence of interactions with resident chaperones.

The assembly of these translocated subunits is facilitated by the molecular chaperone calnexin, a resident of the ER that associates with nascent protein chains.[84,85] Calnexin binds to the HC before association with β2m and peptides, which presumably improves assembly by making the folding of the HC more efficient. However, calnexin is not an absolute requirement for this process within the ER, as demonstrated by normal HC-β2m assembly and expression in calnexin-negative cell lines. Another chaperone, the immunoglobulin-binding protein (BiP), exhibits specificity for HC similar to that of calnexin and possibly has a similar function. Then, in the presence of β2m, the HC attains its correctly folded confirmation and is released from calnexin association. Alternatively, if misfolding occurs, the HC is targeted for degradation. Subsequently, HC-β2m dimers bind to the calreticulin chaperone, a major ER luminal calcium-binding protein that shares a high degree of homology with calnexin and has a lectin-like specificity for monoglycosylated N-linked glycans present on the HC. Unlike calnexin, which binds to HC before its association with β2m, calreticulin binds only to HC-β2m dimers. Thus, the correct assembly of MHC class I dimers is under supervision of the "calnexin/calreticulin-based quality control system."[84]

The assembled but empty HC-β2m–calreticulin complex is then able to interact with the transporter associated with antigen processing (TAP), a dimeric protein specialized in the translocation of cytosolic oligopeptides into the ER lumen.[84,86] Calreticulin, together with tapasin, a TAP-associated glycoprotein, forms important intermediates with HC-β2m dimers in steps to facilitate the generation of the MHC class I–TAP complex; otherwise the class I dimer may be degraded in the ER. Peptide capture by assembled class I dimers may also be helped by their interaction with TAP.[87,88] However, it must be noted that in TAP-deficient mice, MHC class I molecules are nonetheless loaded with peptides present in the ER lumen.[84,86] The native TAP complex is a dimer formed by two MHC-encoded polypeptides TAP1 and TAP2. Both subunits are located in the ER and in the cis-Golgi and contain domains spanning the ER membrane, with small peptide loops within the ER lumen and a larger portion, including an ATP-binding cassette, resident on the cytosolic side of the ER membrane. TAP preferentially transports peptides of suitable length for direct binding to MHC class I molecules in an ATP-dependent fashion. Usually, TAP prefers peptides of 8 to 15 residues but also shorter (hexamers) and much longer (30 to 40-mer) peptides can be translocated, with human TAP being promiscuous concerning peptide sequence specificity.[89,90] Additionally, it must be noted that not all MHC class I alleles interact equally well with the TAP complex, suggesting that MHC class I molecules display different efficiencies of TAP binding.[91] As mentioned earlier, TAP-independent presentation of endogenous proteins has been observed, indicating that epitope-containing peptides have natural access into the ER lumen, alternatively, to be purposely targeted there. Last, within the ER lumen, proteases are detected that are believed to be involved in the final trimming of peptides for peptide loading.[92] Although their population is structurally diverse, bound peptides usually display a narrow length distribution, encompassing 8 to 11 amino acids. In the absence of foreign antigens, MHC class I molecules are usually occupied by peptides derived from self-proteins.[84,90] Then, peptide-loaded but also empty class I dimers transit from the ER to the cell surface. However, empty MHC class I molecules turn over rapidly and are returned to the peptide-loading compartments. This recycling mechanism may help compensate for MHC class I haplotypes that seem to load with peptides less efficiently by giving them several rounds of exposure to the peptide-loading compartments.[93,94] The macromolecular complexes created by TAP, the various chaperones, newly assembled HC-β2m dimers, and the vesicle recycling system carrying these molecules represent the means whereby oligopeptides are trapped and brought to the cell surface.

In general, the cytosol appears to be the main, but not the exclusive, source of precursor proteins that supply peptides for MHC class I molecules. The cytosolic concentration of intracellular proteins is regulated not only by their rate of synthesis but also by their rate of degradation. Although protein catabolism may occur by several pathways, proteasomes have been identified as the main protein degradation machines of the cell. These large multicatalytic proteinase complexes, which are highly conserved throughout the evolutionary system, appear to have been annexed by the endogenous antigen-processing system and are the key to the generation of peptides that are eventually bound to MHC class I molecules. They show a heterogeneous subunit composition and, accordingly, have been classified into the 20S proteasome, the 26S proteasome, and the regulatory complex PA28. However, the active proteolytic core of the larger assemblages, the 26S form and the IFN-γ-inducible PA28 complex, is the cylinder-shaped 20S proteasome. The proteolytic capacities of these complexes with protease/peptidase and protein unfolding activities, which are still poorly characterized, are critical determinants in the generation and destruction of antigenic epitopes contained within various proteins.[95] Oligopeptides containing antigenic epitopes as short as 21 residues require proteasome activity for processing and presentation. For endogenous peptides of 17 amino acids or shorter, however, processing and presentation of epitopes contained in these peptides appear to be proteasome-independent.[96] Interestingly, membrane-permeable proteasome inhibitors that have been shown to interfere with MHC class I restricted antigen presentation have little effect on processing of exogenous antigens for MHC class II presentation. Also, conventional inhibitors of vacuolar cysteine proteases have little effect on MHC class I processing.[97] It has been suggested that long peptides, generated by degradation of native proteins by the 26S proteasome, are then transported to the 20S–PA28 proteasome complex for further, more coordinated processing by a chaperone-assisted pathway resulting in the optimized production of antigenic epitopes.[95] In conclusion, there is good circumstantial evidence that the cleavage preferences of proteasomes control the generation of antigenic epitopes in qualitative and quantitative terms.

The generally held view has been that the MHC class I pathway is exclusively devoted to sampling endogenously synthesized proteins of the cell, whereas the class II pathway surveys exogenous antigens. However, additional data have accumulated showing that a large number of exogenous antigens of different nature, i.e., denatured proteins, soluble antigens associated with cellular debris, apoptotic cells, lipid compounds, or bacteria and parasites that do not enter the cytoplasm, can be processed by APC, especially DC, for MHC class I-dependent T cell priming.[98–100] This function is particularly important for in vivo priming of CTL responses to antigens that are not synthesized by professional APC.[101] Although antigen processing in endosomes or phagosomes following endocytic or phagocytic uptake, respectively, for peptide presentation in the context of MHC class I was long considered an exclusive feature of DC and macrophages,[98,99] recent findings have demonstrated that this pathway also operates in mast cells[102] and B cells.[103] Especially DC, which are considered to be the most potent type of APC to prime naive T cells, can process phagocytosed as well as endocytosed antigens for both MHC class I- and II-restricted epitope presentation.[98,99,104–107] For the processing of exogenous antigen to be presented by MHC class I, two pathways can be distinguished: a cytosolic, TAP-dependent pathway and an endosomal, TAP-independent pathway. Unlike the classical cytosolic processing pathway, processing of exogenous antigen via an alternative MHC class I processing pathway is resistant to proteasome inhibitors and to inhibitors of trans-Golgi vesicle traffic.[98,99,108,109] The exact pathway which internalized extracellular proteins take before they appear as MHC class I bound peptides remains unclear and appears to involve either transfer to the cytosol for conventional MHC class I processing or processing in alternative compartments, such as the cell surface or vesicular compartments like the ER lumen, endosomes, and lysosomes. As mentioned earlier, immature DC are phagocytic, although less so than macrophages, and have a high level of constitutive macropinocytosis. Interestingly, phagocytosis and macropinocytosis have been shown to deliver exogenous antigen via endosomes, phagosomes, and lysosomes into the cytosol for processing and presentation on class I molecules by the classical proteasome and TAP-dependent MHC class I processing pathway.[98,99,110,111] When compared to macrophages, DC were found to be much more efficient in presenting soluble protein antigen on class I molecules, possibly because of their high level of macropinocytosis. Also, the transfer of peptides and proteins between lysosomes and the cytosol, partially mediated by stress proteins, has been demonstrated.[98,99,112,113] Alternatively, some peptides generated in the endocytic pathway may be "regurgitated" and bind to MHC class I molecules, involving the sensitization of bystander cells.[98,99,114] Furthermore, the external exchange of peptides already bound to surface MHC class I molecules in a dissociation/reassociation cycle, which was shown to be regulated by exogenous $\beta 2m$, can result in the presentation of exogenous peptides.[115] On the other hand, exogenous proteins may be presented by MHC class I using a pathway similar to that operating in MHC class II antigen presentation, since this pathway is TAP-independent and is blocked by agents that target endodomal acidification or inhibit vesicular trafficking. Moreover, the Ii, used for directing MHC class II traffic, has been shown to direct a subset of MHC class I molecules to the endocytic compartment.[98,99,116]

Taken together, MHC class I dimers encounter processed peptides of defined length. The peptides are generated in a compartment (usually the cytosol) completely separate from the ER, where initial assembly of MHC class I dimers takes place, and are transported into the ER by specific peptide transporters. The crystal structure of peptide-stabilized MHC class I molecules reveals a peptide-binding groove restricted to peptide lengths of 8 to 11 amino acids. While MHC class I dimers may capture and protect ER peptides from terminal degradation, they do not contribute appreciably to peptide generation. In contrast, for MHC class II-restricted antigen presentation, endosomal proteins destined to generate antigenic epitopes are fragmented by proteases residing in the same compartments as the MHC class II dimers themselves. Moreover, these dimers can bind a wide variety of partially fragmented and denatured proteins. The crystal structure of MHC class II reveals a rather open peptide-binding groove, which allows considerable variation in length of bound peptides. Once bound to MHC class II dimers, which themselves are remarkably resistant to proteolysis, protein fragments can be repeatedly nicked by endosomal proteases to yield a final antigen, the core epitope being completely protected from proteolysis by the MHC binding groove itself. This process may account for the quite variable length (12 to 24 amino acids) of peptides eluted from purified, surface MHC class II dimers. This means that MHC class II dimers may themselves directly participate in processing of antigens, explaining the ability of individuals to display antigenic diversity to a common protein even though the basic enzymes responsible for proteolysis are virtually the same for everyone, a phenomenon probably underlying susceptibility to infection and autoimmune disease.

C. Antigen Processing and Presentation by CD1 Molecules

CD1 molecules constitute a family of nonpolymorphic proteins with five isotypes in humans, namely, CD1a to CD1e. Although not encoded within the MHC but on chromosome 1, their noncovalent association with $\beta 2m$ relates them structurally to MHC proteins, with which they also share limited but significant sequence homology.[117] Human epidermal Langerhans cells express high levels of CD1a and variable amounts of CD1c, while CD1b has been reported on dermal and migrating LC. CD1b and CD1c are expressed on DC in a variety of tissues, including the dermis of the skin, lung, kidney, liver, and lymphoid organs.[118–120] Also, in vitro-generated human DC can express CD1a, CD1b, and CD1c, depending on the culture conditions.[121–123] The recent description of the crystal structure of murine CD1 identified all characteristic features of class I molecules highlighting its MHC-like structure.[124] The binding site is extremely hydrophobic suggesting microbial lipids and glycolipids, but also hydrophobic peptides, to be suitable ligands for antigen presentation.[117,124–126] For example, CD1b could present (glyco-)lipid antigens, such as mycolic acid,[127] lipoarabinomannans,[128] and glucose monomycolate[129] from mycobacteria, and

CD1c has also been shown to bind lipoarabinomannans[130] for presentation in a MHC-independent but CD1-restricted fashion.

CD1 molecules behave like MHC class I molecules in their biosynthesis and transport to the cell surface, but like MHC class II molecules in their subsequent sequestration into acidic endocytic compartments to sample exogenous antigens for presentation which is TAP independent.[117,131] In immature DC, it has been demonstrated that a cytoplasmic sequence of CD1 facilitates its targeting into the endocytic pathway accessing the MIIC via clathrin-coated pits.[132,133] Moreover, very recently it was reported that in immature DC lipoarabinomannans, following their uptake by the MR, could be detected in MIIC colocalized with CD1b, suggesting MIIC to be the antigen-loading compartment of CD1 molecules.[28] The acidic milieu of MIIC also may be important since it promotes a conformational change in CD1b that increases accessibility to the hydrophobic interior of the protein and thereby facilitates binding of lipid ligands.[134] In addition, MIIC are well equipped with degradative enzymes, which may be involved in the trimming of large glycan components of some antigens, i.e., lipoarabinomannans, for presentation by CD1.[28,128] However, it needs to be elucidated in more detail whether this process occurs directly from the Golgi apparatus or via endocytosis from the cell surface and whether additional factors are required for CD1 loading. Furthermore, the function of the other CD1 isotypes, especially CD1a, remains to be established.

IV. SWITCHING FROM CAPTURE MODE TO T CELL-STIMULATORY MODE

A striking characteristic of LC and of in vitro-generated immature DC is their capacity to respond to inflammatory stimuli such as TNF-α, IL-1, and LPS by switching from the Ag-capture mode to the T cell-stimulatory mode. These stimuli induce the loss of macropinocytosis ability and FcR expression (i.e., FcγRII, FcγRIII, FcϵRI), downregulate the MR and CD1a, but, at the same time, increase adhesion and costimulatory molecules[13,14] and induce the expression of CD44 variants implicated in cell migration.[135,136] Indeed, in vivo it was demonstrated that TNF-α, IL-1, and LPS can deplete LC and DC from nonlymphoid organs, i.e., the skin.[137] The capacity to coordinately regulate antigen capture, migration, and T cell stimulation, following contact with inflammatory cytokines, appears to be a key feature of DC and allows them maximal opportunity to present foreign, i.e., infectious, antigens in vivo.

It is now generally accepted that T cells require two signals from APC, i.e., LC, for optimal activation, proliferation, cytokine production, and effector function. The first signal is antigen-specific and provided when antigenic peptides bound to MHC molecules are engaged with the peptide-specific T cell receptor (TCR)/CD3 complex. The second signal is mediated by additional costimulatory signals delivered to the T cell via a number of accessory molecules (i.e., CD28, CD152, and CD154) which serve as receptors for specific antigen-independent ligands expressed on APC (i.e., CD80, CD86, and CD40, respectively).[138] Furthermore, it is well known that MHC class II molecules on APC interact with CD4 on T cells and MHC class I molecules with CD8, respectively, which does not interfere with the peptide-binding domains of both MHC molecules and the TCR. These interactions lead to MHC class II-restricted T helper cell responses and cytotoxic T cell responses restricted to peptides presented on MHC class I molecules. Thus, both T cell receptors, CD4 and CD8, respectively, modulate TCR recognition of antigen and the outcome of immune responses with distinct effector functions.[139]

T cell recognition of CD1 molecules remains a major question. It is known that human T cells can interact with human CD1a, CD1b, and CD1d in an CD1-restricted, antigen-independent manner. Such CD1-reactive T cells are usually double-negative for CD4 and CD8, suggesting that they belong to a different developmental linage compared to most MHC-restricted T cells. Moreover, in humans antigen-dependent, CD1-restricted but MHC-independent T cell responses against mycobacterial (glyco-)lipid antigens could be observed which were also mediated by double-negative T cells. However, mouse CD1 can react with CD4+ and CD8+ T cells. In addition, a murine CD1-reactive T cell subset has been identified characterized by the natural killer cell-associated marker

NK1.1. These NK1.1+ T cells express an invariant TCRα-chain that appears to be highly reactive with mouse CD1d molecules, and their localization correlates with the tissue distribution of CD1d. Similarily, in humans such a CD1d-reactive T cell subset was found recently.[117] Taken together, the structural and functional knowledge on the CD1 family of lipid antigen-presenting molecules reveals important differences from MHC-dependent peptide antigen presentation.

Although the working principles of DC, especially LC, are increasingly understood, we still need more information on the molecular mechanisms of DC function in order to be able to fully exploit their therapeutic potential. It is also important to understand how the mechanisms of antigen capture, processing, and presentation are regulated by cytokines under physiological conditions and how they may be subverted by pathogens or in autoimmune and neoplastic disease. At present, this area of research has entered the exciting stage where knowledge can be applied in vivo, i.e., in clinical trials.[140]

REFERENCES

1. Steinman, R. M., The dendritic cell system and its role in immunogenicity, *Annu. Rev. Immunol.*, 9, 271, 1991.
2. Steinman, R., Hoffman, L., Pope, M., Maturation and migration of cutaneous dendritic cells, *J. Invest. Dermatol.*, 105(1 Suppl), 2S, 1995.
3. Banchereau, J., Steinman, R. M., Dendritic cells and the control of immunity, *Nature*, 392, 245, 1998.
4. Langerhans, P., Über die Nerven der menschlichen Haut, *Virchows Arch. (Pathol. Anat.)*, 44, 325, 1868.
5. De Panfilis, G., Paul Langerhans sesquicentennial, July 23rd, 1997, *J. Invest. Dermatol.*, 109, 120, 1997.
6. Frelinger, J. G., Hood, L., Hill, S., Frelinger, J.A., Mouse epidermal Ia molecules have a bone marrow origin, *Nature*, 282, 321, 1979.
7. Katz, S. I., Tamaki, K., Sachs, D. H., Epidermal Langerhans cells are derived from cells originating in bone marrow, *Nature*, 282, 324, 1979.
8. Stingl, G., Tamaki, K., Katz, S. I., Origin and function of epidermal Langerhans cells, *Immunol. Rev.*, 53, 149, 1980.
9. Steinman, R., Swanson, J., The endocytic activity of dendritic cells, *J. Exp. Med.*, 182, 283, 1995.
10. Pure, E., Inaba, K., Crowley, M. T., Tardelli, L., Witmer-Pack, M. D., Ruberti, G., Fathman, G., Steinman, R. M., Antigen processing by epidermal Langerhans cells correlates with the level of biosynthesis of MHC class II molecules and expression of invariant chain, *J. Exp. Med.*, 172, 1459, 1990.
11. Stossel, H., Koch, F., Kämpgen, E., Stoger, P., Lenz, A., Heufler, C., Romani, N., Schuler, G., Disappearance of certain acidic organelles (endosomes and Langerhans cell granules) accompanies loss of antigen processing capacity upon culture of epidermal Langerhans cells, *J. Exp. Med.*, 172, 1471, 1990.
12. Kämpgen, E., Koch, N., Koch, F., Stoger, P., Heufler, C., Schuler, G., Romani, N., Class II MHC molecules of murine dendritic cells: synthesis, sialylation of invariant chain, and antigen processing capacity are down-regulated upon culture, *Proc. Natl. Acad. Sci. U.S.A.*, 88, 3014, 1991.
13. Sallusto, F., Lanzavecchia, A., Efficient presentation of soluble antigen by cultured human dendritic cells is maintained by GM-CSF plus IL-4 and downregulated by TNF-α, *J. Exp. Med.*, 179, 1109, 1994.
14. Sallusto, F., Cella, M., Danieli, C., Lanzavecchia, A., Dendritic cells use macropinocytosis and the mannose receptor to concentrate macromolecules in the MHC class II compartment: downregulation by cytokines and bacterial products, *J. Exp. Med.*, 182, 389, 1995.
15. Geissmann, F., Prost, C., Monnet, J. P., Dy, M., Brousse, N., Hermine, O., TGF-β1, in the presence of GM-CSF and IL-4, induces differentiation of human peripheral blood monocytes into dendritic Langerhans cells, *J. Exp. Med.*, 187, 961, 1998.
16. Watts, C., Capture and processing of exogenous antigens for presentation on MHC molecules, *Annu. Rev. Immunol.*, 15, 821, 1997.
17. Brossart, P., Bevan, M. J., Presentation of exogenous protein antigens on MHC class I molecules by dendritic cells: pathway of presentation and regulation by cytokines, *Blood*, 90, 1594, 1997.

18. Lutz, M. B., Rovere, P., Kleijmeer, M., Rescigno, M., Assmann, C., Oorschot, V., Geuze, H. J., Trucy, J., Demandolx, D., Davoust, J., Ricciardi-Castagnoli, P., Intracellular routes and selective retention of antigens in mildly acidic cathepsin D/lysosome-associated membrane protein-1/MHC class II-positive vesicles in immature dendritic cells, *J. Immunol.*, 159, 3707, 1997.

19. Esposito-Farese, M. E., Sautes, C., de la Salle, H., Latour, S., Bieber, T., de la Salle, C., Ohlmann, P., Fridman, W. H., Cazenave, J. P., Teillaud, J. L., et al., Membrane and soluble Fc gamma RII/III modulate the antigen-presenting capacity of murine dendritic epidermal Langerhans cells for IgG-complexed antigens, *J. Immunol.*, 155, 1725, 1995.

20. Stingl, G., Maurer, D., IgE-mediated allergen presentation via Fc epsilon RI on antigen-presenting cells, *Int. Arch. Allergy Immunol.*, 113, 24, 1997.

21. Bieber, T., Fc epsilon RI on human epidermal Langerhans cells: an old receptor with new structure and functions, *Int. Arch. Allergy Immunol.*, 113, 30, 1997.

22. Kraft, S., Wessendorf, J. H., Hanau, D., Bieber, T., Regulation of the high affinity receptor for IgE on human epidermal Langerhans cells, *J. Immunol.*, 161, 1000, 1998.

23. Reis e Sousa, C., Stahl, P. D., Austyn, J. M., Phagocytosis of antigens by Langerhans cells in vitro, *J. Exp. Med.*, 178, 509, 1993.

24. Larsson, M., Berge, J., Johansson, A. G., Forsum, U., Human dendritic cells handling of binding, uptake and degradation of free and IgG-immune complexed dinitrophenylated human serum albumin in vitro, *Immunology*, 90, 138, 1997.

25. Stahl, P. D., Ezekowitz, R. A., The mannose receptor is a pattern recognition receptor involved in host defense, *Curr. Opin. Immunol.*, 10, 50 1998.

26. Engering, A. J., Cella, M., Fluitsma, D., Brockhaus, M., Hoefsmit, E. C., Lanzavecchia, A., Pieters, J., The mannose receptor functions as a high capacity and broad specificity antigen receptor in human dendritic cells, *Eur. J. Immunol.*, 27, 2417, 1997.

27. Tan, M. C., Mommaas, A., Drijfhout, J., Jordens, R., Onderwater, J., Verwoerd, D., Mulder, A., van der Heiden, A., Scheidegger, D., Oomen, L., Ottenhoff, T., Tulp, A., Neefjes, J., Koning, F., Mannose receptor-mediated uptake of antigens strongly enhances HLA class II-restricted antigen presentation by cultured dendritic cells, *Eur. J. Immunol.*, 27, 2426, 1997.

28. Prigozy, T. I., Sieling, P. A., Clemens, D., Stewart, P. L., Behar, S. M., Porcelli, S. A., Brenner, M. B., Modlin, R. L., Kronenberg, M., The mannose receptor delivers lipoglycan antigens to endosomes for presentation to T cells by CD1b molecules, *Immunity*, 6, 187, 1997.

29. Jiang, W., Swiggard, W. J., Heufler, C., Peng, M., Mirza, A., Steinman, R. M., Nussenzweig, M. C., The receptor DEC-205 expressed by dendritic cells and thymic epithelial cells is involved in antigen processing, *Nature*, 375, 151, 1995.

30. Kato, M., Neil, T., Clark, G., Morris, C., Sorg, R., Hart, D., cDNA cloning of human DEC-205, a putative antigen-uptake receptor on dendritic cells, *Immunogenetics*, 47, 442, 1998.

31. Schmid, S. L., Clathrin-coated vesicle formation and protein sorting: an integrated process, *Annu. Rev. Biochem.*, 66, 511, 1997.

32. Moll, H., Fuchs, H., Blank, C., Rollinghoff, M., Langerhans cells transport Leishmania major from the infected skin to the draining lymph node for presentation to antigen-specific T cells, *Eur. J. Immunol.*, 23, 1595, 1993.

33. Inaba, K., Inaba, M., Naito, M., Steinman, R. M., Dendritic cell progenitors phagocytose particulates, including bacillus Calmette-Guerin organisms, and sensitize mice to mycobacterial antigens in vivo, *J. Exp. Med.*, 178, 479, 1993.

34. Greenberg, S., Chang, P., Silverstein, S. C., Tyrosine phosphorylation of the gamma subunit of Fc gamma receptors, p72syk, and paxillin during Fc receptor-mediated phagocytosis in macrophages, *J. Biol. Chem.*, 269, 3897, 1994.

35. Scheicher, C., Mehlig, M., Dienes, H. P., Reske, K., Uptake of microparticle-adsorbed protein antigen by bone marrow-derived dendritic cells results in up-regulation of IL-1α and IL-12 p40/p35 and triggers prolonged, efficient antigen presentation, *Eur. J. Immunol.*, 25, 1566, 1995.

36. Filgueira, L., Nestle, F. O., Rittig, M., Joller, H. I., Groscurth, P., Human dendritic cells phagocytose and process *Borrelia burgdorferi*, *J. Immunol.*, 157, 2998, 1996.

37. Cox, D., Chang, P., Zhang, Q., Reddy, P., Bokoch, G., Greenberg, S., Requirements for both Rac1 and Cdc42 in membrane ruffling and phagocytosis in leukocytes, *J. Exp. Med.*, 186, 1487, 1997.

38. Cresswell, P., Assembly, transport, and function of MHC class II molecules, *Annu. Rev. Immunol.*, 12, 259, 1994.
39. Wolf, P. R., Ploegh, H. L., How MHC class II molecules acquire peptide cargo: biosynthesis and trafficking through the endocytic pathway, *Annu. Rev. Cell Dev. Biol.*, 11, 267, 1995.
40. Mellman, I., Endocytosis and molecular sorting, *Annu. Rev. Cell Dev. Biol.*, 12, 575, 1996.
41. van den Elsen, P. J., Gobin, S. J. P., van Eggermond, M. C., Peijnenburg, A., Regulation of MHC class I and II gene transcription: differences and similarities, *Immunogenetics*, 48, 208, 1998.
42. Otten, L. A., Steimle, V., Bontron, S., Mach, B., Quantitative control of MHC class II expression by the transactivator CIITA, *Eur. J. Immunol.*, 28, 473, 1998.
43. Cresswell, P., Invariant chain structure and MHC class II function, *Cell*, 84, 505, 1996.
44. Saudrais, C., Spehner, D., de la Salle, H., Bohbot, A., Cazenave, J. P., Goud, B., Hanau, D., Salamero, J., Intracellular pathway for the generation of functional MHC class II peptide complexes in immature human dendritic cells, *J. Immunol.*, 160, 2597, 1998.
45. Kleijmeer, M. J., Oorschot, V. M., Geuze, H. J., Human resident langerhans cells display a lysosomal compartment enriched in MHC class II, *J. Invest. Dermatol.*, 103, 516, 1994.
46. Kleijmeer, M. J., Ossevoort, M. A., van Veen, C. J., van Hellemond, J. J., Neefjes, J. J., Kast, W. M., Melief, C. J., Geuze, H. J., MHC class II compartments and the kinetics of antigen presentation in activated mouse spleen dendritic cells, *J. Immunol.*, 154, 5715, 1995.
47. Nijman, H., Kleijmeer, M., Ossevoort, M., Oorschot, V., Vierboom, M., van de Keur, M., Kenemans, P., Kast, W., Geuze, H., Melief, C., Antigen capture and MHC class II compartments of freshly isolated and cultured human blood dendritic cells, *J. Exp. Med.*, 182, 163, 1995.
48. Mommaas, A., Mulder, A., Out, C., Girolomoni, G., Koerten, H., Vermeer, B., Koning, F., Distribution of HLA class II molecules in epidermal Langerhans cells in situ, *Eur. J. Immunol.*, 25, 520, 1995.
49. Kleijmeer, M., Morkowski, S., Griffith, J., Rudensky, A., Geuze, H., MHC class II compartments in human and mouse B lymphoblasts represent conventional endocytic compartments, *J. Cell Biol.*, 139, 639, 1997.
50. Pierre, P., Turley, S. J., Gatti, E., Hull, M., Meltzer, J., Mirza, A., Inaba, K., Steinman, R. M., Mellman, I., Developmental regulation of MHC class II transport in mouse dendritic cells, *Nature*, 388, 787, 1997.
51. Rovere, P., Zimmermann, V. S., Forquet, F., Demandolx, D., Trucy, J., Ricciardi-Castagnoli, P., Davoust, J., Dendritic cell maturation and antigen presentation in the absence of invariant chain, *Proc. Natl. Acad. Sci. U.S.A.*, 95, 1067, 1998.
52. Brachet, V., Raposo, G., Amigorena, S., Mellman, I., Ii chain controls the transport of MHC class II molecules to and from lysosomes, *J. Cell Biol.*, 137, 51, 1997.
53. Villadangos, J., Riese, R., Peters, C., Chapman, H., Ploegh, H., Degradation of mouse invariant chain: roles of cathepsins S and D and the influence of MHC polymorphism, *J. Exp. Med.*, 186, 549, 1997.
54. Coulombe, R., Grochulski, P., Sivaraman, J., Menard, R., Mort, J., Cygler, M., Structure of human procathepsin L reveals the molecular basis of inhibition by the prosegment, *EMBO J.*, 15, 5492, 1996.
55. Sealy, L., Mota, F., Rayment, N., Tatnell, P., Kay, J., Chain, B., Regulation of cathepsin E expression during human B cell differentiation in vitro, *Eur. J. Immunol.*, 26, 1838, 1996.
56. Riese, R. J., Wolf, P. R., Bromme, D., Natkin, L. R., Villadangos, J. A., Ploegh, H. L., Chapman, H. A., Essential role for cathepsin S in MHC class II-associated invariant chain processing and peptide loading, *Immunity*, 4, 357, 1996
57. Riese, R. J., Mitchell, R. N., Villadangos, J. A., Shi, G. P., Palmer, J. T., Karp, E. R., De Sanctis, G. T., Ploegh, H. L., Chapman, H. A., Cathepsin S activity regulates antigen presentation and immunity, *J. Clin. Invest.*, 101, 2351, 1998.
58. Cella, M., Engering, A., Pinet, V., Pieters, J., Lanzavecchia, A., Inflammatory stimuli induce accumulation of MHC class II complexes on dendritic cells, *Nature*, 388, 782, 1997.
59. Flohe, S., Lang, T., Moll, H., Synthesis, stability, and subcellular distribution of MHC class II molecules in Langerhans cells infected with Leishmania major, *Infect. Immun.*, 65, 3444, 1997.
60. Pierre, P., Mellman, I., Developmental regulation of invariant chain proteolysis controls MHC class II trafficking in mouse dendritic cells, *Cell*, 93, 1135, 1998.
61. Maurer, D., Fiebiger, E., Reininger, B., Ebner, C., Petzelbauer, P., Shi, G. P., Chapman, H. A., Stingl, G., Fc epsilon receptor I on dendritic cells delivers IgE-bound multivalent antigens into a cathepsin S-dependent pathway of MHC class II presentation, *J. Immunol.*, 161, 2731, 1998.

62. Sukhova, G. K., Shi, G. P., Simon, D. I., Chapman, H. A., Libby, P., Expression of the elastolytic cathepsins S and K in human atheroma and regulation of their production in smooth muscle cells, *J. Clin. Invest.*, 102, 576, 1998.

63. Bevec, T., Stoka, V., Pungercic, G., Dolenc, I., Turk, V., MHC class II-associated p41 invariant chain fragment is a strong inhibitor of lysosomal cathepsin L, *J. Exp. Med.*, 183, 1331, 1996.

64. Fineschi, B., Sakaguchi, K., Appella, E., Miller, J., The proteolytic environment involved in MHC class II-restricted antigen presentation can be modulated by the p41 form of invariant chain, *J. Immunol.*, 157, 3211, 1996.

65. Nakagawa, T., Roth, W., Wong, P., Nelson, A., Farr, A., Deussing, J., Villadangos, J. A., Ploegh, H., Peters, C., Rudensky, A. Y., Cathepsin L: critical role in Ii degradation and CD4 T cell selection in the thymus, *Science*, 280, 450, 1998.

66. Cresswell, P., Proteases, processing, and thymic selection, *Science*, 280, 394, 1998.

67. Liou, W., Geuze, H. J., Geelen, M. J., Slot, J. W., The autophagic and endocytic pathways converge at the nascent autophagic vacuoles, *J. Cell Biol.*, 136, 61, 1997.

68. Cuervo, A. M., Dice, J. F., A receptor for the selective uptake and degradation of proteins by lysosomes, *Science*, 273, 501, 1996.

69. Roche, N., Chinet, T. C., Huchon, G. J., Allergic and nonallergic interactions between house dust mite allergens and airway mucosa, *Eur. Respir. J.*, 10, 719, 1997.

70. Lehrer, S. B., Reese, G., Recombinant proteins in newly developed foods: identification of allergenic activity, *Int. Arch. Allergy Immunol.*, 113, 122, 1997.

71. Kropshofer, H., Arndt, S., Moldenhauer, G., Hammerling, G., Vogt, A., HLA-DM acts as a molecular chaperone and rescues empty HLA-DR molecules at lysosomal pH, *Immunity*, 6, 293, 1997.

72. Kropshofer, H., Hammerling, G., Vogt, A., How HLA-DM edits the MHC class II peptide repertoire: survival of the fittest?, *Immunol. Today*, 18, 77, 1997.

73. Fung-Leung, W., Surh, C., Liljedahl, M., Pang, J., Leturcq, D., Peterson, P., Webb, S., Karlsson, L., Antigen presentation and T cell development in H2-M-deficient mice, *Science*, 271, 1278, 1996.

74. Miyazaki, T., Wolf, P., Tourne, S., Waltzinger, C., Dierich, A., Barois, N., Ploegh, H., Benoist, C., Mathis, D., Mice lacking H2-M complexes, enigmatic elements of the MHC class II peptide-loading pathway, *Cell*, 84, 531, 1996.

75. Denzin, L. K., Hammond, C., Cresswell, P., HLA-DM interactions with intermediates in HLA-DR maturation and a role for HLA-DM in stabilizing empty HLA-DR molecules, *J. Exp. Med.*, 184, 2153, 1996.

76. Ramachandra, L., Kovats, S., Eastman, S., Rudensky, A. Y., Variation in HLA-DM expression influences conversion of MHC class II αβ:class II-associated invariant chain peptide complexes to mature peptide-bound class II αβ dimers in a normal B cell line, *J. Immunol.*, 156, 2196, 1996.

77. Denzin, L. K., Sant'Angelo, D. B., Hammond, C., Surman, M. J., Cresswell, P., Negative regulation by HLA-DO of MHC class II-restricted antigen processing, *Science*, 278, 106, 1997.

78. Kropshofer, H., Vogt, A. B., Thery, C., Armandola, E. A., Li, B. C., Moldenhauer, G., Amigorena, S., Hammerling, G. J., A role for HLA-DO as a co-chaperone of HLA-DM in peptide loading of MHC class II molecules, *EMBO J.*, 17, 2971, 1998.

79. Thery, C., Brachet, V., Regnault, A., Rescigno, M., Ricciardi-Castagnoli, P., Bonnerot, C., Amigorena, S., MHC class II transport from lysosomal compartments to the cell surface is determined by stable peptide binding, but not by the cytosolic domains of the α- and β-chains, *J. Immunol.*, 161, 2106, 1998.

80. Pond, L., Watts, C., Characterization of transport of newly assembled, T cell-stimulatory MHC class II-peptide complexes from MHC class II compartments to the cell surface, *J. Immunol.*, 159, 543, 1997.

81. Raposo, G., Nijman, H., Stoorvogel, W., Liejendekker, R., Harding, C., Melief, C., Geuze, H., B lymphocytes secrete antigen-presenting vesicles, *J. Exp. Med.*, 183, 1161, 1996.

82. Wubbolts, R., Fernandez-Borja, M., Oomen, L., Verwoerd, D., Janssen, H., Calafat, J., Tulp, A., Dusseljee, S., Neefjes, J., Direct vesicular transport of MHC class II molecules from0 lysosomal structures to the cell surface, *J. Cell Biol.*, 135, 611, 1996.

83. Lindner, R., Unanue, E. R., Distinct antigen MHC class II complexes generated by separate processing pathways, *EMBO J.*, 15, 6910, 1996.

84. Pamer, E., Cresswell, P., Mechanisms of MHC class I-restricted antigen processing, *Annu. Rev. Immunol.*, 16, 323, 1998.

85. Prasad, S., Yewdell, J., Porgador, A., Sadasivan, B., Cresswell, P., Bennink, J., Calnexin expression does not enhance the generation of MHC class I-peptide complexes, *Eur. J. Immunol.*, 28, 907, 1998.

86. Elliott, T., How does TAP associate with MHC class I molecules?, *Immunol. Today*, 18, 375, 1997.

87. Ortmann, B., Copeman, J., Lehner, P., Sadasivan, B., Herberg, J., Grandea, A., Riddell, S., Tampe, R., Spies, T., Trowsdale, J., Cresswell, P., A critical role for tapasin in the assembly and function of multimeric MHC class I-TAP complexes, *Science*, 277, 1306, 1997.

88. Solheim, J., Harris, M., Kindle, C., Hansen, T., Prominence of β2-microglobulin, class I heavy chain conformation, and tapasin in the interactions of class I heavy chain with calreticulin and the transporter associated with antigen processing, *J. Immunol.*, 158, 2236, 1997.

89. Androlewicz, M. J., Cresswell, P., How selective is the transporter associated with antigen processing?, *Immunity*, 5, 1, 1996.

90. Koopmann, J. O., Hammerling, G. J., Momburg, F., Generation, intracellular transport and loading of peptides associated with MHC class I molecules, *Curr. Opin. Immunol.*, 9, 80, 1997.

91. Neisig, A., Wubbolts, R., Zang, X., Melief, C., Neefjes, J., Allele-specific differences in the interaction of MHC class I molecules with transporters associated with antigen processing, *J. Immunol.*, 156, 3196, 1996.

92. Hughes, E. A., Ortmann, B., Surman, M., Cresswell, P., The protease inhibitor, N-acetyl-L-leucyl-L-leucyl-leucyl-L-norleucinal, decreases the pool of MHC class I-binding peptides and inhibits peptide trimming in the endoplasmic reticulum, *J. Exp. Med.*, 183, 1569, 1996.

93. Bresnahan, P. A., Barber, L., Brodsky, F. M., Localization of class I histocompatibility molecule assembly by subfractionation of the early secretory pathway, *Hum. Immunol.*, 53, 129, 1997.

94. Machold, R., Ploegh, H., Intermediates in the assembly and degradation of class I MHC molecules probed with free heavy chain-specific monoclonal antibodies, *J. Exp. Med.*, 184, 2251, 1996.

95. Baumeister, W., Walz, J., Zuhl, F., Seemuller, E., The proteasome: paradigm of a self-compartmentalizing protease, *Cell*, 92, 367, 1998.

96. Yang, B., Hahn, Y. S., Hahn, C. S., Braciale, T. J., The requirement for proteasome activity class I MHC antigen presentation is dictated by the length of preprocessed antigen, *J. Exp. Med.*, 183, 1545, 1996.

97. Lee, D. H., Goldberg, A. L., Proteasome inhibitors: valuable new tools for cell biologists, *Trends Cell Biol.*, 8, 397, 1998.

98. Rock, K. L., A new foreign policy: MHC class I molecules monitor the outside world, *Immunol. Today*, 17, 131, 1996.

99. Jondal, M., Schirmbeck, R., Reimann, J., MHC class I-restricted CTL responses to exogenous antigens, *Immunity*, 5, 295, 1996.

100. Albert, M. L., Sauter, B., Bhardwaj, N., Dendritic cells acquire antigen from apoptotic cells and induce class I-restricted CTLs, *Nature*, 392, 86, 1998.

101. Carbone, F. R., Kurts, C., Bennett, S. R., Miller, J. F., Heath, W. R., Cross-presentation: a general mechanism for CTL immunity and tolerance, *Immunol. Today*, 19, 368, 1998.

102. Malaviya, R., Twesten, N., Ross, E., Abraham, S., Pfeifer, J. D., Mast cells process bacterial Ags through a phagocytic route for class I MHC presentation to T cells, *J. Immunol.*, 156, 1490, 1996.

103. Ke, Y., Kapp, J. A., Exogenous antigens gain access to the MHC class I processing pathway in B cells by receptor-mediated uptake, *J. Exp. Med.*, 184, 1179, 1996.

104. Bachmann, M. F., Lutz, M. B., Layton, G. T., Harris, S. J., Fehr, T., Rescigno, M., Ricciardi-Castagnoli, P., Dendritic cells process exogenous viral proteins and virus-like particles for class I presentation to CD8+ cytotoxic T lymphocytes, *Eur. J. Immunol.*, 26, 2595, 1996.

105. Shen, Z., Reznikoff, G., Dranoff, G., Rock, K. L., Cloned dendritic cells can present exogenous antigens on both MHC class I and class II molecules, *J. Immunol.*, 158, 2723, 1997.

106. Svensson, M., Stockinger, B., Wick, M. J., Bone marrow-derived dendritic cells can process bacteria for MHC-I and MHC-II presentation to T cells, *J. Immunol.*, 158, 4229, 1997.

107. Mitchell, D. A., Nair, S. K., Gilboa, E., Dendritic cell/macrophage precursors capture exogenous antigen for MHC class I presentation by dendritic cells, *Eur. J. Immunol.*, 28, 1923, 1998.

108. Song, R., Harding, C. V., Roles of proteasomes, transporter for antigen presentation (TAP), and beta 2-microglobulin in the processing of bacterial or particulate antigens via an alternate class I MHC processing pathway, *J. Immunol.*, 156, 4182, 1996.

109. Wick, M. J., Pfeifer, J. D., MHC class I presentation of ovalbumin peptide 257-264 from exogenous sources: protein context influences the degree of TAP-independent presentation, *Eur. J. Immunol.*, 26, 2790, 1996.

110. Norbury, C., Chambers, B., Prescott, A., Ljunggren, H., Watts. C., Constitutive macropinocytosis allows TAP-dependent MHC class I presentation of exogenous soluble antigen by bone marrow-derived dendritic cells, *Eur. J. Immunol.*, 27, 280, 1997.

111. Rescigno, M., Citterio, S., Thery, C., Rittig, M., Medaglini, D., Pozzi, G., Amigorena, S., Ricciardi-Castagnoli, P., Bacteria-induced neo-biosynthesis, stabilization, and surface expression of functional class I molecules in mouse dendritic cells, *Proc. Natl. Acad. Sci. U.S.A.*, 95, 5229, 1998.

112. Nieland, T. J., Tan, M. C., Monne-van Muijen, M., Koning, F., Kruisbeek, A. M., van Bleek, G. M., Isolation of an immunodominant viral peptide that is endogenously bound to the stress protein GP96/GRP94, *Proc. Natl. Acad. Sci. U.S.A.*, 93, 6135, 1996.

113. Suto, R., Srivastava, P. K., A mechanism for the specific immunogenicity of heat shock protein-chaperoned peptides, *Science*, 269, 1585, 1995.

114. Schirmbeck, R., Reimann, J., 'Empty' Ld molecules capture peptides from endocytosed hepatitis B surface antigen particles for MHC class I-restricted presentation, *Eur. J. Immunol.*, 26, 2812, 1996.

115. Cook, J., Myers, N., Hansen, T., The mechanisms of peptide exchange and beta 2-microglobulin exchange on cell surface Ld and Kb molecules are noncooperative, *J. Immunol.*, 157, 2256, 1996.

116. Vigna, J. L., Smith, K. D., Lutz, C. T., Invariant chain association with MHC class I: preference for HLA class I/beta 2-microglobulin heterodimers, specificity, and influence of the MHC peptide-binding groove, *J. Immunol.*, 157, 4503, 1996.

117. Porcelli, S. A., Segelke, B. W., Sugita, M., Wilson, I. A., Brenner, M. B., The CD1 family of lipid antigen-presenting molecules, *Immunol. Today*, 19, 362, 1998.

118. Furue, M., Nindl, M., Kawabe, K., Nakamura, K., Ishibashi, Y., Sagawa, K., Epitope mapping of CD1a, CD1b, and CD1c antigens in human skin: differential localization on Langerhans cells, keratinocytes, and basement membrane zone, *J. Invest. Dermatol.*, 99, 23S, 1992.

119. Meunier, L., Gonzalez-Ramos, A., Cooper, K. D., Heterogeneous populations of class II MHC+ cells in human dermal cell suspensions. Identification of a small subset responsible for potent dermal antigen-presenting cell activity with features analogous to Langerhans cells, *J. Immunol.*, 151, 4067, 1993.

120. Elder, J. T., Reynolds, N. J., Cooper, K. D., Griffiths, C. E., Hardas, B. D., Bleicher, P. A., CD1 gene expression in human skin, *J. Dermatol. Sci.*, 6, 206, 1993.

121. Kasinrerk, W., Baumruker, T., Majdic, O., Knapp, W., Stockinger, H., CD1 molecule expression on human monocytes induced by GM-CSF, *J. Immunol.*, 150, 579, 1993.

122. Herbst, B., Kohler, G., Mackensen, A., Veelken, H., Kulmburg, P., Rosenthal, F. M., Schaefer, H. E., Mertelsmann, R., Fisch, P., Lindemann, A., In vitro differentiation of CD34+ hematopoietic progenitor cells toward distinct dendritic cell subsets of the birbeck granule and MIIC-positive Langerhans cell and the interdigitating dendritic cell type, *Blood*, 88, 2541, 1996.

123. Caux, C., Massacrier, C., Vanbervliet, B., Dubois, B., Durand, I., Cella, M., Lanzavecchia, A., Banchereau, J., CD34+ hematopoietic progenitors from human cord blood differentiate along two independent dendritic cell pathways in response to GM-CSF plus TNF-α: II. Functional analysis, *Blood*, 90, 1458, 1997.

124. Zeng, Z., Castano, A., Segelke, B., Stura, E., Peterson, P., Wilson, I., Crystal structure of mouse CD1: an MHC-like fold with a large hydrophobic binding groove, *Science*, 277, 339, 1997.

125. Castano, A., Tangri, S., Miller, J. E., Holcombe, H. R., Jackson, M. R., Huse, W., Kronenberg, M., Peterson, P. A., Peptide binding and presentation by mouse CD1, *Science*, 269, 223, 1995.

126. Fairhurst, R. M., Wang, C. X., Sieling, P. A., Modlin, R. L., Braun, J., CD1-restricted T cells and resistance to polysaccharide-encapsulated bacteria, *Immunol. Today*, 19, 257, 1998.

127. Beckman, E. M., Porcelli, S. A., Morita, C. T., Behar, S. M., Furlong, S. T., Brenner, M. B., Recognition of a lipid antigen by CD1-restricted αβ+ T cells, *Nature*, 372, 691, 1994.

128. Sieling, P. A., Chatterjee, D., Porcelli, S. A., Prigozy, T. I., Mazzaccaro, R. J., Soriano, T., Bloom, B. R., Brenner, M. B., Kronenberg, M., Brennan, P. J., et al., CD1-restricted T cell recognition of microbial lipoglycan antigens, *Science*, 269, 227, 1995.

129. Moody, D., Reinhold, B. B., Guy, M., Beckman, E. M., Frederique, D. E., Furlong, S. T., Ye, S., Reinhold, V. N., Sieling, P. A., Modlin, R. L., Besra, G., Porcelli, S. A., Structural requirements for glycolipid antigen recognition by CD1b-restricted T cells, *Science*, 278, 283, 1997.

130. Beckman, E. M., Melian, A., Behar, S. M., Sieling, P. A., Chatterjee, D., Furlong, S. T., Matsumoto, R., Rosat, J. P., Modlin, R. L., Porcelli, S. A., CD1c restricts responses of mycobacteria-specific T cells. Evidence for antigen presentation by a second member of the human CD1 family, *J. Immunol.*, 157, 2795, 1996.

131. Sugita, M., Porcelli, S. A., Brenner, M. B., Assembly and retention of CD1b heavy chains in the endoplasmic reticulum, *J. Immunol.*, 159, 2358, 1997.

132. Sugita, M., Jackman, R. M., van Donselaar, E., Behar, S. M., Rogers, R. A., Peters, P. J., Brenner, M. B., Porcelli, S. A., Cytoplasmic tail-dependent localization of CD1b antigen-presenting molecules to MIICs, *Science*, 273, 349, 1996.

133. Jackman, R. M., Stenger, S., Lee, A., Moody, D. B., Rogers, R. A., Niazi, K. R., Sugita, M., Modlin, R. L., Peters, P. J., Porcelli, S. A., The tyrosine-containing cytoplasmic tail of CD1b is essential for its efficient presentation of bacterial lipid antigens, *Immunity*, 8, 341, 1998.

134. Ernst, W. A., Maher, J., Cho, S., Niazi, K. R., Chatterjee, D., Moody, D. B., Besra, G. S., Watanabe, Y., Jensen, P. E., Porcelli, S. A., Kronenberg, M., Modlin, R. L., Molecular interaction of CD1b with lipoglycan antigens, *Immunity*, 8, 331, 1998.

135. Weiss, J. M., Sleeman, J., Renkl, A. C., Dittmar, H., Termeer, C. C., Taxis, S., Howells, N., Hofmann, M., Kohler, G., Schöpf, E., Ponta, H., Herrlich, P., Simon, J. C., An essential role for CD44 variant isoforms in epidermal Langerhans cell and blood dendritic cell function, *J. Cell Biol.*, 137, 1137, 1997.

136. Ingulli, E., Mondino, A., Khoruts, A., Jenkins, M. K., In vivo detection of dendritic cell antigen presentation to CD4(+) T cells, *J. Exp. Med.*, 185, 2133, 1997.

137. Roake, J., Rao, A., Morris, P., Larsen, C., Hankins, D., Austyn, J., Dendritic cell loss from nonlymphoid tissues after systemic administration of LPS, TNF, and IL-1, *J. Exp. Med.*, 181, 2237, 1995.

138. Thompson, C. B., Allison, J. P., The emerging role of CTLA-4 as an immune attenuator, *Immunity*, 7, 445, 1997.

139. Shaw, A. S., Dustin, M. L., Making the T cell receptor go the distance: a topological view of T cell activation, *Immunity*, 6, 361, 1997.

140. Nestle, F. O., Alijagic, S., Gilliet, M., Sun, Y., Grabbe, S., Dummer, R., Burg, G., Schadendorf, D., Vaccination of melanoma patients with peptide- or tumor lysate-pulsed dendritic cells, *Nat. Med.*, 4, 328, 1998.

9 The Keratinocyte in Cutaneous Irritation and Sensitization

Alain Coquette, Nancy Berna, Yves Poumay, and Mark R. Pittelkow

CONTENTS

I. INTRODUCTION

Epithelial tissues, including epidermis, tracheobronchial epithelium of lung, gastrointestinal epithelium, and uterine cervical epithelium, play a critical role in protecting man and other mammals from external environmental threats. Epithelial cells such as epidermal keratinocytes have long been known to provide a relatively impermeable barrier to outside factors that challenge the structural integrity and resilience of epidermis and other epithelia. However, only more recently have we discovered the active role played by the keratinocyte in initiating, modulating, and regulating responses of the skin as well as organism to the multitude of irritant or allergic (sensitizing) reactions that are part of daily existence. Keratinocytes express and, in some cases, secrete a plethora of biologically active molecules that mediate these responses. As the identification and biological function(s) of factors produced by keratinocytes continue to expand, the complexity and functional sophistication of epidermis become more apparent.

This chapter provides an overview and update on the role of the keratinocyte in cutaneous irritant and sensitization reactions. These findings significantly impact how skin reactions in dermal and transdermal delivery can be biochemically modulated. We also summarize various models that have been developed to better assess and predict epidermal irritation and sensitization. The cellular and molecular mechanisms mediating these responses in man will also be delineated.

The epidermis is a multilayered squamous epithelium that forms the interface between the organism and its environment. It is composed of several types of specialized resident or transient epithelial, neuroectodermal, and bone marrow-derived cells. These include epidermal keratinocytes to generate the protective barrier and provide for repair and regeneration of the epidermis, Langerhans cells, and T lymphocytes (T cells) for immunologic defense, melanocytes for pigment production and protection from ultraviolet radiation, and Merkel cells for neurocutaneous sensibility. Keratinocytes constitute the major cell type (>90%) and thus have the primary biologic role in providing both physical and biochemical attributes that maintain epidermal integrity and homeostasis. Epidermal keratinocytes also create a sentry function and compose the first level of communication with neighboring skin cells as well as other distant organs.[1]

The keratinocyte elaborates its protective function by undergoing a complex and finely coordinated program of cellular differentiation.[2] The basal layer consists of a single layer of proliferative and noncommitted keratinocytes, a fraction of which are functionally stem cells. The basal cell layer is anchored to the basal lamina via hemidesmosomes. These basal cells produce daughter cells that can either continue to populate the germinative layer or exit the basal layer to undergo terminal differentiation as they migrate to the epidermal surface. The spinous layer, constituting several or more cell layers, is located immediately above the basal layer and is characterized by the presence of extensive desmosomal connections between cells. The next morphologic layer, the granular layer, is distinguished by the presence of keratohyalin granules within the cytoplasm of the keratinocyte. Keratohyalin granules contain products of keratinocyte differentiation, such as loricrin, filaggrin, cystatin-α, and lipids that are used in the assembly of the corneocyte membrane and intercellular compartment. Another subcellular organelle, the keratinosome or lamellar body, is a specialized secretory vesicle present in the upper spinous and granular layers. Enzymes such as glucosylceramide synthase, lipid substrates/products such as glucocylceramides and sphyingolipids, as well as specialized proteins such as corneodesmosin that make up the corneodesmosomes of the cornified layers, are also present in keratinosomes.[3,4] The transition zone delineates the region between nucleated and anucleate cells in upper epidermal layers. Within this region, selected cellular organelles and nucleic acids are targeted for elimination by the action of specific proteases, nucleases, and other enzymes. The final stage in keratinocyte terminal differentiation results in the formation of the cornified layer. This outermost layer is made up of corneocytes or "bricks" that form a packaged, stabilized array of keratin filaments, proteins, peptides, and other breakdown products contained within a cross-linked protein envelope and united by a lipid-rich intercellular "mortar."

Each stage of epidermal differentiation is characterized by specific biomarkers of gene expression. During normal epidermal differentiation, keratins 5 (K5) and 14 (K14) are expressed in the basal keratinocyte layer, while keratin 1 (K1) and 10 (K10) are expressed in the suprabasal layers. Involucrin is expressed in the late spinous layers and granular layers, and loricrin and filaggrin are specific markers of granular layers.

In the last decade, it has become clear that keratinocytes are not simply a mechanical barrier to the external environment, but are also able to produce a number of cytokines and other mediators with immunologic, inflammatory, and cell-adaptive (e.g., proliferative) properties. Cytokines are relatively small, soluble (glyco)proteins which are synthesized and secreted by various cells, bind to specific receptors, and regulate activation, proliferation, and differentiation of immune as well as nonimmune cells. They include several subclasses, designated: (1) interleukins (IL), (2) colony-stimulating factors (CSF), (3) interferons (IFN), (4) tumor necrosis factor (TNF) family members, (5) growth factors, and (6) suppressor factors.[5,6] Selected cytokines produced by keratinocytes in sensitization or irritation reactions will be reviewed here as well as in Chapter 12. We also will briefly review other keratinocyte-produced factors that mediate these responses. These include arachidonic acid and metabolites, biogenic amines, small molecular weight factors, and second-messenger molecules, as well as nitric oxide (NO) and reactive oxygen species (ROS). Together, these constitutive or inducible gene products and cellular metabolites of the keratinocyte directly or indirectly regulate the epidermal response to irritant or allergic agents contacting skin.

Figure 1 provides a schematic framework depicting the sequence of cellular and biochemical events that induce irritant or sensitization reactions in epidermis. The keratinocyte plays a central role in controlling and coordinating cutaneous responses by other immune and inflammatory cells within and between the epidermis, dermis, and microvasculature.

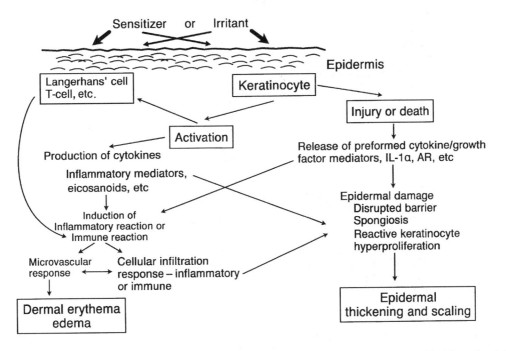

Figure 1   Sequence of events following irritant or sensitizer exposure to epidermis. (Modified from Corsini and Galli, *Toxicol. Lett.*, 102–103, 277–82, 1998.

Numerous protein and nonprotein factors are synthesized and secreted or released by keratinocytes that become "activated" by an irritant or allergen. A current, but inevitably incomplete list of these biologically active factors is presented in Table 1. The function(s) of some of these factors are well characterized while others are less well defined.

An important concept still to be comprehensively addressed for keratinocyte function in irritation and sensitization reactions is the hierarchy and ordering of events that take place within a single cell and the tissue to produce a given response. This concept is also critical for many other epidermal reactions to disease (e.g., psoriasis,[7] dermatitis, viral infections [verrucae-human papillomavirus, etc.]) In this context, some cytokines, such as IL-1 and TNF-α, have been considered to be "primary" cytokines, whereas others, such as IL-6, IL-8, and GM-CSF, are "secondary" since they are insufficient to induce an inflammatory response in the absence of other stimuli or primary cytokines.[8] However, the biological circuitry is no doubt much more complex and will likely require sophisticated mathematical modeling and application of neural network theory to fully describe the biological "output" of the keratinocyte that has been stimulated by an irritant or allergic "input."[9]

II. KERATINOCYTE IRRITATION OR SENSITIZATION:
THE INTEGRATED CELL RESPONSE

As depicted in Figure 1, irritants and allergens (haptens) have the ability to initiate similar responses in epidermis. In fact, irritants and sensitizers have the potential to overlap in their activity profiles; that is, some sensitizers also have irritant properties. The difference lies in the ability of a sensitizer

TABLE 1
Keratinocyte Mediators of Irritation and Sensitization

Cytokines

Primary	C-C chemokines
IL-1α	MCP-1
IL-1β	MIP-1α
TNF-α	RANTES
Humoral/cellular immune regulation	Growth factors
IL-10	TGF-α
IL-12	AR
IL-18	HB-EGF
IFN-α	NDF
IFN-β	VEGF
T cell growth	PDGF
IL-7	NGF
IL-15	FGFs
Colony-stimulating activity	Neurotrophin
IL-6	Suppressive/antagonist
G-CSF	IL-IRA
M-CSF	TGF-β
GM-CSF	IL-10
C-X-C chemokines	
IL-8	
Gro-α, -β, -γ	
IP-10	

Neuroendocrine

α-MSH

Eicosenoids

Arachidonate	12-HETE
PGE-2	LTB$_4$

Oxygen-derived

Nitric oxide (NO)	Superoxide ($O_2{}^{\bullet-}$)
Hydrogen peroxide (H_2O_2)	

to induce a specific immune response with immunological "memory." By contrast, cutaneous irritation is a nonimmunologic, reversible, local inflammatory reaction that induces edema and erythema following a single or repeated epicutaneous exposure to the chemical at a defined skin site.

Upon exposure of the keratinocyte to an irritant or sensitizer, cell injury or cell death (due to sufficiently severe damage induced by agents such as nitrogen or sulfa mustard agents[10]) occurs and triggers a set of responses in the keratinocyte and epidermis. Key to this response is IL-1α release. Loss of barrier function by irritants, such as acetone, a strong delipidizing solvent, also can trigger rapid increase in expression of specific growth factors, such as amphiregulin (AR) and nerve growth factor (NGF).[11]

The keratinocyte becomes "activated" in response to irritant or sensitizer exposure. Specific sets of cytokines, as well as arachidonic acid metabolites and other inflammatory mediators, are expressed and secreted to trigger and modulate the inflammatory reaction. The ability of the keratinocyte to participate in generating effective signals for recruitment of Langerhans cells and T cells and propagating the afferent immune response places it within the central hub of the skin immune system (SIS).

Whether induced by an irritant or a sensitizer, similar morphologic and histologic features of erythema, edema, and epidermal scaling and thickening (acanthosis) are observed. Chapters 6, 7, and 10 delineate the unique roles of the Langerhans cell and the T cell in the epidermal immune response and allergic contact dermatitis.

In addition to expressing and releasing potent cytokines and other inflammatory mediators, the keratinocyte also modulates expression of various immune and nonimmune related cell surface receptors, cell adhesion molecules, and extracellular matrix (ECM) factors. These cell-associated molecules likely play important roles in orchestrating the keratinocyte response during irritant and sensitization reactions. These gene products include ICAM-1, HLA-DR, receptors of growth factor and other cytokine families, integrins, cadherins, fibronectin, heparin sulfate and related proteoglycans, and numerous other cell–cell and ligand–receptor factors.

Intracellular signaling pathways of the keratinocyte are only beginning to be identified, assembled, and integrated into an intricate stimulus–response network that mediates irritant and sensitizer reactions in skin. The keratinocyte has the potential to either upregulate or downregulate a specific cutaneous response. For example, ultraviolet (UV) radiation induces cytokine cascades that have the ability to induce systemic immune suppression.[12] We have recently shown that H_2O_2 and other ROS induced in human keratinocytes by UVB rapidly, but transiently, enhance epidermal growth factor (EGF) receptor phosphorylation and differentially activate downstream protein kinase signaling pathways, including extracellular regulated kinase (ERK), p38, and c-jun N-terminal kinase (JNK), critical kinases of mitogen- and stress-related cascades in keratinocytes.[13,14] These pathways, in part, terminate in the nucleus where specific transcription factors such as activator protein (AP)-1, AP-2, γ-interferon activation site (GAS), NF-κβ, EGR, etc. regulate gene expression within the keratinocyte and many other cell types. In this regard, glucocorticoids are also known to be potent inhibitors of the inflammatory response. Recent studies have demonstrated that these steroid hormones strongly inhibit AP1, GAS, and NF-κβ DNA-binding activities and induction of the arachidonic acid metabolizing enzyme, cyclooxygenase-2 (COX-2), in IL-1β-stimulated keratinocytes.[15]

These findings link cytokines and other inflammatory mediators to signaling pathways that "activate" the keratinocyte, but also demonstrate that keratinocyte responses can be downregulated by UV or glucocorticoids, well known and potent modulators of cutaneous irritation and sensitization (see also Chapters 15 and 20).

In the following sections, we provide a concise review of selected cytokines and other inflammatory mediators produced by keratinocytes that regulate cutaneous sensitization and irritancy. This chapter also examines the progress and comparative evaluation of in vitro models to test irritants and sensitizers using keratinocytes or more complex multicellular systems.

III. KERATINOCYTE ELABORATED MEDIATORS

A. INTERLEUKIN 1 (IL-1)

IL-1 was originally described as a lymphocyte-activating factor produced only by monocytes. However, it is now well established that many cells, including epithelial cells, endothelial cells, fibroblasts, and various tumor cells, produce IL-1.[16] Two different forms of IL-1, IL-1α and IL-1β, encoded by distinct genes, have been identified. These two forms bind to the same two IL-1 receptor types, suggesting they have similar biological activities. IL-1α and IL-1β are synthesized as larger "pro-interleukins," which in the case of IL-1β must be cleaved by a specific converting enzyme to the shorter biologically active form. IL-1α is also cleaved, but this does not seem to be necessary for its activity. Keratinocytes are able to synthesize and secrete both forms of IL-1, but the predominant biologically active form released by keratinocytes is IL-1α,[17] since keratinocytes lack constitutive IL-1β converting enzyme (ICE) activity. However, ICE activity is induced in keratinocytes by both irritant chemicals and sensitizers, such as urushiol.[18] IL-1β activation may be induced in epidermis in vivo by a non-ICE mechanism.[19] This contrasts with observations in vitro suggesting lack of IL-1β processing.[20] IL-1α appears to be retained intracellularly or in a membrane-bound form. As long as the epidermis is intact, IL-1 is eliminated by normal desquamation. Because IL-1 lacks a hydrophobic leader sequence necessary for transmembrane secretion, it has been proposed that it only can be released after some type of cell injury or membrane perturbation.[16] In human skin, the levels of IL-1 are 100 to 1000 times higher than in most other tissues. Keratinocytes are able to produce it constitutively without stimulation. Upregulation of IL-1 synthesis has been observed upon stimulation with lipopolysaccharides (LPS), phorbol myristic acetate (PMA), physical, chemical, or thermal injury, ultraviolet irradiation, and a variety of cytokines (i.e., GM-CSF, TNF-α, IL-6, TGF-α, and IL-1α and IL-1β itself).[21] Interestingly, IL-β appears to be specifically induced by hapten within 1 to 3 h of exposure, whereas IL-1α mRNA is not induced by either hapten or primary irritants, as measured by reverse transcriptase-polymerase chain reaction (RT-PCR).[22] Furthermore, IL-1β induces Langerhans cell migration out of epidermis and neutralizing antibody to IL-β, but not IL-1α, TNF-α, or GM-CSF, prevented allergen-induced migration of Langerhans cells, suggesting that IL-1β plays a role in irritation of contact hypersensitivity.[23] The effects of IL-1 are highly pleiotropic and space limits delineation of all of its biological effects. For further detailed information on IL-1, see Chapter 12.

IL-1 is a proinflammatory cytokine. It is chemotactic for monocytes, lymphocytes, and neutrophils. It stimulates the proliferation, differentiation, and activation of various cells and the production of other cytokines such as GM-CSF, IL-6, and IL-8. Keratinocytes, in addition to producing IL-1, express large amounts of specific IL-1 receptors and IL-1 receptor antagonists (IL-1ra).[24] This antagonist binds to the same receptor as IL-1, but it does not produce cell activation and so acts as a competitive inhibitor to prevent IL-1 effects unless IL-1 exceeds certain threshold levels. The reader is referred to Chapter 14 for further information on IL-1 and IL-1ra effects.

B. INTERLEUKIN 6 (IL-6)

IL-6 is a multifunctional cytokine released by many different cells, including monocytes, fibroblasts, endothelial cells, keratinocytes, and different tumor cells.[25] Unstimulated keratinocytes usually produce low levels of IL-6, but expression can be upregulated by the addition of stimulants such as IL-1, LPS, PMA, or UV-B irradiation, TNF-α, GM-CSF, IL-4, TGF-β, and injury.[6] Like IL-1, IL-6 has a variety of biological activities on different target cells. Many biological effects of IL-1 and IL-6 overlap. IL-6 may augment proliferation of keratinocytes. Moreover, some evidence suggests that IL-6 plays a role as mediator in inflammatory skin diseases such as psoriasis.[21] Compared to other cytokines and growth factors, the potency of IL-6 in these responses is less pronounced and likely secondary.

C. INTERLEUKIN 8 (IL-8)

In addition to monocytes, a variety of cells including endothelial cells, keratinocytes, fibroblasts, and T lymphocytes produce IL-8.[26] Keratinocytes do not produce IL-8 constitutively, but the production is stimulated by other cytokines (IL-1α, IL-1β, TNF-α, and IFN-γ), LPS, and phorbol esters.[27] IL-8 is strongly chemotactic for polymorphonuclear neutrophils and lymphocytes, increases cytosolic free calcium, and induces granule exocytosis.[28] IL-8 is also chemotactic for human basophils and stimulates them to release histamine.[27] Therefore, IL-8 is also classified as a potent chemokine of the C-X-C class.[26]

D. INTERLEUKIN 10 (IL-10)

Originally described as a product of bone marrow-derived cells, IL-10 is also produced by activated murine keratinocytes.[29] IL-10 is known to be an anti-inflammatory cytokine and may act as a suppressor factor of immune reactions. IL-10 expression is enhanced in UV-treated keratinocytes, and hapten-specific tolerance induced by UVB is mediated by IL-10.[30] It may inhibit the production of cytokines such as IFN-γ, IL-1, and TNF-α. By inhibiting IFN-γ production by Th1 cells, it promotes induction of a Th2 response. One role of IL-10 may be to prevent severe damage to the skin by reducing the risk of necrosis by an ongoing inflammatory process.

E. INTERLEUKIN 12 (IL-12)

IL-12 is a heterodimeric protein and a potent costimulator of Th1 cells that are involved in cutaneous sensitization responses. Keratinocytes constitutively express the lower Mr (35 kDa) chain of IL-12 and are induced to express the 40-kDa chain following exposure to contact allergen, but not irritants.[31] IL-12 strongly stimulates T cell proliferation and mediates the primary immune response in skin.

F. INTERLEUKIN 15 (IL-15)

IL-15 has recently been shown to be induced in epidermal keratinocytes by culture and selected cytokines. IL-15 is a potent immunomodulator of T cell-mediated immune responses, similar in function to IL-2, and attracts and activates antigen-specific Th1 cells. IL-15 also stimulates the proinflammatory and antimicrobial properties of neutrophils. Both UVB exposure and corticosteroids downregulate IL-15 expression in keratinocytes.[32]

G. TUMOR NECROSIS ALPHA (TNF-α)

TNF-α is a pleiotropic proinflammatory cytokine that mediates a range of biological responses, including proliferation, apoptosis, and inducing gene responses in TNF receptor-bearing cells. TNF-α also induces inflammation in skin following local synthesis and release or by injection as well as inducing ICAM-1 expression in keratinocytes.[33] Irritants such as SDS and PMA also have been shown to rapidly induce TNF-α expression as well as subsequent inflammation and edema in skin.[34] Selected allergens such as nickel and DNFB also induce TNF-α gene expression and protein in epidermis of sensitized animals.[35]

H. CHEMOKINES — IP-10 ETC.

Chemokines such as interferon-induced protein (IP)-10 and macrophage chemotactic protein (MCP)-1 have been shown to be upregulated in cutaneous delayed-type hypersensitivity reactions and other epidermal responses. Chemokines play an important role in inflammation via T cell chemotactic and adhesion-promoting activities . Interferon-γ strongly stimulates expression of IP-10 in keratinocytes.[36] IP-10 and other selected chemokines expressed by keratinocytes function in the epidermal signaling network to localize and induce specific responses that mediate cutaneous allergic and irritant reactions.

I. MISCELLANEOUS MEDIATORS

Products of the arachidonic acid metabolic pathway (termed "eicosenoids"), as well as arachidonate itself, are potent regulators of inflammation and allergic or irritant epidermal responses. The polyunsaturated fatty acid precursor, arachidonic acid, is produced by the enzymatic action of phospholipases (A_2 or C) on lipids of the cell membrane. In addition to the well-known actions of the cyclooxygenase, lipoxygenase, and monooxygenase metabolites of arachidonate in skin, arachidonic acid itself has been shown to trigger keratinocyte stress-activated responses, such as JNK activation.[37,38] A variety of the early events in skin inflammation are mediated by arachidonic acid and its metabolites. Tumor promoters and other irritants induce arachidonic acid metabolism in skin which may be used as relevant markers for cutaneous irritation.[39,40]

The keratinocyte also generates various free radicals following stimulation by chemical agents, UV radiation, etc. We have recently shown that superoxide and H_2O_2 are rapidly produced and eliminated in keratinocytes following exposure to UVB[13,14] and other agents. These ROS potently regulate levels and activity of phosphorylated proteins and protein kinases within keratinocytes. These mediators may therefore be considered as second messengers mediating irritant or toxic responses in the epidermis.

IV. MODELS OF KERATINOCYTE IRRITANCY AND SENSITIZER TESTING

Human skin irritation and allergic contact dermatitis are common occupational and environmental health problems, resulting from skin exposure to man-made chemicals, waste products, and/or commercially marketed products such as solvents, soaps, organic dyes, cosmetics, pharmaceuticals, and skin protectants. Consequently, it is vital that the potential of a chemical compound to cause dermal irritancy and/or sensitization must be assessed accurately. For this purpose, various animal testing methods have been developed over the decades and have served industry very well. The most widely applied bioassays have been the rabbit skin irritation test,[41] the guinea pig maximization test,[42] the occluded patch test of Buehler,[43] the local lymph node assay,[44] and the mouse ear swelling test.[45] However, major problems of in vivo assays have been identified, including the (1) structural and physiological differences between the skin of rabbit, guinea pig or mouse, and human skin, (2) extrapolation from testing at fixed dose and time of application to the variable conditions of human exposure, (3) subjective nature of multi-end point assessment which can lead to interlaboratory differences, and (4) false-positive and false-negative responses.[46] Finally, when systemic effects of a product are estimated following topical exposure in vivo, metabolism in skin must also be considered. The general lack of data in this category is due to the difficulty in measuring skin metabolism in vivo that requires sampling from skin. Consequently, because of the multitude of problems associated with in vivo protocols as well as other restrictions emerging from ethical issues of animal use, the validity and propriety of in vivo testing methods have been increasingly challenged. As a consequence, in vitro methods offer alternatives to evaluate the interactions between chemical substances and a biological system such as skin and epidermis. Different types of excised skin have been used for in vitro screening studies to test a variety of biological properties, such as percutaneous absorption.[47,48] The major drawback of using this particular model for routine screening purposes is the time necessary to acquire both the specimens and data and the equipment needed to prepare the skin. Therefore, the development of new in vitro models and methods has become a focus of many academic and commercial laboratories. In this review, the usefulness of in vitro skin equivalent models will be illustrated and our experience with a system of human epidermis reconstructed on an inert filter substrate will be summarized.

Keratinocytes grown submerged in culture medium have often been used as in vitro alternatives for testing cutaneous toxicity, and a good correlation between skin irritation, cytotoxicity, and proinflammatory mediators release has been demonstrated.[49,50] However, under these conditions, keratinocytes organize to flattened, loosely associated layers, synthesize a different pattern of polypeptides, only sporadically form keratohyalin granules, and rarely contain lamellar bodies.[51] They lack a normal stratum corneum that acts as a barrier to chemical toxicity and, consequently, fall far short of simulating the in vivo situation. Moreover, these culture models are typically limited to water-soluble compounds.

The development of keratinocyte culture systems using de-epidermized dermis,[52,53] collagen matrix (with or without fibroblasts),[54-56] or inert filters (with or without fibroblasts),[57,58] coupled with living keratinocytes that undergo maturation to form a stratified epidermal tissue at the air–liquid interface, has led to the production of functional human skin equivalent models. They exhibit a considerable greater degree of tissue organization that closely resembles the in vivo state.[51,57,59-61] Over the past few years, different commercially available cultured human skin models have been developed and studied, including: (1) EpiDerm (MatTek Corporation, Ashland, MA), (2) Episkin (SADUC, Chaponost, France), the human reconstructed epidermis from SkinEthic (SkinEthic, Nice, France) with no fibroblasts, (4) Living Skin Equivalent (Organogenesis, Cambridge, MA), and (5) Skin2 (Advanced Tissue Sciences, La Jolla, CA), which are composed of both epithelial cells and fibroblasts.[58,62-65] These cultures exhibit a well-stratified epithelium and cornified epidermis with significantly improved barrier function and metabolic activity.[57,66–68] The presence of a stratum corneum makes it possible to apply topically a wide variety of products and/or complex formulations. Differentiation markers such as suprabasal keratins, integrin $\beta4$, integrin $\alpha6$, fibronectin, involucrin, filaggrin, trichohyalin, type I, III, IV, V, and VII collagen, laminin, heparan sulfate, and membrane-bound transglutaminase have been found to be expressed similar to those of the epidermis.[58,69–71] Moreover, keratin synthesis and the production of cornified envelopes parallels that found in vivo. Spinous cells display abundant glycogen deposit, and keratohyalin granules are more abundant in the granular layer. Both the size and number of hemidesmosomes increase during maturation in vitro and anchoring fibrils are observed.[58,66,69,72–74]

Percutaneous penetration studies performed with human skin recombinant models have revealed that the stratum corneum forms a substantial barrier to ^{3}H-water,[53,63] pindolol, calcitonin,[75] toluene, carbazole, benzopyrene,[63] testosterone,[55,76,77] estradiol,[55] hydrocortisone,[55,76,78] benzoic acid,[15,77] cyclosporine,[79] salicylic acid, provitamin B5, theophylline, and scopolamine.[77] The results obtained are more consistent and reproducible than cadaver skin[79] and correlate well with those recorded for hairless guinea pig skin.[75] Nevertheless, the relative permeability of normal human skin compared to reconstructed skin is different and is likely to vary considerably from one compound to another. A good correlation for one class of chemicals is not necessarily indicative of a similar relationship for other chemicals.[53,55,63,77] This points to an impaired barrier function of reconstructed epidermis in vitro. In fact, despite the similarity in tissue architecture, reconstructed epidermis exhibits some deviations from normal epidermis, depending on the tissue culture method and the source of keratinocytes. Reduction of ceramides 4 to 7 and 6 to 7, integrin overexpression, premature expression of specific differentiation markers, and abnormal lipid composition have been observed under normal in vitro culture conditions.[71,80,81] By using freeze-fracture electron microscopy,[82] X-ray diffraction,[83,84] and confocal laser scanning microscopy,[85] it has been shown that, in some cases, reconstructed epidermis displays abnormalities in lamellar body delivery and extrusion, which manifests itself by a disturbance of the transformation of lamellar bodies into lamellar lipid bilayers by impaired structural organization and distribution of epidermal lipids into the intercellular space.[86,87] Furthermore, by using small-angle X-ray diffraction techniques, it has been shown that the stratum corneum lipids appear to be organized in multilamellar structures with a periodicity of 12 nm[87] in contrast to native epidermis, in which two lamellar phases with periodicities of 6.4 and 13.4 nm are typically detected.[83] Consequently, whereas for native epidermis the penetration pathway is confined only to the extracellular space, diffusion within the stratum corneum in the reconstructed epidermis likely occurs via both extracellular and intracellular pathways.[85] These findings may partially explain the divergent results obtained from various percutaneous penetration studies.

Improvements in the culture conditions, such as maintaining the cultures in delipidized serum, reduction of the relative humidity,[53] and use of chemically defined medium,[57,88] has led to further optimization of these models. Epidermal tissues generated at 33°C in absence of epidermal growth factor,[52,71] and in the presence of vitamin C[71] but absence of retinoic acid,[57,88] improves the stratum corneum architecture and lipid profile. In vitamin C-supplemental medium, the content of glucosylceramides and of ceramides 6 and 7 is markedly increased.[71] In absence of serum, the relative amounts of ceramides, free fatty acids, and cholesterol are comparable to native epidermis.[52] Epidermis reconstructed on fibroblast-populated collagen at 37°C in the presence of EGF has a similar morphology to that of native epidermis. However, irrespective of the culture conditions, involucrin is aberrantly expressed. EGF supplementation has a deleterious effect on epidermal morphogenesis and differentiation. The synthesis of K1 and K10 is suppressed on both protein and mRNA levels.[71]

Since 1990, a fully differentiated epithelium having the features of in vivio epidermis has been obtained in vitro by culturing second-passage normal human keratinocytes in a retinoic acid-free, chemically defined medium MCDB 153 on inert filter substrates exposed to the air–liquid interface for 14 days.[57] In this model, the basal cells synthesize and secrete all major markers of hemidesmosomes as well as components of the lamina lucida. Hemidesmosomes with major dense plaques and anchoring filaments and a basement membrane-like structure were identified, suggesting that the presence of serum and dermal factors is not required.[58] Because of the restricted presence of exogenous growth factors and protein in the medium, this in vitro human living epidermis is approaching the most suitable system for detecting and testing the effects of any product that has the potential to be in contact with epidermis.[58,89]

An advantage of in vitro-reconstructed skin equivalents is the possibility of incorporating various additional cell types alone or in combination with keratinocytes. Recently, the introduction of melanocytes into epidermal reconstructs has expanded potential applications of these models.[90] As in the in vivo state, melanocytes appear as dendritic cells and are located in the basal keratinocyte layer. Melanin has been detected in both the melanocytes and the neighboring keratinocytes. Following UV radiation, increase in the number of dopa-positive melanocytes in the basal layer has been shown that results in increased pigmentation of the irradiated skin equivalent. More recent advances in culture techniques have made it possible to develop reconstructed epidermis containing not only keratinocytes but melanocytes and Langerhans cells as well. Cord blood-derived CD34+ hematopoietic progenitor cells induced to differentiate by GM-CSF and TNF-α were seeded onto a reconstructed epidermis composed of keratinocytes and melanocytes. This culture system gives rise to a reconstructed in vitro model displaying a pigmented epidermis with melanocytes in the basal layer and resident epidermal Langerhans cells located suprabasally and expressing major histocompatibility complex class II, CD1 antigen, and Birbeck granules.[91] It provides an attractive in vitro system to study the regulation of melanogenesis and melanocyte–keratinocyte interactions, and to investigate in a more defined model how these processes are affected by UV irradiation. In addition, this epidermal model can be used to test the phototoxic or photoprotective potential of various compounds as well as sunscreens, which is a distinct advantage over other animal models.

In vitro reconstructed epidermis allows testing of products at concentrations and in formulations that would be used in vivo. In addition, the dose–response relationship can be examined over a wide range of concentrations. Furthermore, the lower part of the tissue is bathed in the culture medium that can be withdrawn for analysis of released mediators. They provide quantifiable and objective end point measurements compared to those in vivo studies where more subjective parameters, such as erythema and edema, are often used. For these reasons, reconstructed human epidermis can be widely exploited for various research purposes, including studies of cutaneous biogenesis and skin wound healing, investigation of the regulation of keratinocyte differentiation, pharmaceutical agent metabolism studies and absorption properties,[63,79,92–95] assessment of cutaneous immunotoxicological response,[61] and responses to irritants[56,58,62,65,69,96–98] and to sensitizers.[99,100]

The end points most frequently used include histological analysis of tissue damage, cell membrane damage estimated by measuring leakage of enzymes such as lactate dehydrogenase (LDH);[56] cell viability determination by MTT conversion[62,65,89,96,101,102] or Neutral Red assay;[101] the modulation of the stratum barrier function and the release of proinflammatory mediators, such as IL-1α,[56,61,62,89,96,103,104] IL-1β, and IL-6,[56,103] IL-8;[56] TNF-α[61] prostaglandins;[56,62,96,105,106] hydroxyeicosanotretaeno (HETEs) and leukotriene B$_4$ (LTB$_4$);[107] plasminogen activator;[96] cytokine mRNA expression;[108–111] antileukoproteinase synthesis;[112] ICAM-1 expression;[81] integrin receptor modulation;[81] measure of intracellular ATP[113] and corneosurfametry.[114]

Upon reaching the living layers of the epidermis, irritant and sensitizing agents modulate cell membrane integrity. Irritation in vivo modulates integrin expression.[81] Keratinocytes in the basal layer of healthy epidermis express four different integrins, namely, $\alpha 2\beta 1$, $\alpha 3\beta 1$, $\alpha 6\beta 4$, and $\alpha_v\beta 5$; they participate in keratinocyte adhesion to the basement membrane that separates the epidermis from the dermis. Integrins have been shown to be involved in keratinocyte differentiation and activation, cell–cell adhesion between keratinocytes, and keratinocyte migration on extracellular matrix proteins.[115] Under inflammatory conditions, upregulation and suprabasal expression of these integrins coupled with the induction of $\alpha 5\beta 1$ and intercellular adhesion molecule-1 (ICAM-1), a specific ligand for $\beta 2$ integrins, have been demonstrated.[116] Finally, in skin reconstructed in vitro, UVB exposure leads to major epidermal developmental changes characterized by a downregulation of major markers of keratinocyte differentiation such as keratin 10, loricrin, filaggrin, and keratinocyte transglutaminase (Type I).[117]

Irritants and sensitizing agents also trigger cutaneous responses by inducing epidermal keratinocytes to elaborate and/or to release proinflammatory cytokines at both the protein and mRNA levels. These cytokines activate dermal microvascular endothelial cells and induce accumulation of specific mononuclear cells in vivo, and they, therefore, are considered as critical signaling molecules in the cascade of events leading to in vivo skin irritation and/or sensitization.[28,29,56,118] Consequently, the expression and/or release of cytokines by human skin equivalent models have been proposed as reliable markers to predict in vivo toxicological effects.[56,65,119,120] Although the complexity of the skin response to injury has created significant challenges in the discrimination of irritant from sensitizing agents by in vitro methods exclusively, it is now evident that analysis of the cytokine mRNA expression and protein release by epidermal keratinocyte cells may provide one possible approach to detect which agents are irritants or sensitizers.

Cultured keratinocytes synthesize constitutively, or can be induced to produce a variety of cytokines, including IL-1α, -6, -8, and -10, GM-CSF, TGF-α, and TGF-β, TNF-α, monocyte chemotaxis and activating factor (MCAF), IP-10, and macrophage inflammatory protein 2 (MIP-2).[29,121] Cultured keratinocytes exposed to contact allergens exhibit a rapid increase in mRNAs for IL-1α, -8, -6, and -1β, GM-CSF, TNF-α, IP-10, and MIP-2,[28,29,122] with subsequent release of keratinocyte-derived IL-10, -8, -6, and TNF-α.[28,118,123]

Studies have shown that skin equivalent models constitutively express mRNAs for inflammatory and immunomodulatory cytokines. The MatTek model expresses mRNAs for IL-1α, -1β, -8, -6, and -15, GM-CSF, and TNF-α.[124] In vitro epicutaneous contact with irritants leads to mRNAs expression of IL-1α, -1β, -6, -8, and -10, GM-CSF, TNF-α, TGF-β, and IL-12.[109] In this case, the mRNA levels for IL-6 and IL-8 are higher. This may well be due to the presence of fibroblasts.[125,126] Finally, experiments performed on reconstituted human epidermis have shown that both the skin irritant sodium lauryl sulfate (SLS) and the sensitizing agent 1-chloro-2,4-dinitrobenzene (DNCB) induce an increase in IL-1α and IL-8 release. However, DNCB only upregulates TNF-α release. Constitutive message was expressed for IL-1α, IL-8, and IL-10 but not for IL-1β. Both DNCB and SLS increased message for IL-1α. The in vitro-reconstituted human epidermis, EPISKIN, was used to assess the molecular mechanisms of skin irritation and sensitization.[127] Studies were performed to assess the ability of irritants and contact allergens to modulate cytokine message in SKIN2™ and EpiDerm cultures and determine if a cytokine or panel of cytokines would identify and contact allergen and differentiate it from an irritant. For the EpiDerm model, two different irritants were evaluated, benzalkonium chloride and nonanoic acid, along with two moderate allergens, TNCB and Oxazolone. Both irritants and allergens increased steady-state message levels for IL-8 and decreased message levels for IL-1β in the epithelial cells. Only irritants increased message levels for TFN-α, whereas the allergens produced either no change or a decrease in TNF-α message. Effects on the message levels of IL-6 and IL-1α differed for each chemical in magnitude, timing, and concentration.[99]

For the SKIN2™, the irritants BC, SLS, and nonanoic acid (NA) were evaluated along with three contact allergens TNCB, DNCB, and oxazolone. All three irritants increased steady-state message levels for IL-6, IL-8, and TNF-α. The allergens DNCB and oxazolone increased message levels for IL-6, IL-8, and GM-CSF, whereas TNCB only increased message for IL-8. The steady-state level of IL-15 was increased by NA only.[100] These results suggest that different patterns of epidermal cytokines are stimulated during in vitro irritation and/or sensitization processes. Consequently, it should be possible to distinguish between skin sensitizing agents and irritants by investigating the differential upregulation and modulation of epidermal cytokines by keratinocytes. In this respect, the roles of IL-1α and IL-8 may be particularly relevant. IL-1α is produced by keratinocytes and sequestered in the epidermis. During irritation, the release of IL-1α causes autocrine regulation of epidermal cytokine synthesis which, in turn, induces accumulation of dendritic cells in lymph nodes, draining the site of irritation, and stimulates the maturation of Langerhans cells.[127,128] Moreover, previous experiments have demonstrated that allergens induce expression and release of IL-8 mRNA, which is a potent chemoattractant for polymorphonuclear neutrophils and T lymphocytes.[28,129]

Recently, a model of reconstructed human epidermis (RHE) was used as an in vitro skin model to discriminate the effects of Tween 80, Triton X100, and benzalkonium chloride (BC) as irritants and 1-chloro-2,4-dinitrobenzene (DNCB) as a sensitizing agent.[131] It is based on the model developed by Rosdy and Cross[59] and consists of a mitotically and metabolically active culture of human-derived epidermal keratinocytes that are differentiated into basal, spinous, granular, and cornified layers analogous to those found in vivo.[58] Specific markers of epidermal differentiation such as keratins 1/10, involucrin, filagrin, loricrin, and transglutaminase have been localized. The lipid profile analysis shows that this model contains free fatty acids and all classes of ceramides. These cultures exhibit barrier function and metabolic activity which allow direct application of the product to be tested, thus simulating in vivo human topical exposure and an in vivo skin irritation/sensitization test.[58,89] In the experiment, the extent of epidermal irritation and sensitization was evaluated morphologically and amounts of intracellular and extracellular of IL-1α and IL-8 were assayed. The corresponding constitutive mRNA levels of these interleukins were quantified and the cytotoxic response was assessed by a MTT assay. The RHE resembled normal human epidermis with all typical epidermal layers. Keratin 10 was typically confined to the suprabasal layers of the tissue, suggesting normal epidermal terminal differentiation. Topical application of each of the three surfactants resulted in significant changes of tissue morphology and was coupled with different dose-dependent decreases in cell viability corresponding to their in vivo irritant potency.[119,130,131] IL-1α release was shown to increase inversely with decrease in cell viability, but interestingly, the surfactants did not stimulate increase in IL-8 levels. In contrast, DNCB did not induce elevated IL-1α release, although it induced a rapid dose-dependent decrease in cell viability. By contrast, DNCB increased IL-8 release. RT-PCR demonstrated the presence of mRNA for IL-1α and for IL-8 as previously described in vivo.[132,133] IL-1α was the most abundant cytokine transcript. BC, Triton X100, and DNCB upregulated IL-8 mRNA expression, while only BC induced a significant increase in IL-1α mRNA expression. The results demonstrate that the production of IL-1α and its release into the extracellular medium were due not only to specific cytotoxicity, but also to the extent of direct epidermal tissue stimulation. Conversely, the production of IL-8 did not directly correlate with cytotoxicity but may be linked to the type of product applied and classified as either irritant or sensitizer. These findings emphasize the requirement to use substances of the same class as standard controls in order to test unknown compounds that will be coupled with the investigation of multiple end points. Our data demonstrate that divergence of the IL-1α and IL-8 releases profiles and corresponding mRNA upregulation differentiates between specific responses to irritants or allergens. These findings suggest that it may be possible in a single integrated assay to classify and discriminate between irritant and sensitizing agents as a function of patterns of induced cytokine production and cell viability measurements. It has not been determined which mechanism is responsible for the change in cytokine mRNA expression, but we have observed that mRNA levels do not necessarily correlate with protein expression, and we also find that the type of product appears to determine the pattern of cell mediator expression and release. This could explain the disparate results obtained with the EpiDerm or the Skin2 models where only mRNA expression was investigated.[100] Our results suggest that skin allergens and skin irritants could stimulate variable patterns of epidermal cytokine production in RHE. The stimulation seems to be nonspecific in terms of mRNA signal strength, but specific in terms of protein production and release. In fact, if the cytokine levels (intracellular vs. extracellular) are plotted, a strong correlation for IL-1α ($R = 0.999$) is observed, suggesting a direct relationship among synthesis, storage, and release. By contrast, we observe for IL-8 that BC and Triton X100 induces synthesis and storage without significant release, while DNCB induces a rapid synthesis and release of IL-8 without storage (Figure 2). These observations highlight the complexity of biochemical pathways underlying cytokine production, and suggest interactions with different specific cellular target sites.

Functional mitochondria seem to be required in keratinocytes for *de novo* IL-1α synthesis.[134] In fact, tributyltin, a well-known skin irritant in rodent and human, causes disturbance in the

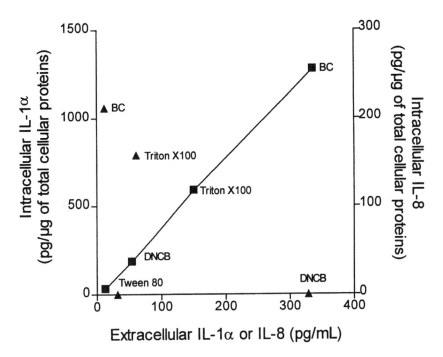

Figure 2   Correlation between the intra- and extracellular levels of IL-1α (■) and IL-8 (▲) in the RHE after topical application of Tween 80, Triton X100, BC, and DNCB (20 h, 37°C, 5%CO_2).

respiratory chain of mitochondria, probably by production of reactive oxygen intermediates at the ubiquinone site which activates transcription factor and promotes IL-1α synthesis.[134,135] In our experiments, the RHE treatments with Triton X100, BC, and DNCB reduce mitochondrial function as demonstrated by decreased MTT conversion and could partially explain the results. However, the release observed with DNCB suggests that mechanisms other than mitochondrial activity may be involved in the RHE cytokine production. In fact, DNCB increases NADPH oxidase enzymatic activity, producing reactive oxygen intermediates that mediate effects of this hapten on cells in vivo.[136] In addition, human keratinocyte IL-8 synthesis may be either positively or negatively regulated by protein kinase C depending on the stimulus.[137]

In conclusion, the reconstructed human epidermal equivalents more closely resemble native tissue in terms of their biosynthetic, morphological, and barrier properties than conventional submerged ones and than animal skins do. Due to the presence of the stratum corneum, water-insoluble as well as solid materials can be applied topically and are better suited than conventional cultures for predicting the irritation and sensitization potentials of topically applied agents. Divergent cytokine secretion profiles characterize the RHE response to irritants and sensitizers, suggesting that it is a complex array of signals that determines the type of protein released, not only in terms of mRNA upregulation, but above all in terms of interaction with the signal transduction. The combination of cell viability measurement with the quantification of IL-1α and IL-8 allows the classification and discrimination between irritant and sensitizing agents. The low interexperimental variations, irrespective of whether the experiments are performed on RHE derived from cells of the same or different donors, indicate that the RHE grown in defined medium represent a very useful in vitro model for toxicological studies which correlates with in vivo results. However, the number of products is not actually sufficient to extend the correlation across different classes of chemicals. The possibility that other irritant or sensitizing agents from different classes may exhibit specific patterns of inflammatory mediators would provide for the validation of in vitro models as alternatives to animal testing.

REFERENCES

1. Pittelkow, M. R., *Principles and Practice of Endocrinology and Metabolism*, 2nd ed., Becker, K. L., Ed., Lippincott, Williams and Wilkens, Philadelphia, PA, 1995, 1526.
2. Eckert, R. L., Structure, function, and differentiation of the keratinocyte, *Physiol. Rev.*, 69, 1316, 1989.
3. Watanabe, R., Wu, K., Paul, P., Marks, D. L., Kobayashi, T., Pittelkow, M. R., and Pagano, R. E., Up-regulation of glucosylceramide synthase expression and activity during human keratinocyte differentiation, *J. Biol. Chem.*, 273, 9651, 1998.
4. Guerrin, M., Simon, M., Montezin, M., Haftek, M., Vincent, C., and Serre, G., Expression of cloning of human corneodesmosin proves its identity with the product of the S gene and allows improved characterization of its processing during keratinocyte differentiation, *J. Biol. Chem.*, 273, 22640, 1998.
5. Sauder, D. N., The role of epidermal cytokines in inflammatory skin diseases, *J. Invest. Dermatol.*, 95, 27S, 1990.
6. Luger, T. A. and Schwartz, T., *Epidermal Growth Factors and Cytokines*, 1st ed., Luger, T. A. and Schwartz, T., Eds., Marcel Dekker, New York, 1994.
7. Pittelkow, M. R., *Psoriasis*, 3rd ed., Roenigk, H. H., Jr. and Maibach, H. I., Eds., Marcel Dekker, New York, 1998, 225.
8. Kupper, T. S., The activated keratinocyte: a model for inducible cytokine production by non-bone marrow-derived cells in cutaneous inflammatory and immune responses, *J. Invest. Dermatol.*, 94, 146S, 1990.
9. Bhella, U. S. and Iyengar, R., Emergent properties of networks of biological signaling pathways, *Science*, 283, 381, 1999.
10. Smith, K. J., Smith, W. J., Hamilton, T., Skelton, H. G., Graham, J. S., Okerberg, C., Moeller, R., and Hackley, B. E., Histopathologic and immunohistochemical features in human skin after exposure to nitrogen and sulfur mustard, *Am. J. Dermatopathol.*, 20, 22, 1998.
11. Liou, A., Eliase, P. M., Granfeld, C., Feingold, K. R., and Wood, L. C., Amphiregulin and nerve growth factor expression are regulated by barrier status in murine epidermis, *J. Invest. Dermatol.*, 108, 73, 1997.
12. Shreedhar, V., Giese, T., Sung, V. W., and E, U. S., A cytokine cascade including prostaglandin E2, IL-4, and IL-10 is responsible for UV-induced systemic immune suppression, *J. Immunol.*, 160, 3783, 1998.
13. Peus, D., Vasa, R. A., Meves, A., Pott, M., Beyerle, A., Squillace, K., and Pittelkow, M. R., H_2O_2 is an important mediator of UVB-induced EGF-receptor phosphorylation in cultured keratinocytes, *J. Invest. Dermatol.*, 110, 966, 1998.
14. Peus, D., Vasa, R. A., Beyerle, A., Meves, A., Krautmacher, C., and Pittelkow, M. R., UVB activates ERK1/2 and p38 signaling pathways via reactive oxygen species in cultured kerationcytes, *J. Invest. Dermatol.*, 112, 751, 1999.
15. Lukiw, W. J., Pelaez, R. P., Martinez, J., and Bazan, N. G., Budesonide epimer R or dexamethasone selectively inhibit platelet-activating factor-induced or interleukin 1beta-induced DNA binding activity of cis-acting transcription factors and cyclooxygenase-2 gene expression in human epidermal keratinocytes, *Proc. Natl. Acad. Sci. U.S.A.*, 95, 3914, 1998.
16. Dinarello, C. A., Interleukin-1, interleukin-1 receptors and interleukin-1 receptor antagonist, *Int. Rev. Immunol.*, 16, 457, 1998.
17. Kupper, T. S. and Groves, R. W., The interleukin-1 axis and cutaneous inflammation, *J. Invest. Dermatol.*, 105, 62S, 1995.
18. Zepter, K., Haffner, A., Soohoo, L. F., DeLuca, D., Tang, H. P., Fisher, P., Chavinson, J., and Elmets, C. A., Induction of biologically active IL-1 beta-converting enzyme and mature IL-1 beta in human keratinocytes by inflammatory and immunologic stimuli, *J. Immunol.*, 159, 6203, 1997.
19. Nylander-Lundqvist, E., Back, O., and Egelrud, T., IL-1 beta activation in human epidermis, *J. Immunol.*, 15, 1699, 1996.
20. Mizutani, H., Black, R., and Kupper, T. S., Human keratinocytes produce but do not process pro-interleukin-1 (IL-1) beta. Different strategies of IL-1 production and processing in monocytes and keratinocytes, *J. Clin. Invest.*, 87, 1066, 1991.
21. Ansel, J., Cytokine modulation of keratinocyte cytokines, *J. Invest. Dermatol.*, 94, 101s, 1990.

22. Matsunga, T., Katayama, I., Yokozeki, H., and Nishioka, K., Epidermal cytokine mRNA expression induced by hapten differs from that induced by primary irritant in human skin organ culture system, *J. Dermatol.,* 25, 421, 1998.

23. Rambukkana, A., Pistoor, F. H., Bos, J. D., Kapsenberg, M. L., and Das, P. K., Effects of contact allergens on human Langerhans' cells in skin organ culture: migration, modulation of cell surface molecules, and early expression of interleukin-1 beta protein, *Lab. Invest.,* 74, 422, 1996.

24. Phillips, W. G., Feldmann, M., Breathnach, S. M., and Brennan, F. M., Modulation of the IL-1 cytokine network in keratinocytes by intracellular IL-1 alpha and IL-1 receptor antagonist, *Clin. Exp. Immunol.,* 101, 177, 1995.

25. Akira, S., Taga, T., and Kishimoto, T., Interleukin-6 in biology and medicine, *Adv. Immunol.,* 54, 1, 1993.

26. Proost, P., Wuyts, A., and van Damme, J., The role of chemokines in inflammation, *Int. J. Clin. Lab. Res.,* 26, 211, 1996.

27. Wilmer, J. L. and Luster, M. I., Chemical induction of interleukin-8, a proinflammatory chemokine, in human epidermal keratinocyte cultures and its relation to cytogenetic toxicity, *Cell. Biol. Toxicol.,* 11, 37, 1995.

28. Barker, J. N. W. N., Mitra, R. S., Griffiths, C. E. M., Dixit, V. M., and Nickoloff, B. J., Keratinocytes as initiators of inflammation, *Lancet,* 337, 211, 1991.

29. Enk, A. H. and Katz, S. I., Early molecular events in the induction of contact sensitivity, *Proc. Natl. Acad. Sci. U.S.A.,* 89, 1398, 1992a.

30. Niizeki, H. and Streilein, J. W., Hapten-specific tolerance induced by acute, low-dose ultraviolet B radiation of skin is mediated via interleukin-10, *J. Invest. Dermatol.,* 109, 25, 1997.

31. Muller, G., Saloga, J., Germann, T., Bellinghausen, I., Mohamadzadeh, M., Knop, J., and Enk, A. H., Identification and induction of human keratinocyte-derived IL-12, *J. Clin. Invest.,* 94, 1799, 1994.

32. Blauvelt, A., Asada, H., Klaus-Kovtun, V., J, A. D., Lucey, D. R., and I, K. S., Interleukin-15 mRNA is expressed by human keratinocytes Langerhans cells, and blood-derived dendritic cells and is downregulated by ultraviolet B radiation, *J. Invest. Dermatol.,* 106, 1047, 1996.

33. Kondo, S. and Sauder, D. N., Tumor necrosis factor (TNF) receptor type 1 (p55) is a main mediator for TNF-alpha-induced skin inflammation, *Eur. J. Immunol.,* 27, 1713, 1997.

34. Lisby, S., Muller, K. M., Jongeneel, C. V., Saurat, J. H., and Hauser, C., Nickel and skin irritants up-regulate tumor necrosis factor-alpha mRNA in keratinocytes by different but potentially synergistic mechanisms, *Int. Immunol.,* 7, 343, 1995.

35. Little, M. C., Gawkrodger, D. J., and MacNiel, S., Chromium- and nickel-induced cytotoxicity in normal and transformed human keratinocytes: an investigation of pharmacological approaches to the prevention of Cr(VI)-induced cytotoxicity, *Br. J. Dermatol.,* 134, 199, 1996.

36. Boorsma, D. M., Flier, J., Sampat, S., Ottevanger, C., de Haan, P., Hooft, L., Willemze, R., Tensen, C. P., and Stoof, T. J., Chemokine IP-10 expression in cultured human keratinocytes, *Arch. Dermatol. Res.,* 190, 335, 1998.

37. Pentland, A. P., *Fitzpatrick's Dermatology in General Medicine,* Vol. 1, 5th ed., Freedberg, I. M., Eisen, A. Z., Wolff, K., Austen, K. F., Goldsmith, L. A., Katz, S. I., and Fitzpatrick, T. B., Eds., McGraw-Hill, New York, 1999, 432.

38. Meves, A., Peus, D., and Pittelkow, M. R., Arachidonic acid-induced generation of superoxide anion and lipid peroxidation mediates c-jun-N-terminal kinase activation in cultured keratinocytes, *J. Invest. Dermatol.,* 112, 533, 1999.

39. Muller-Decker, K., Heinzelmann, T., Furstenberger, G., Kecskes, A., Lehmann, W. D., and Marks, F., Arachidonic acid metabolism in primary irritant dermatitis produced by patch testing of human skin with surfactants, *Toxicol. Appl. Pharmacol.,* 153, 159, 1998.

40. Li-Stiles, B., Lo, H. H., and Fischer, S. M., Differential activation of keratinocyte phospholipase A2S by tumor promoters and other irritants, *Adv. Exp. Med. Biol.,* 407, 117, 1997.

41. Draize, J. H., Woodard, G., and Calvery, H. O., Methods for the study of irritation and toxicity of substances applied topically to the skin and mucous membranes, *J. Pharmacol. Exp. Ther.,* 82, 377, 1994.

42. Magnusson, B. and Kligman, A. M., The identification of contact allergens by animal assay. The guinea pig maximization test, *J. Invest. Dermatol.,* 52, 268, 1969.

43. Buehler, E. V., Delayed contact hypersensitivity in the guinea pig, *Arch. Dermatol.,* 91, 171, 1965.

44. Kimber, I. and Weisenberger, C., A murine local lymph node assay for the identification of contact allergens. Assay development and results of an initial validation study, *Arch. Toxicol.*, 63, 274, 1989.

45. Gad, S. C., Dunn, B. J., Dobbs, D. W., Reilly, C., and Walsh, R. D., Development and validation of an alternative dermal sensitization test: the mouse ear swelling test (MEST), *Toxicol. Appl. Pharmacol.*, 84, 93, 1986.

46. Nixon, G. A., Tyson, C. A., and Wertz, W. D., Interspecies comparison of skin irritancy, *Toxicol. Appl. Pharmacol.*, 31, 481, 1975.

47. Riviere, J. E., Sage, B. H., and Monterio, N. A., Transdermal lindocaine iontophoresis in isolated perfuse porcine skin, *J. Toxicol. Cut. Ocular. Toxicol.*, 8, 493, 1990.

48. Ahmed, S., Imai, T., and Otagiri, M., Stereoselectivity in cutaneous hydrolysis and transdermal transport of propranolol prodrug, *Enantiomer*, 2, 181, 1997.

49. De Leo, V. A., Harber, L. C., Kong, B. M., and S.J., D. S., Surfactant-induced alteration of arachidonic acid metabolism of mammalian cells in culture, *Proc. Soc. Exp. Biol. Med.*, 184, 477, 1987.

50. Brosin, A., Wolf, W., Mattheus, A., and Heise, H., Use of XTT-assay to assess the cytotoxicity of different surfactants and metal salts in human keratinocytes (HACAT) — A feasible method for in vitro testing of skin irritants, *Acta. Dermatol. Venereol.*, 77, 26, 1997.

51. Holbrook, K. A. and Hennings, H., Phenotype expression of epidermal cell in vitro: a review, *J. Invest Dermatol.*, 81, 11S, 1983.

52. Gibbs, S., Vicanova, J., Bouwstra, J., Valstar, D., Kempenaar, J., and Ponec, M., Culture of reconstructed epidermis in a defined medium at 33 degrees C shows a delayed epidermal maturation, prolonged lifespan and improved stratum corneum, *Arch. Dermatol. Res.*, 289, 585, 1997.

53. Regnier, M., Caron, D., Reichert, U., and Schaeffer, H., Reconstructed human epidermis: a model to study in vitro the barrier function of the skin, *Skin Pharmacol.*, 5, 42, 1992.

54. Augustin, C., Collombel, C., and Damour, O., Measurements of the protective effect of topically applied sunscreens using in vitro three-dimensional dermal and skin equivalents, *Photochem. Photobiol.*, 66, 853, 1997.

55. Ernesti, A. M., Swiderek, M., and Gay, R., Absorption and metabolism of topically applied testosterone in organotypic skin culture, *Skin Pharmacol.*, 5, 146, 1992.

56. Ponec, M. and Kempenaar, J., Use of human skin recombinants as an in vitro model for testing the irritation potential of cutaneous irritants, *Skin Pharmacol.*, 8, 49, 1995.

57. Rosdy, M. and Clauss, L. C., Terminal epidermal differentiation of human keratinocytes grown in chemically defined medium on inert filter substrates at the air-liquid interface, *J. Invest. Dermatol.*, 95, 409, 1990.

58. Rosdy, M., Pisani, A., and Ortonne, J. P., Production of basement membrane components by a reconstructed epidermis cultured in the absence of serum and dermal factors, *Br. J. Dermatol.*, 129, 227, 1993.

59. Prunieras, M., Schweizer, J., Michel, S., Bailly, C., and Prunieras, M., Methods for cultivation of keratinocytes with an air-liquid interface, *J. Invest. Dermatol.*, 81, 28S, 1983.

60. Harriger, M. D. and Hull, B. E., Cornification and basement membrane formation in a bilayered human skin equivalent maintained at an air-liquid interface, *J. Burn Care Rehabil.*, 13, 187, 1992.

61. Rheins, L. A., Edwards, S. M., Mia, O., and Donelly, T. A., Skin 2TM: an in vitro model to assess cutaneous immunotoxocity, *Toxicol. In Vitro*, 8, 1007, 1994.

62. Gay, R. S. M., Nelson, D., and Ernesti, A., The living skin equivalent as a model in vitro for ranking the toxic potential of dermal irritants, *Toxicol. In Vitro*, 6, 303, 1992.

63. Yang, J. J. and Krueger, A., Evaluation of two commercial human skin cultures for in vitro percutaneous absorption, *In Vitro Toxicol.*, 5, 211, 1992.

64. Slivka, S. R., Testosterone metabolism in an in vitro skin model, *Cell. Biol. Toxicol.*, 8, 267, 1992.

65. De Wever, B. and Rheins, L. A., Skin 2TM: an in vitro skin analog, *Alt. Meth. Toxicol.*, 10, 121, 1994.

66. Parnigotto, P. P., Bernuzzo, S., Bruno, P., Conconi, M. T., and Montesi, F., Characterization and applications of human epidermis reconstructed in vitro in de-epidermized derma, *Farmaco*, 53, 125, 1998.

67. Slivka, S. R., Laudeen, L. L., Zimber, M. P., and Bartel, R. L., Biochemical characterization barrier function and drug metabolism in an in vitro skin model, *J. Cell Biol.*, 115, 2072, 1991.

68. Geesin, J. C., Brown, L. J., Liu, Z. Y., and Berg, R. A., Development of a skin model based on insoluble fibrillar collagen, *J. Biomed. Mater. Res.*, 33, 1, 1996.

69. Fleischmajer, R., MacDonald, E. D., Contard, P., and Perlish, J. S., Immunochemistry of a keratinocyte-fibroblast co-culture model for reconstruction of human skin, *J. Histochem. Cytochem.*, 41, 1359, 1993.

70. Rosdy, M., Fartasch, M., and Darmon, M., Normal permeability barrier to tritiated water in reconstituted human epidermis, 1997.

71. Ponec, M., Gibbs, S., Weerheim, A., Kempenaar, J., Mulder, A., and Mommaas, A. M., Epidermal growth factor and temperature regulate keratinocyte differentiation, *Arch. Dermatol. Res.*, 289, 317, 1997.

72. Vicanova, J., Mommaas, A. M., Mulder, A. A., Koerten, H. K., and Ponec, M., Impaired desquamation in the in vitro reconstructed human epidermis, *Cell Tissue Res.*, 186, 115, 1996.

73. Stoppie, P., Borghraef, P., De Wever, B., Geysen, J., and Borgers, M., The epidermal architecture of an in vitro reconstructed human skin equivalent (Advanced Tissue Sciences Skin2 Models ZK 1300/2000), *Eur. J. Morphol.*, 31, 26, 1993.

74. van de Sandt, J. J., Bos, T. A., and Rutten, A. A., Epidermal cell proliferation and terminal differentiation in skin organ culture after topical exposure to sodium dodecyl sulphate, *In Vitro Cell Dev. Biol. Anim.*, 31, 761, 1995.

75. Hager, D. F., Mancuso, F. A., Nazareno, J. P., Sharkey, J. W., and Siverly, J. R., Evaluation of Testskin TM as a model membrane, *Proc. Int. Symp. Control. Rel. Bioact. Mater.*, 19, 487, 1992.

76. Regnier, M., Caron, D., Reichert, U., and Schaeffer, H., Barrier function of human skin and human reconstructed epidermis, *J. Pharm. Sci.*, 82, 404, 1993.

77. Doucet, O., Garcia, N., and Zastrow, L., Skin culture model: a possible alternative to the use of excised human skin for assessing in vitro percutaneous absorption, *Toxicol. In Vitro*, 12, 423, 1998.

78. Godwin, D. A., Michniak, B. B., and Creek, K. E., Evaluation of transdermal enhancers using a novel skin alternative, *J. Pharmaceutical. Sci.*, 86, 1001, 1997.

79. Vickers, A. E. M., Biggi, W. A., Dannecker, R., and Fisher, V., Uptake and metabolism of cyclosporin A and SDZ IMM 125 in the human in vitro Skin 2TM dermal and barrier function models, *Life Sci.*, 57, 215, 1995.

80. Nickoloff, B. J. and Naidu, Y., Perturbation of epidermal barrier function correlates with initiation of cytokine cascade in human skin, *J. Am. Acad. Dermatol.*, 30, 535, 1994.

81. von den Driesch, P., Fartasch, M., Huner, A., and Ponec, M., Expression of integrin receptors and ICAM-1 on keratinocytes in vivo and in an in vitro reconstructed epidermis: effects of sodium dodecyl sulphate, *Arch. Dermatol. Res.*, 287, 249, 1995.

82. Bodde, H. E., Holman, B., Spies, F., Weerheim, A., Kempenaar, J., Mommaas, M., and Ponec, M., Freeze-fracture electron microscopy on in vitro reconstructed epidermis, *J. Invest. Dermatol.*, 95, 108, 1990.

83. Bouwstra, J. A., Gooris, G. S., van der Spek, J. A., and Bras, W., Structural investigations of human stratum corneum by small-angle x-ray scattering, *J. Invest. Dermatol.*, 97, 1007, 1991.

84. Bouwstra, J. A., Gooris, G. S., Salomon-de Vries, M. A., van der Spek, J. A., and Bras, W., Structure of human stratum corneum as a function of temperature and hydration: A wide-angle x-ray diffraction study, *Int. J. Pharmaceutics*, 84, 205, 1991.

85. Simonetti, O., Hoogstraate, A. J., Bialik, W., Kempenaar, J. A., Schrijvers, A. H. G. J., Bodde, H. E., and Ponec, M., Visualization of diffusion pathways across the stratum corneum of native and in vitro reconstructed epidermis by confocal laser scanning microscopy, *Arch. Dermatol. Res.*, 1995.

86. Fartasch, M. and Ponec, M., Improved barrier structure formation in air-exposed human keratinocyte culture systems, *J. Invest. Dermatol.*, 102, 366, 1994.

87. Ponec, M., Bouwstra, J., and Fartasch, M., *Prediction of Percutaneous Penetration*, Vol. 3b, Brain, K. R., James, V. J., and Walters, K. A., Eds., STS Publishing, Cardiff, U.K., 1993, 428.

88. Rosdy, M., Fartasch, M., and Ponec, M., Structurally and biochemically normal permeability barrier of human epidermis reconstituted in chemically defined medium, *J. Invest. Dermatol.*, 107, 664, 1996.

89. Doucet, O., Robert, C., and Zastrow, L., Use of a serum-free reconstituted epidermis as a skin pharmacological model, *Toxicol. In Vitro*, 10, 305, 1996.

90. Todd, C., Hewitt, S. D., Kempenaar, J., Noz, K., Thody, A. J., and Ponec, M., Co-culture of melanocytes and keratinocytes at the air-liquide interface, *Arch. Dermatol. Res.*, 285, 455, 1993.

91. Regnier, M., Staquet, M. J., Schmitt, D., and Schmidt, R., Integration of Langerhans' cells into a pigmented reconstructed human epidermis, *J. Invest. Dermatol.*, 109, 510, 1997.

92. Boyce, S., Michel, S., Reichert, U., Schroot, B., and Schmidt, R., Reconstructed skin from cultured human keratinocytes and fibroblasts on a collagen-glycosaminoglycan biopolymer substrate, *Skin Pharmacol.*, 3, 136, 1990.

93. Ponec, M., Wauben-Penris, P. J., Burger, A., Kempenaar, J., and Bodde, H. E., Nitroglycerin and sucrose permeability as quality markers for reconstructed human epidermis, *Skin Pharmacol.*, 3, 126, 1990.

94. Lapiere, C. M. and Nusgens, B. V., The various uses of in-vitro reconstituted skin, *Bull. Mem. Acad. R. Med. Belg.*, 145, 235, 1990.

95. Magnaldo, T., Bernerd, F., Asslineau, D., and Darmon, M., Expression of loricrin is negatively controlled by retinoic acid in human epidermis reconstructed in vitro, *Differentiation*, 49, 39, 1992.

96. Slivka, S. R. and Zeigler, F., Use of an in vitro skin model for determining epidermal and dermal contributions to irritant response, *J. Toxicol. Cut. Ocular Toxicol.*, 12, 49, 1993.

97. Nickoloff, B. J., The cytokine network in psoriasis, *Arch. Dermatol.*, 127, 871, 1991.

98. Kubilus, J., Cannon, C., and Neal, P., Response of the EpiDerm skin model to topically applied irritants and allergens, *Toxicol. In Vitro*, 9, 157, 1996.

99. Sikorski, E. E., Gerberick, G. F., and Limardi, L. C., Evaluation of cytokine message levels in the EpiDerm TM in vitro skin model following application of contact allergens and skin irritants, *J. Invest. Dermatol.*, 108, 662, 1997.

100. Sikorski, E. E., Gerberick, G. F., and Limardi, L. C., Evaluation of a human skin equivalent model as a potential in vitro system to predict the contact sensitization potential of chemicals, 106, 939, 1996.

101. Triglia, D., Braa, S. S., Yonan, C., and Naughton, G. K., Cytotoxicity testing using neutral red and MTT assays on a three-dimensional human skin substrate, *Toxicol. In Vitro*, 5, 573, 1991.

102. Edwards, S. M., Donnelly, T. A., Sayre, R. M., and Rheins, L. A., *European Medicines Research*, Fracchia, G. N., Ed., IOS Press, 1994, 106.

103. Arlian, L. G., Vyszenskimoher, D. L., Rapp, C. M., and Hull, B. E., Production of IL-1-alpha and IL-1-beta by human skin equivalents parasitized by sarcoptes scobiei, *J. Parasitol.*, 82, 719, 1996.

104. Noelhudson, M. S., Brautboucher, F., Robert, M., Aubrey, M., and Wepierre, J., Comparison of six different methods to assess UVA cytotoxicity on reconstructed epidermis-relevance of a fluorimetric assay (the calcein-am) to evaluate the photoprotective effects of alpha-tocopherol, *Toxicol. In Vitro*, 11, 645, 1997.

105. Roguet, R., Dossou, K. G., and Rougier, A., *In Vitro Skin Toxicology: Irritation, Phototoxicity, Sensitization*, Rougier, A., Goldberg, A. M., and Maibach, H. I., Eds., Mary Ann Liebert, New York, 1994, 141.

106. Sato, T., Kirimura, Y., and Mori, Y., The co-culture of dermal fibroblasts with human epidermal keratinocytes induces increased prostaglandin E2 production and cyclooxygenase 2 activity in fibroblasts, *J. Invest. Dermatol.*, 109, 334, 1997.

107. Dykes, P. J., Edwards, M. J., Donovani, M. R., Merrett, V., Morgan, H. E., and Marks, R., In vitro reconstruction of human skin: The use of skin equivalents as potential indicators of cutaneous toxicity, *Toxicol. In Vitro*, 5, 1, 1991.

108. Corsini, E., Terzoli, A., Bruccoleri, A., Marinovich, M., and Galli, C. L., Induction of tumor necrosis factor-alpha in vivo by a skin irritant, tributyltin, through activation of transcription factors: its pharmacological modulation by anti-inflammatory drugs, *J. Invest. Dermatol.*, 108, 892, 1997.

109. Burleson, F. G., Limardu, L. C., Sikorski, E. E., Rheins, L. A., Donnelly, T. A., and Gerberick, G. F., Cytokine mRNA expression in an in vitro human skin model SKIN2(TM), *Toxicol. In Vitro*, 10, 513, 1996.

110. Boelsma, E., Tanojo, Bodde, H. E., and Ponec, M., Assessment of the potential irritancy of oleic acid on human skin-evaluation in vitro and in vivo, *Toxicol. In Vitro*, 10, 729ff, 1996.

111. Boelsma, E., Tanojo, H., Bodde, H. E., and Ponec, M., An in vitro study of the use of a human skin equivalent for irritancy screening of fatty acids, *Toxicol. In Vitro*, 11, 365, 1997.

112. Boelsma, E., Gibbs, S., and Ponec, M., Expression of skin-derived antileukoproteinase (SKALP) in reconstructed human epidermis and its value as a marker for skin irritation, *Acta. Derm. Venereol.*, 78, 107, 1998.

113. Buche, P., Violin, L., and Girard, P., Evaluation of the effects of cosmetic or dermo-pharmaceutical products on cutaneous energy metabolism using the Episkin model of reconstructed epidermis, *Cell. Biol. Toxicol.*, 10, 381, 1994.

114. Goffin, V., Paye, M., and Pierard, G. E., Comparison of in vitro predictive tests for irritation induced by anionic surfactants, *Contact Dermatitis,* 33, 38, 1995.

115. Watt, F. M. and Jones, P. H., Expression and function of the keratinocytes integrins, *Development,* Suppl. l, 185, 1993.

116. Kellner, I., Konter, U., and Sterry, W., Overexpression of extracellular matrix receptors (VLA-3,5 and 6) on psoriatic keratinocytes, *Br. J. Dermatol.,* 123, 211, 1991.

117. Bernerd, F. and Asselineau, D., Successive alteration and recovery of epidermal differentiation and morphogenesis after specific UVB damages in skin reconstructed in vitro, *Dev. Biol.,* 183, 123, 1997.

118. Enk, A. H. and Katz, S. I., Identification and induction of keratinocyte-derived IL-10, *J. Immunol.,* 149, 92, 1992b.

119. Roguet, R. D., K.G., and Rougier, A., Use of in vitro skin recombinants to evaluate cutaneous toxicity: a preliminary study, *J. Toxicol. Cut Ocular Toxicol.,* 11, 305, 1994.

120. Dickson, F. M., Lawrence, J. N., and Benford, D. J., Release of inflammatory mediators in human keratinocyte cultures following exposure to a skin irritant, *Toxicol. In Vitro,* 7, 385, 1993.

121. Barker, J. N. W. N., Role of keratinocytes in allergic contact dermatitis, *Contact Dermatitis,* 26, 145, 1992.

122. Knop, J. and Enk, A. H., Cellular and molecular mechanisms in the induction phase of contact sensitivity, *Int. Arch. Allergy Immunol.,* 107, 231, 1995.

123. Holliday, M. R., Dearman, R. J., Corsini, E., Basketter, D. A., and Kimber, I., Selective stimulation of cutaneous interleukin 6 expression by skin allergens, *J. Appl. Toxicol.,* 16, 65, 1996.

124. Limardi, L. C., Sikorski, E. E., and Gerberick, G. F., Cytokine gene expression in the MatTek EpiDerem cultures, *J. Invest. Dermatol.,* 106, 929, 1996.

125. Konstantinove, N., Friant, S., and Hazarika, P., IL-8 release is highly elevated in skin equivalent cultures and is further induced by psoriatic patient fibroblasts, *J. Invest. Dermatol.,* 104, 685, 1995.

126. Waelti, E. R., Inaebit, S. P., and Rast, H. P., Co-culture of human keratinocytes on post-mitotic human dermal fibroblast feeder cells: production of large amount of interleukin-6, *J. Invest. Dermatol.,* 98, 805, 1992.

127. Kupper, T., Interleukin 1 and other human keratinocytes cytokines in inflammation and functional characterization, *Adv. Dermatol.,* 3, 293, 1988.

128. Cumberbatch, M. and Kimber, I., Dermal tumor necrosis factor alpha induces dendritic cell migration to draining lymph nodes and possibly provides one stimulus for Langerhans cell migration, *Immunology,* 75, 257, 1992.

129. Gueniche, A., Viac, J., Lizard, G., Chaveron, M., and Schmitt, D., Effect of different sensitizing haptens on intracellular adhesion molecule-1 expression and cytokine prouction by normal human keratinocytes, *Eur. J. Dermatol.,* 5, 320, 1995.

130. Bettley, F. R., The toxicity of soaps and detergents, *Br. J. Dermatol.,* 80, 635, 1968.

131. Singer, E. J. and Pitts, E. P., *Surfactants in Cosmetics,* Rieger, M., Ed., New York, 1985, 133.

132. Rowbottom, A. W., Norton, J., Riches, P. G., and Sloane, J. P., Cytokine gene expression in skin and lymphoid organs in human graft-versus-host disease, *J. Pathol.,* 169, 150A, 1993.

133. Anttila, H. S. I., Reitamo, S., Erkko, P., Ceska, M., Moser, B., and Baggiolini, M., Interleukin-8 immunoreactivity in the skin of healthy subjects and patients with palmoplantar pustulosis and psoriasis, *J. Invest. Dermatol.,* 98, 96, 1992.

134. Corsini, E., Shubert, C., Marinovich, M., and Galli, C. L., Role of mitochondria in Tributyltin-induced interleukin-1-alpha production in murine keratinocytes, *J. Invest. Dermatol.,* 107, 720, 1996a.

135. Corsini, E., Bruccoleri, A., Marinovich, M., and Galli, C. L., Endogenous interleukin-1-alpha is associated with skin irritation induced by tributyltin, *Toxicol. Appl. Pharmacol.,* 138, 268, 1996b.

136. Arner, E. S. J., Bjornstedt, M., and Holmgren, A., 1-Chloro-2,4-dinitrobenzene is an irreversible inhibitor of human thioredoxin reductase — loss of thioredoxin disulfide reductase activity is accompanied by a large increase in NADPH oxidase activity, *J. Biol. Chem.,* 270, 3479, 1995.

137. Chabot-Fletcher, M., Breton, J., Lee, J., Young, P., and Griswold, D. E., Interleukin-8 production is regulated by protein kinase C in human keratinocytes, *J. Invest. Dermatol.,* 103, 509, 1941.

10 Pathogenesis of Allergic Contact Dermatitis: Role of T Cells*

Richard S. Kalish

CONTENTS

I. OVERVIEW OF ALLERGIC CONTACT DERMATITIS

Allergic contact dermatitis requires prior sensitization of T-lymphocytes. When a hapten contacts the epidermis, it interacts with and covalently binds keratinocyte and Langerhans cell proteins (Table 1). Keratinocytes participate in the reaction by producing inflammatory cytokines such as interleukin-1 (IL-1) and tumor necrosis factor-alpha (TNF-α). These cytokines induce endothelial cells to express adhesion molecules necessary for accumulation of inflammatory cells. Langerhans cells migrate to the lymph nodes where they present antigen (urushiol) to T cells. Activated T cells must then home to the site of inflammation, which is recognized by virtue of the endothelial adhesion molecules, induced by inflammatory cytokines. T cells then reencounter antigen presented by Langerhans cells and induce pathology by a variety of effector mechanisms.

II. THE CHEMISTRY OF CONTACT ALLERGENS

Contact allergens are small molecules, and recognition by the immune system requires that they function as haptens and bind macromolecules. Haptens can be classified by their chemical reactivity.[1] Mechanisms used to bind proteins include nucleophilic substitution, electrophilic reactions, free radical reactions, and chelation of metallic salts. Many allergens, such as dinitrochlorobenzene, are chemically reactive and capable of covalently conjugating proteins. Other allergens, such as nickel and chromium,[2] form noncovalent complexes with proteins. A third class of allergens is

* This work was funded in part by a grant from the Dermatology Foundation supported by Dermik Laboratories.

145

TABLE 1
Overview of Allergic Contact Dermatitis to Urushiol

1. Hapten interacts with both keratinocytes and Langerhans cells.
2. Induction of inflammatory cytokine (e.g., IL-1 and TFN-α) production by keratincytes, or possibly mast cells.
3. Cytokines induce endothelial cell adhesion molecules (e.g., ICAM-1, E-selectin, VCAM-1).
4. Langerhans cells activated, migrate to lymph nodes and present hapten to T cells.
5. T cells home to inflamed skin with aid adhesion molecules induced by inflammatory cytokines.
6. T cells recognized hapten in skin presented by Langerhans cells.
7. T cells induce skin pathology.

"prohaptens." These compounds must be activated to a chemically reactive intermediate before they can conjugate proteins. Urushiol, the immunogenic component of poison ivy resin, is such a prohapten. Oxidation of the catechol group of urushiol to a quinone makes it a target for nucleophilic substitution by amino acid side chains.

Conjugation of haptens to proteins is also a function of the chemical reactivity of the amino acid side chains.[3] Cysteine, lysine, and histidine (least active) are nucleophiles which will take part in nucleophilic substitutions. Aromatic amino acids such as tyrosine, tryptophan, and phenylalanine can act as electron acceptors and react with free radicals. These last reactions are particularly significant for photoallergy reactions.

III. INITIATION OF CONTACT DERMATITIS AND THE ROLE OF KERATINOCYTES

Keratinocytes have an active role in the initiation of both allergic contact and irritant contact dermatitis.[4] Keratinocytes are capable of producing and secreting many cytokines, including interleukin-1 (IL-1), IL-6, IL-8, TNF-α, and GM-CSF.[5–7] Many allergens and irritants have been shown to induce keratinocyte activation with synthesis and secretion of these cytokines.[8] Mast cells are an alternate source of IL-1 and TNF-α during the initiation phase of allergic contact reactions.[9] It is controversial whether the cytokine profile induced by irritants differs from that induced by allergens. IL-1 and TNF-α are induced by urushiol (poison ivy), dinitrofluorobenzene, and croton oil, but not by the tolerizing urushiol derivative, 5-methyl-3-n-pentadecyl-catechol.[10]

These proinflammatory cytokines have a role in the recruitment of inflammatory cells. Both IL-1 and TNF-α induce expression of the adhesion molecules ICAM-1 and E-selectin on endothelial cells.[11–13] These molecules are essential for the homing (migration) of inflammatory cells to the involved epidermis.

IV. THE ROLE OF LANGERHANS CELLS

Langerhans cells are dendritic antigen-presenting cells which serve as the primary antigen-presenting cell of the epidermis.[14–18] As with other "professional" antigen-presenting cells, Langerhans cells constitutively express cell surface MHC class II molecules (e.g., DR).[19] Langerhans cells also express the co-stimulatory molecule B7 (B7-1, CD80; B7-2, CD86) following activation.[20] Upon interaction with a hapten, Langerhans cells become activated, increase their cell surface expression of MHC class II,[21] and migrate to lymph nodes to present antigen to T cells.[22,23]

Unique markers of Langerhans cells include cell surface expression of CD1a[24] and the presence of intracytoplasmic Birbeck granules.[25] CD1a is structurally related to MHC class I molecules[26] and a role for CD1a in antigen presentation is postulated.[26,27] The related molecule CD1b is capable of presenting *Mycobacterium tuberculosis* antigens to T cells.[28] CD1b-restricted T cells with an α/β T cell receptor are capable of recognizing a lipoarabinomannan derived from *Mycobacterium lepra*.[29]

The function of Birbeck granules is not known. Internalized exogenous protein,[30] CD1a,[31] and Ia (MHC class II) molecules[32] are all reported in association with Birbeck granules. It is proposed that Birbeck granules may have a role in antigen processing, although they are not essential for antigen presentation by Langerhans cells.[33] Langerhans cells process and present both exogenous antigens (e.g., soluble protein)[34] and endogenous antigens (e.g., transplantation antigens).[35]

V. PRESENTATION OF HAPTEN TO T CELLS

T lymphocyte antigen receptors recognize peptides presented in the peptide binding groove of major histocompatibility complex (MHC) molecules.[36,37] CD8+ T lymphocytes recognize peptides presented by MHC class I (HLA-A,B,C) molecules and CD4+ T lymphocytes recognize peptides presented by MHC class II (DR, DP, DQ) molecules.[38] Prior to presentation to T lymphocytes, protein antigens are first cleaved into peptides and then bound to the peptide binding grooves of MHC molecules. Contact allergens function as haptens and bind proteins either prior to or after cleavage into peptides.[39] This process of cleaving proteins into peptides and loading the peptides onto MHC molecules is known as antigen processing.[40] Antigen processing is a function of antigen-presenting cells which have the metabolic functions required for processing along with expression of MHC molecules and costimulatory molecules (e.g., B7-1, B7-2).

T cell receptor occupancy alone is not sufficient to induce T cell proliferation. Presentation of antigen to T lymphocytes requires the interactions of multiple adhesion molecules. CD4+ T cell recognition of antigen in the absence of such appropriate costimulatory signals can induce tolerance or anergy.[41,42] The interaction of CD28 and B7-1 (CD80) or B7-2 (CD86) has been shown to deliver such an essential costimulatory signal to both human[43–45] and murine[46,47] CD4+ T cells, as well as human CD8+ hapten specific T cells.[48] CD28 is a T cell antigen and B7-1 is an inducible antigen of antigen-presenting cells, including Langerhans cells. Keratinocytes are capable of expressing B7,[49,50] and keratinocyte B7 expression is observed in inflammatory skin diseases.[51] However, keratinocyte presentation of hapten to T cells for T cell activation has not been demonstrated.

VI. PROCESSING OF PROTEIN HAPTEN CONJUGATES FOR PRESENTATION TO T CELLS

Antigen processing proceeds by different pathways, depending upon whether the antigen is an extrinsic protein or an endogenously synthesized protein.[52–54] Extrinsic antigens are phagocytosed or endocytosed and degraded into peptides within the endosome/lysosome compartment. Processed antigenic peptides associate with class II MHC molecules within the endosome/lysosome compartment for eventual presentation to CD4+ T cells. Newly synthesized MHC class II molecules are prevented from binding peptides prior to transport to the endosomal compartment by association with the invariant chain.[55] Inhibitors which interfere with endosome-dependent protein processing include chloroquine,[56] monensin,[57] leupeptin,[58] and ammonium chloride. Peptides isolated from murine MHC class II molecules include secretory and membrane proteins with access to endosomal compartments.[59] Urushiol (poison ivy) is processed by this pathway for presentation to CD4+ T cells.[60]

In contrast, proteins synthesized endogenously are degraded into peptides and transported into the endoplasmic reticulum where they associate with class I MHC molecules for eventual presentation to CD8+ T cells.[61] Degradation of cytoplasmic proteins into peptides of approximately 9 amino acids in length is believed to be a function of the proteasome complex,[62] a 26S multisubunit complex with protease activity. The genes for several subunits of this complex are linked to the MHC class II region.[63,64] Transport of cytoplasmic peptides into the endoplasmic reticulum is dependent upon transporter proteins which bind ATP and are coded by the Tap-1 and Tap-2 genes which also map within the MHC class II region.[65–68] Class I MHC molecules associate with peptides within the endoplasmic reticulum and are transported to the Golgi for presentation on the cell surface.[69] In addition to its effects on endosomal antigen processing, monensin disrupts the Golgi, inhibiting transport to the plasma membrane.[70] Brefeldin A interferes with transport of proteins from the endoplasmic reticulum to the Golgi,[71] thereby inhibiting presentation of proteins dependent upon the endogenous presentation pathway.[72] By the use of pulsed urushiol, antigen-presenting cells and the above inhibitors it was demonstrated that urushiol is preferentially processed as a cytoplasmic antigen by the endogenous pathway.[73] This suggests that urushiol enters cells and conjugates cytoplasmic proteins, which are subsequently processed by the endogenous pathway. Since CD8+ T cells predominate in the urushiol response, the endogenous pathway may be the preferential pathway for processing of urushiol conjugated proteins.

Thus, small lipid-soluble molecules (e.g., urushiol) are capable of entering the cytoplasm and being presented by the endogenous pathway to CD8+ cells. Polar haptens (e.g., nickel, cobalt) are likely to be presented by the exogenous pathway to CD4+ cells. Haptens that are both chemically reactive and lipid soluble (e.g., DNCB) can react with both exogenous and endogenous proteins and are processed by both pathways for presentation to both CD4+ and CD8+ cells. The murine response to DNCB is marked by a CD8+-mediated production of interferon-γ, and a CD4+-mediated production of immunoregulatory Th2 cytokines,[74] and the response to dinitrofluorobenzene is mediated by CD8+ cells, with CD4+ cells having a suppressive role.[75]

VII. T CELL RESPONSE TO HAPTENS

T helper (inducer) CD4+ lymphocytes are classified by the cytokines they produce into Th1 and Th2 subsets (review in Reference 76). Murine Th1 cells principally produce IL-2, interferon-γ, and GM-CSF, whereas Th2 cells produce IL-3, IL-4, IL-5, and IL-6. Th1 cells are responsible for delayed hypersensitivity reactions and Th2 cells produce IL-4 and additional helper factors for production of IgE and other antibodies.[77] The Th1 cytokine, interferon-γ, is believed to have a key role in allergic contact dermatitis by the induction of ICAM-1 on both endothelium and keratinocytes of involved skin.[78] Both urushiol (poison ivy) and nickel-specific human T cells secrete interferon-γ,[79,80] indicating that allergic contact dermatitis has properties of a Th1 response.

VIII. HOMING OF T LYMPHOCYTES

Homing is the process by which circulating cells recognize and localize to relevant sites. Hapten-conjugated Langerhans cells initially migrate to the lymph node to present antigen to T cells. On primary sensitization, initial recognition of hapten is probably within the lymph node. T cells which become activated following recognition of hapten in the lymph node must then home to the inflamed skin. The proportion of urushiol-specific T lymphocytes in a skin lesion of allergic contact dermatitis to urushiol is less than 1:1000.[81] This represents a severalfold enrichment over the frequency of such T lymphocytes in the peripheral blood, where the frequency is less than 1:5000, and indicates the ability of antigen-specific T lymphocytes to localize at sites of inflammation.

Leukocytes have homing receptors which recognize the endothelium of appropriate tissues.[82] The homing receptor which recognizes the high endothelial venules of lymph nodes is a molecule called L-selectin. This molecule is essential to the homing of lymphocytes to lymph nodes. Addressins are the ligands for homing receptors. Addressins signal the lymphocytes where to exit the circulation. Addressins expressed on dermal endothelial cells include E-selectin and P-selectin.

The ligand for E-selectin (CLA: cutaneous lymphocyte antigen) is believed to be the homing receptor for T lymphocytes that localize in inflamed skin.[83–85] The selectins (E-selectin, P-selectin, and L-selectin) belong to a super-gene family and have considerable homology.[86] Selectins have an N-terminal lectin domain. Lectins are proteins that bind carbohydrate. There is evidence that the ligands for these selectins are carbohydrates. The ligand for E-selectin is a glycoprotein with a carbohydrate group similar to the sLe^x blood group substance.[87] T cells recognizing allergic contact allergens (e.g., nickel) preferentially express the CLA ligand for E-selectin.[88]

Additional adhesion molecule pairs are essential for lymphocyte homing. These include endothelial ICAM-1, which interacts with lymphocyte LFA-1,[89] and endothelial VCAM-1, which interacts with lymphocyte VLA-4.[90] Both LFA-1 and VLA-4 are integrins.

Initial interactions between lymphocytes and endothelial cells are mediated by the selectins (e.g., E-selectin), which induce the lymphocyte to roll along the endothelium.[91] This initial contact permits integrin interactions (e.g., LFA-1) which transmit an activation signal to the cell. The activation signal mediated by integrins induces the cell to flatten out and migrate through the vessel wall into the dermis.[92] Activated T lymphocytes express higher levels of cell surface LFA-1 and VLA-4 and it is probable that activated T lymphocytes home nonspecifically to sites of inflammation.

The adhesion molecules ICAM-1, VCAM-1, and E-selectin are expressed on endothelium of inflamed skin in both irritant and allergic contact dermatitis.[93] Allergens and irritants, including urushiol, have the ability to induce expression of these molecules either by direct action or through induction of proinflammatory keratinocyte cytokines.[94–96]

IX. INDUCTION OF INFLAMMATORY CHANGES

Following homing to skin and recognition of hapten, activated T lymphocytes induce pathology in the dermis and the epidermis. The proportion of T lymphocytes specific for the inciting antigen is less than 1:1000, indicating that T lymphocytes are extremely potent and must evoke significant amplification. Lymphocytes have many potential mechanisms for inducing inflammation. These include cell-mediated cytotoxicity, amplification by autoreactive T cells, recruitment of inflammatory cells, and direct effects of cytokines. TNF-α has a critical role since blocking of TNF-α with antibodies inhibits allergic contact dermatitis.[97]

Lesions of allergic contact dermatitis show increased vascular permeability with alterations of the postcapillary venules that include interendothelial cell gaps and endothelial cell hypertrophy.[98] These changes are associated with diapedesis and perivascular cuffing by inflammatory cells. CD4+ T cells predominate in the dermal infiltrate of allergic contact dermatitis.[99]

X. CLINICAL APPLICATIONS: DEVELOPMENT OF NOVEL TREATMENT MODALITIES FOR INFLAMMATORY DERMATOSES

Recent advances in the understanding of allergic contact dermatitis may be translated into novel treatment modalities. Numerous potential approaches have been explored in murine systems. Ion channel blockers can inhibit both allergic and irritant contact dermatitis in the mouse. Possible mechanisms include interference with antigen processing by altering the pH of lysosomes, and inhibition of cell signaling. Potential targets for cell signaling inhibition include Langerhans cells (migration, upregulation of MHC), keratinocytes (cytokine production), and T cells.

Amiloride inhibits membrane sodium transport. Topical application of 1% cream inhibits mouse ear swelling to allergic contact dermatitis (TNCB) and ultraviolet B.[100] However, structure function studies show inconsistent correlation of inhibitory effects and ability to inhibit Na$^+$/H$^+$ antiport.[101]

Ethacrynic acid also inhibits both induction and elicitation of allergic contact dermatitis in the mouse ear swelling assay.[102] The calcium channel blockers lanthanum and diltiazem inhibit the mouse ear swelling response to DNCB by both topical and systemic application.[103] Changes in Langerhans cell morphology were observed, with a slight decrease in number, and alteration in morphology of dendrites.

Antioxidants may inhibit allergic contact dermatitis by several mechanisms. Antioxidants have been shown to inhibit allergic contact dermatitis of mice to trinitrochlorobenzene[104] and urushiol.[105] Both 10% topical and oral *N*-acetylcysteine were used in the TNCB study. Subcutaneously injected 2-oxo-4-thiazolidine carboxylate was used in the urushiol study. Both these compounds replenish intracellular glutathione levels. One proposed mechanism of action is inhibition of nuclear factor κB, which induces inflammatory cytokines including TNF-α.[106,107] An alternative mechanism is interference with intracellular oxidation of urushiol to reactive intermediates. *N*-Acetylcysteine also inhibits ICAM-1 induction on human keratinocytes, which may interfere with accumulation of inflammatory cells, particularly if it also blocks ICAM-1 expression on endothelium.[108]

Pentoxifylline inhibits TNF-α production, as well as elicitation of allergic and irritant dermatitis.[109] However, no activity was observed against induction of allergic contact dermatitis, suggesting that TNF-α inhibitors may have therapeutic use (elicitation) but not prevent sensitization.

Manipulation of T cell cytokine profiles can alter T cell response. Delayed hypersensitivity and allergic contact dermatitis are mediated by T cells which produce Th1 cytokines (e.g., γ-interferon), whereas IgE production is favored by T cells which produce Th2 cytokines (e.g., IL-4, IL-10).[110] IL-10 inhibits the production of Th1 cytokines,[111,112] and injection of IL-10 inhibits both allergic contact dermatitis and delayed hypersensitivity.[113]

Allergic contact dermatitis can also be inhibited at the level of T cell recognition of antigen. Activation of T cells by antigen-presenting cells requires a costimulatory signal mediated by B7 on the antigen-presenting cell and CD28 on the T cell.[114,115] CTLA4Ig is a recombinant fusion molecule which blocks B7-mediated costimulation of human T cells by CD28.[116] CTLA4Ig also inhibits human T cell response to urushiol (poison ivy), and blocking of costimulation can induce CD8+ T cell tolerance to urushiol.[117] The great promise of such CD28-blocking reagents is the possibility that they can be used to induce antigen-specific tolerance.

The immunosuppressive agent FK506 has been shown to be active when applied topically. FK506 is similar in action to cyclosporin A, and preferentially inhibits the production of IL-2 by activated T cells.[118] Topically applied FK506 inhibits allergic contact sensitivity in both mice[119] and guinea pigs.[120]

XI. SUMMARY

Allergic contact dermatitis requires an interaction of both antigen-specific and nonantigen-specific processes. The nonantigen-specific processes include the initial induction of cytokines from keratinocytes, and/or mast cells. This initial induction of IL-1 and TNF-α induces the endothelial adhesion molecules (e.g., E-selectin, ICAM-1) required for the homing of activated T cells to the involved skin. Antigen specificity is provided by Langerhans cell presentation of hapten to T cells in both lymph nodes and skin. It may be possible to interfere with allergic contact dermatitis at multiple steps, including initial induction of inflammatory cytokines, Langerhans cell activation, antigen presentation, T cell activation, T cell homing, and induction of the inflammatory lesion.

REFERENCES

1. Dupuis G, Benezra C: Chemically reactive functions in haptens and in proteins. In: *Allergic Contact Dermatitis to Simple Chemicals a Molecular Approach*. Marcel Dekker, New York, 1982, pp. 47–84.

2. Romagnoli P, Sinigaglia F. Selective interaction of Ni with an MHC-bound peptide. *EMBO J.* 10:1303–1306, 1991.

3. Dupuis G, Benezra C. Chemically reactive functions in haptens and in proteins. In: *Allergic Contact Dermatitis to Simple Chemicals a Molecular Approach.* Marcel Dekker, New York, 1982, pp. 47–84.

4. Barker JN. Role of keratinocytes in allergic contact dermatitis. *Contact Dermatitis* 26:145–148, 1992.

5. Hauser C, Saurat JH, Schmitt A, et al. Interleukin 1 is present in normal human epidermis. *J. Immunol.* 136:3317–3321, 1986.

6. Kupper TS, Ballard D, Chua AO, et al. Human keratinocytes contain mRNA indistinguishable from monocyte interleukin 1 alpha and beta mRNA. *J. Exp. Med.* 164:2095–2100, 1986.

7. Kupper TS. The activated keratinocyte: a model for inducible cytokine production by non-bone marrow-derived cells in cutaneous inflammatory and immune responses. *J. Invest. Dermatol.* 94:146S–150S, 1990.

8. Soohoo L, Tang H, Haqqi T, Elmets CA. Cytokine RNA profiles in human keratinocytes exposed to the contact allergen urushiol. (Abstr) *J. Invest. Dermatol.* 100:507, 1993.

9. Walsh LJ, Trichieri G, Waldorf HA, Whitaker D, Murphy GF. Human dermal mast cells contain and release tumor necrosis factor α, which induces endothelial leukocyte adhesion molecule 1. *Proc. Natl. Acad. Sci. U.S.A.* 88:4220–4224, 1991.

10. Haas J, Lipkow T, Mohamadzadeh M, Kolde G, Knop J. Induction of inflammatory cytokines in murine keratinocytes upon in vivo stimulation with contact sensitizers and tolerizing analogues. *Exp. Dermatol.* 1:76–83, 1992.

11. Buchsbaum ME, Kupper TS, Murphy GF. Differential induction of intercellular adhesion molecule-1 in human skin by recombinant cytokines. *J. Cutan. Pathol.* 20:21–27, 1993.

12. Xu Y, Swerlick RA, Sepp N, Bosse D, Ades EW, Lawley TJ. Characterization of expression and modulation of cell adhesion molecules on an immortalized human dermal microvascular endothelial cell line (HMEC-1). *J. Invest. Dermatol.* 102:833–837, 1994.

13. Kyan-Aung U, Haskard DO, Poston RN, Thornhill MH, Lee TH. Endothelial leukocyte adhesion molecule-1 and intercellular adhesion molecule-1 mediate the adhesion of eosinophils to endothelial cells in vitro and are expressed by endothelium in allergic cutaneous inflammation in vivo. *J. Immunol.* 146:521–528, 1991.

14. Stingl G, Katz SI, Clement L, Green I, Shevach EM. Immunological functions of Ia-bearing epidermal Langerhans cells. *J. Immunol.* 121:2005–2013, 1978.

15. Stingl G, Gazze-Stingl LA, Aberer W, Wolff K. Antigen presentation by murine epidermal Langerhans cells and its alteration by ultraviolet B light. *J. Immunol.* 127:1707–1713, 1981.

16. Toews GB, Bergstresser PR, Streilein JW. Epidermal Langerhans cell density determines whether contact hypersensitivity or unresponsiveness follows skin painting with DNCB. *J. Immunol.* 124:445–453, 1980.

17. Stingl G, Tamaki K, Katz SI. Origin and function of epidermal Langerhans cells. *Immunol. Rev.* 53:149–174, 1980.

18. Peguet-Navarro J, Moulon C, Schmitt D. The antigen presenting capacity of human epidermal Langerhans cells. *Cell Mol. Biol.* 40 Suppl 1:15–20, 1994.

19. Stingl G, Katz SI, Shevach EM, Wolff-Schreiner E, Green I. Detection of Ia antigens on Langerhans cells in guinea pig skin. *J. Immunol.* 120:570–578, 1978.

20. Girolomoni G, Zambruno G, Manfredini R, Zacchi V, Ferrari S, Cossarizza A, Giannetti A. Expression of B7 costimulatory molecule in cultured human epidermal Langerhans cells is regulated at the mRNA level. *J. Invest. Dermatol.* 103:54–59, 1994.

21. Aiba S, Katz SI. Phenotypic and functional characteristics of in vivo activated Langerhans cells. *J. Immunol.* 145:2791–2796, 1990.

22. Bigby M, Vargas R, Sy MS. Production of hapten-specific T cell hybridomas and their use to study the effect of ultraviolet B irradiation on the development of contact hypersensitivity. *J. Immunol.* 143:3867–3872, 1989.

23. Kripke ML, Munn CG, Jeevan A, Tang JM, Bucana C. Evidence that cutaneous antigen-presenting cells migrate to regional lymph nodes during contact sensitization. *J. Immunol.* 145:2833–2838, 1990.

24. Chu A, Eisinger M, Lee JS, Takezaki S, Kung PC, Edelson RL. Immunoelectron microscopic identification of Langerhans cells using a new antigenic marker. *J. Invest. Dermatol.* 78:177–180, 1982.

25. Caputo R, Peluchetti D, Monti M. Freeze-fracture of Langerhans granules. A comparative study. *J. Invest. Dermatol.* 66:297–301, 1976.

26. Longley J, Kraus J, Alonso M, Edelson R. Molecular cloning of CD1a (T6), a human epidermal dendritic cell marker related to class I MHC molecules. *J. Invest. Dermatol.* 92:628–631, 1989.

27. Moulon C, Peguet-Navarro J, Schmitt D. A potential role for CD1a molecules on human epidermal Langerhans cells in allogeneic T-cell activation. *J. Invest. Dermatol.* 97:524–528, 1991.

28. Porcelli S, Morita CT, Brenner MB. CD1b restricts the response of human CD4⁻8⁻ T lymphocytes to a microbial antigen. *Nature* 360:593–597, 1992.

29. Sieling P, Porcelli S, Chatterjee D, Brennan P, Brenner M, Rea T, Modlin R. CD1-restricted αβ TCR T-cells recognize non-peptide ligands from microbial pathogens (Abstr). *J. Invest. Dermatol.* 104:569, 1995.

30. Bartosik J. Cytomembrane-derived Birbeck granules transport horseradish peroxidase to the endosomal compartment in the human Langerhans cell. *J. Invest. Dermatol.* 99:53–58, 1992.

31. Hanau D, Fabre M, Schmitt DA, Garaud JC, Pauly G, Cazenzve JP. Appearance of Birbeck granule-like structures in anti-T6 antibody-treated human epidermal Langerhans cells. *J. Invest. Dermatol.* 90:298–304, 1998.

32. Bucana CD, Munn G, Song MJ, Dunner K, Kripke ML. Internalization of Ia molecules into Birbeck granule-like structures in murine dendritic cells. *J. Invest. Dermatol.* 99:365–373, 1992.

33. Mommaas M, Mulder A, Vermeer BJ, Koning F. Functional human epidermal Langerhans cells that lack Birbeck granules. *J. Invest. Dermatol.* 103:807–810, 1994.

34. Aiba S, Katz SI. The ability of cultured langerhans cells to process and present protein antigens is MHC-dependent. 146:2479–2487, 1991.

35. Streilein JW, Grammer SF. In vitro evidence that Langerhans cells can adopt two functionally distinct forms capable of antigen presentation to T lymphocytes. *J. Immunol.* 143:3925–3933, 1989.

36. Bjorkman PJ, Sapper MA, Samraoui B, Bennett WS, Strominger JL, Wiley DC. Structure of the human class I histocompatibility antigen, HLA-A2. *Nature* 329:506–512, 1987.

37. Bjorkman PJ, Sapper MA, Samraoui B, Bennett WS, Strominger JL, Wiley DC. The foreign antigen binding site and T cell recognition regions of class I histocompatibility antigens. *Nature* 329:512–518, 1987.

38. Meuer SC, Schlossman SF, Reinherz EL. Clonal analysis of human cytotoxic T lymphocytes: T4+ and T8+ effector T cells recognize products of different major histocompatibility complex regions. *Proc. Natl. Acad. Sci. U.S.A.* 79:4395–4399, 1982.

39. Kalish RS, Wood JA, LaPorte A. Processing of urushiol (poison ivy) hapten by both endogenous and exogenous pathways for presentation to human T-cells. *J. Clin. Invest.* 93:2039–2047, 1994.

40. Kalish RS. Antigen processing: the gateway to the immune response (Review). *J. Am. Acad. Dermatol.* 32:640–652, 1995.

41. Jenkins MK, Schwartz RH. Antigen presentation by chemically modified splenocytes induces antigen-specific T cell unresponsiveness in vitro and in vivo. *J. Exp. Med.* 165:302–319, 1987.

42. Quill H, Schwartz RH. Stimulation of normal inducer T cell clones with antigen presented by purified Ia molecules in planar lipid membranes: specific induction of a long-lived state of proliferative nonresponsiveness. *J. Immunol.* 138:3704–3712, 1987.

43. Jenkins MK, Taylor PS, Norton SD, Urdahl KB. CD28 delivers a costimulatory signal involved in antigen-specific IL2 production by human T cells. *J. Immunol.* 147:2461–2466, 1991.

44. Gimm CD, Freeman GJ, Gribben JG, Sugita K, Freeman AS, Morimoto C, Nadler LM. B-cell surface antigen B7 provides a costimulatory signal that induced T cells to proliferate and secrete interleukin 2. *Proc. Natl. Acad. Sci. U.S.A.* 88:6575–6579, 1991.

45. Freeman GJ, Gribben JG, Boussiotis VA, Ng JW, Restivo VA, Lombard LA, Gray GS, Nadler LM. Cloning of B7-2: A CTLA-4 counter-receptor that costimulates human T cell proliferation. *Science* 262:909–911, 1993.

46. Harding FA, McArthur JG, Groos JA, Raulet DH, Allison JP. CD28-mediated signalling co-stimulates murine T cells and prevents induction of anergy in T-cell clones. *Nature* 356:607–609, 1992.

47. Gross JA, Callas E, Allison JP. Identification and distribution of the costimulatory receptor CD28 in the mouse. *J. Immunol.* 149:380–388, 1992.

48. Kalish RS, Wood JA: Induction of hapten specific tolerance of human CD8+ urushiol (poison ivy) reactive T-cells. *J. Invest. Dermatol.* 108:253–257, 1997.

49. Augustin M, Dietrich A, Niedner R, Knapp A, Schopf E, Ledbettor JA, Brady W, Linsley PS, Simon JC. Phorbol-12-myristate-13-acetate treated human keratinocytes express B7-like molecules that serve a costimulatory role in T-cell activation. *J. Invest. Dermatol.* 100:275–281, 1993.

50. Naisir A, Ferbel B, Gaspari AA. Human keratinocytes regulate their expression of B7/BB-1 antigen by a unique calcium-dependent mechanism. *J. Invest. Dermatol.* 104:763–767, 1995.

51. Simon JC, Dietrich A, Mielke V, Augustin M, Vanscheidt W, Ledbetter JA, Linsley PS, Schopf E, Sterry W. Distribution of the B7 activation AG and its ligand CD28 in T-cell mediated skin diseases (Abstr). *J. Invest. Dermatol.* 100:576, 1993.

52. Germain RN. The ins and outs of antigen processing and presentation. *Nature (Lond.)* 322:687–689, 1986.

53. Sweetser MT, Morrison LA, Braciale VL, Braciale TJ. Recognition of pre-processed endogenous antigen by class I but not class II MHC-restricted T cells. *Nature (Lond.)* 342:180–182, 1989.

54. Nuchtern JG, Bonifacino JS, Biddison WE, Klausner RD. Brefeldin A implicates egress from endoplasmic reticulum in class I restricted antigen presentation. *Nature (Lond.)* 339:223–225, 1989.

55. Teyton L, O'Sullivan D, Dickson PW, Lotteau V, Sette A, Fink P, Peterson PA. Invariant chain distinguishes between the exogenous and endogenous antigen presentation pathways. *Nature (Lond.)* 348:39–44, 1990.

56. Ziegler HK, Unanue ER. Decrease in macrophage antigen catabolism caused by ammonia and chloroquine is associated with inhibition of antigen presentation to T cells. *Proc. Natl. Acad. Sci. U.S.A.* 79:175–178, 1982.

57. Bauer A, Rutenfranz I, Kirchner H. Processing requirements for T cell activation by Mycoplasma arthridis-derived mitogen. *Eur. J. Immunol.* 18:2109–2112, 1988.

58. Michalek MT, Benacerraf B, Rock KL. The class II MHC-restricted presentation of endogenously synthesized ovalbumin displays clonal variation, requires endosomal/lysosomal processing, and is upregulated by heat shock. *J. Immunol.* 148:1016–1024, 1992.

59. Hunt DF, Michel H, Dinckinson TA, Shabanowitz J, Cox AL, Sakaguchi K, Appella E, Grey HM, Sette A. Peptides presented to the immune system by the murine class II major histocompatibility complex molecule I-A^d. *Science* 256:1817–1820, 1992.

60. Kalish RS, Wood JA, LaPorte A. Processing of urushiol (poison ivy) hapten by both endogenous and exogenous pathways for presentation to human T-cells. *J. Clin. Invest.* 93:2039–2047, 1994.

61. Momburg F, Hammerling GJ. Generation and TAP-mediated transport of peptides for major histocompatibility complex class I molecules. *Adv. Immunol.* 68:191–256, 1998.

62. Yang Y, Waters JB, Fruh K, Peterson PA. Proteasomes are regulated by interferon gamma: implications for antigen processing. *Proc. Natl. Acad. Sci. U.S.A.* 89:4928–4932, 1992.

63. Kelly A, Powis SH, Glynne R, Radley E, Beck S, Trowsdale J. Second proteasome-related gene in the human MHC class II region. *Nature (Lond.)* 353:6678–6680, 1991.

64. Martinez CK, Monaco JJ. Homology of proteasome subunits to a major histocompatibility complex-linked LMP gene. *Nature (Lond.)* 353:664–667, 1991.

65. Attaya M, Jameson S, Martinez CK, Hermel E, Aldrich C, Forman J, Lindahl KF, Bevan MJ, Monaco JJ. Ham-2 corrects the class I antigen processing defect in RMA-S cells. *Nature (Lond.)* 355:647–649, 1992.

66. Spies T, Bresnahan M, Bahram S, Arnold D, Blanck G, Mellins E, Pious D, DeMars R. A gene in the human major histocompatibility complex class II region controlling the class I antigen presentation pathway. *Nature (Lond.)* 348:744–747, 1990.

67. Spies T, Cerundolo V, Colonna M, Cresswell P, Townsend A, DeMars R. Presentation of viral antigen by MHC class I molecules is dependent on a putative peptide transporter heterodimer. *Nature (Lond.)* 355:644–646, 1992.

68. Colonna M, Bresnahan M, Bahram S, Strominger JL, Spies T. Allelic variants of the human putative peptide transporter involved in antigen processing. *Proc. Natl. Acad. Sci. U.S.A.* 89:3932–3936, 1992.

69. Cox JH, Yewdell JW, Eisenlohr LC, Johnson PR, Bennink JR. Antigen presentation requires transport of MHC class I molecules from the endoplasmic reticulum. *Science* 247:715–718, 1990.

70. Ledger PW, Tanzer ML. Monensin — a perturbant of cellular physiology. *TIPS* 5:313–314, 1984.

71. Lippincott-Schwartz J, Yuan LC, Bonifacino JS, Klausner RD. Rapid redistribution of golgi proteins into the ER in cells treated with brefeldin A: evidence for membrane cycling from golgi to ER. *Cell* 56:801–813, 1989.

72. Yewdell JW, Bennink JR. Brefeldin A specifically inhibits presentation of protein antigens to cytotoxic T lymphocytes. *Science* 244:1072–1075, 1989.

73. Kalish RS, Wood JA, LaPorte A. Processing of urushiol (poison ivy) hapten by both endogenous and exogenous pathways for presentation to human T-cells. *J. Clin. Invest.* 93:2039–2047, 1994.

74. Xu H, Heeger PS, Fairchild RL. Distinct roles for B7-1 and B7-2 determinants during priming of effector CD8+ Tc1 and regulatory CD4+ Th2 cells for contact hypersensitivity. *J. Immunol.* 159:4217–26, 1997.

75. Bour H, Peyron E, Gaucherand M, Garrigue JL, Desvignes C, Kaiserlian D, Revillard JP, Nicolas JF. Major histocompatibility complex class I-restricted CD8+ T cells and class II-restricted CD4+ T cells, respectively, mediate and regulate contact sensitivity to dinitrofluorobenzene. *Eur. J. Immunol.* 25:3006–3010, 1995.

76. Street NE, Mosmann TR. Functional diversity of T lymphocytes due to secretion of different cytokine patterns. *FASEB J.* 5:171–177, 1991.

77. Coffman RL, Ohara J, Bond MW, Carty J, Zlotnik A, Paul WE. B cell stimulatory factor-1 enhances the IgE response of lipopolysaccharide-activated B cells. *J. Immunol.* 136:4538–4541, 1986.

78. Griffiths CEM, Voorhees JJ, Nickoloff BJ. Characterization of intercellular adhesion molecule-1 and HLA-DR expression in normal and inflamed skin: modulation by recombinant gamma interferon and tumor necrosis factor. *J. Am. Acad. Dermatol.* 20:617–629, 1989.

79. Kapsenberg ML, Wierenga EA, Stiekema FEM, Tiggelman AMBC, Bos JD. Th1 lymphokine production profiles of nickel-specific CD4+ T-lymphocyte clones from nickel contact allergic and non-allergic individuals. *J. Invest. Dermatol.* 98:59–63, 1992.

80. Kalish RS, Morimoto C. Quantitation and cloning of human urushiol specific peripheral blood T-cells: isolation of urushiol specific suppressor T-cells. *J. Invest. Dermatol.* 92:46–52, 1989.

81. Kalish RS, Johnson KL. Enrichment and function of urushiol (poison ivy) specific T-lymphocytes in lesions of allergic contact dermatitis to urushiol. *J. Immunol.* 145:3706–3713, 1990.

82. Foster CA, Dreyfuss M, Mandak B, Meingassner JG, Naegeli HU, Nussbaumer A, Oberer L, Scheel G, Swoboda EM. Pharmacological modulation of endothelial cell-associated adhesion molecule expression: implications for future treatment of dermatological diseases. *J. Dermatol.* 21:847–854, 1994.

83. Picker LJ, Martin RJ, Trumble A, Newman LS, Collins PA, Bergstresser PR, Leung DY. Differential expression of lymphocyte homing receptors by human memory/effector T cells in pulmonary versus cutaneous immune effector sites. *Eur. J. Immunol.* 24:1269–1277, 1994.

84. Picker LJ. Regulation of tissue-selective T-lymphocyte homing receptors during the virgin to memory/effector cell transition in human secondary lymphoid tissues. *Am. Rev. Resp. Dis.* 148:S47–54, 1993.

85. Bos JD, de Boer OJ, Tibosch E, Das PK, Pals ST. Skin-homing T lymphocytes: detection of cutaneous lymphocyte-associated antigen (CLA) by HECA-452 in normal human skin. *Arch. Dermatol. Res.* 285:179–183, 1993.

86. Alon R, Rossiter H, Wang X, Springer TA, Kupper TS. Distinct cell surface ligands mediate T lymphocyte attachment and rolling on P and E selectin under physiological flow. *J. Cell Biol.* 127:1485–1495, 1994.

87. Berg EL, Yoshino T, Rott LS, Robinson MK, Warnock RA, Kishimoto TK, Picker LJ, Butcher EC. The cutaneous lymphocyte antigen is a skin lymphocyte homing receptor for the vascular lectin endothelial cell-leukocyte adhesion molecule 1. *J. Exp. Med.* 174:1461–1466, 1991.

88. Hauser C, Santamaria LF, Babi LJ, Picker LJ, Blaser K. Skin allergy-associated T cell responses in the blood are largely confined to the CLA+ CD45RO+ subset (Abstract). *J. Invest. Dermatol.* 104:555, 1995.

89. Dustin LM, Singer KH, Tuck DT, Springer TA. Adhesion of T lymphoblasts to epidermal keratinocytes is regulated by interferon gamma and is mediated by intercellular adhesion molecule 1 (ICAM-1). *J. Exp. Med.* 167:1323–1340, 1988.

90. Walsh LJ, Murphy GF. Role of adhesion molecules in cutaneous inflammation and neoplasia. *J. Cutan. Pathol.* 19:161–171, 1992.

91. Yago T, Tsukuda M, Yamazaki H, Nishi T, Amano T, Minami M. Analysis of an initial step of T cell adhesion to endothelial monolayers under flow conditions. *J. Immunol.* 154:1216–1222, 1995.

92. Jones DA, McIntire LV, Smith CW, Picker LJ. A two-step adhesion cascade for T cell/endothelial cell interactions under flow conditions. *J. Clin. Invest.* 94:2443–2450, 1994.

93. Das PK, de Boer OJ, Visser A, Verhagen CE, Bos JD, Pals ST. Differential expression of ICAM-1, E-selectin and VCAM-1 by endothelial cells in psoriasis and contact dermatitis. *Acta. Derm. Venereol. Suppl.* 186:21–22, 1994.

94. Cornelius LA, Taylor JT, Degitz K, Li LJ, Lawley TJ, Caughman SW. A 5′ portion of the ICAM-1 gene confers tissue-specific differential expression levels and cytokine responsiveness. *J. Invest. Dermat.* 100:753–758, 1993.

95. Griffiths CEM, Nickoloff BJ. Keratinocyte intracellular adhesion molecule-1 (ICAM-1) expression precedes dermal T lymphocyte infiltration in allergic contact dermatitis (Rhus dermatitis). *Am. J. Path.* 135:1045–1053, 1989.

96. Wildner O, Lipkow T, Knop J. Increased expression of ICAM-1, E-selectin, and VCAM-1 by cultured human endothelial cells upon exposure to haptens. *Exp. Dermatol.* 1:191–198, 1992.

97. Piguet PF, Grau GE, Hauser C, Vassalli P. Tumor necrosis factor is a critical mediator in hapten induced irritant and contact hypersensitivity reactions. *J. Exp. Med.* 173:673–679, 1991.

98. Dvorak AM, Mihm MC Jr, Dvorak HF. Morphology of delayed-type hypersensitivity reactions in man. II. Ultrastructural alterations affecting the microvasculature and the tissue mast cells. *Lab. Invest.* 34:179–191, 1976.

99. Wood GS, Volterra AS, Abel EA, Nickoloff BJ, Adams RM. Allergic contact dermatitis: Novel immunohistologic features. *J. Invest. Dermatol.* 87:688–693, 1986.

100. Gallo RL, Granstein RD. Inhibition of allergic contact dermatitis and ultraviolet radiation-induced tissue swelling in the mouse by topical amiloride. *Arch. Dermatol.* 125:502–506, 1989.

101. Lindgren AM, Granstein RD, Hosoi J, Gallo RL. Structure-function relations in the inhibition of murine contact hypersensitivity by amiloride. *J. Invest. Dermatol.* 104:38–41, 1995.

102. Kalish RS, Wood JA, Kydonieus A, Wille JJ: Prevention of contact hypersensitivity to topically applied drugs by ethacrynic acid: Potential application to transdermal drug delivery. *J. Controlled Release* 48:79–87, 1997.

103. Diezel W, Gruner S, Diaz LA, Anhalt GJ. Inhibition of cutaneous contact hypersensitivity by calcium transport inhibitors lanthanum and diltiazem. *J. Invest. Dermatol.* 93:322–326, 1989.

104. Senaldi G, Pointaire P, Pierre-Francois P, Grau GE. Protective effect of N-acetylcysteine in hapten induced irritant and contact hypersensitivity reactions. *J. Invest. Dermatol.* 102:934–937, 1994.

105. Schmidt RJ, Khan L, Chung LY. Are free radicals and not quinones the haptenic species derived from urushiol and other contact allergenic mono- and dihydric alkylbenzenes? The significance of NADH, glutathione, and redox cycling in the skin. *Arch. Dermatol. Res.* 282:56–64, 1990.

106. Roederer M, Staal FJT, Raju PA, Ela SW, Herzenberg LA, Herzenberg LA. Cytokine-stimulated HIV replication is inhibited by N-acetylcysteine. *Proc. Natl. Acad. Sci. U.S.A.* 87:4884–4888, 1990.

107. Staal FJT, Roederer M, Herzenberg LA, Herzenberg LA. Intracellular thiols regulate activation of nuclear factor kB and transcription of human immunodeficiency virus. *Proc. Natl. Acad. Sci. U.S.A.* 87:9943–9947, 1990.

108. Ikeda M, Schroeder KK, Mosher LB, Woods CW, Akeson AL. Suppressive effect of antioxidants on intracellular adhesion molecule-1 (ICAM-1) expression in human epidermal keratinocytes. *J. Invest. Dermatol.* 103:791–796, 1994

109. Schwarz A, Krone C, Trautinger F, Aragane Y, Neuner P, Luger TA, Schwarz T. Pentoxifylline suppresses irritant and contact hypersensitivity reactions. *J. Invest. Dermatol.* 101:549–552, 1993.

110. Mosmann TR, Cherwinski H, Bond MW, Giedlin MA, Coffman RL. Two types of murine helper T cell clone I. Definition according to profiles of lymphokine activities and secreted proteins. *J. Immunol.* 136:2348–2357, 1986.

111. Fiorentino DF, Bond MW, Mosmann TR. Two types of mouse T helper cell IV. Th2 clones secrete a factor that inhibits cytokine production by Th1 clones. *J. Exp. Med.* 170:2081–2095, 1989.

112. Moore KW, Vieira P, Fiorentino DF, Trounstine ML, Khan TA, Mosmann TR. Homology of cytokine synthesis inhibitory factor (IL10) to the Epstein-Barr virus gene BCRF1. *Science* 248:1230–1233, 1990.

113. Schwarz A, Grabbe S, Riemann H, Aragane Y, Simon M, Manon S, Andrade S, Luger TA, Zlotnik A, Schwarz T. In vivo effects of interleukin-10 on contact hypersensitivity and delayed-type hypersensitivity reactions. *J. Invest. Dermatol.* 103:211–216, 1994.

114. Jenkins MK, Taylor PS, Norton SD, Urdahl KB. CD28 delivers a costimulatory signal involved in antigen-specific IL2 production by human T cells. *J. Immunol.* 147:2461–2466, 1991.
115. Tan P, Anasetti C, Hansen JA, Melrose J, Brunvand M, Bradshaw J, Ledbetter JA, Linsley PS. Induction of alloantigen-specific hyporesponsiveness in human T lymphocytes by blocking interaction of CD28 with its natural ligand B7/BB1. *J. Exp. Med.* 177:165–173, 1993.
116. Schwartz RH. Costimulation of T lymphocytes: the role of CD28, CTLA-4, and B7/BB1 in interleukin-2 production and immunotherapy. *Cell* 71:1065–1068, 1992.
117. Kalish RS, Wood JA: Induction of hapten specific tolerance of human CD8+ urushiol (poison ivy) reactive T-cells. *J. Invest. Dermatol.* 108:253–257, 1997.
118. Tocci MJ, Matkovich D, Collier K, Kwok P, Dumont F, Lin S, Degubicibus S, Siekierka JJ, Chin JJ, Hutchinson N. The immunosuppressant FK 506 selectively inhibits expression of early T cell activation genes. *J. Immunol.* 143:718–726, 1989.
119. Furue M, Osada A, Chang CH, Tamaki K. Immunosuppressive effects of azelastine hydrochloride on contact hypersensitivity and T-cell proliferative response: a comparative study with FK-506. *J. Invest. Dermatol.* 103:49–53, 1994.
120. Duncan J. Differential inhibition of cutaneous T-cell mediated reactions and epidermal cell proliferation by cyclosporin, FK-506, and rapamycin. *J. Invest. Dermatol.* 102:84–88, 1994.

11 Mast Cells Regulate Endothelial Cell Function in Inflammation and Repair*

Marcia R. Monteiro and George F. Murphy

CONTENTS

I. INTRODUCTION

Mast cells are granulated, bone marrow-derived, fixed inhabitants of cutaneous and mucosal tissues that form host–environmental interfaces. For many years, these cells were believed to represent precursors of mobile granulated blood cells, and only recently their true function has been revealed. Insights into the physiologic and pathologic roles of mast cells may be gained through under-standing the significance of their consistent localization to microanatomical compartments rich in nerve fibers and blood vessels. In addition, the metachromatic cytoplasmic granules contained within mast cells and released upon stimulation by a plethora of seemingly unrelated signals also have provided key insights into mast cell function. In this chapter, recent molecular and cell biological data concerning the growing significance of mast cells in health and disease will be reviewed. Insights revealed by current knowledge of mast cell biology have led to development of a model for mast cell function in tissue inflammation as well as in mesenchymal homeostasis, injury, and repair.

II. MAST CELL LOCALIZATION IN TISSUE: CELLULAR AND MOLECULAR INTERACTIONS

Mast cells are consistently observed in close association with nerves and vessels in connective tissue microenvironments that are situated directly beneath epithelial barriers. These structural relationships are preserved by precise molecular interactions that mediate mast cell localization to these specific microanatomical sites. Indeed, there is evidence that the binding of mast cell

* Supported by a grant (R01-CA40358) from the National Institute of Health.

membrane adhesion receptors to specific extracellular matrix (ECM) proteins constitutively present in the perivascular space is responsible for preferential mast cell localization in certain tissues.

The dermal perivascular compartment (DPVC) is composed of a network of fibers, glycoproteins, and mucopolysaccharides; specialized cells such as macrophages, dendritic antigen-presenting cells, and Factor XIIIa-positive dermal dendrocytes; and cell processes such as axons (Figure 1). Through the DPVC, transportation of nutrients and other molecules between the intra- and extravascular spaces occurs. Moreover, the DPVC also provides protection for the delicate vascular tissue which it envelops. Collagens type I, III, IV, V, VI, and VIII are normal components of the perivascular space, as are the glycoproteins fibronectin and laminin, elastin, and certain proteoglycans.[1]

In human skin, mast cells are found within the DPVC in close association with the vascular basement membrane. In the mid 1980s, we and others became interested in the molecular basis for this localization. VLA-6 ($\alpha6\beta1$) is a component of the integrin family, known to be an important receptor for laminin, and is expressed by mouse bone marrow-derived mast cells mediating the adhesion of these cells to laminin.[2] Immunohistochemically, we found that human mast cells stain for the integrin receptor of the basement membrane protein, laminin.[3] Moreover, when mast cells are enzymatically separated from the DPVC, they retain laminin "caps" at sites of previous apposition with basement membrane, indicating persistent interaction between extracellular laminin and its plasma membrane receptor. Moreover, isolated murine[4] and human[3] mast cells adhere to laminin-coated substrates. Degranulation of mast cells decreases their binding to laminin substrates in vitro and correlates with mast cell movement away from their original location in the perivascular space in vivo.[3] This phenomenon appears to be triggered by degranulation-related loss of laminin receptor expression. In addition, the immature human mast cell line, HMC-1, binds spontaneously to fibronectin (FN), laminin (LN), and collagen types I and III,[5] all present in normal DPVC. Upon phorbol myristate acetate (PMA) activation, these same cells are capable of binding to vitronectin (VN) and collagen type IV. It is also known that the binding of these cells to VN and FN involves such integrin receptors as $\alpha5\beta1$ and $\alpha v\beta5$.[6] Human mast cells obtained from adult normal skin are also capable of spontaneously adhering to fibronectin and laminin, and this is mediated by expression of VLA-3, VLA-4, and VLA-5 integrins. Thus, complex interactions between membrane adhesion receptors (integrins) expressed by the mast cells and molecules in the DPVC are involved in the localization of the mast cells.[6]

There is now evidence that specific factors play a role in modulation of integrin expression by mast cells. One example of this is the regulatory effect played by mast cell growth factor (MGF) on the function of mast cell integrins. MGF is a cytokine growth factor produced by fibroblasts, endothelial cells, and epithelial cells which contributes to the regulation of mast cell growth and differentiation. Adhesion of mast cells to fibronectin (FN) is transiently increased by MGF and requires lower concentrations of this cytokine than is required for growth stimulation. In addition, this increase in the binding of mast cells to FN is not related to a change in the quantity of mast cell surface VLA-5 receptors, indicating that MGF probably acts by modifying the affinity or other qualitative characteristics of the receptor.[7]

The observation that mast cells are spatially related to nerve fibers is not new and has been reported previously by many authors.[8,9] This relationship occurs not only in the skin, but in other organs as well, as is evidenced in human intestinal mucosa.[10] The functional significance of this relatively consistent finding appears to relate to the ability of specific neuropeptides such as substance P[11,12] and calcitonin–gene related peptide[13] to be capable of triggering the release of mast cell contents. Indeed, this has led to speculation that there exists neuroimmunomodulation of certain inflammatory responses, such as some forms of dermatitis (psoriasis), asthma, and even gastrointestinal disturbances (ulcerative disorders of the stomach and intestine). With regard to psoriasis, it is known that mast cells and nerves are more closely associated in the dermis of lesional skin from psoriatic patients when compared to nonlesional skin from the same patients, suggesting a role of this anatomical relationship to the pathophysiology of the lesions.[14]

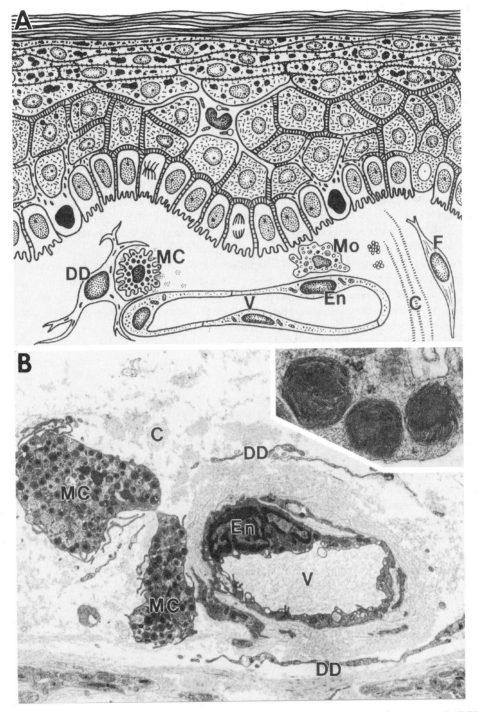

Figure 1   A. Schematic representation of components of the perivascular connective tissue matrix (DPVC). This region is directly beneath the epidermal layer and consists of postcapillary venules (V) lined by endothelial cells (En) and surrounded by mast cells (MC), adjacent dermal dendrocytes (DD), occasional monocyte/macrophages (Mo), fibroblasts (F), and collagen bundles (C). (Illustration by Michael Ioffreda.) B. Transmission electron micrograph depicting some of the constituents of the DPVC of normal adult human skin; inset depicts higher magnification of typical mast cell granules. Although cell bodies of DD are not seen in this section, the thin, enveloping membrane shrouds resembling dendrites in two-dimensional sections are readily apparent.

Egan and co-workers in our laboratory[15] recently have defined a plexus of axons surrounding human dermal mast cells and extending vertically into the overlying epidermis of human and nonhuman primate skin. In the same study, the application of a neuropeptide-releasing agent (capsaicin) at the epidermal surface resulted in mast cell degranulation and subsequent alterations in endothelial cells that promoted inflammation (see below). Furthermore, this cascade could not be triggered without an intact neural plexus within the skin. From these studies, we concluded that agents which act at the epidermal surface may rapidly and efficiently provoke dermal inflammation via axonal "hardwiring" which unifies the epidermal and dermal strata.

In addition to their anatomical and functional relation to vessels and nerves, mast cells also demonstrate a close structural relation with Factor XIIIa (FXIIIa)-containing dermal dendrocytes (especially with the dendrocytes located in the perivascular spaces of normal skin). Three-dimensional reconstructions disclose that membrane flaps of dermal dendrocytes envelop mast cell plasma membranes for 50 to 90% of their perimeter.[16] Moreover, 70% of mast cells located in the upper dermis appear to be related to dermal dendrocytes in this way. Dermal dendrocytes show increased Factor XIIIa expression in response to mast cell secretion, an event that is related to the mast cell liberation of tumor necrosis factor α (TNF-α) upon degranulation.[17]

From these and other studies, we have begun to understand the cellular and molecular basis for mast cell localization about microvessels. Mast cells appear to be tethered to numerous macromolecules in the DPVC via plasma membrane receptors which are regulated by cytokines such as MGF synthesized by surrounding fibroblasts, endothelial cells, and overlying epithelial cells. This localization fosters intimate interactions between mast cells and other cell types, such as endothelial cells and dermal dendrocytes. As will be described in the paragraphs to follow, these phenotypic characteristics have served as a basis for hypotheses that have led to recent novel findings which provide important clues concerning the functional significance of these spatial relationships.

III. MAST CELL CYTOLOGY: EVIDENCE FOR EFFECTOR SECRETORY FUNCTION

Mast cells contain within their cytoplasm numerous granules which characteristically take up metachromatic stains, such as toluidine blue and giemsa. Ultrastructurally, skin mast cell granules are membrane-bound organelles which exhibit different morphologic features that are determined, in part, by their microanatomical localization in tissues (Figure 2).[18] In general, two morphological domains are recognized to compose the internal matrix of mast cell granules: amorphous regions and crystalline regions. The crystalline regions contain scroll-like, lamellar, and grating/lattice-like configurations. It is now known, based on immunoelectron microscopic studies, that there exists a correlation between the subgranular distribution of mast cell serine proteinases with specific granule subcomponents. Chymase and cathepsin-G are localized electron-dense amorphous subregions, whereas tryptase is concentrated in crystalline subregions in the same granule. The finding of a subgranular separation of these enzymes suggests that they can be packaged separately within the same granules and may account for some of the structural features observed by electron microscopy.[19] Moreover, it raises the possibility that mast cell mediators may be differentially stored and secreted.

The content of mast cell protease mediators can vary among mast cells that populate different tissues and thus is one indicator of mast cell heterogeneity. Mast cells may be classified as both tryptase and chymase-positive (MCtc) or tryptase-positive, chymase-negative mast cells (MCt), depending on their mediator content. The MCtc mast cells are predominantly present in the skin, synovium, small intestinal submucosa, and conjunctival substantia propria. In addition to tryptase and chymase, mast cells also contain cathepsin-G-like protease and carboxypeptidase. On the other hand, MCt, which are mostly present in the alveolar walls of the lung and small intestinal mucosa, contain only tryptase, lacking the other components.[20]

The maturation, development, proliferation, and phenotypic differentiation of mast cells are processes regulated by many mast cell growth factors, such as stem cell factor (otherwise known

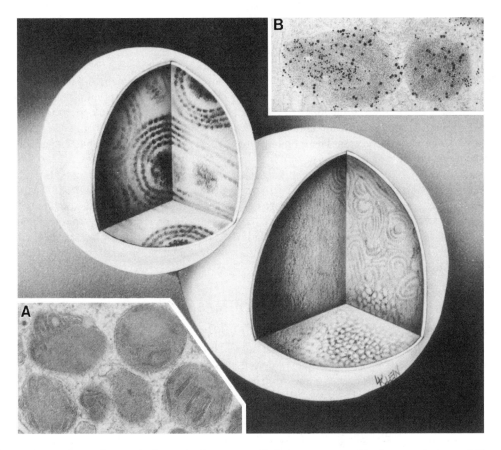

Figure 2   Schematic model of granules from mast cells in human mucosal lamina propria (upper left) and DPVC (lower right); note different granule sizes and internal patterns of subgranular structural domains. Inset A represents ultrastructure of mast cell granules with prominent scroll-like subregions and adjacent electron-dense amorphous domains. Inset B portrays immunoultrastructural restriction of specific chemical components to discrete granule subregions (smaller gold particles = tryptase, larger gold particles = chymase). (Illustration by Lynn Klein.)

as mast cell growth factor, MGF). Indeed, expression of granule proteases is dependent on the cytokine media to which mast cells are exposed.[21] In one in vivo rodent model,[22] local administration of MGF promoted the development of connective tissue-type mast cells (CTMC) in the skin of mice and the systemic administration of SCF induced the development of both CTMC and mucosal mast cells (MMC) in rats. These findings demonstrate that MGF can induce the expansion of both CTMC and MMC populations in vivo.

Two different types of mast cell degranulation patterns are recognized. In the "anaphylactic" type, after an appropriate secretory stimulus, there is rapid fusion of granule membranes with the plasma membrane and between granules themselves to form conduits for the release of stored mediators into the extracellular space.[23] Generally, the stimulus for the release of mast cell contents is the binding of antigen to cell-bound IgE antibody. "Anaphylactic" type of degranulation can be observed after nonimmunological stimuli such as morphine sulfate, calcium ionophore, and compound 48/80, indicating that the structural characteristics of mast cell secretion may depend on factors other than the nature of the stimulus.[24] Indeed, the ultrastructural morphology of this form of secretion is similar, regardless of metachromatic cell type (basophils or mast cells), species, or provocative trigger.

On the other hand, in the "piecemeal" pattern of degranulation, dissipation of granule contents appears to occur more gradually, with shuttling of granule contents to the cell surface via microvesicles. This pattern of mast cell degranulation has been observed in contact allergy,[25] bullous pemphigoid,[26] Crohn's disease,[27] and many other entities.

Kaminer et al.[28] have used electron microscopic analysis of skin biopsies obtained from atopic individuals following positive ragweed intradermal injections to document different forms of degranulation as a consequence of a single stimulus. These data disclosed an initial rapid degranulation event, with a pattern compatible with the anaphylactic type of degranulation, followed after 5 min by a pattern of degranulation similar to the piecemeal type whereby granules appeared to secrete only part of their contents. These findings may reflect time-dependent granule heterogeneity in response to IgE-mediated secretory stimuli.

Dvorak et al.[29] have found that human lung mast cells can reuse their granule membranes and some of the contents after degranulation. These processes are called "conservation" and "reconstitution" and were generally observed in mast cells that showed only partial degranulation. An alternative mechanism for granulopoiesis after secretory discharge is the neosynthesis of mature granules from Golgi-associated "progranules." This mechanism, however, may be utilized predominantly in the process of mast cell differentiation from agranular precursors exposed to specific growth and differentiation factors like MGF.

IV. THE ORIGIN OF MAST CELLS

Mast cells are bone marrow-derived cells[30] which develop, function, and survive as a consequence of precise regulation by growth factors and interleukins. Initial studies performed in murine models demonstrated that recombinant IL-3 is able to promote the proliferation of mouse mast cell lines.[31] Ishizaka and co-workers[32] examined a long-term coculture of mononuclear cells of human umbilical cord blood with mouse embryo-derived 3T3 fibroblasts, and under these conditions documented the development of mast cells that were morphologically and functionally mature cells and clearly different from basophilic granulocytes. These cells contained granules which expressed both chymase and tryptase, resembling mature mast cells in human skin. Furthermore, upon challenge with anti-IgE, the sensitized mast cells released histamine.

Later, other groups developed mast cells from cocultures of CD34+ pluripotent progenitor cells derived from the bone marrow[33] and fetal liver cells [34] by exposing them to 3T3 murine fibroblasts. Based upon such approaches, it was reasoned that there existed a mast cell growth factor present in the supernatant of the 3T3 fibroblast culture which was responsible for the mast cell development. Several groups next performed studies to better characterize and clone this novel cytokine that was called stem cell factor,[35] mast cell growth factor,[36] and kit ligand.[37]

The identification and characterization of the MGF as a potent determinant of mast cell phenotype and function led to several studies that focused on further characterization of the maturation and development of mast cell from their precursors. Several groups used recombinant MGF in animal models to induce proliferation of mast cell populations in vivo,[38,39] and human recombinant MGF was shown to experimentally induce mature mast cells from human umbilical cord blood cells[40] and fetal liver cells.[41] In addition, the interaction of MGF with other interleukins, such as Il-3 and IL-4, has been shown to be synergistic with respect to development and differentiation of murine mast cells.[42] Moreover, MGF also may stimulate directional motility of both mucosal and connective tissue-type mast cells[43] and regulate the survival of mouse mast cells by suppressing apoptosis.[44]

MGF is produced by several cell types in the skin, including fibroblasts,[45] keratinocytes,[46] and endothelial cells.[47] It is a membrane-bound molecule which may be proteolytically cleaved to produce a soluble bioactive form. Although the proteases producing this cleavage are still unknown, Longley et al.[48] recently demonstrated that human mast cell chymase cleaves MGF at a novel site, resulting in a soluble bioactive product that is different than the previously identified soluble MGF. This study suggests a possible autocrine loop in which chymase released from mast cell secretory granules may solubilize MGF bound to the membrane of surrounding stromal cells. The liberated soluble MGF could, in turn, stimulate mast cell proliferation and differentiation, possibly contributing to local accumulation of mast cells in the skin at sites of the initial secretory stimulus.

From the data presented above, it is reasonable to question what role, if any, MGF may play in conditions such as mastocytosis, where mast cells may accumulate in the skin and visceral tissues and result in significant functional impairment and, in some patients, even death. In normal skin, immunoreactive MGF is associated with keratinocytes and some dermal cells, in a cell-bound pattern (membrane-bound pattern). In the setting of mastocytosis, however, lesions as well as normal skin exhibit a staining pattern for MGF, where this factor is apparently within the intercellular spaces that separate keratinocytes and free within the dermis (secretory pattern).[46] These findings suggested the possibility of an altered metabolism of this factor in some patients with mastocytosis, consistent with an abnormal production of its soluble form. This may not account for the entire mechanism underlying human mastocytosis, however, we have recently learned that in some cases, the abnormal mast cells exhibit clonal characteristics characterized by permanent activation of their MGF receptor.[49]

Workers in our laboratory have also found that human skin xenografted to severe combined immunodeficient mice can be used as a model to study human cutaneous mast cell hyperplasia.[50] In this experimental system, patterns of epidermal MGF expression resembling human mastocytosis develop weeks after xenotransplantation, and this event is closely linked to the development of markedly increased numbers of dermal mast cells. While such studies provide potentially important insights into mechanisms that regulate mast cell proliferation, it is equally important from a therapeutic perspective to understand how mast cell number and function may be modulated. It is well recognized that mast cell number is diminished by chronic application of corticosteroids.[51] This action now appears to be the result of downregulation of tissue MGF production required for the survival of local mast cells.[52] The ability to therapeutically modulate MGF and its effects may be of importance in the treatment and management of allergic diseases.

The nerve growth factor (NGF) has also been described as a stimulator of granulocyte colony growth and eosinophils and basophils/mast cell differentiation.[53] Kannan et al.[54] and Matsuda et al.[55] have performed in vitro studies suggesting that NGF may play a role in the development of granulopoiesis and mast cell differentiation via interaction with hemopoietic factors such as IL-3 to increase mast cell colony formation from bone marrow and spleen cells. In addition to its effects in mast cell proliferation, NGF is also capable of inhibiting mast cell apoptosis.[56] It is of interest that mast cells are capable of synthesizing, storing, and releasing NGF,[57] contributing further to the notion that mast cells may play an important role in the interactions between the neural and immune systems that regulate inflammatory and allergic reactions.

V. THE FUNCTION OF MAST CELLS IN HEALTH AND DISEASE

The first clues that provided insight into the functional role of mast cells involved the observations that (1) these cells are consistently situated about superficial post-capillary venules, and (2) mast cells regularly degranulate in a wide variety of inflammatory processes. The role of mast cells in delayed-type hypersensitivity (DTH) reactions was initially suggested by studies that reported that this type of reaction was most easily elicited in mouse skin sites that are rich in mast cells (foot pads and ears) and that reserpine, a drug which depletes mast cells of 5-HT5-hydroxytryptamine (5-HT), abolished the ability of the mouse to present DTH reactions in the skin.[58] Subsequently, two different strains of mice with independent genetic defects that lead to a substantial mast cell deficiency (W/Wv and Sl/Sld) were investigated with regard to their ability to express DTH.[59] The results indicated that the inability of mast cell-deficient mice to express DTH was overcome when sensitized T cells and specific antigen were placed in the extravascular tissues by local passive transfer. It was concluded that local release of vasoactive mediators from mast cells is required in DTH to allow effector T cells to leave the intravascular space, enter the tissues, and become activated by antigen to release chemoattractant lymphokines that recruit a nonspecific infiltrate of leukocytes which then amplify the inflammatory response.

Lewis et al.[60] evaluated challenge reactions elicited by the application of dinitrochlorobenzene to skin of human subjects sequentially over a 96-h period using immunohistochemical and ultrastructural techniques. At 4 h after antigen challenge, the first alteration documented was mast cell degranulation within perivenular foci in the superficial dermis. This was followed by a sparse superficial perivascular T cell infiltrate by 24 h after antigen application. In a follow-up study by Waldorf et al.,[61] which evaluated in greater detail the events occurring at the level of the microvasculature in the cutaneous DTH, mast cell degranulation was followed by elicitation of a cascade of adhesion molecules expressed by microvascular endothelium, including E-selectin. Although it had been recognized for some time that mast cell degranulation accompanied DTH reactions potentially as a result of T cell infiltration,[25] the temporal relationships in these more recent studies led to a novel hypothesis that mast cells might actually trigger T cell infiltration by inducing adhesion molecule expression directly in the adjacent microvessels.

In experimentally induced dermatitis in rodent models, the relationship between mast cell degranulation and dermal inflammation also appears to hold. For example, in a murine model for graft vs. host disease (GVHD),[62] mast cell degranulation is the first pathological alteration noted, whether the disease was mediated by CD4+ or CD8+ T cells. Recently, the involvement of IgE in the pathogenesis of GVHD in a particular strain combination was studied, and the use of a peptide analogue which inhibits IgE-FCεRIα receptor interactions significantly improved the survival of the treated group in comparison to the untreated group.[63]

Ultraviolet B radiation has effects on dermal mast cells in a manner that may provide clues as to their role as potential inflammatory triggers. In irradiated hairless mice, the number of dermal mast cells increased with UVB exposure in a dose-dependent manner.[64] In addition, the expression and distribution of MGF is altered, with an increase in the expression of the MGF by the epidermis and a shift from a cytoplasmic pattern of staining to a membrane-associated or intercellular pattern to resemble that described above for cutaneous mastocytosis. UVB exposure has been recognized for many years as a stimulus for mast cell degranulation in the skin,[65] although the pathological significance and mechanism of this phenomenon remained an enigma. In the early 1990s,[66] we determined that UVB-induced mast cell degranulation in vivo and in skin explants in vitro triggered endothelial activation and E-selectin expression in a manner identical to that seen in the early phases of the cutaneous DTH. The endothelial activation was shown to be independent of any direct effects of UVB on this cell type, and the mast cell–endothelial alterations induced by UVB were inhibited by agents that abrogated degranulation or which blocked UVB penetration at the cutaneous surface. From these and other experiments, it was concluded that mast cell degranulation elicited by a variety of factors may be responsible for rapid induction of endothelial-leukocyte adhesion molecules, such as E-selectin. The "phenotype" of subsequent inflammation would then depend in large part of the nature of circulating cells that the induced cascade of endothelial-leukocyte adhesion molecules would recruit to the dermal microvasculature (memory T cells in DTH, alloreactive cytotoxic cells in GVHD, nonspecific responders such as neutrophils in UVB-elicited injury).

Based upon these and other in vivo observations temporally linking mast cell degranulation to induction of endothelial adhesion molecules, like E-selectin, we hypothesized in the late 1980s that mast cells may actually secrete proinflammatory mediators. Accordingly, we developed a system whereby human skin may be cultured in vitro in order to better assess mast cell–endothelial interactions. We found that after addition of recombinant IL-1 or TNF-α to skin organ cultures, E-selectin is reliably induced only in postcapillary venular endothelium.[67] Moreover, mast cell degranulation provoked in mechanistically different ways by a variety of secretagogues results in nearly identical effects on adjacent endothelium which can be blocked only by antiserum to TNF-α.[68] Based upon these findings, we next established that human dermal mast cells synthesize, store, and release TNF-α upon degranulation which, in turn, induces the expression of E-selectin on dermal postcapillary venules.[69] These data suggested that perivascular mast cells are strategically positioned and functionally capable of acting as "gatekeepers" of the dermal microvasculature, regulating adhesion and influx of leukocytes that possess ligands for membrane glycoproteins like E-selectin displayed during mast cell-induced endothelial activation.

In order to establish the functional validity of this hypothesis, a murine chimeric model for the in vivo experimental manipulation of human skin was established. In this model, human skin was xenotransplanted onto genetically immunodeficient mice (severe combined immunodeficient [SCID] mice). Human cells and structures within the grafts maintained functional integrity for many months and could be experimentally manipulated with microinjected recombinant cytokines which induced endothelial adhesion cascades in a manner analogous to inflamed skin in vivo.[70] Moreover, circulating leukocytes adhered and migrated to graft dermal microvessels so stimulated, and such events could be easily quantified. Mast cell degranulation in the xenografts, as expected, resulted in local TNF-α release, endothelial E-selectin induction, and leukocyte-endothelial binding which could be inhibited by administration of blocking antiserum to E-selectin.[71] In these and other experiments, the functional significance of mast cell degranulation had been established with regard to their contributory role in leukocyte homing and adhesion to microvascular endothelial cells.

Because TNF-α is a pleiotropic cytokine capable of a wide variety of biological actions, it is not surprising that the effects of mast cell degranulation are not restricted to endothelial cells. In skin organ cultures, for example, the integrins α6β4 and α6β1 on epidermal Langerhans cells (LC) are upregulated as a consequence of mast cell degranulation, and this effect also appears to depend on local liberation of TNF-α during the secretory process.[72] Since these integrins serve as receptors that mediate LC interaction with the basement membrane constituent, laminin, such findings may have important implications concerning spatial localization of LC within various cutaneous compartments during immune responses.

There also is evidence that mast cells may contribute to fibrosing processes, particularly in the lung[73] where fibrosis tends to be consistently associated with fields of mast cell hyperplasia. Indeed, histamine has been shown in vitro to increase lung fibroblast proliferation in a dose-dependent manner. Tryptase, a trypsin-like serine proteinase stored in mast cell secretory granules, has recently been recognized as a potent mitogen for fibroblasts in vitro[74] and to induce an increase in the synthesis of collagen in the human lung fibroblast cell line MRC-5.[75] Tryptase has been implicated in upregulation of procollagen mRNA synthesis[76] in a human organotypic skin-equivalent culture system. These data revealed an increase in the type α1(I) procollagen mRNA synthesis by fibroblasts in the presence of degranulating mast cells, and identical results were obtained when tryptase was added to this culture system in the place of mast cells. IgE-dependent activation of mouse mast cells is associated with fibroblast proliferation, and this effect appears in part to be mediated by TNF-α and TGF-β liberated by murine mast cells upon degranulation.[77] Based on these and other experiments, it is clear that mast cells contain an array of potentially fibrogenic mediators that could influence homeostasis within the dermal extracellular matrix, particularly in the setting of chronic or recurrent degranulation stimuli.

Although their function remains to be fully elucidated, we recently have become aware of an additional polydendritic, fibroblast-like cell within the dermal matrix, the "dermal dendrocyte." These cells are relatively abundant in the perivascular space and contain within their cytoplasm the transglutaminase, Factor XIIIa, important in macromolecular cross-linking of fibrin and fibronectin. Release of TNF-α upon mast cell degranulation results in upregulation of FXIIIa expression by dermal dendrocytes in vitro,[17] and serial three-dimensional reconstructions have revealed that intimate spatial relationships exist between these two cell types.[16]

The role of mast cells in angiogenesis has been a topic of active investigation for several decades, and recent data have served to reinforce this association. It is recognized that mast cells accumulate in sites of forming microvessels,[78,79] and insight into this association has been achieved by recent studies by Gruber and co-workers.[80] In this work, transforming growth factor-β, a regulator of angiogenesis, was also shown to serve as a chemotactic factor for mast cells in vitro. Moreover, in mast cell migration assays, the angiogenic factors, platelet-derived growth factor-AB (PDGF-AB), vascular endothelial cell growth factor (VEGF), and basic fibroblast growth factor (βFGF), also are potent stimulators of directed migration of murine mast cells.[81] These data may in part explain the observation that mast cells accumulate in sites of angiogenesis.

Mast cells also contain factors that may act directly on vessels to stimulate the angiogenic response. Mast cell heparin stimulates bovine capillary endothelial cell migration, which can be blocked by specific antagonists of heparin and heparinase.[82] In addition, mast cell histamine has been shown to mediate the proliferation of human endothelial cells in vitro[83] and to stimulate neovascularization via H1 and H2 receptors.[84] βFGF, an angiogenic cytokine that stimulates endothelial capillary growth in vitro and that induces angiogenesis in vivo,[85,86] is now known to be expressed by mast cells.[87,88] Blair et al.[89] recently performed coculture of a human mast cell line (HMC-1) with human dermal microvascular endothelial cells (HDMEC) and obtained a dose–response increase in the network area of vascular tube growth. The extent of in vitro vascular tube formation was enhanced greatly when HMC-1 were degranulated in the presence of HDMEC. When tryptase was directly added to HDMEC, there was a significant increase of tube formation, and tryptase antagonists served to reverse the effects of degranulated mast cells. In aggregate, the observations described above indicate an intimate relationship between mast cells and endothelial cells, and suggest that finely tuned regulatory control may exist between these two cell types which may mediate endothelial proliferation and neovascular morphogenesis.

VI. REGULATION OF MAST CELL SECRETION

Based upon the data presented above, it seems likely that mast cells function in a number of ways which directly affect cells in the immediate DPVC. Acute responses to degranulation may involve induction of endothelial–leukocyte adhesion pathways with elicitation of tissue inflammation, alteration of Langerhans cell integrin expression potentially influencing pathways of antigen presentation, and induction of FXIIIa expression potentially important in cross-linking of transuded fibrin within the extracellular matrix. More chronically, mast cell products appear to play a role in regulation of collagen synthesis and angiogenesis. It is therefore important to identify endogenous factors that influence mast cell activation and secretion.

In 1990 Matis et al.[90] were the first to expose organ cultures of neonatal human foreskins to substance P in order to experimentally assess the effects of this neuronally derived mast cell secretagogue on cells in the DPVC. Superficial venules of explants exposed to substance P showed evidence of E-selectin induction, an effect not obtained when explants were preincubated with an inactive substance P analog which binds to the substance P receptor on mast cells, or after preincubation of explants with the mast cell inhibitor, cromolyn sodium. Based upon these results, it was speculated that substance P endogenously released by dermal nerve fibers may be important in the regulation of endothelial–leukocyte interactions in vivo via induction of mast cell secretion and attendant liberation of TNF-α.[91] Most recently, Egan et al.[15] examined this axis further by evaluating the effects of the chile pepper-derived protein, capsaicin, after topical application to the surface of skin of human volunteers. Capsaicin is a potent stimulus for liberation, including substance P, and, as anticipated, application on the skin induced mast cell degranulation and E-selectin expression on microvessels. The specificity of this phenomenon for initial substance P liberation was next demonstrated in a novel approach where replicate experiments were performed using living human skin xenografted to SCID mice, which is selectively depleted only of neuropeptide-containing intraepidermal and dermal axons as a result of Wallerian degeneration within the otherwise structurally intact human skin grafts. In this setting, the capsaicin application had no effect on mast cells and microvascular endothelium. Such data establish substance P as a potentially important endogenous trigger of mast cell interaction with cells in the DPVC, such as endothelium, and provide further evidence for neurogenic and psychogenic modulation of the inflammatory response. In this regard, direct and indirect mast cell effects on cells in the immediate perivascular environment could have implications in the pathogenesis of disorders as diverse as psoriasis, asthma, peptic ulcer disease, chronic inflammatory bowel disease, and certain forms of alopecia.

VII. CONCLUSIONS

Enormous strides have been made in the past several decades concerning the structure and function of mast cells. The molecular basis for localization of mast cells within the DPVC about vessels is now partially understood, and the functional rationale for these spatial relationships appears to adhere to a strategic rationale involving acute and chronic regulation of tissue inflammation and repair. It is perhaps logical that mast cells subserve this function, since they are (1) "hardwired" to nerves via neuropeptide intermediaries; (2) capable of rapid synthesis and efficient release of a wide array of potent biological mediators; and (3) replenished by an abundant supply of bone marrow-derived precursors upon depletion. Their localization in host–environmental interfaces seems to represent a symbiotic event. After efflux of precursors into the perivascular space, mast cell differentiation and proliferation are nourished by growth factors like MGF, which are plentiful in the fibroblast-rich connective tissue microenvironment as well as within nearby epithelial layers. Once captured by adhesive interactions on the DPVC, mature mast cells are ideally positioned to release molecular cues via secretion, which mediate in part the subsequent behavior of endothelium, fibroblasts, antigen-presenting cells, and dermal dendrocytes (Figure 3). In this setting, mast cells become important targets for future development of therapeutic agents designed to modulate tissue inflammation and repair.

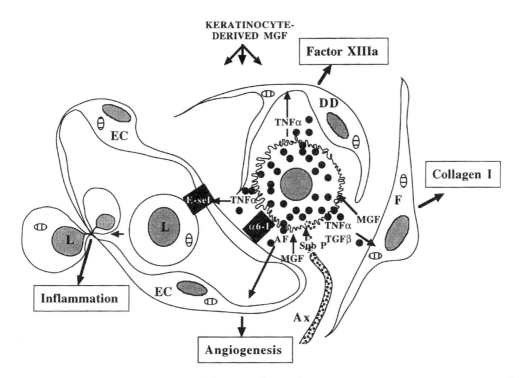

Figure 3   Schematic representation of functional interactions between mast cells (e.g., granulated cell slightly left of center) and related components of the DPVC. MGF originating from keratinocytes, fibroblasts (F), and endothelial cells (EC) promotes local maturation and differentiation of mast cells. Most mast cells in the DPVC are strategically tethered to the pervascular space by binding interactions in part between integrins like α6 and basement membrane components such as laminin (α6-L). Small axons (Ax) containing the mast cell secretagogue, substance P (Sub P), as well as many other endogenous and exogenous factors may trigger mast cell degranulation. TNF-α released upon degranulation contributes to endothelial activation by inducing adhesive glycoproteins, such as E-selectin (E-sel), on EC, thus promoting leukocyte (L) binding and resultant inflammation. Mast cell-derived and secreted angiogenic factors (AF) such as tryptase, histamine, and heparin may provide proliferative stimuli to endothelium. In addition, mast cell TNF-α and TGFβ may induce collagen type I gene transcription in nearby fibroblasts. Finally, Factor XIIIa expression by dermal dendrocytes (DD) is enhanced when TNF-α is liberated as a result of mast cell degranulation.

REFERENCES

1. Voss B., Rauterberg J., Muller K.-M.: The perivascular connective matrix. *Pathol. Res. Pract.* 190: 969, 1994.
2. Fehlner-Gardiner C., Uniyal S., von Ballestrem C., Dougherty G. J., Chan B. M.: Integrin VLA-6 ($\alpha6\beta1$) mediates adhesion of mouse bone marrow-derived mast cells to laminin. *Allergy* 51: 650, 1996.
3. Walsh L. J., Kaminer M. S., Lazarus G. S., Lavker R. M., Murphy G. F.: Role of laminin in localization of human dermal mast cells. *Lab. Invest.* 65: 433, 1991.
4. Thompson H. L., Burbelo P. D., Segui-Real B., Yamada Y., Metcalfe D. D.: Laminin promotes mast cell attachment. *J. Immunol.* 143: 2323, 1989.
5. Kruger-Krasagakes S., Grutzkau A., Baghramian R., Henz B. M.: Interactions of immature human mast cells with extracellular matrix: expression of specific adhesion receptors and their role in cell binding to matrix proteins. *J. Invest. Dermatol.* 106: 538, 1996.
6. Columbo M., Bochner B. S., Marone G.: Human skin mast cells express functional beta 1 integrins that mediate adhesion to extracellular matrix proteins. *J. Immunol.* 154: 6058, 1995.
7. Kinashi T., Springer T. A.: Steel Factor and c-kit ligand regulate cell-matrix adhesion. *Blood* 83: 1033, 1994.
8. Wiesner-Menzel L., Schultz B., Vakilzadeh F., Czarnetzki B. M.: Electron microscopical evidence for a direct contact between nerve fibers and mast cells. *Acta Derm. Venereol. Stockh.* 61: 465, 1981.
9. Newson B., Dahlstom A., Enerback L., Ahlman H.: Suggestive evidence for a direct innervation of mucosal mast cells. *Neuroscience* 10: 565, 1983.
10. Stead R. H., Dixon M. F., Bramwell N. H., Riddell R. H., Bienenstock J.: Mast cells are closely apposed to nerves in the human gastrointestinal mucosa. *Gastroenterology* 97: 575, 1989.
11. Hagermark O., Hokfelt T., Pernow B.: Flare and itch induced by substance P in human skin. *J. Invest. Dermatol.* 71: 233, 1978.
12. Ebertz J. M., Hirshman C. A., Kettelkamp N. S., Uno H., Hanifin J. M.: Substance P-induced histamine release in human cutaneous mast cells. *J. Invest. Dermatol.* 88: 682, 1987.
13. Piotrowski W., Foreman J. C.: Some effects of calcitonin gene-related peptide in human skin and on histamine release. *Br. J. Dermatol.* 114: 37, 1986.
14. Naukkarinen A., Jarvikallio A., Lakkakorpi J., Harvima I. T., Harvima R. J., Horsmanheimo M.: Quantitative histochemical analysis of mast cells and sensory nerves in psoriatic skin. *J. Pathol.* 180: 200, 1996.
15. Egan C. L., Viglione-Schenck M. J., Walsh L. J., Green B., Trojanowski J. Q., Whitaker-Menezes D., Murphy G. F.: Characterization of unmyelinated axons uniting epidermal and dermal immune cells in primate and murine skin. *J. Cutan. Pathol.* 25: 20, 1998.
16. Sueki H., Telegan B., Murphy G. F.: Computer-assisted three-dimensional reconstruction of human dermal dendrocytes. *J. Invest. Dermatol.* 105: 704, 1995.
17. Sueki H., Whitaker D., Buchsbaum M., Murphy G. F.: Novel interactions between dermal dendrocytes and mast cells in human skin. Implications for hemostasis and matrix repair. *Lab. Invest.* 69: 160, 1993.
18. Weidner N., Austen K. F.: Evidence for morphologic diversity of human mast cells. *Lab. Invest.* 60: 63, 1990.
19. Whitaker-Menezes D., Schechter N. M., Murphy G. F.: Serine proteinases are regionally segregated within mast cell granules. *Lab. Invest.* 72: 34, 1995.
20. Irani A. M., Schwartz L. B:. Human mast cell heterogeneity. *Allergy Proc.* 15: 303, 1994.
21. Gurish M. F., Ghildyal N., McNeil H. P., Austen K. F., Gillis S., Stevens R. L.: Differential expression of secretory granule proteases in mouse mast cells exposed to interleukin 3 and c-kit ligand. *J. Exp. Med.* 175: 1003, 1992.
22. Tsai M., Shih L. S., Newlands G. F., Takeishi T., Langley K. E., Zsebo K. M., Miller H. R., Geissler E. N., Galli S., J.: The rat c-kit ligand, stem cell factor, induces the development of connective tissue-type and mucosal mast cells in vivo. Analysis by anatomical distribution, histochemistry, and protease phenotype. *J. Exp. Med.* 174: 125, 1991.
23. Dvorak, A. M: Degranulation of basophils and mast cells, in *Basophil and Mast Cell Degranulation and Recovery* (Dvorak, A. M., Ed.), pp 101-202, Plenum Press, New York, 1991.
24. Kaminer M. S., Lavker R. M., Walsh L. J., Whitaker D., Zweiman B., Murphy G. F.: Extracellular localization of human connective tissue mast cell granule contents. *J. Invest. Dermatol.* 96: 857, 1991.

25. Dvorak A. M., Mihm M. C. Jr., Dvorak H. F.: Morphology of delayed-type hypersensitivity reactions in man II. Ultrastructural alterations affecting the microvasculature and the tissue mast cells. *Lab. Invest.* 34: 179, 1976.

26. Dvorak A. M., Mihm M. C. Jr., Osage J. E., Kwan T. H., Austen K. F., Wintroub B. U.: Bullous pemphigoid, an ultrastructural study of the inflammatory response: eosinophil, basophil and mast cell granule changes in multiple biopsies from one patient. *J. Invest. Dermatol.* 78: 91, 1982.

27. Dvorak A. M.: Mast cell hyperplasia and degranulation in Crohn's disease, in: *The Mast Cell. Its Role in Health and Disease* (J. Pepys and A. M. Edwards, Eds.), pp. 657-662, Pitman Medical Publishing Kent, England, 1979.

28. Kaminer M. S., Murphy G. F., Zweiman B., Lavker R. M.: Connective tissue mast cells exhibit time-dependent degranulation heterogeneity. *Clin. Diag. Lab. Immunol.* 2: 297, 1995.

29. Dvorak A. M., Schleimer R. P., Schulman E. S., Lichtenstein L. M.: Human mast cells use conservation and condensation mechanisms during recovery from degranulation. In vitro studies with mast cells purified from human lungs. *Lab. Invest.* 54: 663, 1986.

30. Kitamura Y., Shimada M., Hatanaka K., Miyano Y.: Development of mast cells from grafted bone marrow cells in irradiated mice. *Nature* 268: 442, 1977.

31. Rennick D. M., Lee F. D., Yokota T., Asai H., Cantor H., Nabel G. J.: A cloned MCGF cDNA encodes a multilineage hematopoietic growth factor: multiple activities of interleukin 3. *J. Immunol.* 139: 910, 1985.

32. Ishizaka T., Furitsu T., Inagaki N.: In vitro development and functions of human mast cells. *Int. Arch. Allergy Appl. Immunol.* 94: 116, 1991.

33. Kirshenbaum A. S., Kessler S. W., Goff J. P., Metcalfe D. D.: Demonstration of the origin of human mast cells from CD 34+ bone marrow progenitor cells. *J. Immunol.* 146: 1410 1991.

34. Irani A. A., Craig S. S., Nilsson G., Ishizaka T., Schwartz L. B.: Characterization of human mast cells developed in vitro from fetal liver cells cocultured with murine 3T3 fibroblasts. *Immunology* 77: 136, 1992.

35. Zsebo K. M., Williams D. A., Geissler E. N., Broudy V. C., Martin F. H., Atkins H. L., Hsu R. Y., Birkett N. C., Okino K. H., Murdock D. C., et al.: Stem cell factor is encoded at the Sl locus of the mouse and is the ligand for the c-kit tyrosine kinase receptor. *Cell* 63: 213, 1990.

36. Anderson D. M., Lyman S. D., Baird A., Wignall J. M., Eisenman J., Rauch C., March C. J., Boswell H. S., Gimpel S. D., Cosman D., et al.: Molecular cloning of mast cell growth factor, a hematopoietin that is active in both membrane bound and soluble forms. *Cell* 63: 235, 1990.

37. Flanagan J. G., Leder P.: The kit ligand: a cell surface molecule altered in steel mutant fibroblasts. *Cell* 63: 185, 1990.

38. Ulich T. R., del Castillo J., Yi E. S., Yin S., McNiece I., Yung Y. P., Zsebo K. M.: Hematologic effects of stem cell factor in vivo and in vitro in rodents. *Blood* 78: 645, 1991.

39. Tsai M., Takeishi T., Thompson H., Langley K. E., Zsebo K. M., Metcalfe D. D., Geissler E. N., Galli S. J.: Induction of mast cell proliferation, maturation, and heparin synthesis by the rat c-kit ligand, stem cell factor. *Proc. Natl. Acad. Sci. U.S.A.* 88: 6382, 1991.

40. Mitsui H., Furitsu T., Dvorak A. M., Irani A. M., Schwartz L. B., Inagaki N.: Development of human mast cells from umbilical cord blood cells by recombinant human and murine c-kit ligand. *Proc. Natl. Acad. Sci. U.S.A.* 90: 735, 1993.

41. Irani A. M., Nilsson G., Miettinen U., Craig S. S., Ashman L. K., Ishizaka T., Zsebo K. M. , Schwartz L. B.: Recombinant human stem cell factor stimulates differentiation of mast cells from dispersed human fetal liver cells. *Blood* 80: 3009, 1992.

42. Tsuji K., Zsebo K. M., Ogawa M.: Murine mast cell colony formation supported by IL-3, IL-4, and recombinant rat stem cell factor, ligand for c-kit. *J. Cell. Physiol.* 148: 362, 1991.

43. Meininger C. J., Yano H., Rottapel R., Bernstein A., Zsebo K. M., Zetter B. R.: The c-kit receptor ligand functions as a mast cell chemoattractant. *Blood* 79: 958, 1992.

44. Iemura A., Tsai M., Ando A., Wershil B. K., Galli S. J.: The c-kit ligand, stem cell factor, promotes mast cell survival by suppressing apoptosis. *Am. J. Pathol.* 144: 321, 1994.

45. Linenberger M. L., Jacobson F. W., Bennett L. G., Broudy V. C., Martin F. H.: Stem cell factor production by human marrow stromal fibroblasts. *Exp. Hematol.* 23: 1104, 1995.

46. Longley B. J. Jr., Morganroth G. S., Tyrrell L., Ding T. G., Anderson D. M., Williams D. E., Halaban R.: Altered metabolism of mast-cell growth factor (c-kit ligand) in cutaneous mastocytosis. *N. Engl. J. Med.* 328: 1302, 1993.

47. Meininger C. J., Brightman S. E., Kelly K. A., Zetter B. R.: Increased stem cell factor release by hemangioma-derived endothelial cells. *Lab. Invest.* 72: 166, 1995.

48. Longley B. J., Tyrrell L., Ma Y., Williams D. A., Halaban R., Langley K., Lu H. S., Schechter N. M.: Chymase cleavage of stem cell factor yields a bioactive, soluble product. *Proc. Natl. Acad. Sci. U.S.A.* 94: 9017, 1997.

49. Longley B. J., Tyrrell L., Lu S., Ma Y., Klump V., Murphy G. F.: Chronically KIT-stimulated clonally-derived human mast cells show heterogeneity in different tissue microenvironments. *J. Invest. Dermatol.* 108: 792, 1997.

50. Christofidou-Solomidou M., Longley B. J., Whitaker-Menezes D., Albelda S. M., Murphy G. F.: Human skin/SCID mouse chimeras as an in vivo model for human cutaneous mast cell hyperplasia. *J. Invest. Dermatol.* 109: 102, 1997.

51. Lavker R. M., Schechter N. M:. Cutaneous mast cell depletion results from topical corticosteroid usage. *J. Immunol.* 135: 2368, 1985.

52. Finotto S., Mekori Y. A., Metcalfe D. D.: Glucocorticoids decrease tissue mast cell number by reducing the production of the c-kit ligand, stem cell factor, by resident cells: in vitro and in vivo evidence in murine systems. *J. Clin. Invest.* 99: 1721, 1997.

53. Matsuda H., Coughlin M. D., Bienenstock J., Denburg J. A.: Nerve growth factor promotes human hemopoietic colony growth and differentiation. *Proc. Natl. Acad. Sci. U.S.A.* 85: 6508, 1988.

54. Kannan Y., Matsuda H., Ushio H., Kawamoto K., Shimada Y.: Murine granulocyte-macrophage and mast cell colony formation promoted by nerve growth factor. *Int. Arch. Allergy Appl. Immunol.* 102: 362, 1993.

55. Matsuda H., Kannan Y., Ushio H., Kiso Y., Kanemoto T., Suzuki H., Kitamura Y.: Nerve growth factor induces development of connective tissue-type mast cells in vitro from murine bone marrow cells. *J. Exp. Med.* 174: 7, 1991.

56. Kawamoto K., Okada T., Kannan Y., Ushio H., Matsumoto M., Matsuda H.: Nerve growth factor prevents apoptosis of rat peritoneal mast cells through the trk proto-oncogene receptor. *Blood* 86: 4638, 1995.

57. Leon A., Buriani A., Dal Toso R., Fabris M., Romanello S., Aloe L., Levi-Montalcini R.: Mast cells synthesize, store, and release nerve growth factor. *Proc. Natl. Acad. Sci. U.S.A.* 91: 3739, 1994.

58. Gershon R. K., Askenase P. W., Gershon M. D.: Requirement for vasoactive amines for production of delayed-type hypersensitvity skin reactions. *J. Exp. Med.* 142: 732, 1975.

59. Askenase P. W., Van Loveren H., Kraeuter-Kops S., Ron Y., Meade R., Theoharides T. C., Nordlund J. J., Scovern H., Gerhson M. D., Ptak W.: Defective elicitation of delayed-type hypersensitivity in W/Wv and SI/SId mast cell-deficient mice. *J. Immunol.* 131: 2687, 1983.

60. Lewis R. E., Buchsbaum M., Whitaker D., Murphy G. F.: Intercellular adhesion molecule expression in the evolving human cutaneous delayed hypersensitivity reaction. *J. Invest. Dermatol.* 93: 672, 1989.

61. Waldorf H. A., Walsh L. J., Schechter N. M., Murphy G. F.: Early cellular events in evolving cutaneous delayed hypersensitivity in humans. *Am. J. Pathol.* 138: 477, 1991.

62. Murphy G. F., Sueki H., Teuscher C., Whitaker D., Korngold R.: Role of mast cells in early epithelial target cell injury in experimental acute graft-versus-host disease. *J. Invest. Dermatol.* 102: 451, 1994.

63. Korngold R., Jameson B. A., McDonnell J. M., Leighton C., Sutton B. J., Gould H. J., Murphy G. F.: Peptide analogs that inhibit IgE-Fc epsilon RI alpha interactions ameliorate the development of lethal graft-versus-host disease. *Biol. Blood Marrow Transplant* 3: 187, 1997.

64. Kligman L. H., Murphy G. F.: Ultraviolet B radiation increases hairless mouse mast cells in a dose-dependent manner and alters distribution of UV-induced mast cell growth factor. *Photochem. Photobiol.* 63: 123, 1996.

65. Gilchrest B. A., Soter N. A., Stoff J. S., Mihm M. C. Jr.: The human sunburn reaction: histologic and biochemical studies. *J. Am. Acad. Dermatol.* 5: 411, 1981.

66. Lavker R. M., Kaminer M. S., Murphy G. F.: Mast cell degranulation results in endothelial activation after acute exposure of human skin to UV irradiation. In: *Environmental Threat to the Skin Proceedings*, (Marks and Plewig, Eds.), London, Martin Dunitz, 1992, pp. 125-129.

67. Messadi D. V., Pober J. S., Fiers W., Gimbrone M. A. Jr., Murphy G. F.: Induction of an activation antigen on postcapillary venular endothelium in human skin organ culture. *J. Immunol.* 139: 1557, 1987.

68. Klein L. M., Lavker R. M., Matis W. L., Murphy G. F.: Degranulation of human mast cells induces an endothelial antigen central to leukocyte adhesion. *Proc. Natl. Acad. Sci. U.S.A.* 86: 8972, 1989.

69. Walsh L. J., Trinchieri G., Waldorf H. A., Whitaker D., Murphy G. F.: Human dermal mast cells contain and release tumor necrosis factor alpha, which induces endothelial leukocyte adhesion molecule 1. *Proc. Natl. Acad. Sci. U.S.A.* 88: 4220, 1991.

70. Pilewski J. M., Yan H. C., Juhasz I., Christofidou-Solomidou M., Williams J., Murphy G. F., Albelda S. M.: Modulation of adhesion molecules by cytokines in vivo using human/severe combined immunodeficient (SCID) mouse chimeras. *J. Clin. Immunol.* 15: 122S, 1995.

71. Christofidou-Solomidou M., Murphy G. F., Albelda S. M.: Induction of E-selectin-dependent leukocyte recruitment by mast cell degranulation in human skin grafts transplanted on SCID mice. *Am. J. Pathol.* 148: 177, 1996.

72. Ioffreda M. D., Whitaker D., Murphy G. F.: Mast cell degranulation upregulates alpha 6 integrins on epidermal Langerhans cells. *J. Invest. Dermatol.* 101: 150, 1993.

73. Jordana M., Befus A. D., Newhouse M. T., Bienenstock J., Gauldie J.: Effect of histamine on proliferation of normal human adult lung fibroblasts. *Thorax* 43: 552, 1988.

74. Ruoss S. J., Hartmann T., Caughey G. H.: Mast cell tryptase is a mitogen for cultured fibroblasts. *J. Clin. Invest.* 88: 493, 1991.

75. Cairns J. A., Walls A. F.: Mast cell tryptase stimulates the synthesis of type I collagen in human lung fibroblasts. *J. Clin. Invest.* 99: 1313, 1997.

76. Gruber B. L., Kew R. R., Jelaska A., Marchese M. J., Garlick J., Ren S., Schwartz L. B., Korn J. H.: Human mast cells activate fibroblasts: tryptase is a fibrogenic factor stimulating collagen messenger ribonucleic acid synthesis and fibroblast chemotaxis. *J. Immunol.* 158: 2310, 1997.

77. Kendall J. C., Li XH., Galli S. J., Gordon J. R.: Promotion of mouse fibroblast proliferation by IgE-dependent activation of mouse mast cells: role for mast cell tumor necrosis factor-alpha and transforming growth factor-beta 1. *J. Allergy Clin. Immunol.* 99: 113, 1997.

78. Mulliken J. B., Zetter B. R., Folkman J.: In vitro characteristics of endothelium from hemangiomas and vascular malformations. *Surgery* 92: 348, 1982.

79. Kessler D. A., Langer R. S., Pless N. A., Folkman J.: Mast cells and tumor angiogenesis. *Int. J. Cancer* 18: 703, 1976.

80. Gruber B. L., Marchese M. J., Kew R. R.: Transforming growth factor-beta 1 mediates mast cell chemotaxis. *J. Immunol.* 152: 5860, 1994.

81. Gruber B. L., Marchese M. J., Kew R.: Angiogenic factors stimulate mast-cell migration. *Blood* 86: 2488, 1995.

82. Azizkhan R. G., Azizkhan J. C., Zetter B. R., Folkman J.: Mast cell heparin stimulates migration of capillary endothelial cells in vitro. *J. Exp. Med.* 152: 931, 1980.

83. Marks R. M., Roche W. R., Czerniecki M., Penny R., Nelson D. S.: Mast cell granules cause proliferation of human microvascular endothelial cells. *Lab. Invest.* 55: 289, 1986.

84. Sorbo J., Jakobsson A., Norrby K.: Mast-cell histamine is angiogenic through receptors for histamine1 and histamine2. *Int. J. Exp. Pathol.* 75: 43, 1994.

85. Schweigerer L., Neufeld G., Friedman J., Abraham J. A., Fiddes J. C., Gospodarowicz D.: Capillary endothelial cells express basic fibroblast growth factor, a mitogen that promotes their own growth. *Nature* 325: 257, 1987.

86. Yang E. Y., Moses H. L.: Transforming growth factor beta 1-induced changes in cell migration, proliferation, and angiogenesis in chicken chorioallantoic membrane. *J. Cell. Biol.* 111: 731, 1990.

87. Reed J. A., Albino A. P., McNutt N. S.: Human cutaneous mast cells express basic fibroblast growth factor. *Lab. Invest.* 72: 215, 1995.

88. Qu Z., Liebler J. M., Powers M. R., Galey T., Ahmadi P., Huang X. N., Ansel J. C., Butterfield J. H., Planck S. R., Rosenbaum J. T.: Mast cells are a major source of basic fibroblast growth factor in chronic inflammation and cutaneous hemangioma. *Am. J. Pathol.* 147: 564, 1995.

89. Blair R. J., Meng H., Marchese M. J., Ren S., Schwartz L. B., Tonnesen M. G., Gruber B. L.: Human mast cells stimulate vascular tube formation. Tryptase is a novel, potent angiogenic factor. *J. Clin. Invest.* 99: 2691, 1997.

90. Matis W. L., Lavker R. M., Murphy G. F.: Substance P induces the expression of an endothelial-leukocyte adhesion molecule by microvascular endothelium. *J. Invest. Dermatol.* 94: 492, 1990.

91. Murphy G. F.: The secret of NIN: a novel neural-immunological network potentially integral to immunologic function in human skin, in *Dermal Immune System* (Nickoloff, B. J, Ed.), CRC Press, Boca Raton, FL, 1993, chap 12.

12 Interleukin-1 Receptors and Signal Transduction*

Charles A. Dinarello

CONTENTS

I. INTRODUCTION

Interleukin-1 (IL-1) is the prototypic proinflammatory cytokine. There are two forms of IL-1, IL-1α and IL-1β, and in most studies, their biological activities are indistinguishable. IL-1 affects nearly every cell type, often in concert with another proinflammatory cytokine, tumor necrosis factor (TNF). The synthesis, processing, secretion, and activity of IL-1, particularly IL-1β, are tightly regulated events. Studies have revealed that IL-1 signal transduction is also shared with another cytokine, IL-18. Both cytokines have ligand binding chains which form a heterodimer with a nonligand binding, signaling chain. This signaling chain is essential for biological activity and the the cytoplasmic domain contains unique "Toll-like protein." In fact, IL-1/IL-18 receptors and signaling are part of a larger family of Toll-like protein receptors, of which one member is also the signaling chain for the endotoxin receptor. A unique aspect of cytokine biology is the naturally occurring IL-1 receptor antagonist (IL-1Ra). IL-1Ra is structurally similar to IL-1β but, lacking agonist activity, is used in clinical trials to reduce disease severity. In addition, regulation

---

* These studies are supported by NIH Grant AI-15614.

of IL-1 activity extends to low numbers of surface receptors, circulating soluble receptors, and a cell surface "decoy" receptor to downregulate responses to IL-1β. This review updates the current knowledge on IL-1.

The intron–exon organization of the three IL-1 genes (IL-1α, IL-1β, and IL-1Ra) suggests duplication of a common gene some 350 million years ago. Before this common IL-1 gene, there may have been an ancestral gene from which fibroblast growth factor (FGF) also evolved, since IL-1 and FGF share significant amino acid homologies, lack a signal peptide, and form an all β–pleated sheet tertiary structure. IL-18 may also be derived from this same ancestral gene since it also shares the β–pleated sheet structure with IL-1β[1] and lacks a signal peptide. IL-1α and β are synthesized as precursors without leader sequences. The molecular weight of each precursor is 31 kDa. Processing of IL-1α or IL-1β to "mature" forms of 17 kDa requires specific cellular proteases. In contrast, IL-1Ra evolved with a signal peptide and is readily transported out of the cells and termed "secreted IL-1Ra" (sIL-1Ra).

There are two primary cell surface binding proteins (IL-1 receptors) for IL-1. IL-1 type I receptor (IL-1RI) transduces a signal, whereas the type II receptor (IL-1RII) binds IL-1 but does not transduce a signal. In fact, IL-1RII acts as a sink for IL-1β and has been termed a "decoy" receptor, which is somewhat unique to cytokine biology.[2] When IL-1 binds to IL-1RI, a complex is formed which then binds to the IL-1R accessory protein (IL-1R–AcP) resulting in high affinity binding.[3] The IL-1R–AcP itself does not bind IL-1. It is likely that the heterodimerization of the cytosolic domains of IL-1RI and IL-1R–AcP triggers IL-1 signal transduction.

As with other cytokines, importance in embryonic development and in health has been revealed using targeted gene disruption in mice. Gene expression and synthesis of IL-1α, IL-1β, or IL-1Ra has been shown in ovarian granulosa and theca cells as well as in the dividing embryo. Although IL-1 is found in placental trophoblasts and appears to play a role in embryonic development, implantation, birth, and neonatal development of mice deficient in IL-1β, IL-1β converting enzyme (ICE), or IL-1RI suggests that ovulation, fertilization, implantation, and parturition either do not require IL-1 receptor signaling or that compensatory cytokines are used by these mice. In addition, mice deficient in IL-1β, ICE, or IL-1RI are not susceptible to infection in the standard animal facility, which is in sharp contrast to mice deficient in IL-10 or transforming growth factor-β (TGF-β).

II. IL-1 AND CONTACT DERMATITIS

IL-1 is a highly inflammatory molecule and as such is often implicated in a variety of inflammatory diseases, including skin diseases. IL-1α is constitutively expressed in the skin of healthy humans and a skin-specific chymase cleaves proIL-1β different from that of the ICE cleavage site. This skin-derived chymase from mast cells results in biologically active IL-1β.[4] It is unclear whether IL-1α plays a role as a growth factor for skin and whether IL-1β acts as a proinflammatory molecule, but mice deficient in IL-1RI have normal skin. Therefore, if IL-1α acts through the IL-1RI, this is not an essential growth factor for the skin.

In mice deficient in IL-1β, the contact hypersensitivity which follows the application of trinitrochlorobenzene is impaired.[5] The defect can be overcome by increasing the amount of the sensitizing antigen or by local instillation of IL-1β prior to the application of trinitrochlorobenzene. Thus, there is a role for IL-1β early in the development of contact dermatitis.

In 15 human subjects with known allergies to common household antigens, IL-1sRI was injected together intradermally with different allergens. A placebo group was also used (saline rather than IL-1sRI). On the contralateral arm, the antigens were injected without saline or IL-1sRI. After 8 hours, induration, erythema, and itching were reduced in subjects given the soluble receptor compared to the placebo. Most interesting, there was a reduction in the reaction even in the contralateral side,[6] suggesting that systemic levels of the soluble receptor were sufficient to suppress the reaction on the contralateral side.

A role for IL-1β in irritant dermatitis is supported by a study in which human skin was obtained after irritant as well as allergic contact dermatitis. IL-1β mRNA increased in both types of contact dermatitis, but the highest levels were observed after irritant dermatitis. The draining lymph nodes also contained elevated levels of IL-1β mRNA.[7]

III. IL-1 RECEPTORS

A. IL-1 RECEPTOR COMPLEX

Two primary IL-1 binding proteins (receptors) have been identified and one receptor accessory protein (IL-1R–AcP).[3,8] The extracellular domains of the two receptors and the IL-1R–AcP are members of the immunoglobulin superfamily; they are each comprised of three IgG-like domains and share a significant homology to each other. The two IL-1 receptors are distinct gene products, and in humans the genes for IL-1RI and IL-1RII are located on the long arm of chromosome 2.[9] The binding of the IL-1RI (low affinity) plus the formation of a complex with the nonbinding IL-1R–AcP forms the heterodimer of high affinity and initiates signal transduction.

B. IL-1R TYPE I

IL-1RI is an 80-kDa glycoprotein found prominently on endothelial cells, smooth muscle cells, epithelial cells, hepatocytes, fibroblasts, keratinocytes, epidermal dendritic cells, and T lymphocytes. IL-1RI is heavily glycosylated, and blocking the glycosylation sites reduces the binding of IL-1.[10] Surface expression of this receptor is likely on most IL-1-responsive cells, as biological activity of IL-1 is a better assessment of receptor expression than ligand binding. Failure to show specific and saturable IL-1 binding is often due to the low numbers of surface IL-1RI on primary cells.[11] In cell lines, the number of IL-1RI can reach 5000 per cell, but primary cells usually express fewer than 200 receptors per cell. In some primary cells there are less than 50 per cell, and IL-1 signal transduction has been observed in cells expressing less than 10 type I receptors per cell. The low number of IL-1RI on cells and the discrepancy between binding affinities and biological activities can be explained by the increased binding affinity of IL-1 in the complex with the IL-1R–AcP.[3]

As shown in Figure 1, IL-1RI has a single transmembrane segment and a cytoplasmic domain. Using specific neutralizing antibodies, IL-1RI but not IL-1RII is the primary signal-transducing receptor (reviewed in Reference 8). Antisense oligonucleotides directed against IL-1RI block IL-1 activities in vitro and in vivo.[12] The cytoplasmic domain of IL-1RI has no apparent intrinsic tyrosine kinase activity, but tyrosine phosphorylation of the MAP p38 kinase is certainly part of the IL-1 signal transduction pathway.[13] Of considerable importance is the finding that the cytosolic domain of IL-1RI has a 45% amino acid homology with the cytosolic domain of the *Drosophila Toll* gene.[14] Toll is a transmembrane protein which acts like a receptor, although the specific ligand for the Toll protein is unknown. Gene organization and amino acid homology suggest that the IL-1RI and the cytosolic Toll-like protein are derived from a common ancestor and trigger similar signals.[15] In fact, if the specific sequences of the Toll-like protein domain in the IL-1RI are deleted, there is no signal transduction.[15] This sequence is commonly called the Heguy sequence. The Heguy sequence is also present in the IL-1R–AcP.[3]

In addition to the importance of the Toll-like protein sequence for IL-1 signaling, the signaling chain of the endotoxin receptor (previously unknown) is also a member of the Toll-like receptor (TLR) family.[16] What is the connection? At present, there are at least five TLRs expressed in human cells[17] and function during immune responses.[18] In the endotoxin signaling TLP-2, a segment of its cytoplasmic domain is homologous to a segment in the IL-1RI cytoplasmic domain, which is required for IL-1 signaling.[15] In fact, the specific domain of the IL-1R that is responsible for the recruitment of the IL-1R-activating kinase (IRAK)[19,20] and also for the recruitment of MyD88[21] is the same domain in the TLR-2 that is required for signal transduction by endotoxin.[16]

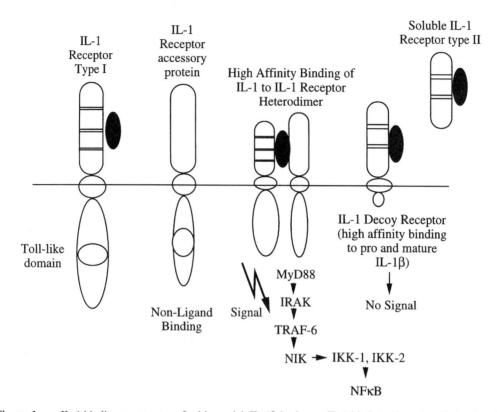

Figure 1   IL-1 binding to receptors. In this model, IL-1β is shown. IL-1 binds to the extracellular domain of either type I (IL-1RI) or type II (IL-1RII). Although there is preferential binding of IL-1β to IL-1RII, this receptor, lacking a cytosolic segment, does not transduce a signal but rather acts as a decoy receptor or a "sink" for IL-1β. Following low affinity binding of IL-1β to the IL-1RI, there is a structural change in the third IgG-like domain of this receptor. This structural change allows for the IL-1R accessory protein (IL-1RAcP) to form a compex with the low affinity IL-1β/IL-1RI. This results in a high affinity complex (IL-1R–AcP/IL-1β/IL-1RI) and in signal transduction. MyD88 binds to the complex and acts to assist the recruitment of the IL-1R activating kinase (IRAK). IRAK phosphorylates the TNF-receptor activating factor-6 (TRAF) which, in turn, phosphorylates the NFκB-inducing factor (NIK). NIK then acts to phosphorylate the inhibitory κB kinases (IKK-1 and IKK-2). Once phosphorylated, IκB is rapidly degraded by a ubiquitin pathway liberating NFκB which translocates to the nucleus for gene transcription.

For endotoxin, biological activity depends on two nonsignaling molecules: the constitutive serum protein "lipopolysaccharide binding protein" (LBP) which binds endotoxin's lipid chains and then presents this complex to another protein, membrane CD14.[22] Although membrane CD14 does not have a cytoplasmic domain for signal transduction, expression of membrane CD14 is optimal for cell responses to endotoxin. In cells lacking CD14, the addition of LBP does not restore the response to endotoxin, but in cells expressing membrane CD14, soluble LBP greatly enhances signal transduction by endotoxin. Clearly, the existence of a signaling chain for endotoxin was predicted and, in fact, Lei and Morrison described an endotoxin receptor on the cell surface with a molecular weight of 80,000.[23] It is likely that TLR-2 is the 80,000 MW endotoxin receptor. Therefore, LBP binds endotoxin and allows for the coupling of TLR-2. This binding results in limited signal transduction. Although the binding of endotoxin to TLR-2 is of very low affinity (500 to 900 nM),[16] signaling is greatly enhanced by the presence of CD14 on the cell. One can now envisage the optimal endotoxin signaling complex to be TLR-2/endotoxin/CD14. Of related interest, the endotoxin-resistant mouse strain C3H/HeJ has a mutation in another Toll-like protein, TLR-4.[24] Thus, there is a clear relationship between IL-1 signaling receptors and those of endotoxin.

As described below, IL-18 signaling also uses structurally related receptors which recruit similar intracellular kinases to the cytoplasmic domains which function to activate a cascade of kinases.

As shown in Figure 1, like other models of two-chain receptors, IL-1 binds first to the IL-1RI with a low affinity. The crystal structure of the IL-1RI complexed with IL-1β has been reported and sheds light on the changes that take place after the low affinity binding.[25] The two receptor binding sites of IL-1β have been reported using specific mutations. The crystal structure reveals that both receptor binding sites contact the IL-1RI at the first and third domains.[25] Upon contact with the first domain, there appears to be a change in the rigidity of the third domain to encounter contact with the second binding site of IL-1β. IL-1β itself does not undergo a structural change. IL-1Ra has only one binding site[26] and its absence prevents contact with the third domain. Hence the critical contact point appears to be at the third domain. Since this contact is likely to be absent in complexes with the IL-1Ra,[27] the structural change in the IL-1RI third domain may allow docking of the IL-1R–AcP with the IL-1RI/IL-1β complex. Without the complex of IL-1R–AcP/IL-1RI/IL-1β, there is no signal transduction.[3]

C. IL-1R–AcP

Antibodies to the type I receptor and to the IL-1R–AcP block IL-1 binding and activity.[3] The IL-1R–AcP is essential to IL-1 signaling; in cells deficient of the IL-1R–AcP, no IL-1-induced activation of the stress kinases takes place, but this response is restored upon transfection with a construct expressing the IL-1R–AcP.[28] Affinity purified antibodies to the IL-1R–AcP third domain amino acids preferentially block IL-1β activity,[29] suggesting that the docking of the IL-1R–AcP with the IL-1RI takes place with the third domain of each receptor.

Similar to IL-1RI and IL-1RII, a soluble form of the IL-1R–AcP exists. Unlike the soluble forms of the IL-1RI and IL-1RII, the soluble IL-1R–AcP is not formed by proteolytic cleavage of the full length accessory protein, but rather by alternate splicing of RNA. Since the IL-1R–AcP does not bind IL-1,[3] the effect of the soluble IL-1R–AcP on the binding of IL-1 remains unclear. As discussed above and shown in Figure 1, IL-1Ra does not form a complex with the IL-1RI and this likely explains how the IL-1Ra can bind so tightly to the IL-1RI and yet not exhibit any agonist activity. One thus concludes that the IL-1RI/IL-1/IL-1R–AcP complex triggers the cell and without the IL-1R–AcP participation, the IL-1 signal via the IL-1RI is weak or nonexistent. Studies deleting the Heguy sequence from the IL-1RI which result in loss of functional activity suggest that the Toll-like protein on both chains of the IL-1R complex must participate in the recruitment of kinases. As described below, that indeed is the case.

D. IL-1R Type II, a Decoy Receptor

There is a third IL-1R which is unique. The IL-1RII has a short cytosolic domain consisting of 29 amino acids. The type II receptor actually acts as "decoy" molecule, particularly for IL-1β. The receptor binds IL-β tightly, thus preventing binding to the signal transducing type I receptor.[2] It is the lack of a signal transducing cytosolic domain which makes the type II receptor a functionally negative receptor. For example, when the extracellular portion of the type II receptor is fused to the cytoplasmic domain of the type I receptor, a biological signal occurs.[30] The extracellular portion of the type II receptor is found in body fluids where it is termed "IL-1 soluble receptor type II (IL-1sRII)." It is assumed that a proteolytic cleavage of the extracellular domain of the IL-1RII from the cell surface is the source of the IL-1sRII. A splice variant may also exist. It is likely that as cell-bound IL-1RII increases, there is a comparable increase in soluble forms.[31]

E. Soluble IL-1R

Similar to soluble receptors for TNF, the extracellular domain of the type I and type II IL-1R is found as "soluble" molecules in the circulation and urine of healthy subjects and in inflammatory synovial and other pathologic body fluids.[32-34] In healthy humans, the circulating levels of IL-1sRII are 100 to 200 pM. The rank of affinities for the two soluble receptors is remarkably different for each of the three IL-1 molecules. The rank for the three IL-1 ligands binding to IL-1sRI is IL-1Ra > IL-1α > IL-1β, whereas for IL-1sRII, the rank is IL-1β > IL-1α > IL-1Ra. In fact, the binding of IL-1Ra to IL-1sRI is considered irreversible.

Elevated levels of IL-1sRII are found in the circulation of patients with sepsis[35] and in the synovial fluid of patients with active rheumatoid arthritis,[34] whereas the elevations of soluble type I receptor in these fluids are tenfold lower. To date the highest levels of IL-1sRII have been found in patients with hairy cell leukemia.[36] In addition, patients undergoing repair of thoraco-abdominal aneurysm have markedly elevated levels, likely due to the ischemia associated with this procedure.[37]

Unlike other cytokine receptors, in cells expressing both IL-1 type I and type II receptors, there is competition to bind IL-1 first. This competition between signaling and nonsignaling receptors for the same ligand appears unique to cytokine receptors, although it exists for atrial natriuretic factor receptors. Since the type II receptor is more likely to bind to IL-1β than IL-1α, this can result in a diminished response to IL-1β. The soluble form of IL-1sRII circulates in healthy humans at molar concentrations which are tenfold greater than those of IL-1β measured in septic patients and 100-fold greater than the concentration of IL-1β following intravenously administration.[38,39] Why do humans have a systemic response to an infusion of IL-1β? One concludes that binding of IL-1β to the soluble form of IL-1R type II exhibits a slow "on" rate compared to the cell IL-1RI. An alternative explanation is that in vivo, the type II soluble IL-1R is occupied by IL-1β or, more likely, proIL-1β. However, there are no studies to examine this possibility.

IV. SIGNAL TRANSDUCTION

A. EARLY EVENTS IN IL-1 SIGNAL TRANSDUCTION

Within a few minutes following binding to cells, IL-1 induces several biochemical events (reviewed in References 40 to 44). It remains unclear which is the most "upstream" triggering event or whether several occur at the same time. No sequential order or cascade has been identified, but several signaling events appear to be taking place during the first 2 to 5 min. Some of the biochemical changes associated with signal transduction are likely cell specific. Within 2 min, hydrolysis of GTP, phosphotidylcholine, phosphotidylserine, or phosphotidylethanolamine,[45] and release of ceramide by neutral,[46] not acidic, sphingomyelinase[47] have been reported. In general, multiple protein phosphorylations and activation of phosphatases can be observed with 5 min[48] and some are thought to be initiated by the release of lipid mediators. The release of ceramide has attracted attention as a possible early signaling event.[49] Phosphorylation of phospholipase A_2 (PLA_2) activating protein also occurs in the first few minutes,[50] which would lead to a rapid release of arachidonic acid. Multiple and similar signaling events have also been reported for TNF.

Of special consideration to IL-1 signal transduction is the unusual discrepancy between the low number of receptors (<10 in some cells) and the low concentrations of IL-1 which can induce a biological response. This latter observation, however, may be clarified in studies on high affinity binding with the IL-1R–AcP complex. A rather extensive "amplification" step(s) takes place following the initial postreceptor binding event. The most likely mechanism for signal amplification is multiple and sequential phosphorylations (or dephosphorylations) of kinases which result in nuclear translocation of transcription factors and activation of proteins participating in translation of mRNA. IL-1RI is phosphorylated following IL-1 binding. It is unknown whether the IL-1R–AcP is phosphorylated during receptor complex formation. In primary cells, the number of IL-1RI type I is very low (<100 per cell) and a biological response occurs when only as few as 2 to 3% of IL-1RI receptors are occupied.[51,52] In IL-1-responsive cells, one assumes that there is constitutive expression of the IL-1R–AcP.

With few exceptions, there is general agreement that IL-1 does not stimulate hydrolysis of phosphatidylinositol nor an increase in intracellular calcium. Without a clear increase in intracellular calcium, early postreceptor binding events nevertheless include hydrolysis of a GTP with no associated increase in adenyl cyclase, activation of adenyl cyclase,[53,54] hydrolysis of phospholipids,[11,55] release of ceramide,[56] and release of arachidonic acid from phopholipids *via* cytosolic PLA$_2$ following its activation by PLA$_2$-activating protein.[50] Some IL-1 signaling events are prominent in different cells. Postreceptor signaling mechanisms may therefore provide cellular specificity. For example, in some cells, IL-1 is a growth factor and signaling is associated with serine/threonine phosphorylation of the MAP kinase p42/44 in mesangial cells.[57] The MAP p38 kinase, another member of the MAP kinase family, is phosphorylated in fibroblasts,[13] as is the p54α MAP kinase in hepatocytes.[58]

B. CHARACTERISTICS OF THE CYTOPLASMIC DOMAIN OF THE IL-1RI

The cytoplasmic domain of the IL-1RI does not contain a consensus sequence for intrinsic tyrosine phosphorylation, but deletion mutants of the receptor reveal specific functions of some domains. There are four nuclear localization sequences which share homology with the glucocorticoid receptor. Three amino acids (Arg-431, Lys-515, and Arg-518), also found in the Toll protein, are essential for IL-1–induced IL-2 production.[15] However, deletion of a segment containing these amino acids did not affect IL-1-induced IL-8.[59] There are also two cytoplasmic domains in the IL-1RI which share homology with the IL-6-signaling gp130 receptor. When these regions are deleted, there is a loss of IL-1-induced IL-8 production.[59]

The C-terminal 30 amino acids of the IL-1RI can be deleted without affecting biological activity.[60] Two independent studies have focused on the area between amino acids 513 to 529. Amino acids 508 to 521 contain sites required for the activation of NFκB. In one study, deletion of this segment abolished IL-1–induced IL-8 expression and in another study, specific mutations of amino acids 513 and 520 to alanine prevented IL-1-driven E-selectin promoter activity. This area is also present in the Toll protein domain associated with NFκB translocation and previously shown to be part of the IL-1 signaling mechanism. This area (513 to 520) is also responsible for activating a kinase which associates with the receptor. This kinase, termed "IL-1RI associated kinase" phosphorylates a 100-kDa substrate. Others have reported a serine/threonine kinase which co-precipitates with the IL-1RI.[61] Amino acid sequence comparisons of the cytosolic domain of the IL-1RI have revealed similarities with a protein kinase C (PKC) acceptor site. Because PKC activators usually do not mimic IL-1–induced responses, the significance of this observation is unclear.

C. GTPASE

Hopp reported a detailed sequence and structural comparison of the cytosolic segment of IL-1RI with the *ras*-family of GTPases.[62] In this analysis, the known amino acid residues for GTP binding and hydrolysis by the GTPase family were found to align with residues in the cytoplasmic domain of the IL-1RI. In addition, Rac, a member of the Rho family of GTPases, was also present in the binding and hydrolytic domains of the IL-1RI cytosolic domain. These observations are consistent with the observations that GTP analog undergoes a rapid hydrolysis when membrane preparations of IL-1RI are incubated with IL-1. Amino acid sequences in the cytosolic domain of the IL-1R–AcP also align with the same binding and hydrolytic regions of the GTPases (T. P. Hopp, personal communication). A protein similar to G-protein activating protein has been identified which associates with the cytosolic domain of the IL-1RI.[63] This finding is consistent with the hypothesis that an early event in IL-1R signaling involves dimerization of the two cytosolic domains, activation of putative GTP binding sites on the cytosolic domains, binding of a G-protein, hydrolysis of GTP, and activation of a phospholipase. In then follows that hydrolysis of phospholipids generates diacylglycerol or phosphatidic acids.

D. RECRUITMENT OF MYD88 AND IL-1 RECEPTOR-ACTIVATING KINASE

An event that may be linked to the binding of G-proteins to the IL-1 receptor complex is the recuitment of the cytosolic protein MyD88. This small protein has many of the characteristics of cytoplasmic domains of receptors, but MyD88 lacks any known extracellular or transmembrane structure. It is unclear exactly how this protein functions since it does not have any known kinase activity. However, it may assist in the binding of IRAK to the complex and hence has been said to function as an adapter molecule. The binding of IRAK to the IL-1R complex appears to be a critical step in the activation of NFκB.[60] The IL-1R–AcP is essential for the recruitment and activation of IRAK.[20,28] In fact, deletion of specific amino acids in the IL-1R–AcP cytoplasmic domain results in loss of IRAK association.[28] In addition, the intracellular adapter molecule termed MyD88 appears to dock to the complex allowing IRAK to become phosphorylated.[60,64] IRAK then dissociates from the IL-1R complex and associates with TNF receptor-associated factor-6 (TRAF-6).[19] TRAF-6 then phosphorylates NIK[65] and NIK phosphorylates the inhibitory κB kinases (IKK-1 and IKK-2).[66] Once phosphorylated, IκB is rapidly degraded by a ubiquitin pathway liberating NFκB, which translocates to the nucleus for gene transcription.

E. IL-1 AND IL-18 SIGNALING ARE SIMILAR

A full review of the biology of IL-18 has been published.[67] There are both high (0.4 nM) and low (40 nM) affinity binding sites for IL-18 in murine primary T cells.[68] Clearly there are two chains to the IL-18 receptor complex. Similar to the nomenclature for other heterodimeric receptors, there is an α chain which functions as a ligand binding chain and a β chain, which is the signaling chain. For IL-18, the ligand binding chain was isolated and found to be a member of the IL-1R family. Hence the IL-18Rα had been previously cloned and called the IL-1R–related protein IL-1Rrp.[69] This receptor remained an orphan receptor until the work by Torigoe et al.[70] The binding of a second chain would explain the higher affinity. This "other" receptor chain has been identified as the "accessory protein-like (AcPL) receptor,"[71] and is related to the IL-1 accessory protein identified by Greenfeder et al.[3] Like the IL-1 accessory protein, the IL-18 AcPL does not bind to its ligand, but rather binds to the complex formed by IL-18 with the IL-18Rα chain.[71] This heterodimeric form is likely the high affinity complex.

Therefore, it is likely that the IL-18 receptor complex is comprised of a ligand binding chain of IL-1Rrp (IL-18Rα), with the second chain being the non–IL-18 binding AcPL (IL-18Rα).[71] An IL-18 binding protein (IL-18BP) has been purified from human urine and cloned.[72] But a transmembrane form of the IL-18BP has not been isolated to date despite murine cDNA cloning and human genomic analyses.[72] Thus, the IL-18BP is a third gene product and appears to be the "decoy" receptor of IL-18, similar to the IL-1R type II which is the decoy receptor for IL-1.

IRAK also associates with the IL-18R complex.[73,74] This was demonstrated using IL-12–stimulated T cells followed by immunoprecipitation with anti–IL-18R or anti-IRAK.[73] Furthermore, IL-18 triggered cells also recruited TRAF-6.[73] Like IL-1 signaling, MyD88 has a role in IL-18 signaling. MyD88-deficient mice do not produce acute phase proteins and have diminished cytokine responses. Recently, Th1-developing cells from MyD88-deficient mice were unresponsive to IL-18–induced activation of NFκB and c-Jun N-terminal kinase (JNK).[75] Thus, MyD88 is an essential component in the signaling cascade that follows IL-1 receptor as well as IL-18 receptor binding. It appears that the cascade of sequential recruitment of MyD88, IRAK, and TRAF-6 followed by the activation of NIK and degradation of IκBK and release of NFκB are nearly identical for IL-1 as well as for IL-18. Indeed, in cells transfected with IL-18Rα (IL-1Rrp) and then stimulated with IL-18, translocation of NFκB is observed using electromobility shift assay.[70] In U1 macrophages which already express the gene for IL-1Rrp, there is translocation of NFκB and stimulation of the human immunodeficiency virus-type 1 (HIV-1) production.[76]

F. Activation of MAP Kinases Following IL-1 Receptor Binding

As shown in Figure 2, multiple phosphorylations take place during the first 15 min following IL-1 receptor binding. Most consistently, IL-1 activates protein kinases which phosphorylate serine and threonine residues, targets of the MAP kinase family. An early study reported an IL-1–induced serine/threonine phosphorylation of a 65-kDa protein clearly unrelated to those phosphorylated via PKC.[77] As reviewed by O'Neill,[78] prior to IL-1 activation of serine/threonine kinases, IL-1 receptor binding results in the phosphorylation of tyrosine residues.[13,58] Tyrosine phosphorylation induced by IL-1 is likely due to activation of MAP kinase which then phosphorylates tyrosine and threonine on MAP kinases.

Following activation of MAP kinases, there are phosphorylations on serine and threonine residues of the epidermal growth factor receptor, heat-shock protein p27, myelin basic protein, and serine 56 and 156 of β–casein, each of which has been observed in IL-1–stimulated cells;[79] Guesdon, 1993. TNF also activates these kinases. There are at least three families of MAP kinases. The p42/44 MAP kinase family is associated with signal transduction by growth factors including ras-raf-1 signal pathways. In rat mesangial cells, IL-1 activates the p42/44 MAP kinase within 10 min and also increases *de novo* synthesis of p42.[57]

G. p38 MAP Kinase Activation

The stress-activated protein kinase (SAPK), which is molecularly identified as JNK, is phosphorylated in cells stimulated with IL-1.[80] In addition to p42/44, two members of the MAP kinase family (p38 and p54) have been identified as part of an IL-1 phosphorylation pathway and are responsible for phosphorylating hsp 27.[13,58] In rabbit primary liver cells, IL-1 selectively activates JNK without apparent activation of p38 or p42 p38 MAP kinases.[81] These MAP kinases are highly conserved proteins homologous to the *HOG-1* stress gene in yeasts. In fact, when *HOG-1* is deleted, yeasts fail to grow in hyperosmotic conditions; however, the mammalian gene coding for the IL-1–inducible p38 MAP kinase[58] can reconstitute the ability of the yeast to grow in hyperosmotic conditions.[82] In cells stimulated with hyperosmolar NaCl, LPS, IL-1, or TNF, indistinguishable phosphorylation of the p38 MAP kinase takes place.[83] In human monocytes exposed to hyperosmolar NaCl (375 to 425 mosm/l), IL-8, IL-1β, IL-1α, and TNF-α gene expression and synthesis take place which are indistinguishable from that induced by LPS or IL-1.[84,85] Thus, the MAP p38 kinase pathways involved in IL-1, TNF, and LPS signal transductions share certain elements that are related to the primitive stress-induced pathway. The dependency of Rho members of the GTPase family (see above) for IL-1-induced activation of p38 MAP kinases has been demonstrated.[86] This latter observation links the intrinsic GTPase domains of IL-1RI and IL-1R–AcP with activation of the p38 MAP kinase.

H. Inhibition of p38 MAP Kinase

The target for pyridinyl imidazole compounds has been identified as a homologue of the *HOG-1* family;[87] its sequence is identical to that of the p38 MAP kinase-activating protein-2.[88] Inhibition of the p38 MAP kinase is highly specific for reducing LPS- and IL-1–induced cytokines.[87] IL-1-induced expression of HIV-1 is suppressed by specific inhibition using pyridinyl imidazole compounds.[89] As expected, this class of imidazoles also prevents the downstream phosphorylation of hsp 27.[90] Compounds of this class appear to be highly specific for inhibition of the p38 MAP kinase in that there was no inhibition of 12 other kinases. Using one of these compounds, both hyperosmotic NaCl- and IL-1α–induced IL-8 synthesis were inhibited.[85] It has been proposed that MAP kinase-activating protein-2 is one of the substrates for the p38 MAP kinases and that MAP kinase-activating protein-2 is the kinase which phosphorylates hsp-27[90] (Figure 2).

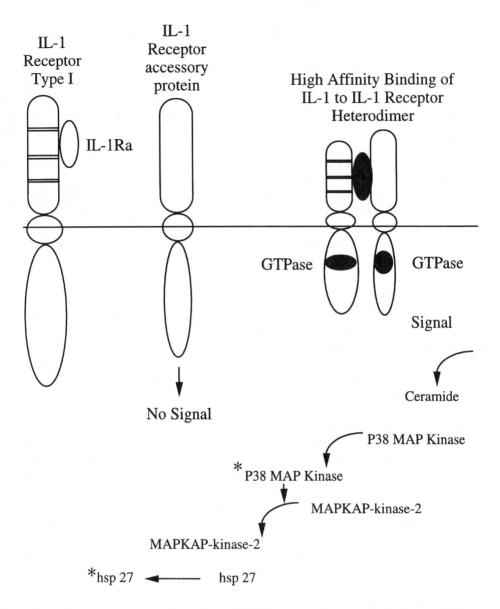

Figure 2   IL-1 postreceptor phosphorylation of MAP kinases. Lacking a second binding site, IL-1 receptor antagonist (IL-1Ra) binds primarily to IL-1RI but does not result in a structural change in the receptor. Hence the IL-1R–AcP does not form a high affinity complex with the IL-1/IL-1R, no signal is transduced, and there is no biological response. Signal transduction appears to require the formation of a heterodimer of IL-1RI with IL-1R–AcP. The cytoplasmic domain of the IL-1RI contains areas with putative GTPase activity. The proximity of the two cytoplasmic domains likely initiates signal transduction which may include hydrolysis of GTP by the intrinsic GTPase activity of the cytoplasmic domains and GTPase activating protein. This is followed by activation of low molecular weight GTP-binding proteins, liberation of ceramide. Phosphorylation of kinases such a c-JUN N-terminal kinase (JNK) and the p38 MAP kinase is known to take place as well as downstream phosphorylation of MAPKAP-kinase-2 and phosphorylation of hsp 27. Asterisks indicate phosphorylations.

I. TRANSCRIPTION FACTORS

The cytosolic domain of IL-1RI shares significant homology to the receptor-like *Toll* gene and suggests that both molecules signal similar events. Following IL-1 stimulation, phosphorylation of inhibitory κB (IκB) takes place, and this is rapidly degraded within the proteosome.[91] Translocation of NFκB to the nucleus is then observed.[92,93] A substrate for the β-casein kinase in IL-1– and TNF–activated cells[94] has been identified as the p65 subunit of NFκB.[95] Most of the biological effects of IL-1 take place in cells following nuclear translocation of NFκB and activating protein-1 (AP-1),[43,80] two nuclear factors common to many IL-1–induced genes. In T lymphocytes and cultured hepatocytes, the addition of IL-1 increases nuclear binding of *c-jun* and *c-fos*, the two components of AP-1.[96] Similar to NFκB, AP-1 sites are present in the promoter regions of many IL-1–inducible genes. IL-1 also increases the transcription of *c-jun* by activating two novel nuclear factors (jun-1 and jun-2) which bind to the promoter of the *c-jun* gene and stimulate *c-jun* transcription.[97]

REFERENCES

1. Bazan, J. F., J. C. Timans, and R. A. Kaselein. A newly defined interleukin-1? *Nature* 379, 591, 1996.
2. Colotta, F., F. Re, M. Muzio, R. Bertini, N. Polentarutti, M. Sironi, J. Giri, S. K. Dower, J. E. Sims, and A. Mantovani. Interleukin-1 type II receptor: a decoy target for IL-1 that is regulated by IL-4. *Science 261*, 472, 1993.
3. Greenfeder, S. A., P. Nunes, L. Kwee, M. Labow, R. A. Chizzonite, and G. Ju. Molecular cloning and characterization of a second subunit of the interleukin-1 receptor complex. *J. Biol. Chem.* 270, 13757, 1995.
4. Mizutani, H., N. Schecter, G. Zazarus, R. A. Black, and T. S. Kupper. Rapid and specific conversion of precursor interleukin-1β to an active IL-1 species by human mast cell chymase. *J. Exp. Med. 174*, 821, 1991.
5. Shornick, L. P., P. De Togni, S. Mariathasan, J. Goellner, J. Strauss-Schoenberger, R. W. Karr, T. A. Ferguson, and D. D. Chaplin. Mice deficient in IL-1beta manifest impaired contact hypersensitivity to trinitrochlorobenzone. *J. Exp. Med. 183*, 1427, 1996.
6. Mullarkey, M. F., K. M. Leiferman, M. S. Peters, I. Caro, E. R. Roux, R. K. Hanna, A. S. Rubin, and C. A. Jacobs. Human cutaneous allergic late-phase response is inhibited by soluble IL-1 receptor. *J. Immunol. 152*, 2033, 1994.
7. Brand, C. U., T. Hunziker, N. Yawalkar, and L. R. Braathen. IL-1 beta protein in human skin lymph does not discriminate allergic from irritant contact dermatitis. *Contact Dermatitis 35*, 152, 1996.
8. Sims, J. E., J. G. Giri, and S. K. Dower. The two interleukin-1 receptors play different roles in IL-1 activities. *Clin. Immunol. Immunopathol. 72*, 9, 1994.
9. Sims, J. E., S. L. Painter, and I. R. Gow. Genomic organization of the type I and type II IL-1 receptors. *Cytokine 7*, 483, 1995.
10. Mancilla, J., I. Ikejima, and C. A. Dinarello. Glycosylation of the interleukin-1 receptor type I is required for optimal binding of interleukin-1. *Lymphokine Cytokine Res. 11*, 197, 1992.
11. Rosoff, P. M., N. Savage, and C. A. Dinarello. Interleukin-1 stimulates diacylglycerol production in T lymphocytes by a novel mechanism. *Cell 54*, 73, 1988.
12. Burch, R. M., and L. C. Mahan. Oligonucleotides antisense to the interleukin-1 receptor mRNA block the effects of interleukin-1 in cultured murine and human fibroblasts and in mice. *J. Clin. Invest. 88*, 1190, 1991.
13. Freshney, N. W., L. Rawlinson, F. Guesdon, E. Jones, S. Cowley, J. Hsuan, and J. Saklatvala. Interleukin-1 activates a novel protein cascade that results in the phosphorylation of hsp27. *Cell 78*, 1039, 1994.
14. Gay, N. J., and F. J. Keith. Drosophila *Toll* and IL-1 receptor. *Nature 351*, 355, 1991.
15. Heguy, A., C. T. Baldari, G. Macchia, J. L. Telford, and M. Melli. Amino acids conserved in interleukin-1 receptors and the *Drosophila Toll* protein are essential for IL-1R signal transduction. *J. Biol. Chem. 267*, 2605, 1992.

16. Yang, R. B., M. R. Mark, A. Gray, A. Huang, M. H. Xie, M. Zhang, A. Goddard, W. I. Wood, A. L. Gurney, and P. J. Godowski. Toll-like receptor-2 mediates lipopolysaccharide-induced cellular signalling. *Nature 395*, 284, 1998.

17. Rock, F. L., G. Hardiman, J. C. Timans, R. A. Kastelein, and J. F. Bazan. A family of human receptors structurally related to Drosophila Toll. *Proc. Natl. Acad. Sci. U.S.A. 95*, 588, 1998.

18. Medzhitov, R., P. Preston-Hurlburt, and C. A. Janeway, Jr. A human homologue of the Drosophila Toll protein signals activation of adaptive immunity. *Nature 388*, 394, 1997.

19. Cao, Z., J. Xiong, M. Takeuchi, T. Kurama, and D. V. Goeddel. Interleukin-1 receptor activating kinase. *Nature 383*, 443, 1996.

20. Huang, J., X. Gao, S. Li, and Z. Cao. Recruitment of IRAK to the interleukin 1 receptor complex requires interleukin 1 receptor accessory protein. *Proc. Natl. Acad. Sci. U.S.A. 94*, 12829, 1997.

21. Medzhitov, R., P. Preston-Hurlburt, E. Kopp, A. Stadlen, C. Chen, S. Ghosh, and C. A. Janeway, Jr. MyD88 is an adaptor protein in the hToll/IL-1 receptor family signaling pathways. *Mol. Cell 2*, 253, 1998.

22. Ulevitch, R. J., and P. S. Tobias. Recognition of endotoxin by cells leading to transmembrane signaling. *Curr. Opin. Immunol. 6*, 125, 1994.

23. Lei, M. G., and D. C. Morrison. Specific endotoxic lipopolysaccharide-binding proteins on murine splenocytes. II. Membrane localization and binding characteristics. *J. Immunol. 141*, 1006, 1988.

24. Du, X., P. Thompson, E. K. L. Chan, J. Ledesma, B. Roe, S. Clifton, S. N. Vogel, and B. Beutler. Genetic and physical mapping of the Lps locus: identification of the Toll-4 receptor as a candidate gene in the critical region. *Blood Cells Mol. Dis. 24*, 340, 1998.

25. Vigers, G. P. A., L. J. Anderson, P. Caffes, and B. J. Brandhuber. Crystal structure of the type I interleukin-1 receptor complexed with interleukin-1β. *Nature 386*, 190, 1997.

26. Evans, R. J., J. Bray, J. D. Childs, G. P. A. Vigers, B. J. Brandhuber, J. J. Skalicky, R. C. Thompson, and S. P. Eisenberg. Mapping receptor binding sites in the IL-1 receptor antagonist and IL-1β by site-directed mutagenesis: identification of a single site in IL-1ra and two sites in IL-1β. *J. Biol. Chem. 270*, 11477, 1994.

27. Schreuder, H., C. Tardif, S. Trump-Kallmeyer, A. Soffientini, E. Sarubbi, A. Akeson, T. Bowlin, S. Yanofsky, and R. W. Barrett. A new cytokine-receptor binding mode revealed by the crystal structure of the IL-1 receptor with an antagonist. *Nature 386*, 194, 1997.

28. Wesche, H., C. Korherr, M. Kracht, W. Falk, K. Resch, and M. U. Martin. The interleukin-1 receptor accessory protein is essential for IL-1-induced activation of interleukin-1 receptor-associated kinase (IRAK) and stress-activated protein kinases (SAP kinases). *J. Biol. Chem. 272*, 7727, 1997.

29. Yoon, D. Y., and C. A. Dinarello. Antibodies to domains II and III of the IL-1 receptor accessory protein inhibit IL-1 beta activity but not binding: regulation of IL-1 responses is via type I receptor, not the accessory protein. *J. Immunol. 160*, 3170, 1998.

30. Heguy, A., C. T. Baldari, S. Censini, P. Ghiara, and J. L. Telford. A chimeric type II/I interleukin-1 receptor can mediate interleukin-1 induction of gene expression in T cells. *J. Biol. Chem. 268*, 10490, 1993.

31. Giri, J., R. C. Newton, and R. Horuk. Identification of soluble interleukin-1 binding protein in cell-free supernatants. *J. Biol. Chem. 265*, 17416, 1990.

32. Symons, J. A., J. A. Eastgate, and G. W. Duff. Purification and characterization of a novel soluble receptor for interleukin-1. *J. Exp. Med. 174*, 1251, 1991.

33. Symons, J. A., P. A. Young, and G. W. Duff. The soluble interleukin-1 receptor: ligand binding properties and mechanisms of release. *Lymphokine Cytokine Res. 12*, 381, 1993.

34. Arend, W. P., M. Malyak, M. F. Smith, T. D. Whisenand, J. L. Slack, J. E. Sims, J. G. Giri, and S. K. Dower. Binding of IL-1α, IL-1β, and IL-1 receptor antagonist by soluble IL-1 receptors and levels of soluble IL-1 receptors in synovial fluids. *J. Immunol. 153*, 4766, 1994.

35. Giri, J. G., J. Wells, S. K. Dower, C. E. McCall, R. N. Guzman, J. Slack, T. A. Bird, K. Shanebeck, K. H. Grabstein, J. E. Sims, and M. R. Alderson. Elevated levels of shed type II IL-1 receptor in sepsis. *J. Immunol. 153*, 5802, 1994.

36. Barak, V., B. Nisman, A. Polliack, E. Vannier, and C. A. Dinarello. Correlation of serum levels of interleukin-1 family members with disease activity and response to treatment in hairy cell leukemia. *Eur. Cytokine Netw. 9*, 33, 1998.

37. Pruitt, J. H., M. B. Welborn, P. D. Edwards, T. R. Harward, J. W. Seeger, T. D. Martin, C. Smith, J. A. Kenney, R. I. Wesdorp, S. Meijer, M. A. Cuesta, A. Abouhanze, E. M. Copeland, J. Giri, J. E. Sims, L. L. Moldawer, and H. S. Oldenburg. Increased soluble interleukin-1 type II receptor concentrations in postoperative patients and in patients with sepsis syndrome. *Blood 87*, 3282, 1996.

38. Crown, J., A. Jakubowski, N. Kemeny, M. Gordon, C. Gasparetto, G. Wong, G. Toner, B. Meisenberg, J. Botet, J. Applewhite, S. Sinha, M. Moore, D. Kelsen, W. Buhles, and J. Gabrilove. A phase I trial of recombinant human interleukin-1β alone and in combination with myelosuppressive doses of 5-fluoruracil in patients with gastrointestinal cancer. *Blood 78*, 1420, 1991.

39. Crown, J., A. Jakubowski, and J. Gabrilove. Interleukin-1: biological effects in human hematopoiesis. *Leuk. Lymphoma 9*, 433, 1993.

40. Mizel, S. B. IL-1 signal transduction. *Eur. Cytokine Netw. 5*, 1994.

41. Rossi, B. IL-1 transduction signals. *Eur. Cytokine Netw. 4*, 181, 1993.

42. Kuno, K., and K. Matsushima. The IL-1 receptor signaling pathway. *J. Leukoc. Biol. 56*, 542, 1994.

43. O'Neill, L. A. J., and C. Greene. Signal transduction pathways activated by the IL-1 receptor family: ancient signaling machinery in mammals, insects, and plants. *J. Leukoc Biol. 63*, 650, 1998.

44. Martin, M. U., and W. Falk. The interleukin-1 receptor complex and interleukin-1 signal transduction. *Eur. Cytokine Netw. 8*, 5, 1997.

45. Rosoff, P. M. Characterization of the interleukin-1-stimulated phospholipase C activity in human T lymphocytes. *Lymphokine Res. 8*, 407, 1989.

46. Schutze, S., T. Machleidt, and M. Kronke. The role of diacylglycerol and ceramide in tumor necrosis factor and interleukin-1 signal transduction. *J. Leukoc. Biol. 56*, 533, 1994.

47. Andrieu, N., R. Salvayre, and T. Levade. Evidence against involvement of the acid lysosomal shingomyelinase in the tumor necrosis factor and interleukin-1-induced sphigomyelin cycle and cell proliferation in human fibroblasts. *Biochem. J. 303*, 341, 1994.

48. Bomalaski, J. S., M. R. Steiner, P. L. Simon, and M. A. Clark. IL-1 increases phospholipase A_2 activity, expression of phospholipase A_2-activating protein, and release of linoleic acid from the murine T helper cell line EL-4. *J. Immunol. 148*, 155, 1992.

49. Kolesnick, R., and D. W. Golde. The sphingomyelin pathway in tumor necrosis factor and interleukin-1 signalling. *Cell 77*, 325, 1994.

50. Gronich, J., M. Konieczkowski, M. H. Gelb, R. A. Nemenoff, and J. R. Sedor. Interleukin-1α causes a rapid activation of cytosolic phospholipase A_2 by phosphorylation in rat mesangial cells. *J. Clin. Invest. 93*, 1224, 1994.

51. Ye, K., K.-C. Koch, B. D. Clark, and C. A. Dinarello. Interleukin-1 down regulates gene and surface expression of interleukin-1 receptor type I by destabilizing its mRNA whereas interleukin-2 increases its expression. *Immunology 75*, 427, 1992.

52. Gallis, B., K. S. Prickett, J. Jackson, J. Slack, K. Schooley, J. E. Sims, and S. K. Dower. IL-1 induces rapid phosphorylation of the IL-1 receptor. *J. Immunol. 143*, 3235, 1989.

53. Mizel, S. B. Cyclic AMP and interleukin-1 signal transduction. *Immunol. Today 11*, 390, 1990.

54. Munoz, E., U. Beutner, A. Zubiaga, and B. T. Huber. IL-1 activates two separate signal transduction pathways in T helper type II cells. *J. Immunol. 144*, 964, 1990.

55. Kester, M., M. S. Siomonson, P. Mene, and J. R. Sedor. Interleukin-1 generate transmembrane signals from phospholipids through novel pathways in cultured rat mesangial cells. *J. Clin. Invest. 83*, 718, 1989.

56. Mathias, S., A. Younes, C.-C. Kan, I. Orlow, C. Joseph, and R. N. Kolesnick. Activation of the sphingomyelin signaling pathway in intact EL4 cells and in a cell-free system by IL-1β. *Science 259*, 519, 1993.

57. Huwiler, A., and J. Pfeilschifter. Interleukin-1 stimulates de novo synthesis of mitogen-activated protein kinase in glomerular mesangial cells. *FEBS Lett. 350*, 135, 1994.

58. Kracht, M., O. Truong, N. F. Totty, M. Shiroo, and J. Saklatvala. Interleukin-1α activates two forms of p54α mitogen-activated protein kinase in rabbit liver. *J. Exp. Med. 180*, 2017, 1994.

59. Kuno, K., S. Okamoto, K. Hirose, S. Murakami, and K. Matsushima. Structure and function of the intracellular portion of the mouse interleukin-1 receptor (Type I). *J. Biol. Chem. 268*, 13510, 1993.

60. Croston, G. E., Z. Cao, and D. V. Goeddel. NFkB activation by interleukin-1 requires an IL-1 receptor-associated protein kinase activity. *J. Biol. Chem. 270*, 16514, 1995.

61. Martin, M., G. F. Bol, A. Eriksson, K. Resch, and R. Brigelius-Flohe. Interleukin-1-induced activation of a protein kinase co-precipitating with the type I interleukin-1 receptor in T-cells. *Eur. J. Immunol.* *24*, 1566, 1994.

62. Hopp, T. P. Evidence from sequence information that the interleukin-1 receptor is a transmembrane GTPase. *Protein Sci. 4*, 1851, 1995.

63. Mitchum, J. L., and J. E. Sims. IIP1: a novel human that interacts with the IL-1 receptor. *Cytokine 7*, 595(abstr), 1995.

64. Cao, Z. Signal transduction of interleukin-1. *Eur. Cytokine Netw. 9*, 378(abstr), 1998.

65. Malinin, N. L., M. P. Boldin, A. V. Kovalenko, and D. Wallach. MAP3K-related kinase involved in NF-kappaB induction by TNF, CD95 and IL-1. *Nature 385*, 540, 1997.

66. DiDonato, J. A., M. Hayakawa, D. M. Rothwarf, E. Zandi, and M. Karin. A cytokine-responsive I kappaB kinase that activates the transcription factor NF-kappaB. *Nature 388*, 548, 1997.

67. Dinarello, C. A. Interleukin-18: a Th1-inducing, proinflammatory cytokine and new member of the IL-1 family. *J. Allergy Clin. Immunol.* In press.

68. Yoshimoto, T., K. Takeda, T. Tanaka, K. Ohkusu, S. Kashiwamura, H. Okamura, S. Akira, and K. Nakanishi. IL-12 upregulates IL-18 receptor expression on T cells, Th1 cells and B cells: synergism with IL-18 for IFNγ production. *J. Immunol. 161*, 3400, 1998.

69. Parnet, P., K. E. Garka, T. P. Bonnert, S. K. Dower, and J. E. Sims. IL-1Rrp is a novel receptor-like molecule similar to the type I interleukin-1 receptor and its homologues T1/ST2 and IL-1R AcP. *J. Biol. Chem. 271*, 3967, 1996.

70. Torigoe, K., S. Ushio, T. Okura, S. Kobayashi, M. Taniai, T. Kunikate, T. Murakami, O. Sanou, H. Kojima, M. Fuji, T. Ohta, M. Ikeda, H. Ikegami, and M. Kurimoto. Purification and characterization of the human interleukin-18 receptor. *J. Biol. Chem. 272*, 25737, 1997.

71. Born, T. L., E. Thomassen, T. A. Bird, and J. E. Sims. Cloning of a novel receptor subunit, AcPL, required for interleukin-18 signaling. *J. Biol. Chem. 273*, 29445, 1998.

72. Novick, D., S.-H. Kim, G. Fantuzzi, L. Reznikov, C. A. Dinarello, and M. Rubinstein. Interleukin-18 binding protein: a novel modulator of the Th1 cytokine response. *Immunity 10*, 127, 1999.

73. Kojima, H., M. Takeuchi, T. Ohta, Y. Nishida, N. Arai, M. Ikeda, H. Ikegami, and M. Kurimoto. Interleukin-18 activates the IRAK-TRAF6 pathway in mouse EL-4 cells. *Biochem. Biophys. Res. Commun. 244*, 183, 1998.

74. Robinson, D., K. Shibuya, A. Mui, F. Zonin, E. Murphy, T. Sana, S. B. Hartley, S. Menon, R. Kastelein, F. Bazan, and A. O'Garra. IGIF does not drive Th1 development but synergizes with IL-12 for interferon-γ production and activates IRAK and NFκB. *Immunity 7*, 571, 1997.

75. Adachi, O., T. Kawai, K. Takeda, M. Matsumoto, H. Tsutsui, M. Sakagami, K. Nakanishi, and S. Akira. Targeted disruption of the MyD88 gene results in loss of IL-1– and IL-18–mediated function. *Immunity 9*, 143, 1998.

76. Shapiro, L., A. J. Puren, H. A. Barton, D. Novick, R. L. Peskind, M. S.-S. Su, Y. Gu, and C. A. Dinarello. Interleukin-18 stimulates HIV type 1 in monocytic cells. *Proc. Natl. Acad. Sci. U.S.A. 95*, 12550, 1998.

77. Matsushima, K., Y. Kobayashi, T. D. Copeland, T. Akahoshi, and J. J. Oppenheim. Phosphorylation of a cytosolic 65-kDa protein induced by interleukin-1 in glucocorticoid pretreated normal human peripheral blood mononuclear leukocytes. *J. Immunol. 139*, 3367, 1987.

78. O'Neill, L. A. J. Towards and understanding of the signal transduction pathways for interleukin-1. *Biochim. Biophys. Acta 1266*, 31, 1995.

79. Bird, T. A., P. R. Sleath, P. C. de Roos, S. K. Dower, and G. D. Virca. Interleukin-1 represents a new modality for the activation of extracellular signal-related kinases/microtubule-associated protein-2 kinases. *J. Biol. Chem. 266*, 22661, 1991.

80. Stylianou, E., and J. Saklatvala. Interleukin-1. *Int. J. Biochem. Cell Biol. 30*, 1075, 1998.

81. Finch, A., P. Holland, J. Cooper, J. Saklatvala, and M. Kracht. Selective activation of JNK/SAPK by interleukin-1 in rabbit liver is mediated by MKK7. *FEBS Lett. 418*, 144, 1997.

82. Galcheva-Gargova, Z., B. Dérijard, I.-H. Wu, and R. J. Davis. An osmosensing signal transduction pathway in mammalian cells. *Science 265*, 806, 1994.

83. Han, J., J.-D. Lee, L. Bibbs, and R. J. Ulevitch. A MAP kinase targeted by endotoxin and hyperosmolarity in mammalian cells. *Science 265*, 808, 1994.

84. Shapiro, L., and C. A. Dinarello. Cytokine expression during osmotic stress. *Exp. Cell Res. 231*, 354, 1997.

85. Shapiro, L., and C. A. Dinarello. Osmotic regulation of cytokine synthesis in vitro. *Proc. Natl. Acad. Sci. U.S.A. 92*, 12230, 1995.

86. Zhang, S., J. Han, M. A. Sells, J. Chernoff, U. G. Knaus, R. J. Ulevitch, and G. M. Bokoch. Rho family GTPases regulate p38 mitogen-activated protein kinase through the downstream mediator Pak 1. *J. Biol. Chem. 270*, 23934, 1995.

87. Lee, J. C., J. T. Laydon, P. C. McDonnell, T. F. Gallagher, S. Kumar, D. Green, D. McNulty, M. J. Blumenthal, J. R. Heys, S. W. Landvatter, J. E. Strickler, M. M. McLaughlin, I. R. Slemens, S. M. Fisher, G. P. Livi, J. R. White, J. L. Adams, and P. R. Young. A protein kinase involved in the regulation of inflammatory cytokine biosynthesis. *Nature 372*, 739, 1994.

88. Han, J., B. Richter, Z. Li, V. V. Kravchenko, and R. J. Ulevitch. Molecular cloning of human p38 MAP kinase. *Biochim. Biophys. Acta 1265*, 224, 1995.

89. Shapiro, L., K. A. Heidenreich, M. K. Meintzer, and C. A. Dinarello. Role of p38 mitogen-activated protein kinase in HIV type 1 production in vitro. *Proc. Natl. Acad. Sci. U.S.A. 95*, 7422, 1998.

90. Cuenda, A., J. Rouse, Y. N. Doza, R. Meier, P. Cohen, T. F. Gallagher, P. R. Young, and J. C. Lee. SB 203580 is a specific inhibitor of a MAP kinase homologue which is stimulated by stresses and interleukin-1. *FEBS Lett. 364*, 229, 1995.

91. DiDonato, J. A., F. Mercurio, and M. Karin. Phosphorylation of IκBα precedes but is not sufficient for its dissociation from NFκB. *Mol. Cell Biol. 15*, 1302, 1995.

92. Shirakawa, F., and S. B. Mizel. In vitro activation and nuclear translocation of NF-kappa B catalyzed by cyclic AMP-derived protein kinase and protein kinase C. *Mol. Cell Biol. 9*, 2424, 1989.

93. Stylianou, E., L. A. J. O'Neill, L. Rawlinson, M. R. Edbrooke, P. Woo, and J. Saklatvala. Interleukin-1 induces NFkB through its type I but not type II receptor in lymphocytes. *J. Biol. Chem. 267*, 15836, 1992.

94. Guesdon, F., R. J. Waller, and J. Saklatvala. Specific activation of β-casein kinase by the inflammatory cytokines interleukin-1 and tumour necrosis factor. *Biochem. J. 304*, 761, 1994.

95. Bird, T. A., H. Downey, and G. D. Virca. Interleukin-1 regulates casein kinase II-mediated phosphorylation of the p65 subunit of NGκB. *Cytokine 7*, 603(abstr), 1995.

96. Muegge, K., T. M. Williams, J. Kant, M. Karin, R. Chiu, A. Schmidt, U. Siebenlist, H. A. Young, and S. K. Durum. Interleukin-1 costimulatory activity on the interleukin-2 promoter via AP-1. *Science 246*, 249, 1989.

97. Muegge, K., M. Vila, G. L. Gusella, T. Musso, P. Herrlich, B. Stein, and S. K. Durum. IL-1 induction of the c-jun promoter. *Proc. Natl. Acad. Sci. U.S.A. 90*, 7054, 1993.

13 Proinflammatory Mediators of the Arachidonic Acid Cascade

Kouichi Ikai

CONTENTS

I. INTRODUCTION

Metabolites of arachidonic acid (eicosanoids), including the prostaglandins (PGs), thromboxanes (TXs), leukotrienes (LTs), and hydroxyeicosatetraenoic acids (HETEs), have been implicated as mediators or modulators of a number of physiological functions and pathologic conditions (Figure 1).[1-3] Eicosanoids are actively synthesized and degraded in the skin[4,5] and contribute to the pathogenesis of a number of skin diseases, such as ultraviolet-dermatitis,[6] atopic dermatitis,[7] urticaria,[8] and psoriasis.[9] Eicosanoids have generally been regarded as the mediators of inflammatory conditions, including those in the skin.[10] This traditional approach resulted in the establishment of therapeutic procedures using nonsteroidal anti-inflammatory drugs (NSAIDs), which are inhibitors of the enzymes involved in eicosanoid synthesis, such as aspirin or indomethacin. However, it has been postulated that most eicosanoids show reciprocal pharmacological actions; in other words, they are both pro- and anti-inflammatory, and act synergistically with other mediators, growth factors, and cytokines. In addition, eicosanoids play an important role in the skin, not only under pathological conditions, but also in normal body functions such as tissue protection,[11] immune regulation,[12] carcinogenesis,[13] differentiation,[14] and wound healing.[15] With the rapid progress on the molecular biology of eicosanoids, investigations on eicosanoids and related compounds in the skin have now been revisited. From these points of view, the traditional concept that eicosanoids are mediators of inflammation should be reevaluated. Therefore, apart from NSAIDs, the treatment of various diseases, including skin diseases, with eicosanoid analogs or derivatives may be the ultimate therapeutic benefit derived from studies on eicosanoid in the skin, as has already been exemplified in the treatment of gastric ulcers with stable prostaglandin derivatives.[11] Moreover, special drug delivery systems for eicosanoid-related compounds should be devised to specifically deliver these compounds to targeted organs or tissues such as the skin.[16] This review will focus on the recent progress on the pathophysiological functions of eicosanoids in the skin, and will discuss eicosanoid derivatives as novel drugs for skin diseases.

0-8493-2117-4/00/$0.00+$.50
© 2000 by CRC Press LLC

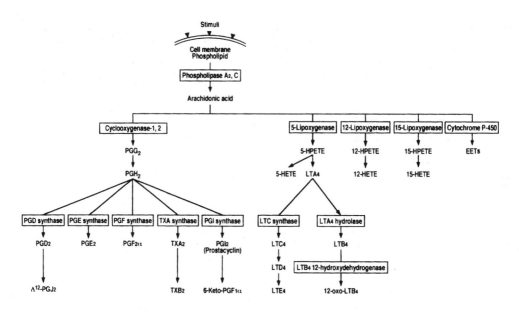

Figure 1   Arachidonic acid cascade; various eicosanoids are synthesized via the cyclooxygenase and lipoxygenase pathways.

II. ARACHIDONIC ACID CASCADE AND EICOSANOIDS

Arachidonic acid (5,8,11,14-eicosatetraenoic acid, C20:4, n6), a long-chain polyunsaturated fatty acid, is released from the plasma membrane by the action of phospholipases on membrane phospholipids such as phosphatidyl choline, phosphatidyl inositol, and phosphatidyl ethanolamine. The release of arachidonic acid is triggered by a variety of physiological or pathological stimuli. The physiological stimuli include hormones such as bradykinin, angiotensin II or epinephrine, antigen–antibody complexes, and proteases such as thrombin. The pathological stimuli include mechanical damage, ischemia/hypoxia, hypoglycemia, membrane active toxins such as mellitin, Ca^{2+} ionophores such as ionophore A23187, and tumor promotors such as phorbol myristate acetate. The major enzyme responsible for stimulation-evoked arachidonic acid release in various tissues is believed to be cytosolic, high-molecular weight, and micromolar order Ca^{2+}-required phospholipase A_2 (PLA_2), which translocates from the cytosol to the membrane upon activation by Ca^{2+} and phosphorylation by the MAP kinase cascade.[17,18] In the skin, Ilchysyn et al.[19] reported that the PLA_2 levels were elevated in psoriatic epidermis. However, transgenic mice which overexpress human group II PLA_2 show epidermal hyperplasia without any dermal inflammatory infiltration.[20] In cytosolic PLA_2-deficient mice, the eicosanoid production was markedly decreased, but no significant skin changes could be observed, although the anaphylactic responses were significantly reduced and bronchial hyperreactivity was completely diminished.[21] Annexin I (lipocortin I) was initially proposed to be one of the anti-inflammatory proteins induced by corticosteroids to inhibit PLA_2.[22] Subsequent studies have demonstrated that annexin I can associate with phospholipid vesicles in a Ca^{2+}-dependent manner, and that the PLA_2 inhibitory action was due to an interaction of annexin I with its phospholipid substrates rather than to a direct inhibition of the enzyme. Although several studies on annexin I in the skin have been carried out,[23,24] the in vivo functions of annexin I are not yet fully understood.

The second rate-limiting step in arachidonic acid metabolism involves fatty acid oxygenation. Free arachidonic acid undergoes enzymatic oxygenation by different enzymatic pathways and is converted to biologically active eicosanoids.[2,3] A schematic diagram of arachidonic acid metabolism (arachidonic acid cascade) is shown in Figure 1. The cyclooxygenase (COX) pathway involves a

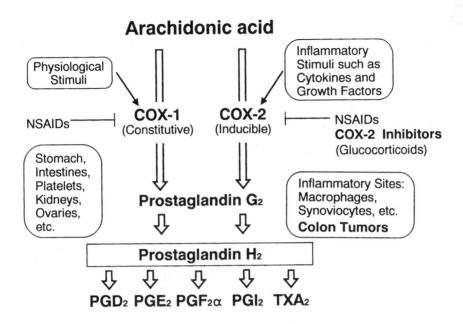

Figure 2   The two cyclooxygenases.

series of peroxidations and cyclizations of arachidonic acid, leading initially to unstable intermediates (PGG$_2$ and PGH$_2$) (Figure 1). The subcellular localization of the cyclooxygenases is in the
microsomal fraction of the epidermal cells. Recently, two COX isozymes, COX-1 and COX-2, have
been identified (Figure 2). The former is a constitutive enzyme, whereas COX-2 can be induced
by cytokines, growth factors, and tumor promoters.[25] We have examined the expression of COX-
1 and COX-2 in human skin by immunohistochemistry and Western blotting using isozyme-specific
antibodies.[26] In normal human skin, COX-1 immunostaining can be observed throughout the
epidermis, whereas COX-2 immunostaining is localized to the suprabasilar keratinocytes and basal
cells. In the involved skin of patients with psoriasis, COX-1 immunostaining can be observed
throughout the epidermis, whereas COX-2 immunostaining is not detectable. Western blotting
demonstrated that transformed human cultured keratinocytes expressed COX-1 constitutively. In
contrast, the expression of COX-2 was barely detectable but was inducible upon the addition of
phorbol myristate acetate. These data confirmed the previous reports[27,28] and suggest that the
expression of COX-2 in human skin is at least partly related to epidermal differentiation as well
as to the pathogenesis of psoriasis.

The unstable intermediates (PGG$_2$ and PGH$_2$) then undergo isomerizations and reductions and
are converted to PGD$_2$, PGE$_2$, PGF$_2\alpha$, PGI$_2$, and TXA$_2$ by the action of PGD synthase, PGE
synthase, PGF synthase, PGI synthase, and TXA$_2$ synthase, respectively[2,3,29] (Figure 1). In contrast
to the COXs, these eicosanoid synthases show a unique localization mainly in the cytoplasm. For
example, PGD synthase is localized in the cytoplasm of Langerhans cells in the epidermis, and
macrophages, mast cells, and fibroblasts in the dermis.[30,31] Ultraviolet-B irradiation suppresses PGD
synthase activity in rat skin.[32] The cellular distribution of PGE synthase, PGF synthase, PGI
synthase, and TXA$_2$ synthase was also examined.[29]

With respect to the degradation of prostanoids, the two enzymes most prominently involved in
prostanoid biodegradation are 4,5-hydroxyprostaglandin dehydrogenase and 9-keto prostaglandin
reductase. These enzymes are present in the cytosolic fraction of the epidermis of human skin.[33]
Apart from these degradation systems, PGD$_2$ and PGE$_2$ are nonenzymatically hydrolyzed by
albumin, and are converted to Δ^{12}-PGJ$_2$ and PGA$_2$, respectively.[34–36] These cyclopentenone prostaglandins have been demonstrated to inhibit cell growth and proliferation both in vitro and in vivo.

The prostaglandins produced are then released outside the cells by various stimuli (Figure 3). Prostaglandins and thromboxanes have individual receptor systems that are coupled to the G-protein system (Figure 4).[37] Their cDNAs have been cloned, and their structure has been studied extensively. Most recently, knockout mice lacking prostanoid receptors have also been developed.[38,39]

The lipoxygenase pathway begins with the oxidation of arachidonic acid to hydroperoxide, which is then transformed either enzymatically or spontaneously. Within the hydroperoxide molecule, the peroxidation can occur at different sites, thus generating 5-, 12-, or 15-HPETEs. The enzyme 5-lipoxygenase catalyzes the first two steps of the 5-lipoxygenase pathway.[40] The first step results in the conversion of free arachidonic acid to 5-HPETE. The second converts 5-HPETE to

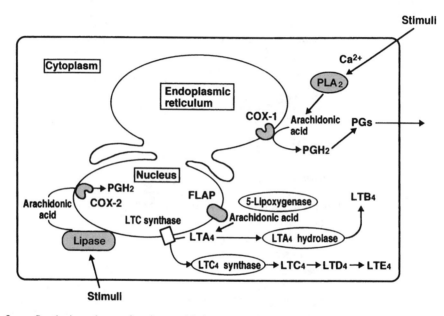

Figure 3   Synthetic pathways for eicosanoids in mammalian cells.

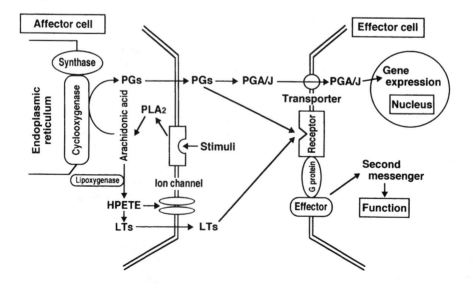

Figure 4   Mechanism of action of the eicosanoid.

LTA_4. LTA_4 is the pivotal intermediate from which all other leukotrienes are synthesized. The activation of 5-lipoxygenase in intact cells appears to be regulated by intracellular Ca^{2+} and 5-lipoxygenase activating protein (FLAP) (Figure 3). The 5-lipoxygenase and FLAP are localized in the nuclear envelope under activated cell conditions.[41] It is still controversial whether the 5-lipoxygenase activity is present in epidermal keratinocytes. Although some authors have reported that epidermal keratinocytes have significant 5-lipoxygenase activity,[42] others have claimed that several kinds of cells, such as endothelial cells and keratinocytes, lack 5-lipoxygenase activity.[43] There are two subsequent metabolic routes from LTA_4 that lead to the production of biologically active compounds (Figures 1 and 3). The first route involves LTA_4 hydrolase, which is the rate-limiting enzyme for LTB_4 biosynthesis. The LTA_4 hydrolase has been reported to be ubiquitously distributed and is found in large amounts in blood cells such as human leukocytes, erythrocytes, and neutrophils.[44] The LTA_4 hydrolase has been recognized as a Zn^{2++}-metallohydrolase possessing intrinsic amino-peptidase activity, and its activity can be inhibited by bestatin and captopril, which are inhibitors of aminopeptidase.[45] LTA_4 hydrolase activity is localized in the skin[46] and is elevated in peripheral blood leukocytes from patients with atopic dermatitis.[47]

The second enzymatic route for LTA_4 metabolism involves conjugation with glutathione by the enzyme LTC_4 synthase to produce LTC_4.[48,49] LTC_4 can then be metabolized through the cleavage of a glutamic acid by a membrane-bound γ-glutamyl transferase to produce LTD_4. LTD_4 in turn can be converted to LTE_4, the cysteinyl conjugate, by a specific membrane-bound peptidase with a loss of glycine. Although it has been reported that human epidermal keratinocytes can synthesize LTB_4, LTC_4, and LTD_4 from arachidonic acid,[50] and that the synthesis of cysteinyl leukotrienes is enhanced in the urine and blood cells from patients with psoriasis[51] and atopic dermatitis,[52,53] the details of the biosynthesis and degradation of these leukotrienes in the epidermis have not been definitely established. LTC_4 synthase can be detected in the microsomal fraction from human epidermal[50] and melanoma cells,[54] but no significant 5-lipoxygenase activity was found in these cells.

As described above, LTB_4 can be converted from LTA_4 by LTA_4 hydrolase in keratinocytes.[46] If the keratinocytes lack 5-lipoxygenase activity as claimed by Breton et al.,[43] then the actual substrate, LTA_4, should not be present in the keratinocytes. The question then arises as to where the LTA_4 comes from. Most probably, the LTA_4 is transferred from other cells such as neutrophils or macrophages to the keratinocytes by unknown mechanisms.

Considerable enzyme activity of LTB_4 12-hydroxydehydrogenase,[55] which converts LTB_4 into 12-oxo-LTB_4, a biologically less active compound, has been detected in the cytosolic from human foreskin epidermis.[50]

Although the products of 5-lipoxygenase have attracted much attention, arachidonic acid can also be oxidized by 12-lipoxygenase in the skin. Hammarström et al.[56] reported that the quantity of free arachidonic acid and 12-HETE in the involved skin of psoriasis patients was elevated 25- and 80-fold, respectively, as compared to the uninvolved skin. In contrast, the amount of PGE_2 and $PGF_{2\alpha}$ was increased by only 40 and 86%, respectively. This increase in 12-HETE may be due to increased arachidonic acid levels, but not to elevated 12-lipoxygenase activity, because 12-lipoxygenase activity is increased only 1.5-fold in the uninvolved skin in psoriasis as compared to the normal skin.[57] There are two isoforms of 12-lipoxygenase: a platelet type and a leukocyte type.[58] The platelet 12-lipoxygenase results in the formation of 12-HPETE, which is rapidly reduced to form 12-HETE, mainly as the 12*(S)*-HETE isomer. Takahashi et al. demonstrated that keratinocytes have a potent 12-lipoxygenase activity, which forms 12*(S)*-HETE, and that the platelet and epidermal 12-lipoxygenases are identical.[59] However, Woollard[60] reported that 12-HETE derived from the lesional scales of patients with psoriasis was stereochemically distinct from the platelet 12*(S)*-enantiomer, as its derivative co-chromatographed with the 12*(R)*-diastereomer. The enantiomer of 12*(R)*-HETE increased in the psoriatic scales and can be detected naturally in the rat liver and sea urchin. This stereochemical difference may be biologically significant, because the 12*(R)*-HETE form is more chemotactic than the 12*(S)* form in vitro,[61,62] suggesting that the 12*(R)*-HETE in psoriatic scales is not a product of the epidermal 12-lipoxygenase. However, Hussain et al.[63] reported that the epidermis contains the platelet type of 12-lipoxygenase, which is overexpressed in the germinal keratinocytes in psoriasis. On the other hand, Baer et al.[64] reported that the incubation of psoriatic scales with arachidonic acid resulted in a 5:7 ratio of 12*(R)*-HETE and 12*(S)*-HETE formed. With respect to the biosynthesis of 12*(R)*-HETE, it may be formed by a 12*(R)*-HETE-specific 12-lipoxygenase or cytochrome P-450,[65] but the exact mechanism remains unknown.[66] However, the skin also has significant activity of cytochrome P-450 (epoxygenase), which produces several types of epoxyeicosatrienoic acid (EET).[67] The origin, function, and metabolism of 12*(R)*-HETE in psoriatic scales are very interesting.

The initial step in the 15-lipoxygenase pathway is the oxygenation of arachidonic acid at C-15, resulting in the formation of 15-HPETE, which can be reduced to form 15-HETE. Several cell types found in the skin contain 15-lipoxygenase.[68,69] The activation of the 15-lipoxygenase pathway is poorly understood, but in contrast to 5-lipoxygenase, 15-lipoxygenase activation is dependent on the presence of exogenous arachidonic acid.[70] Although 15-HETE possesses no proinflammatory activity different from PGE_2, LTB_4, or 12-HETE,[68] it can modulate the enzyme activities of the arachidonic acid cascade. Leukocyte 5-lipoxygenase and platelet 12-lipoxygenase are also more sensitive to inhibition by 15-HETE than cyclooxygenase.[71]

Recently, the lipoxins, a new series of triple oxygenation products, have been identified. These metabolites are formed by the interactions of the 5- and 15-lipoxygenase pathways under in vitro conditions.[72] The function of these lipoxins in the skin has not been discovered yet in vivo.

III. BIOLOGICAL FUNCTION OF EICOSANOIDS IN THE SKIN

Human skin can generate eicosanoids, and the eicosanoids thus formed exert proinflammatory and immunoregulatory actions by their effects on blood vessels and inflammatory cells; they are also involved in the regulation of growth and differentiation of the epithelia. Eicosanoids present in both normal and diseased skin can be produced by intrinsic skin cell types such as epidermal keratinocytes, melanocytes, macrophages, Langerhans cells, fibroblasts, mast cells, and endothelial cells. Furthermore, neutrophils and monocytes are the primary source of eicosanoids in inflammatory skin conditions. It is also important to note that eicosanoids may be formed by multiple cell types acting in concert.[4,5]

A. PROSTAGLANDINS

The intradermal injection of E-type prostaglandins causes vasodilation and increase cutaneous blood flow. Furthermore, PGE_2 can potentiate the vascular permeability changes induced by other mediators.[73] These responses appear to be due to a direct effect of PGE_2 on the blood vessels. Specific and high affinity binding sites for PGE_2 have been reported to be located on the membrane fraction of human epidermal cells. The proinflammatory properties of PGE_2 stand in contrast to its potential immunosuppressive effects. Following stimulation of adenyl cyclase and the elevation in intracellular cyclic-AMP levels, PGE_2 may exert inhibitory effects on lymphocytes and monocytes.[12] In contrast to these findings, prostaglandins do not seem to play a central role in the cause of inflammatory skin diseases. This claim is supported by the clinical lack of therapeutic efficacy of NSAIDs in some inflammatory skin diseases. Instead, the administration of NSAIDs induces an exacerbation of the psoriasis[74] and urticaria.[75] Recently, knockout mice lacking cyclooxygenase have been developed,[76] but these mice had apparently normal skin.

PGD_2 is a naturally occurring prostanoid that shows various kinds of pharmacological activity.[77] In the skin, PGD_2 is known to be actively produced by mast cells during IgE stimulations and to modify the anaphylactic process, thus suggesting that PGD_2 contributes to the development of various skin diseases.[78]

Cyclopentenone prostaglandins such as Δ^{12}-PGJ_2 and PGA_2 have no cell surface receptors, but are actively transported into cells where they accumulate in the nuclei and act as potent inducers of cell growth inhibition and cell differentiation.[34–36] Forman et al.[79] and Kliewer et al.[80] reported that PGJ_2 and its derivatives are efficacious activators of peroxisome proliferator-activated receptors α and γ (PPARα and PPARγ, respectively); these receptors are orphan nuclear receptors that have been implicated in lipid homeostasis and adipocyte differentiation. These data provide strong evidence that PGJ_2 and its derivatives can function as adipogenic agents through direct interactions with $PPAR_\gamma$, and further suggest a novel mechanism for the actions of cyclopentenone prostaglandins. These experimental results indicate that cyclopentenone prostaglandins are not only anticancer agents, but also play an important pathophysiological role. Hirata et al.[81] developed a highly sensitive and specific solid-phase enzyme immunoassay for Δ^{12}-PGJ_2, and demonstrated the natural occurrence of Δ^{12}-PGJ_2 in human urine using this method. Δ^{12}-PGJ_2 may play a significant role in the regulation of the proliferation of epidermal cells in vivo through the induction of heat shock proteins or via cytoskeletal damage.[82] Furthermore, the mechanisms of action of the cyclopentenone prostaglandins are notably different from other anticancerous drugs such as 5-fluorouracil or bleomycin,[34–36] thus suggesting that cyclopentenone prostaglandins may be promising antineoplastic agents. Cyclopentenone PGs also show antiviral actions against herpes simplex and HIV infection.[83,84] A number of clinical studies are presently ongoing,[34–36] and in vivo experiments on human skin cancer are currently in progress.

B. Leukotrienes

LTB_4 has been established as a mediator of skin inflammation in vivo and appears to be a potent proinflammatory agent. LTB_4 is one of the most powerful chemotactic and chemokinetic agents, and in neutrophils it causes degranulation, cation fluxes, and enhanced binding to endothelial cells.[1,2,85] LTB_4, through binding to its receptor, stimulates neutrophil activity such as chemokinesis, aggregation, degranulation, adhesion to the endothelium, etc. Recently, Yokomizo et al. have succeeded in cloning the complementary DNA encoding a cell-surface LTB_4 receptor which is coupled to the G-protein system.[86] The topical application of nanogram amounts of LTB_4 to normal human skin results in erythema and edema lasting several days. Histologically, this reaction is characterized by epidermal neutrophil microabscesses.[87] The intradermal injection of LTB_4 causes local edema, vasoconstriction, and perivascular neutrophil accumulation in humans.[88] The erythema and edema produced by LTB_4 are potentiated by a concomitant injection of PGE_2.[89] The inflammatory skin response to a topical application of LTB_4 is also accompanied by epidermal hyperproliferation, which is similar to a psoriatic lesion.[87,90] This effect on the epidermal keratinocytes may be secondary to the inflammatory response, but it can also be caused by a direct effect via receptors specific for LTB_4 on the keratinocytes (Figure 4).[91] LTB_4 can also induce pigmentation in human melanocytes,[92] and therefore LTB_4 has been suspected to play an important role in the pathogenesis of various inflammatory and allergic diseases, including skin diseases such as psoriasis[9] or atopic dermatitis.[7] Based on its chemotactic activity, the topical application of LTB_4 is effective against tinea pedis.[93] LTC_4, LTD_4, and LTE_4 are known as the sulfidopeptide leukotrienes, and collectively account for the biological activity originally described as the slow-reacting substance of anaphylaxis (SRS-A)(Figure 1).[1,2,85] Leukotrienes are vasoactive compounds, and LTC_4 increases both vascular permeability and blood flow. The intradermal injection of LTC_4 in normal human skin produces erythema and a flare reaction.[73] These leukotrienes have been implicated as potentially important mediators of immediate hypersensitivity reactions and allergic conditions of the skin.[94] In contrast, mice deficient for 5-lipoxygenase are indistinguishable in growth and size from control mice, although knockout mice are unable to synthesize detectable levels of leukotrienes.[95]

C. 12-HETE and Other Eicosanoids

12-HETE, particularly in its *R*-form, is chemotactic for neutrophils and is present in psoriatic scales, although it is far less potent than LTB_4. Previously, the actions of 12(*R*) and (*S*)-HETE were believed to be mediated by the LTB$_4$ receptor, since no 12-HETE receptors have been found in epidermal cells. However, Arenberger et al. demonstrated that the number of binding sites for 12-HETE in both the involved and uninvolved epidermis from psoriatic patients was increased as compared to normal controls, but no significant difference in the affinity of the receptor was found.[96] The significance of these data remains unknown.

Recently, Antón et al.[97] found that the normal human epidermis produces relatively high amounts of hepoxilins and trioxilins in vitro. The levels of biologic activities of the hepoxilins indicated that they could amplify and maintain the inflammatory response, suggesting that these compounds could play a role as mediators in the inflammatory response of the skin, particularly in psoriasis.

IV. THERAPEUTIC TRIALS AND DRUG DELIVERY OF EICOSANOID-RELATED COMPOUNDS IN SKIN DISEASES

As described above, eicosanoids are not only mediators of inflammation, but are also important modulators of physiological and pathological conditions, especially for defensive functions such as tissue protection, immune regulation, and wound healing. Apart from inhibitors of eicosanoid synthesis (NSAIDs), eicosanoid analogs and derivatives are widely used for various diseases, including skin diseases. Moreover, special drug delivery systems (dermal and transdermal delivery) for eicosanoid-related compounds should be devised to deliver these compounds to targetted organs such as the skin.[16,98]

PGE$_1$ and PGI$_2$ have potent vasodilatory and antithrombotic actions, and both oral and injective forms of these prostaglandins have been widely used for circulatory disturbances of the lower limbs in various collagen diseases, Buerger disease, etc. These prostaglandins are also widely used in skin ulcers due to diabetes mellitus, bed sores, collagen diseases, and obstructive arterial diseases. Since PGE$_1$ and its analogs are rapidly inactivated in the lung, the arterial administration route has been previously used. However, the newly developed lipo-PGE$_1$ is not inactivated in the lung, and intraveous lipo-PGE$_1$ has now been established and used. The oral administration of PGE$_1$ has been used for skin ulcer and collagen diseases. Topical PGE$_1$ ointment has also been developed for skin ulcers, and its efficacy has been thoroughly evaluated because the topical application is free from systemic side effects.[99]

Besides the improvement in blood flow, prostaglandins can modulate immune function. From this point of view, novel strategies for the use of prostaglandins in the treatment of various allergic diseases are under investagation. PGI$_2$ is more potent but more unstable than PGE$_1$, and new and more stable PGI$_2$ analogs are being developed and used for various types of ulcers.

Cyclopentenone prostaglandins such as Δ^{12}-PGJ$_2$ and PGA$_2$ act as potent inducers of cell growth inhibition and cell differentiation. The mechanisms of action of the cyclopentenone prostaglandins are notably different from other anticancerous drugs such as 5-fluorouracil or bleomycin, thus suggesting that cyclopentenone prostaglandins may be promising antineoplastic agents. Prior to their clinical application in skin cancer treatment, further investigation of the mechanisms of action of cytotoxic prostaglandins on epidermal cells is necessary. In vivo experiments on human skin cancers are currently in progress in our laboratory. These anticancerous prostaglandins are also effective against viral diseases such as herpes simplex[83] or AIDS.[84]

V. CONCLUSION

In this review, recent progress on the pathophysiological significance of eicosanoids in the skin was described. Eicosanoids are closely related to the pathogenesis of a number of skin diseases, but the demonstration of their precise relationship is not feasible at present. Eicosanoids probably function as one of the predisposing factors such as cytokines or growth factors, or may act as synergistic factors with these compounds. Many eicosanoid-related compounds, including the eicosanoids themselves, their analogs, and inhibitors of eicosanoid synthesis, are frequently used for the treatment of various skin diseases, and it is expected that new drugs related to the eicosanoids will be developed.

REFERENCES

1. Samuelsson, B., Leukotrienes: mediators of immediate hypersensitivity reactions and inflammation, *Science*, 220, 568, 1983.
2. Needleman, P., Turk, J., Jakschick, B. A., Morrison, A. R., and Lefkowith, J. B., Arachidonic acid metabolism, *Annu. Rev. Biochem.*, 55, 69, 1986.
3. Smith, W. L., Prostanoid biosynthesis and mechanisms of action, *Am. J. Physiol.*, 263, F181, 1992.
4. Ruzicka, T., The physiology and pathophysiology of eicosanoids in the skin, *Eicosanoids*, 1, 59, 1988.
5. Ruzicka, T., *Eicosanoids and the Skin*, CRC Press, Boca Raton, FL, 1990, 24.
6. Miller, C. C., Hale, P., and Pentland, A. P., Ultraviolet B injury increases prostaglandin synthesis through a tyrosine kinase-dependent pathway, *J. Biol. Chem.*, 269, 3529, 1994.
7. Ikai, K. and Imamura, S., Role of eocosanpoids in the pathogenesis of atopic dermatitis, *Pros. Leuko. Ess. Fatty Acid*, 48, 409, 1993.
8. Sabroe, R. A. and Greaves, M. W., The pathogenesis of chronic idiopathic urticaria, *Arch. Dermatol.*, 133, 1003, 1997.
9. Ikai, K., Role of eicosanoids in the pathogenesis of psoriasis, *J. Dermatol. Sci.*, in press.
10. Goldyne, M. E., Prostaglandins and cutaneous inflammation, *J. Invest. Dermatol.*, 64, 377, 1975.
11. Robert, A., Current history of cytoprotection, *Prostaglandins*, 21, 89, 1980.
12. Goodwin, J. S. and Ceuppens, J., Regulation of the immune response by prostaglandins, *J. Clin. Immunol.*, 3, 295, 1983.
13. Lupulescu, A., Prostaglandins, their inhibitors and cancer, *Pros. Leuko. Ess. Fatty Acid*, 54, 83, 1996.
14. Evans, C. B., Pillai, S., and Goldyne, M. E., Endogenous prostaglndin E_2 modulates calcium-induced differentiation in human skin keratinocytes, *Pros. Leuko. Ess. Fatty Acid*, 49, 777, 1993.
15. Zhou, L. J., Inoue, M., Gunji, H., Ono, I., and Kaneko, F., Effects of prostaglandin E_1 on cultured dermal fibroblasts from normal and hypertrophic scarred skin, *J. Dermatol. Sci.*, 14, 217, 1997.
16. Ledger, P. W., Gale, R., and Yum, S. I., *Pharmacology of the Skin*, CRC Press, Boca Raton, FL, 1992, 73.
17. Prescott, S. M., A thematic series on phospholipases, *J. Biol. Chem.*, 272, 15043, 1997.
18. Leslie, C. C., Properties and regulation of cytosolic phospholipase A_2, *J. Biol. Chem.*, 272, 16709, 1997.
19. Ilchysyn, A., Ilderton, E., Kingsbury, J. A., and Yardley, H. J., Evidence that raised levels of phospholipase A_2 in uninvolved epidermis of psoriasis are caused by hyperphosphorylation of an inhibitor. *Br. J. Dermatol.*, 111, 721, 1984.
20. Grass, D. S., Felkner, R. H., Chiang M. Y., Wallace, R. E., Nevalainen, T. J., Bennett, C. F., and Swanson, M. E., Expression of human group II PLA_2 in transgenic mice results in epidermal hyperplasia in the absence of inflammatory infiltrate, *J. Clin. Invest.*, 97, 2233, 1996.
21. Uozumi, N., Kume, K., Nagase, T., Nakatani, N., Ishii, S., Tashiro, F., Komagata, Y., Maki, K., Ikuta, K., Ouchi, Y., Miyazaki, J. I. and Shimizu, T., Role of cytosolic phospholipase A_2 in allergic response and parturition, *Nature*, 390, 618, 1997.
22. Raynal, P. and Pollard, H. B., Annexins: the problem of assessing the biological role for a gene family of multifunctional calcium- and phospholipid-binding proteins, *Biochim. Biophys. Acta*, 1197, 63, 1994.
23. Kitajima, Y., Owada, M. K., Mitsui, H., and Yaoita, H., Lipocortin I (annexin I) is preferentially localized on the plasma membrane in keratinocytes of psoriatic lesional epidermis as shown by immunofluorescence microscopy, *J. Invest. Dermatol.*, 97, 1032, 1991.
24. Ikai, K., Shimizu, K., Ando, Y., Furukawa, F., Imamura, S., and Kannagi, R., Immunohistochemical localization of lipocortins in normal and psoriatic human skin, *Arch. Dermatol. Res.*, 285, 296, 1993.
25. DeWitt, D. L., Prostaglandin endoperoxide synthase: regulation of enzyme expression, *Biochim. Biophys. Acta*, 1083, 121, 1991.

26. Ikai, K., Ishii, A., Tanaka, T., and Nomura, A., Expression of cyclooxygenases in human skin, *J. Invest. Dermatol.,* 110, 536, 1998.

27. Scholz, K., Fürstenberger, G., Müller-Decker, K., and Marks, F., Differential expression of prostaglandin-H synthase isozymes in normal and activated keratinocytes in vivo and in vitro, *Biochem. J.,* 309, 263, 1996.

28. Leong J., Hughes-Fulford, M., Rakhlin, N., Habib, A., Maclouf, J., and Goldyne, M. E., Cyclooxygenases in human and mouse skin and cultured human keratinocytes: association of COX-2 expression with human keratinocyte differentiation, *Exp. Cell Res.,* 224, 79, 1996.

29. Urade, Y., Watanabe, K., and Hayaishi, O., Prostaglandin D, E, and F synthetases, *J. Lipid Mediat. Cell Signal.,* 12, 257-273, 1995.

30. Ruzicka, T. and Auböck, J., Arachidonic acid metabolism in guinea pig Langerhans cells: studies on cyclooxygenase and lipoxygenase pathways, *J. Immunol.,* 138, 539, 1987.

31. Ujihara, M., Horiguchi, Y., Ikai, K., and Urade, Y., Characterization and distribution of prostaglandin D synthetase in rat skin, *J. Invest. Dermatol.,* 90, 448, 1988.

32. Ikai, K., Ujihara, M., Kanauchi, H., and Urade, Y., Effect of ultraviolet irradiation on the activity of rat skin prostaglandin D synthetase, *J. Invest. Dermatol.,* 93, 345, 1989.

33. Camp, R. and Greaves, M. W., The catabolism of prostaglandins by rat skin, *Biochem. J.,* 186, 153, 1980.

34. Fukushima, M., Sasaki, H., and Fukushima, S., Prostaglandin J_2 and related compounds, *Ann. New York Acad. Sci.,* 744, 161, 1994.

35. Negishi, M., Koizumi, T., and Ichikawa, A., Biological actions of Δ^{12}-PGJ_2, *J. Lipid Mediat. Cell Signal.,* 12, 443, 1995.

36. Suzuki, M., Mori, M., Niwa, T., Hirata, R., Furuta, K., Ishikawa, T., and Noyori, R., Chemical implications for antitumor and antiviral prostaglandins: reaction of Δ^7-prostaglandin A_1 and prostaglandin A_1 methyl esters with thiols, *J. Am. Chem. Soc.,* 119, 2376, 1997.

37. Negishi, M., Sugimoto, Y., and Ichikawa, A., Molecular mechanisms of diverse actions of prostanoid receptors, *Biochim. Biophys. Acta,* 1259, 109, 1995.

38. Murata, T., Ushikubi, F., Matsuoka, T., Hirata, M., Yamasaki, A., Sugimoto, Y., Ichikawa, A., Aze, Y., Tanaka, T., Yoshida, N., Ueno, A., Ohishi, S., and Narumiya, S., Altered pain perception and inflammatory response in mice lacking prostacyclin receptor, *Nature,* 388, 678, 1997.

39. Sugimoto, Y., Yamasaki, A., Segi, E., Tsuboi, K., Aze, Y., Nishimura, T., Oida, H., Yoshida, N., Tanaka, T., Katsuyama, M., Hasumoto, K., Murata, T., Hirata, M., Ushikubi, F., Negishi, M., Ichikawa, A., and Narumiya, S., Failure of parturition in mice lacking the prostaglandin F receptor, *Science,* 277, 681, 1997.

40. Ford-Hutchinson, A. W., Gresser, M., and Young, R. N., 5-Lipoxygenase, *Annu. Rev. Biochem.,* 63, 383, 1994.

41. Woods, J. W., Evans, J. F., Ethier, D., Scott, S., Vickers, P. J., Hearn, L., Heibein, J. A., Charleson, S., and Singer, I. I., 5-Lipoxygenase and 5-lipoxygenase-activating protein are localized in the nuclear envelope of activated human leukocytes, *J. Exp. Med.,* 178, 1935, 1993.

42. Janssen-Timmen, U., Vickers, P. J., Wittig, U., Lehmann, W. D., Stark, H. J., Fusenig, N. E., Rosenbach, T., Rådmark, O., Samuelsson, B., and Habenicht, A. J. R., Expression of 5-lipoxygenase in differentiating human skin keratinocytes, *Proc. Natl. Acad. Sci. U.S.A.,* 92, 6966, 1995.

43. Breton, J., Woolf, D., Young, P., and Chabot-Fletcher, M., Human keratinocytes lack the components to produce leukotriene B_4, *J. Invest. Dermatol.,* 106, 162, 1996.

44. Ohishi, N., Minami, M., Kobayashi, J., Seyama, Y., Hata, J., Yotsumoto, H., Takaku, F., and Shimizu, T., Immunological quantification and immunohistochemical localization of leukotriene A_4 hydrolase in guinea pig tissues, *J. Biol. Chem.,* 265, 7520, 1990.

45. Minami, M., Mutoh, H., Ohishi, N., Honda, Z., Bito, H., and Shimizu, T., Amino-acid sequence and tissue distribution of guinea-pig leukotriene A_4 hydrolase, *Gene,* 161, 249, 1995.

46. Ikai, K., Okano, H., Horiguchi, Y., and Sakamoto, Y., Leukotriene A_4 hydrolase in human skin, *J. Invest. Dermatol.,* 102, 253, 1994.

47. Okano-Mitani, H., Ikai, K., and Imamura, S., Leukotriene A_4 hydrolase in peripheral leukocytes of patients with atopic dermatitis, *Arch. Dermatol. Res.,* 288, 168, 1996.

48. Welsh, D. J., Creely, D. P., Hauser, S. D., Mathis, K. L., Krivi, G. G., and Isakson, P. C., Molelular cloning and expression of human leukotriene-C_4 synthase. *Proc. Natl. Acad. Sci. U.S.A.*, 91, 9745, 1994.

49. Penrose, J. F., Spector, J., Baldasaro, M., Xu, K. Boyce, J., Arm, J. P., Austen, K. F., and Lam, B. K., Molecular cloning of the gene for human leukotriene C_4 synthase. Organization, nucleotide sequence, and chromosomal localization to 5q35, *J. Biol. Chem.*, 271, 11356, 1996.

50. Ikai, K., Mitani, H., and Tanaka, T., Generation and degradation of leukotrienes in human keratinocytes, *J. Invest. Dermatol.*, 105, 471, 1995.

51. Fauler, J., Neumann, C., Tsikas, D., and Frölich, J., Enhanced synthesis of cysteinyl leukotrienes in psoriasis, *J. Invest. Dermatol.*, 99, 8, 1992.

52. Sampson, A. P., Thomas, R. U., and Costello, J. F., Enhanced leukotriene synthesis in leukocytes of atopic and asthmatic subjects, *Br. J. Clin. Pharmacol.*, 33, 423, 1992.

53. Fauler, J., Neumann, C., Tsikas, D., and Frölich, J. C., Enhanced synthesis of cysteinyl leukotrienes in atopic dermatitis, *Br. J. Dermatol.*, 128, 627, 1993.

54. Okano-Mitani, H., Ikai, K., and Imamura, S., Human melanoma cells generate leukotriene B_4 and C_4 from leukotriene A_4, *Arch. Dermatol. Res.*, 289, 331, 1997.

55. Yokomizo, T., Ogawa, Y., Uozumi, N., Kume, K., Izumi, T., and Shimizu, T., cDNA cloning, expression, and mutagenesis study of leukotriene B_4 12-hydroxydehydrogenase, *J. Biol. Chem.*, 271, 2844, 1996.

56. Hammarström, S., Hamberg, M., Samuelsson, B., Duell, E. A., Stawiski, M., and Voorhees, J. J., Increased concentrations of nonesterified arachidonic acid, 12L-hydroxy-5,8,10,14-eicosatetraenoic acid, prostaglandin E_2, and prostaglandin $F_{2\alpha}$ in epidermis of psoriasis, *Proc. Natl. Acad. Sci. U.S.A.*, 72, 5130, 1975.

57. Kragballe, K., Desjarlais, L., Duell, E. A., and Voorhees, J.J., In vitro synthesis of 12-hydroxy-eicosatetraenoic acid is increased in uninvolved psoriatic epidermis, *J. Invest. Dermatol.*, 87, 47, 1986.

58. Yamamoto, S., Suzuki, H., and Ueda, N., Arachidonate 12-lipoxygenases, *Prog. Lipid Res.*, 36, 23, 1997.

59. Takahashi, Y., Reddy, G. R., Ueda, N., Yamamoto, S., and Arase, S., Arachidonate 12-lipoxygenase of platelet-type in human epidermal cells, *J. Biol. Chem.*, 268, 16443, 1993.

60. Woollard, P. M., Stereochemical difference between 12-hydroxy- 5,8,10,14-eicosatetraenoic acid in platelets and psoriatic lesions, *Biochem. Biophys. Res. Commun.*, 136, 169, 1986.

61. Cunningham, F. M. and Woollard, P. M., 12(R)-hydroxy-5,8,10,14-eicosatetraenoic acid is a chemoattractant for human polymorphonuclear leucocytes in vitro, *Prostaglandins*, 34, 71, 1987.

62. Fretland, D. J., Widomski, D. L., Zemaitis, J.M., Tsai, B.S., Djuric, S.W., Penning, T. D., Miyashiro, J. M., and Bauer, R.F., 12(R)-hydroxy-eicosatetraenoic acid is a neutrophil chemoattractant in the cavine, lapine, murine and canine dermis, *Pros. Leuko. Ess. Fatty Acid*, 37, 79, 1989.

63. Hussain, H., Shornick, L. P., Shannon, V. R., Wilson, J. D., Funk, C. D., Pentland, A. P., and Holtzman, M. J., Epidermis contains platelet-type 12-lipoxygenase that is overexpressed in germinal keratinocytes in psoriasis, *Am. J. Physiol.*, 266, C243, 1994.

64. Baer, A.N., Costello, P.B., and Green, F.A., Stereospecificity of the products of the fatty acid oxygenases derived from psoriatic scales, *J. Lipid Res.*, 32, 341, 1991.

65. Fitzpatrick, F. A. and Murphy, R. C., Cytochrome P-450 metabolism of arachidonic acid: formation and biological actions of "epoxygenase"-derived eicosanoids, *Pharmacol. Rev.*, 40, 229, 1989.

66. Holtzman, M. J., Turk, J., and Pentland, A., A regiospecific monooxygenase with novel stereopreference is the major pathway for arachidonic acid oxygenation in isolated epidermal cells, *J. Clin. Invest.*, 84, 1446, 1989.

67. Keeney, D. S., Skinner, C., Wei, S., Friedberg, T., and Waterman, M. R., A keratinocyte-specific epoxygenase, CYP2B12, metabolizes arachidonic acid with unusual selectivity, producing a single major epoxyeicosatrienoic acid, *J. Biol. Chem.*, 273, 9279, 1998.

68. Ford-Hutchinson, A. W., Arachidonate 15-lipoxygenase; characteristics and potential biological significance, *Eicosanoids*, 4, 65, 1991.

69. Brash, A. R., Boeglin, W. E., and Chang, M. S., Discovery of a second 15S-lipoxygenase in humans, *Proc. Natl. Acad. Sci. U.S.A.*, 94, 6148, 1997.

70. Heitmann, J., Iversen, L., Kragballe, K., and Ziboh, V. A., Incorporation of 15-hydroxyeicosatrienoic acid in specific phospholipids of cultured human keratinocytes and psoriatic plaques, *Exp. Dermatol.*, 4, 74, 1995.

71. Green, F. A., Transformations of 5-HETE by activated keratinocyte 15-lipoxygenase and the activation mechanism, *Lipids*, 25, 618, 1990.

72. Samuelsson, B., Dahlén, D. A., Lindgren, C. A., Rouzer, C. A., and Serhan, C. N., Leukotrienes and lipoxins: structures, biosynthesis, and biological effects, *Science*, 237, 1171, 1987.

73. Soter, N. A., Lewis, R. A., Corey, E. J., and Austen, K. F., Local effects of synthetic leukotrienes (LTC$_4$, LTD$_4$, LTE$_4$, and LTB$_4$) in human skin, *J. Invest. Dermatol.*, 80, 115, 1983.

74. Voorhees, J. J., Leukotrienes and other lipoxygenase products in the pathogenesis and therapy of psoriasis and other dermatoses, *Arch. Dermatol.*, 119, 541, 1983.

75. James, J. and Warin, R. P., Chronic urticaria: the effect of aspirin, *Br. J. Dermatol.*, 82, 204, 1970.

76. Langenbach, R., Morham, S. G., Tiano, H. F., Loftin, C. D., Ghanayem, B. I., Chulada, P. C., Mahler J. F., Lee, C. A., Goulding E, H., Kluckman, K. D., Kim, H. S., and Smithies, O., Prostaglandin synthase 1 gene dusruption in ice reduced arachidonic acid-induced inflammation and indomethacin-induced gastric ulceration, *Cell*, 83, 483, 1995.

77. Ito, S., Narumiya, S., and Hayaishi, O., Prostaglandin D$_2$: a biochemical perspective, *Pros. Leuko. Ess. Fatty Acid*, 37, 219, 1989.

78. Ikai, K. and Imamura, S., Prostaglandin D$_2$ in the skin, *Int. J. Dermatol.*, 27, 141, 1988.

79. Forman, B. M., Tontonoz, P., Chen, J., Brun, R. P., Spiegelman, B. M., and Evans, R. M., 15-Deoxy-Δ12, 14-prostaglandin J$_2$ is a ligand for the adipocyte determination factor PPARγ, *Cell*, 83, 803, 1995.

80. Kliewer, S. A., Lenhard, J. M., Willson, T. M., Patel, I., Morris, D. C., and Lehmann, J. M., A prostaglandin J$_2$ metabolite binds peroxisome proliferator-activated receptor gamma and promotes adipocyte differentiation, *Cell,* 83, 813, 1995.

81. Hirata, Y., Hayashi, H., Ito, S., Kikawa, Y., Ishibashi, M., Sudo, M., Miyazaki, H., Fukushima, M., Narumiya, S., and Hayaishi, O., Occurrence of 9-deoxy-Δ^9, Δ^{12} -13, 14-dihydroprostaglandin D$_2$ in human urine, *J. Biol. Chem.*, 263, 16619, 1988.

82. Ikai, K., Shimizu, K., Furukawa, F., and Fukushima, M., Induction of 72-kD heat shock protein and cytoskeleton damage by cytotoxic prostaglandin, Δ^{12}-PGJ$_2$ in transformed human epidermal cells in culture, *J. Invest. Dermatol.*, 98, 890, 1992.

83. Yamamoto, N., Rahman, M. M., Fukushima, M., Maeno, K., and Nishiyama, Y., Involvement of prostaglandin-induced proteins in the inhibition of herpes simplex virus replication, *Biochem. Biophys. Res. Commun.*, 158, 189, 1989.

84. Rozera C., Carattoli, A., De Marco, A., Amici, C., Giorgi, C., and Santoro, M. G., Inhibition of HIV-1 replication by cyclopentenone prostaglandins in acutely infected human cells, *J. Clin. Invest.*, 97, 1795, 1996.

85. Henderson, W. R., The role of leukotrienes in inflammation, *Ann. Intern. Med.*, 121, 684, 1994.

86. Yokomizo, T., Izumi T., Chang K., Takuwa, Y., and Shimizu, T., A G-protein-coupled receptor for leukotriene B$_4$ that mediates chemotaxis, *Nature,* 387, 620, 1997.

87. Camp, R. D. R., Russel, J. R., Brain, D., and Woollard, P. M., Production of intraepidermal micro-abscesses by topical application of leukotriene B, *J. Invest. Dermatol.*, 82, 202, 1984.

88. Camp, R. D. R., Coutts, A. A., Greaves, M. W., and Walport, M. J., Responses of human skin to intradermal injection of leukotrienes C$_4$, D$_4$, and B$_4$, *Br. J. Pharmacol.* 80, 497, 1983.

89. Archer, C. B., Page, C. P., Juhlin, L., Morley, J., and MacDonald, D. M., Delayed-onset synergism between leukotriene B$_4$ and prostaglandin E$_2$ in human skin, *Prostaglandins*, 33, 799, 1987.

90. Bauer, F. W., van de Kerkhof, P. C. M., and Maassen-de Grood, R. M., Epidermal hyperproliferation following the induction of microabscesses by leukotriene B$_4$, *Br. J. Dermatol.*, 114, 409, 1986.

91. Reusch, M. K. and Wastek, G. J., Human keratinocytes in vitro have receptors for leukotriene B, *Acta Dermatol. Venereol. (Stockh.)*, 69, 429, 1989.

92. Medrano, E. E., Farooqui, J. Z., Boissy, R. E., Boissy, Y. L., Akadiri, B., and Nordlund, J. J., Chronic growth stimulation of human adult melanocytes by inflammatory mediators in vitro: implication for nevus formation and initial steps in melanocyte oncogenesis, *Proc. Natl. Acad. Sci. U.S.A.*, 90, 1790, 1993.

93. Katayama, H., The treatment of tinea with topically applied leukotriene B$_4$, *Prostaglandins*, 34, 797, 1987.

94. Talbot, S. F., Atkins, P. C., Goetzl, E. J., and Zweiman, B., Accumulation of leukotriene C_4 and histamine in human allergic skin reactions, *J. Clin. Invest.*, 76, 650, 1985.

95. Goulet, J. L., Snouwaert, J. N., Latour, A. M., Coffman, T. M., and Koller, B. H., Altered inflammatory responses in leukotriene-deficient mice, *Proc. Natl. Acad. Sci. U.S.A.*, 91, 12852, 1994.

96. Arenberger, P., Kemény, L., and Ruzicka, T., Defect of epidermal 12*(S)*-hydroxyeicosatetraenoic acid receptors in psoriasis, *Eur. J. Clin. Invest.*, 22, 235, 1992.

97. Antón, R., Puig, L., Esgleyes, T., de-Moragas, J. M., and Vila, L., Occurrence of hepoxilins and trioxilins in psoriatic lesions, *J. Invest. Dermatol.*, 110, 303, 1998.

98. Mizushima, Y., Lipo-prostaglandin preparations, *Pros. Leuko. Ess. Fatty Acid*, 42, 1, 1991.

99. Gunji, H., Ono, I., Tateshita, T., and Kaneko, F., Clinical effectiveness of an ointment containing prostaglandin E1 for the treatment of burn wounds, *Burn*, 22, 399, 1996.

Section III

Biochemical Modulators and Modes of Action

14 Modulation of Skin Reactions: A General Overview

Agis F. Kydonieus and John J. Wille

CONTENTS

I. INTRODUCTION

Development of an irritant or allergic skin reaction to drugs often occurs in patients receiving systemic drug therapy via a transdermal drug patch and is, therefore, a major obstacle to the further development of novel transdermal drug delivery systems. For example, delayed hypersensitivity reactions (contact allergic dermatitis) have been reported to occur to both topically applied dermal antihistaminic drugs (e.g., diphenhydramine), and transdermally delivered drugs (clonidine). The list of known sensitizing drugs and drug classes extends to most beta-blockers (nadolol), antiasthmatics (albuterol), and antihistamines (chlorpheniramine).

The skin functions as an immune organ. It has its own immune surveillance system with locally acting lymphoid cell and humoral components which protect the body from potentially harmful agents that penetrate the skin. This immune system includes the Langerhans cells, which are professional antigen-processing and antigen-presenting cells of the skin. The Langerhans cells pick up foreign antigens, process and place them on their cell surface, and convey them to appropriate MHC class II T cells in local lymph nodes. These early immune events are part of the induction phase of the sensitization response. They hinge on the formation of proper cell–cell interactions, including the coordinated synthesis and release of cytokines among the network of cytokine producing and responding cell types, including epidermal keratinocytes, Langerhans cells, and specific T lymphocyte subsets. Although the detailed mechanisms are not totally understood, the science is presented in Chapters 7 through 13 and will not be considered further in this chapter.

Due to the extent of the scientific literature, we decided in this overview to concentrate on the patent literature and, more specifically, on the patent literature pertaining to the application of topical and transdermal drugs, as well as cosmetics, to the skin. We also felt that this approach would minimize duplication with the work presented in the following nine chapters. We also hope that this overview will allow one to see the pragmatic aspects of this subject: how did the practitioner in the field of topical drug delivery and cosmetics address this important issue in the past, and now that some of the secrets of the science of contact dermatitis are being elucidated.

II. STRATEGIES FOR THE ABROGATION OF CONTACT DERMATITIS

A. Trial and Error Approaches

Since abrogation of irritation and sensitization was not well understood, the initial approach was to try different polymeric formulations, excipients, enhancers, and drugs and determine by actual in vivo testing which formulations were not irritating or sensitizing. For example, European Patent Application 066,411,9A2 describes 21 formulations containing different polymers such as acrylic, polyisobutylene, styrene–isoprene–styrene copolymer, and hygroscopic materials such as pectin, dextrin, gelatin, and sodium carboxymethylcellulose.[1] The irritation caused by these formulations while delivering propranolol, indomethacin, or ketoprofen was determined using human volunteers. The hygroscopic materials were shown to improve irritation, presumably due to the absorption of the transepidermal water loss. The simple testing performed was not adequate to show, for example, that propranolol is a contact sensitizer.[48]

Canadian Patent Application 2,058,059 exhibited the testing of several formulations of albuterol and the effect of several enhancers, such as ethanol and Azone®, on permeation through mouse skin.[2] The formulations were tested for irritation and sensitization. Irritation was tested on rabbits and it was shown that albuterol causes slight erythema and slight edema. The guinea pig skin sensitization studies showed that albuterol was not a sensitizer. Albuterol is now known to be a sensitizer.[3,4] Guinea pig testing was developed for testing strong sensitizers and it is not able to discern the sensitization potential of most drugs which are weak sensitizers. This inability allowed a clonidine patch to be introduced in the marketplace, although it sensitizes more than 20% of the users. More sensitive methods have since been developed as described in Chapters 4 and 5.

World Patent Publication 9,402,176 pertains to specific polymers and other excipients which enhance skin penetration of drugs, especially salicylic acid, with significantly reduced irritation, especially in compositions requiring a low pH.[5] It is claimed that a formulation containing a high molecular weight cationic polymer, a nonionic surfactant, and an alkoxylated ether increases permeation with a reduction in skin irritation.

U.S. Patent 5,308,625 discloses formulations and enhancers to increase skin permeation of molsidomine without irritation.[6] From the many enhancers tested, monoalkyl phosphates were shown to increase permeation of molsidomine with very mild irritation.

Many pharmaceutical agents are weak organic acids or bases able to ionize in the physiologic pH range and, due to their hydrophilic nature, they are not able to penetrate through the lipophilic heterogeneous stratum corneum and, due to their low or high pH, they can cause irritation. U.S. Patent 5,374,645 addresses this issue by the use of a pH-controlled aqueous isopropanol counterion composition.[7] The counterion increases the lipophilicity of the drug to increase permeation through the skin and controls the pH to improve the skin irritation profile.

Antihistamines are known to be irritants and sensitizers. Sequeira tested 18 antihistamines for irritation and sensitization to determine if any of them had an acceptable profile for transdermal delivery.[8] His studies indicated that only Azatadine had adequate permeation and an acceptable skin irritation profile.

B. Prodrug Development

Another approach used to minimize irritation and sensitization in topical delivery is to form salts of the basic drug or form some other prodrug. The concept is to prevent the reaction of the drug (hapten) with epidermal proteins to give a complete antigen. Protein groups capable of forming strong covalent bonds with a hapten (electrophilic drugs) produce the antigen, a modified protein.[9]

U.S. Patent 5,075,340 describes the use of retinoic acid glucuronide to eliminate retinoid dermatitis, an objectionable side effect of topical application of retinoid compounds.[10] Retinoids are used to treat acne and aging skin and to reverse the structural damage of skin caused by photoaging. In many trials (up to 7 months) described in the patent, mainly to treat acne, it was shown that 0.1% retinoic acid and retinoic acid glucuronide had the same effectiveness. However, 100% of the retinoic acid patients showed skin irritation, but none of the patients treated with retinoic acid glucuronide.

A method for delivering irritating amines to the skin in a minimally or nonirritating composition is described, without reducing the transdermal flux rate.[11,12] The method involves providing the amine as a nonirritating salt of a stochiometric molar excess of a fatty acid of from 8 to 22 carbon atoms, in a nonpolar, nonvolatile solvent. It is important that, for each amine, the following four factors be simultaneously considered: (1) a complexing agent for the physiologically active amine, (2) a solvent for the complexed amine, (3) the amount of solvent used for the complexed amine, and (4) the amount of the complexing agent used in relation to the amine. Irritating amines disclosed include chlorpheniramine, dexbrompheniramine, clonidine, nicotine, diphenhydramine, and scopolamine. Complexing agents include undecylenic acid and isostearic acid. Appropriate solvents include isopropyl myristate and isopropyl oleate.

European Patent Application 0,245,126A describes methods for reducing the irritation caused by acidic drugs, such as anti-inflammatory or analgesic drugs having carboxylic acid groups.[13] The invention involves the preparation of calcium salts of said anti-inflammatory or analgesic drugs. The calcium salts in a medium of propylene glycol or polyethylene glycol or dimethylsulfoxide provide therapeutically effective concentrations with less irritating action to skin. Indomethacin, mefenamate, ketoprofen, flufenamate, diclofenac, alclofenac, and bendazac are disclosed as active agents for appropriate use with the invention.

C. Plant Extracts

Natural products, specifically plant extracts, have been used in cosmetic formulations, as well as in other topical applications, to avoid irritation, including the sensation of stinging, itching, and burning, as well as the clinical signs of redness and peeling. U.S. Patent 5,393,526 describes rosmarrinic acid as an anti-irritant for alpha hydroxy carboxylate compounds such as lactic acid, glycolic acid, and hydroxycaprilic acid.[14] The overall stinging response to a 10% lactic acid formulation was reduced by more than threefold by the addition of 5% rosmarrinic acid (as a sage extract).

Hydroalcoholic extracts of *Cola nitida* have also been used to prevent or treat both irritation and sensitization. In European Patent Application 0,354,554A2, it is recommended that the *Cola nitida* extract be applied half an hour before or half an hour after the application of topical cosmetic and pharmaceutical formulations or physical irritants (e.g., skin waxing).[15] A 10% *Cola nitida* extract formulation gave excellent results against two known irritants, para-aminobenzoic acid and balsam of Peru.

The oil extracted from the yerba plant (*Eriodictyon californicum*) has also been claimed to minimize or completely eliminate the irritation and sensitization that accompanies topical, transdermal, or transmucosal drug delivery. World Patent Application WO 9,114,441 uses formulations containing eriodictyon fluid extract (fluid extracted from dried yerba santa leaves) to minimize irritation and sensitization of topically applied substances such as dihydroergotamine mesylate, acetaminophen, oxymetazoline, diphenhydramine, nystatin, clindamycin, and para aminobenzoic acid.[16]

U.S. Patent 4,908,213 pertains to antipruritics to be codelivered with nicotine.[17] Nicotine patches are used to minimize withdrawal symptoms during smoking cessation, but are known to cause minor irritation and itching. Among other antipruritics, oil of chamomile, chamazulene, and bis-abolol are claimed in the above-mentioned patent. Oil of chamomile is extracted from the dried flower heads of *Anthemis nobilis*. Chamazulene (7-ethyl-1,4-dimethylylazulene) is an anti-inflammatory compound found in chamomile, wormwood, and yarrow.

Many studies in the scientific literature have also investigated the anti-irritant and countersensitizer effects of plant extracts. Pretreatment of the skin with a *Ginkgo biloba* extract mitigated contact dermatitis to the allergens nickel sulfate, balsam of Peru, and methyl-isothiazolinone.[18]

D. Glucocorticoids

Steroids are well known for their anti-inflammatory and immunosuppressive properties, and formulations containing 0.5 and 1.0% hydrocortisone are standard remedies for treating skin irritation and inflammatory responses caused by allergens such as poison oak.[19] However, their ability to prevent irritation and the induction of sensitization had not been studied until recently. A series of patents by Alza studied the effect of steroids on the induction phase of sensitization for both intact epidermal skin, and mucosal membranes.[20,21] Coadministration, as well as pretreatment with hydrocortisone, was studied with positive results. Steroids, as well as steroid esters, were found to be suitable and they include hydrocortisone, hydrocortisone ester, betamethasone, betamethasone valerate, fluocinonide, and triamcinolone. In a human test on 80 volunteers (40 subjects each), dex-chlorpheniramine maleate administered transdermally sensitized 16 subjects. When it was codelivered with 2% hydrocortisone, only two subjects were sensitized. In a separate experiment, it was shown that hydrocortisone did not affect the elicitation phase of sensitization — i.e., once sensitized, the presence of hydrocortisone did not prevent a skin reaction in allergic individuals. Two other Alza patents pertain to induction of skin immune tolerance to a sensitizing drug when the drug is delivered both transdermally or through the mucosal membrane.[22,23] Skin immune tolerance is the state of prolonged unresponsiveness to a specific antigen when the antigen is repeatedly applied to the skin. Tolerance to skin sensitization has been induced with repeated doses of UV irradiation and by application to the skin of agents that suppress the immune system, prior to the application of the sensitizer.[24,25] Alza's patents disclose the induction of tolerance in humans to sensitizing drugs such as dex-chlorpheniramine maleate (DCPM) through its coextensive coadministration with hydrocortisone. None of the subjects treated with hydrocortisone experienced sensitization reactions to DCPM, vs. 15% for the control group. Drugs that could be delivered transdermally, due to the development of immune tolerance, included naloxone, clonidine, nicotine, tetracaine, and scopolamine.

U.S. Patent 5,028,431 used a medium potency steroid to minimize the irritation and sensitization caused by several transdermally administered drugs, such as guanfacine, clonidine, fluphenazine, trifluoperazine, and timolol.[26] Fluocinonide, a medium potency steroid, was coadministered from polyvinyl chloride patches. From patches containing 10% clonidine, the codelivery of fluocinonide reduced significantly erythema and blistering caused by clonidine to an individual previously sensitized to clonidine (Table 1). In a separate experiment with patches containing 35% fluphenazine, the codelivery of 1% fluocinonide almost completely blocked the erythema and blistering caused by fluphenazine to an individual previously sensitized to fluphenazine (Table 2). It is of interest to note that the results from patches codelivering 5% fluocinonide were not as good as

TABLE 1
Reduction in Allergic Contact Dermatitis Response to Clonidine by the Codelivery of Fluocinonide from a 7-Day Patch

Patch Concentration (%)		Inflammatory Response	
Clonidine	Fluocinonide	7 Days	8 Days
10	0	4+	4+
10	2	1+	1+
0	0	0	0

Adapted from Reference 26.

TABLE 2
Reduction in Allergic Contact Dermatitis Response to Fluphenazine by the Codelivery of Fluocinonide from a 48-H Patch

Patch Concentration (%)		Inflammatory Response (hours)		
Fluphenazine	Fluocinonide	48	72	96
35	0	4+	4+	4+
35	1	+/-	0	0
35	5	1+	+/-	+/-

Adapted from Reference 26.

TABLE 3
Reduction in Irritant Contact Dermatitis Response to RO 22-1327 by the Codelivery of Fluocinonide from an 8-H Patch

Fluocinonide Concentration (%)	Inflammatory Response	
	8 hours	24 hours
0	3+	2+
0.1	3+	1+
1.0	+/-	0
5.0	1+	+/1

Adapted from Reference 26.

those codelivering 1%. This may not be too surprising, considering that steroids not only suppress, but also direct and enhance immune functions.[27] Irritant contact dermatitis was also reduced by the use of fluocinonide. Four polyvinyl chloride patches containing the irritant antihypertensive (5Z, 13E, 15R, 16R)-16-fluoro-15-hydroxy-9-osoprosta-5-dienoic acid (RO 22-1327) and different concentrations of fluocinonide were tested on a human subject not previously exposed to this drug. The incorporation of 1% fluocinonide in the patch resulted in significant reduction of irritant contact dermatitis (Table 3). The grading system for the experiments, shown in Tables 1 to 3, was

+/- Faint, or spotty, pink color within test site
1   Uniform pink color covering all of test site
2   Uniform pink-to-red color covering all of test site
3   Uniform bright red color covering all of test site
4   Uniform bright red color covering all of test site with edema, blisters, or weeping

U.S. Patent 4,897,260 and World Patent WO 8807371 describe glucocorticoid carboxylic acid esters to suppress cutaneous delayed hypersensitivity.[28,29] The advantage of the carboxylic acid esters is that, in contrast to steroids, they do not cause epidermal atrophy and other adverse systemic effects such as suppression of plasma B. The glucocorticoid carboxylic acid esters and, more specifically, triamcinolone acetonide 21-oic methyl ester at a permeation rate of 100 mcg/24 h can specifically, temporarily, and locally suppress the cutaneous immune system to the coadministered allergen. The carboxylic acid esters were shown to prevent allergic reactions and also the induction phase of sensitization which must precede the allergic state. Moreover, their effects were shown to be confined to the site of application, so that other areas of the body surface remained armed.

Two other patents discuss the use of steroids for the prevention of pruritis caused by the transdermal administration of nicotine and the prevention of irritation in the delivery of polypeptides through mucosal membranes.[30,31]

E. IMMUNOSUPPRESSIVE AGENTS

World Patent Application WO 9,600,058 teaches methods for site-specific immunosuppression using topical formulations containing immunosuppressants such as cyclosporins, rapamycins, FK-506 derivatives, and combinations thereof.[32] The methods and formulations described affect site-specific immune suppression of local inflammatory/immune responses in mammalian tissue for the treatment of many autoimmune and T cell-mediated diseases, including inhibition of contact hypersensitivity. The major advantage of the topical delivery is that it eliminates the concerns of systemic administration of immunosuppressants with its many side effects, i.e., kidney and liver damage. Cyclosporine A and hydrocortisone produce a synergistic combination to attack multiple disease mechanisms at a local site-specific level.

F. ARACHIDONIC ACID CASCADE MODULATORS

European Patent Application EP 0314528A describes inhibitors of the arachidonic acid cascade to prevent contact dermatitis associated with transdermal delivery.[33] They claim that agents which inhibit the key enzymes in the process (e.g., phospholipase A_2, 5-lipoxygenase, 12-lipoxygenase, or cyclooxygenase) or block the end response (e.g., receptor antagonists) are effective in treating contact dermatitis, both irritant or allergic. Since the transformation of the arachidonic acid to its metabolic products (leucotrienes, prostaglandins), which are responsible for the inflammatory reaction, is an enzyme-catalyzed free radical oxidative process, free radical scavengers could be used to reduce the inflammatory reactions. Such free radical scavengers disclosed include hindered phenols such as 2,6-ditertiarybutyl-para-cresol (BHT), p-tertiarybutyl catechol, hydroquinone, benzoquinone, and N,N-diethylhydroxyamine. Materials that compete with the arachidonic acid biotransformation are also disclosed as anti-irritants because they allow less arachidonic acid to be transformed into irritating products such as leucotrienes and prostaglandins with four double bonds. Chemicals that compete with arachidonic acid and which byproducts are not irritating include eicosatetraenoic acid, eicosapentanoic acid, and dihomolinoleic acid.

Omega-9-unsaturated fatty acids and especially the cis isomers have been shown to prevent or alleviate the inflammatory symptoms of allergic contact dermatitis.[34] Previous work had shown that synthesis of leucotriene B_4 is inhibited when rats were fed omega-9-unsaturated fatty acids. The inventors studied several unsaturated fatty acids and found the omega-9 gave the best suppression of delayed allergy reactions. The effective omega-9-unsaturated fatty acids had a minimum of 2 double bonds and 18 to 22 carbon atoms. Specific fatty acids claimed include 6,9-octadecadienoic acid, 8,11-eicosadienoic acid, and 5,8,11-eicosatrienoic acid. Mice fed 5,8,11-eicosatrienoic acid for 1 week showed a 50% reduction of footpad swelling over the control mice sensitized to sheep red blood cells.

G. Lipid Mediators

The irritation caused by aqueous detergents selected from the group consisting of anionic, cationic, nonionic, and amphoteric organic detergents was substantially improved by incorporating in the formulation up to 10% of an additive comprising the polymerized product of 2 to 4 molecules of a monomeric C_{12} to C_{26} fatty acid, said additive containing 2 to 4 carboxyl or carboxyl salt groups.[35] It was proposed that the detergent degrades the protein molecules of the keratin layer, thus exposing the living cells to the detergent and other irritating molecules in the formulation. The lipid additives stabilize the keratin layer and protect the living tissue. The preferred lipid additives are ethylenically unsaturated fatty acids polymerized into dimers, trimers, and tetramers, which result in a cyclo aliphatic ring structure. The only lipid modifier shown in the examples was the dimer of linoleic acid, and it was tested with several detergents including sodium lauryl sulphate, alkyl benzene sulfonate, linear alkane sulfonate, and N-coco-β-aminopropionic acid. U.S. Patent 4,076,799 comes from the same laboratory as the above-mentioned work and used similar lipid modifiers to reduce the inflammatory response of allergic contact dermatitis during challenge. The method comprises applying to the skin lipid modifiers, which are organic compounds having at least two polar, e.g., carboxyl groups, separated by a chain of at least 15 atoms, the majority of which are carbon atoms, and containing a cyclic moiety of at least five atoms, prior to contact of the skin with the allergenic agent.[36] Lipid modifiers used in the examples were bis(hydroxyethyl) dimerate (esterification of dimerized linoleic acid with ethylene glycol) and bis(triethanolamine salt) dimerate.

Cis and trans traumatic acid salts have been claimed for the treatment of many skin diseases, including itching and allergic dermatitis.[37] Traumatic acid or 10-dodecendioic acid is a linear long chain carboxylic acid having 12 carbon atoms and an unsaturated bond. The anti-irritant activity of traumatic acid is claimed to be due to the carboxylic group distribution along the carbon chain.[38]

The topical application of *cis*-9-heptadecenoic acid has been shown to be useful in the prophylaxis and treatment of skin diseases including contact allergies.[39] In vitro tests showed that *cis*-9-heptadecenoic acid suppresses the release of important triggering mediators, such as TNF-α, which is important in the prophylaxis and treatment of skin diseases including allergies. Heptadecenoic acid also showed significant inhibition of mitogen-induced proliferation of lymphocytes and, therefore, should also have anti-inflammatory immunomodulating potency.

Sphingosine and other aliphatic aminodiol lipids have been shown to provide long-term anti-irritant activity when formulated into cosmetic compositions containing irritants such as lactic, hydroxybenzoic, or retinoic acids.[40] Comparative data show a beneficial control of long-term irritation induced by several weeks of daily use of a variety of skin-renewal stimulating acids, as mentioned above. In contrast to the aliphatic aminodiol lipids, the incorporation into the formulations of other skin lipids such as phospholipids, cerobrosides, and ceramides had little activity in controlling long-term irritation. In addition to sphingosine, phytosphingamine and dihydrosphingosine are claimed as anti-irritants, together with their analogs, homologs, and derivatives.

H. Antioxidants

Antioxidants and free radical scavengers have been considered in the patent literature for eliminating or minimizing irritation and sensitization in transdermal delivery. European Patent EP 0,314,528A1 claims that irritation mechanisms involve inflammatory reaction of skin caused by the metabolic products of arachidonic acid transformations, (leucotrienes, 12-hydroxyeicosatetraenoic acid, and prostaglandins).[41] The enzymatic transformations (lipoxygenase and cyclo-oxygenase) are catalyzed by free radical oxidative processes which can be minimized by the presence in the skin of antioxidants and free radical scavengers. Some free radical scavengers mentioned include hindered phenols such as BHT, *p*-tertiarybutyl catechol, hydroquinone, benzoquinone, and N,N-diethylhydroxyamine. Vitamin E and nordihydroguaiaretic acid are also disclosed as antioxidants that minimize irritation when used as pretreaments or codelivered with the transdermal drug.

Ascorbic acid (vitamin C) has also been found to decrease skin irritation caused by topical administration of active ingredients. U.S. Patent 5,516,793 indicates that ascorbic acid, provided in topical application in as low as 5% concentration from a separate solution or by admixture with a cosmetically acceptable vehicle, is effective in reducing the irritation caused by many cosmetic and pharmaceutical ingredients.[42] Examples of such ingredients include α-hydroxy acids, benzoyl peroxide, retinol (vitamin A), retinoic acid, quaternary ammonium lactates, and salicylic acid.

U.S. Patent 5,545,407 and German Patent DE 3,522,572 pertain to the use of vitamin E to protect skin and reduce irritation caused by actives and, more specifically, of benzoyl peroxide for the treatment of acne and other skin lesions.[43,44] Tocopherol acetate, tocopherol sorbate, tocopherol linoleate, and mixtures thereof are disclosed as useful vitamin E analogs. α-Tocopherol has also been shown to reduce irritation.[44,45] U.S. Patent 5,252,604 discloses liquid compositions for topical applications containing up to 5% α-tocopherol for the reduction of irritation caused by retinoic acid.[45] Topical α-tocopherol was shown to reduce, in a dose-response fashion, the irritation caused by repeated applications of retinoic acid. Inflammatory response was measured by MPO activity (MPO is a neutrophil enzyme marker), which is directly proportioned to the increase in neutrophils. Inhibition levels of 20 and 70% were observed with 0.01 and 5% concentrations of α-tocopherol, respectively.

Methyl nicotinate has also been shown to reduce irritation of transdermally administered drugs, as well as reduce the elicitation response of sensitization.[46] The methyl nicotinate is coadministered with the irritant or sensitizer at preferred concentrations of 0.5 to 5%. Methyl nicotinate was tested against the irritant chloroquine and the sensitizers propranolol, ketoprofen, and tetracaine.

In the case of ketoprofen, 2% hydroxyethylcellulose alcoholic gels were prepared and placed in Finn chambers and applied on the backs of ten hairless guinea pigs. After 24 h, the chambers were removed and the intensity of the reaction scored for edema and erythema at 24 and 48 h. The average visual score for erythema and edema was greater at 24 and 48 h for the formulations that did not contain methyl nicotinate.

I. PANTHENOL AND ITS DERIVATIVES

Panthenol and its analogs and derivatives such as pantothenic acid, pantetheine, and pantethine, have been claimed as anti-irritants for formulations containing up to 20% of benzoyl peroxide.[47] The formulations are gels that exhibit low skin irritation and are useful for topical application to human skin for the treatment of acne and other skin lesions. U.S. Patent 4,908,213 discloses D-panthenol as an antipruritic, in formulations containing nicotine for the treatment of symptoms associated with tobacco smoking cessation.[48] Dexpanthenol has also been claimed as an enhancer/anti-irritant useful with many drug families, including opioids, calcium antagonists, beta-blockers, and antihypertensives.[49] Specific drugs claimed include hydromorphon, biperiden, and gallopamil. Several formulations containing 15% gallopamil and 15% dexpanthenol were shown to produce substantially less irritation than the control formulations without the dexpanthenol.

J. REDUCTION OF ELECTROTRANSPORT IRRITATION

Iontophoresis and electroporation are two processes studied extensively to increase the permeation of drugs through intact skin. By applying electric current through the skin, the irritation issues are amplified in comparison to those of passive transdermal delivery.[50] World Patent WO 9,506,497 discloses an electrotransport device with a cathodic reservoir containing the agent to be delivered and an anodic reservoir and an electrical power source to apply a voltage across the reservoirs. It is claimed that when the anodic reservoir is maintained at a pH above 4 (4 to 10) and the cathodic reservoir at a pH below 4 (2 to 4), the irritation is minimized.[51] U.S. Patent 5,221,254 describes methods for reducing the sensations (pain) during iontophoretic drug delivery by delivering the therapeutic agent with a multivalent ion.[52] Their experimental work indicated that the preferred multivalent ions to mitigate the iontophoretic sensations were calcium, magnesium, phosphate, and zinc. At high iontophoretic current density, $600 \, \mu A/cm^2$, the ranking from best to worst was calcium, phosphate, chloride, acetate, citrate, sulfate, potassium, and sodium.

K. METABOLIC MODULATORS/LYSOSOME MODIFIERS

U.S. Patents 4,885,154 and 5,304,379 pertain to methods and devices for the reduction of sensitization and irritation caused by transdermally delivered drugs, wherein one or more metabolic modulators is coadministered with the sensitizing or irritating drug.[53,54] Metabolic modulators affect the enzymes in the skin and thus modify the metabolism of the drug, so as to inhibit the formation of reactive or irritating metabolites. An irritant reaction occurs if irritating metabolites are formed which can react adversely with cellular components, and sensitization occurs when the reactive metabolites formed provide a configuration capable of activating the immune system. Enzymes present in the skin include monoamine oxidases, peroxidases, decarboxylases, carboxyl esterases, and alcohol dehydrogenases. Monoamine oxidases are probably the most important as they can deaminate transdermally delivered amine drugs such as beta-blockers, antihistamines, and local anesthetics. Metabolic modulators that can modify monoamine oxidase activity include harmine, benzyl alcohol, tranylcypromine, phenylhydrazine, 2-phenyl-1-ethanol, and cinnamyl alcohol. Examples showed that 2-phenyl-1-ethanol prevented the induction of sensitization to tetracaine and completely prevented the inflammatory response of already sensitized subjects.

U.S. Patents 5,120,545 and 5,149,539 disclose methods for preventing induction of sensitization and treating the inflammatory response upon elicitation.[55,56] The method involves the coadministration to the skin or mucosa of a sensitizing drug together with an antigen processing–inhibiting agent. Events that lead to the association of the antigens with the cell surface of a class II MHC molecule are referred to as antigen processing. The above-mentioned association is required for the occurrence of presentation of the antigen by the Langerhans cells to T cells. Presentation is required for both the induction and the elicitation step of the sensitization process. Antigen-processing inhibitors include ionophores and weak base compounds such as ammonium chloride. The processing inhibitors prevent the processing of the drug in the lysosome due to the increase in pH; thus the proteases in the lysosome are not able to chemically alter the drug into the proper antigenic form for class II MHC association. Excellent data were obtained for two sensitizing drugs, propranolol and tetracaine. Over 90% reduction in inflammatory response to propranolol was obtained with a formulation containing 4% ammonium chloride (Table 4).

TABLE 4
Sensitization Response to Propranolol and Modulation by Ammonium Chloride

Time after Removal (Days)	Ammonium Chloride Concentration (%)			
	0	2	4	8
0	0.7[a]	0.7	0.7	0.7
4	6.3	4.0	1.0	4.8
7	7.2	4.7	1.2	4.1
11	2.8	1.5	0.7	1.5

[a] Evaluated using Minolta chromameter.

Adapted from Reference 55.

In U.S. Patents 5,160,741 and 5,130,139, the reduction in irritation caused by drugs that are weak bases, such as the beta-adrenergic antagonist propranolol and the antimalarial chloroquine, are described.[57,58] Weak bases are known to accumulate in lysosomes due to the low intralysosomal pH.[59] The weak bases can permeate the lysosomal membranes at their uncharged molecular form; however, the low pH of the lysosomes favors protonation and the charged weak bases are now relatively membrane impermeable and less able to pass back through the lysosomal membrane. Ionophores have also been shown to accumulate in lysosome membranes and thus increase the pH of the lysosomes.[60] The invention pertains to the use of ionophores to increase the pH, as mentioned above, and the use of competitive weak bases which would also increase the lysosomal pH. The increased pH would reduce the protonation of the weak base drug and thus reduce its accumulation in the lysosome and reduce irritation. Ionophores suitable for the invention include monensin, nigericin, valinomycin, and gramicidin. Competitive weak bases include ammonia, ammonium chloride, methylamine, ethanolamine, and tromethamine. A formulation containing 5% ammonium chloride reduced tenfold the irritation caused by 2% chloroquine or 2% propranolol.

L. Mast Cell Cytokine Release Modifiers

European Patent Application 5,612,525A pertains to the use of mast cell degranulators to abrogate the induction step of delayed hypersensitivity in the dermal or transdermal delivery of drugs.[61] The mast cell degranulators are also capable of inducing a state of immunological tolerance to the skin when the sensitizing agent is delivered prior to, or at the onset of, transdermal administration. *cis*-Urocanic acid and its analogs, capsaicin, chloroquine, an antihuman IgE antibody, compound 48/80, morphine sulfate, and substance P, are shown to be appropriate mast cell-degranulating agents. *cis*-Urocanic acid was able to reduce in Balb/c mice the sensitization to DNCB, in dose response fashion. This technology is discussed in detail in Chapter 17.

Topical application of *p*-substituted phenoxy alkanols jointly with an agent that causes irritation or contact sensitization modifies and mitigates such irritation or sensitization.[62] The lead compound is chlorphenesin, a phenoxy propanol originally described as a muscle relaxant. Chlorphenesin inhibits histamine from human leukocytes and inhibits the degranulation of the rat mast cells mediated by IgE/anti-IgE reactions.[63,64] It is claimed that *p*-phenoxy alkanols inhibit irritation and sensitization by inhibiting the release of chemical mediators that are responsible for the symptoms of allergic diseases and inflammation. These mediators are histamine and the IgE-mediated cytokines. In an experiment using Balb/c mice already sensitized to dinitrofluorobenzene, a 2% solution of chlorphenesin reduced by 100% the ear swelling of the mice upon challenge. The use of nitric oxide synthase inhibitors has also been disclosed to reduce the skin irritant effects of topically applied cosmetics and pharmaceutical components.[65] This is in accordance with the observation that nitric oxide directly inhibits the IgE-mediated secretory function of mast cells.[66] Nitric oxide synthase inhibitors useful with the teachings of this patent include *N*-monomethyl-*L*-arginine, *N*-nitro-*L*-arginine, *N*-amino-*L*-arginine and *N,N*-dimethyl-arginine. The nitric oxide synthase inhibitors are useful in reducing the irritation caused by retinoic acid, salicylic acid, and vitamin D and its derivatives.

U.S. Patent 5,162,361 discloses the use of aromatic diamidines to control diseases in which a diminution of IL-1 is beneficial, including skin hypersensitivity.[67] The inventors have also shown for the first time that aromatic diamidines block the secretion of IL-6 and tumor necrosis factor from cells producing these cytokines. The lead diamidine is 1,5-bis(4-amidinophenoxy) pentane (pentamidine) or its imidazoline-substituted derivatives. In experiments with already sensitized mice to oxazolone, pentamidine was able to reduce the inflammatory response upon challenge in a dose-dependent fashion. Immediate ear pretreatment with 20 μg per ear of pentamidine reduced ear swelling by 50% over the positive control. Application of 80 μg pentamidine per ear reduced ear swelling about 75%.

M. Ion Channel Modulators

Ion channel modulators have been studied extensively, and they have been shown to modulate both the induction and elicitation steps of the sensitization response. The mechanism of modulation has not been elucidated. One could hypothesize that, by modulating the ion channels on the cell surface, you alter the permeation of small molecules into the cells which then interfere with signal transduction as well as cell-to-cell communication.

Bristol-Myers Squibb was recently issued four U.S. Patents addressing the abrogation of sensitization, as well as pure irritation, by the use of ion channel modulators.[68–71] Since this is the subject of Chapter 16 in this book, we will only briefly summarize the work here. U.S. Patent 5,686,100 describes loop diuretics, such as ethacrynic acid for the prevention and/or treatment of adverse reactions of the skin, to the presence of a skin sensitizing or irritating substance. Ethacrynic acid was shown to be effective against the classical sensitizers, such as DNCB and oxazolone, as well as the important sensitizing drugs albuterol, nadolol, clonidine, and chlorpheniramine. U.S. Patent 5,716,987 pertains to nondiuretic analogs of ethacrynic acid as modulators of irritation and sensitization. The analogs include phenoxyacetic acid and its lower alkyl esters such as phenoxyacetic acid methyl ester. In general, the analogs were as effective as ethacrynic acid. U.S. Patent 5,618,557 pertains only to the prophylactic treatment of allergic contact dermatitis by the use of potassium-sparing diuretics, and it is specifically positioned for the prevention of sensitization in the dermal and transdermal delivery of drugs. Granstein and Gallo had previously shown in WO 9,009,792 that amiloride, a potassium-sparing diuretic, and its analogs were able to treat the inflammation caused by a sensitizer applied to the skin of previously sensitized subjects.[72] The last Bristol-Myers Squibb patent WO 9,718,782 pertains to the use of calcium channel blockers, such as nifedipine and verapamil, to prevent or treat reactions of the skin to the presence of a skin-sensitizing agent.[71] Calcium channel blockers were shown to be effective against DNCB, as well as the beta adrenergic agonist nadolol. Patents U.S. 5,202,130 and South African ZA 9,006,583 also teach the treatment of contact sensitization with calcium flux inhibitors.[73,74] In the South African patent, the use of nifedipine was shown to significantly reduce the inflammation caused by 3% oxazolone to already sensitized mice. Diltiazem, a calcium channel blocker, was shown to effectively treat the inflammation caused by DNCB to already sensitized mice.[73] One significant contribution of this patent pertains to the use of lanthanum ions, from lanthanum chloride or lanthanum citrate, to treat sensitization. Lanthanum ions are competitors to calcium ions for the inhibition of calcium channels. A German (East) patent claims that magnesium ions, optionally together with lanthanum ions, are suitable for the treatment of allergic inflammations.[75] Magnesium chloride (28%) was effective in treating the inflammation caused by 0.5% DNCB.

Several other patents have been issued using metal ions to reduce irritation and sensitization. World Patent WO 9,619,181 provides formulations containing aqueous soluble monovalent potassium cations or monovalent lithium ions to reduce irritation and the itch sensation of topically applied formulations.[76] These ions affect the sensory nerves and prevent the transmission of sensory impulses and the desire to scratch. Chapter 18 discusses this technology in detail. French Patent 2,740,341 pertains to the use of metallic salts such as lanthanides, tin, cobalt, barium, manganese, strontium, zinc, and others for the treatment of cutaneous pain and prevention of irritation among other cutaneous disorders.[77] They claim that the metal salts are substance P antagonists and thus are useful in reducing or preventing irritant effects of cosmetics and dermatological and pharmaceutical compositions. In U.S. Patent 5,708,023 the use of zinc gluconate is claimed as an irritant-inactivating agent.[78] A method is also disclosed of inactivating irritants in a fluid contacting skin, comprising applying the composition containing zinc gluconate to the skin. U.S. Patent 5,489,441 discloses the use of ruthenium red as an immunosuppressant which, among other uses, is useful in alleviating contact dermatitis.[79] Ruthenium red is an inorganic hexavalent polycationic dye which has been used to stain complex polysaccharides. These dyes have also been shown to affect calcium ion transport in pig stomach cells and in rat liver cells.[80,81] Ruthenium red reduced significantly, and in a dose–response fashion, the inflammation caused by trinitrochlorobenzene on previously sensitized mice.

N. LOCAL ANESTHETICS

Topical anesthetics could be considered ion channel modulators because their action is probably similar in nature to that of diuretics. Local anesthetics block conduction of the nerve impulse by preventing the large transient increase in the permeability of excitable membranes to Na^+ ions. This action is due to the direct interaction of the anesthetic with the voltage-sensitive Na^+ ion channels. Local anesthetics can also bind to other membrane-bound proteins and they can block K^+ ion channels as well.[82]

Topical anesthetics, in concentrations up to 25%, have been used in formulations containing capsaicin to inhibit the local topical irritant effect of capsaicin.[83] The formulations containing up to 1% capsaicin were used to treat superficial pain syndromes. Benzocaine and lidocaine were the local anesthetics of choice. The local anesthetics lidocaine, benzocaine, lignocaine, methocaine, butylaminobenzoate, and procaine have also been disclosed as anti-irritants in transdermal formulations containing nicotine.[84] The once-daily transdermal formulations containing nicotine are being used to treat symptoms associated with tobacco smoking cessation.

O. OTHER ANTI-IRRITANT TECHNOLOGIES

Glycerin has been disclosed as an anti-irritant for reducing the skin irritation of transdermal drug/enhancer compositions.[85] The method involves treating the skin with glycerin, prior to or concurrently with the administration of the drug/enhancer composition. It is effective in reducing the irritation caused by drugs such as pindolol and enhancers such as ethanol, propylene glycol, dimethyl sulfoxide, and Azone™.

Aluminum chlorhydrate has also been shown to prevent, as well as treat, allergic contact dermatitis caused by urushiol oil, poison ivy, or poison oak.[86] Treatment with an aerosol solution of 25% aluminum chlorhydrate was effective in relieving the symptoms in the infected area and preventing further spread of the dermatitis.

A method for preventing or treating irritation or itching of the skin is disclosed where the active ingredient is 1-[3-4-(diphenylmethyl)-1-piperazinyl] propyl]-1H-benzimidazole.[87] The product is recommended for use in cosmetics including sunscreens, antiwrinkle products, shampoos, shaving creams, diaper rash, face masks, deodorants, and aftershaves.

Topical compositions containing capsazepine have been shown to be suitable for treating neurogenic skin disorders and diseases.[88] In particular, the compositions are useful for preventing and/or controlling skin and eye irritation, itching, and erythema, as well as for reducing the irritancy of an active substance having an irritant side effect. Actives with irritant side effects include alpha and beta hydroxyacids, beta ketoacids, retinoids, anthralins, anthranoids, peroxides, minoxidil, lithium salts, vitamin D, surfactants, and reducing and oxidizing agents, as well as strong acids and bases.

Patent Application EP 0,723,774A discloses antagonists of CGRP (calcitonin gene-related peptide) to prevent and treat irritation and sensitization.[89] Compounds disclosed as anti-irritants include CGRP 8-37 and antibodies of anti-CGRP. These compounds have been used successfully in cosmetic, pharmaceutical, and dermatological compositions.

U.S. Patent 5,578,300 claims a method of treatment of allergic contact dermatitis, which comprises treating a patient with a formulation capable of inducing oxidative stress and a heat shock response so as to convert the allergic reaction of the allergic contact dermatitis to an irritant reaction.[90] Oxidative stress is induced, preferably by hydrogen peroxide, through a polymeric precursor such as chitin, gelatin, pectin, and sodium carboxymethylcellulose.

Use of superoxide dismutase (SOD) as an agent for the protection of the skin against inflammatory reactions associated with chemical irritation has also been disclosed in the patent literature.[91]

SOD is an oxygen-free radical scavenger that had been previously shown to suppress carrageenan-induced inflammation in the rat.[92] It is claimed that SOD eliminates the superoxide anion radicals, hydrogen peroxide, and hydroxyl radical formation and thus reduces the damage to cells and irritation from diverse classes of chemical irritants including inorganic and organic peroxides, acids, and bases. The formulation containing the SOD, from 1 to 1000 CIU/cm^2 (CIU is defined as the cytochrome inhibition unit), is applied topically 5 to 10 min before exposure to chemical irritants. Examples with sodium lauryl sulfate, lauric acid, cinnamaldehyde, benzoyl peroxide, sodium hydroxide, and eugenol are presented.

III. SUMMARY

The mechanisms of irritant, as well as allergic contact, dermatitis are still not totally understood, although a lot of progress has been made during the last few years as demonstrated by the advances presented in Chapters 7 through 13 of this volume.

It is not, therefore, surprising that the patent literature reviewed in this chapter involves, to a large degree, inventions based on observation and trial and error approaches. The methodology and results presented in most cases would not pass peer review. The quality of the patent literature has improved in the last few years, as the science of immunology is making progress in understanding the mechanisms involved in these processes. The sections on Metabolic Modulators, Ion Channel Modulators, and Mast Cell Degranulators are based on the latest understanding of science which is still evolving. Alza, Bristol-Myers, and L'Oreal appear to be in the forefront in trying to apply the latest scientific breakthroughs to the delivery of drugs and cosmetics to skin with reduced skin reactions.

It is reasonable to assume that, as the science improves, so will the approaches of abrogating contact dermatitis.

REFERENCES

1. Mitsuhico, H., European Patent Application 06,641,191, assigned to Nitto Denko, Tape for transdermal use easily detachable from skin (January 1995).
2. Farhadieh, B., Gokhale, R., Vallner, J., and Berger, H., Canadian Patent Application 2,058,059 assigned to G.D. Searle, Single layer transdermal administration system (November 1991).
3. Kydonieus, A., Unpublished data.
4. Kalish, R., Wood, J., Kydonieus, A., and Wille, J., Prevention of contact hypersensitivity to topically applied drugs by ethacrynic acid, *J. Control Rel.*, 48, 79, 1997.
5. Bloom, R. C. and Deckner, G. E., World Patent Application WO 9,402,176 assigned to Procter and Gamble, Pharmaceutical composition for topical use containing a cross-linked cationic polymer and an alkoxylated ether (February 1994).
6. Wong, O. and Nguyen, T., U.S. Patent 5,308,625 assigned to Cygnus, Enhancement of transdermal drug delivery using monoalkyl phosphates and other absorption promoters (May 1994).
7. Bergstrom, J. K. and Liu, P., U.S. Patent 5,374,645 assigned to Ciba Geigy, Transdermal administration of ionic pharmaceutically active agents via aqueous isopropanol (December 1994).
8. Sequeira, J. A., U.S. Patent 4,834,980 assigned to Schering Plough, Transdermal delivery of azatadine (May 1989).
9. Benerza, C., Sigman, C., Bagheri, D., Fraginals, R., and Maibach, H., Molecular aspects of allergic contact dermatitis, in *Textbook of Contact Dermatitis*, Rycroft, R., Menne, T., Frosch, P., and Benezra, C., Eds., p. 105–119 (1992).
10. Barua, A. B., Gunning, D., and Olson, J. A., U.S. Patent 5,075,340 assigned to Iowa State University, Retinoic acid glucuronide preparations for application to the skin (December 1991).
11. Brown, L. R., Cline, J. F., and Davidson, J., U.S. Patent 5,422,118 assigned to Pure Pak, Inc., Transdermal administration of amines with minimal irritation and high transdermal flux rate (June 1995).

12. Brown, L. R., Cline, J. F., and Davidson, J., European Patent Application 0,267,051A assigned to Moleculon, Transdermal administration of amines (November 1987).

13. Taro, O., European Patent Application 0,245,126A assigned to Maruho Co, Percutaneous absorption preparation and process for preparing same (April 1987).

14. Castro, J. R., U.S. Patent 5,393,526 assigned to Elizabeth Arden, Cosmetic Compositions (February 1995).

15. Smith, W. P., Pelliccione, N. J., Marenus, K. D., and Maes, D. H., European Patent Application 0,354,554A assigned to Estee Lauder, Anti-irritant and desensitizing compositions and methods of their use (August 1989).

16. Parnell, F., World Patent Application WO 9,114,441 assigned to Parnell Pharma, Eriodictyon drug delivery systems (October 1991).

17. Govil, S. K. and Kohlman, P., U.S. Patent 4,908,213 assigned to Schering Plough, Transdermal delivery of nicotine (March 1990).

18. Castelli, D., Colin, L., Camel, E., and Ries, G., Pretreatment of skin with a *Ginkgo biloba* extract/sodium carboxymethyl-β-1, 3-glucan formulation appears to inhibit the elicitation of allergic contact dermatitis in man, *Contact Dermatitis,* 38, 123–126, 1998.

19. Cupps., T. R. and Fauci, A. S., *Immunol. Rev.,* 65, 133–135, 1982.

20. Amkraut, A. and Shaw, J., U.S. Patent 5,077,054 assigned to Alza, Prevention of contact allergy by coadministration of a corticosteroid with a sensitizing drug (December 1991).

21. Amkraut, A. and Shaw, J., U.S. Patent 5,000,596 assigned to Alza, Prevention of contact allergy by coadministration of a corticosteroid with a sensitizing drug (March 1991).

22. Amkraut, A., U.S. Patent 5,049,387 assigned to Alza, Inducing skin tolerance to a sensitizing drug (September 1991).

23. Amkrout, A., U.S. Patent 5,118,509 assigned to Alza, Inducing skin tolerance to a sensitizing drug (June 1992).

24. Cruz, A. et al., *Photodermatology,* 5, 126–132, 1988.

25. Rheins, B. and Nordlund, H., *J. Immunol.,* 136(3), 867–876, 1986.

26. Franz, T. J., Shah, K., and Kydonieus, A., U.S. Patent 5,028,431 assigned to Hercon Labs, Article for the delivery to animal tissue of a pharmacologically active agent (July 1991).

27. Wilckens, T. and DeRijk, R., Glucocorticoids and immune function: unknown dimensions and new frontiers, *Immunol. Today,* 18(9), 418, 1997.

28. Ross, P. M., U.S. Patent 4,897,260 assigned to Rockefeller University, Compositions that affect suppression of cutaneous delayed hypersensitivity and products including same (January 1990).

29. Ross, P. M., World Patent Application WO 8,807,371 assigned to Rockefeller University, Prevention and treatment of the deleterious effects of exposing skin to the sun, and compositions thereof (October 1988).

30. Govil, S. K. and Kohlman, P., U.S. Patent 4,908,213 assigned to Schering Plough, Transdermal administration of nicotine (March 1990).

31. Wang, Y. J., Lee, W. A., and Narog, B., World Patent Application WO 9,009,167 assigned to California Biotechnology, Composition and method for administration of pharmaceutically active substances (August 1990).

32. Hewitt, C. W. and Black, K. S., World Patent Application WO 9,600,058 assigned to the University of California, Methods for inducing site-specific immunosuppression and compositions of site-specific immunosuppressants (January 1996).

33. Franz, T. J., Shah, K., and Kydonieus, A., European Patent Application 0,314,528A assigned to Hercon Labs, Article for controlled release and delivery of substances to animal tissues (October 1988).

34. Akimoto, K., Kawashima, H., Hamazaki, T., and Sawazaki, S., European Patent Application 0,704,211A to Suntory Ltd, Preventive or alleviating agent for medical symptoms caused by delayed allergy reactions (August 1995).

35. Kelly, R. and Ritter, E. J., U.S. Patent 3,538,009 assigned to Cincinnati Milacron, Method of reducing skin irritation in detergent compositions (November 1970).

36. Willer, S. G., Yusf, P., and Kelly, R., U.S. Patent 4,076,799 assigned to Cincinnati Milacron, Method of inhibiting skin irritation (February 1978).

37. Della Valle, F. and Marcolongo, G., European Patent Application 0,599,188A assigned to Lifegroup, Trans and cis traumatic acid salts having cicatrizant activity (November 1993).

38. Goldberg, R. L. et al., Reduction of topical irritation, *J. Chem. Soc.,* 28, 667–679, 1977.
39. Degwert, J., Jacob, J., and Steckel, F., U.S. Patent 5,708,028 assigned to Beiersdorf AG, Use of cis-9-heptadecenoic acid for treating psoriasis and allergies (January 1998).
40. Herstein, M., World Patent Application WO 9,503,028., Cosmetic skin-renewal stimulating composition with long term irritation control (February 1995).
41. Franz, T. et al., European Patent Application EP 0,314,528A assigned to Hercon Labs, Article for the controlled release and delivery of substances to animal tissue (October 1988).
42. Duffy, J., U.S. Patent 5,516,793 assigned to Avon Products, Use of ascorbic acid to reduce irritation of topically applied active ingredients (May 1996).
43. Hall, B. J., Baur, J. A., and Deckner, G. E., U.S. Patent 5,545,407 assigned to Proctor and Gamble, Dermatological compositions and methods of treatment of skin lesions therewith using benzoyl peroxide and tocopherol esters (August 1996).
44. Roshdy, I., German Patent DE 3,522,572., Mittel zum Schutz und Behandlung der Haut (February 1987).
45. Nagy, C. F., Quick, T. W., and Shapiro, S. S., U.S. Patent 5,252,604 assigned to Hoffman LaRoche, Compositions of retinoic acids and tocopherol for prevention of dermatitis (October 1993).
46. Cormiez, M., Amkraut, A., and Ledger, P. W., U.S. Patent 5,451,407 assigned to Alza, Reduction or prevention of skin irritation or sensitization during transdermal administration of an irritating or sensitizing drug (September 1995).
47. Hall, B. J., Baur, J. A., and Deckner, G. E., U.S. Patent 5,445,823 assigned to Proctor and Gamble, Dermatological compositions and methods of treatment of skin lesions therewith (August 1995).
48. Govil, S. K. and Kohlman, P., U.S. Patent 4,908,213 assigned to Schering Plough, Transdermal delivery of nicotine (March 1990).
49. Kolter, K., European Patent Application 0,380,989A assigned to Knoll, Pflaster zur transdermalen Andwendung (January 1990).
50. Ledger, P., Skin biological issues in electronically enhanced transdermal delivery, *Adv. Drug Del. Rev.,* 9, 289–307, 1992.
51. Cormiez, M., Ledger, P., Johnson, J., and Phipps, J., World Patent Application WO 9,506,497 assigned to Alza, Reduction of skin irritation and resistance during electrotransport (March 1995).
52. Phipps, J. B., U.S. Patent 5,221,254 assigned to Alza, Method for reducing sensation in iontophoretic drug delivery (June 1993).
53. Cormiez, M., Ledger, P., Amkraut, A., and Marty, J., U.S. Patent 4,885,154 assigned to Alza, Method for reducing sensitization in transdermal drug delivery and means thereof (December 1989).
54. Cormiez, M., Ledger, P., Amkraut, A., and Marty, J., U.S. Patent 5,304,739 assigned to Alza, Method for reducing sensitization in transdermal drug delivery and means thereof (April 1994).
55. Ledger, P. W., Cormiez, M., and Amkraut, A., U.S. Patent 5,120,545 assigned to Alza, Reduction or prevention of sensitization to drugs (June 1992).
56. Ledger, P., Cormiez, M., and Amkraut, A., U.S. Patent 5,149,539 assigned to Alza, Reduction or prevention of sensitization to drugs (September 1992).
57. Cormiez, M., Ledger, P., and Amkraut, A., U.S. Patent 5,160,741 assigned to Alza, Reduction or prevention of skin irritation to drugs (November 1992).
58. Cormiez, M., Ledger, P., and Amkraut, A., U.S. Patent 5,130,139 assigned to Alza, Reduction or prevention of skin irritation to drugs (July 1992).
59. MacIntyre, H. et al., *Biopharm. Drug Disposition,* 9, 513, 1988.
60. Maxfield, L., *J. Cell Biol.,* 95, 676, 1982.
61. Wille, J. and Kydonieus, A., European Patent Application 5,612,525 assigned to Bristol-Myers Squibb, Transdermal treatment with mast cell degranulating agents for drug-induced hypersensitivity (February 1994).
62. Berger, F. M., U.S. Patent 5,008,293., Process for the treatment of the skin to alleviate skin diseases arising from contact sensitization or irritation utilizing p-substituted phenoxy alcanols (April 1991).
63. Lichtenstein, J. et al., *J. Immunol.,* 103, 866, 1969.
64. Kimura, J. et al., *Immunology,* 26, 983, 1974.
65. Giacomoni, P. and Andral, C., World Patent Application WO 9,626,711 assigned to L'Oreal, Nitric oxide synthase inhibitors (September 1996).

66. Eastmond, N. C., Banks, M., and Coleman, J., Nitric oxide inhibits IgE- mediated degranulation of mast cells and is the principal intermediate in IFN-gamma-induced suppression and exocytotis, *J. Immunol.*, 159, 1444–1450, 1997.

67. Rosenthal, G. J., Kouchi, Y., Corsini, E., Blaylock, B., Comment, C., Luster, M., Craig, W., and Taylor, M., U.S. Patent 5,162,361 assigned to U.S. Government, Method of treating diseases associated with elevated levels of Interleukin 1 (November 1992).

68. Wille, J. and Kydonieus, A., U.S. Patent 5,686,100 assigned to Bristol-Myers Squibb, Prophylactic and therapeutic treatment of skin sensitization and irritation (November 1997).

69. Wille, J., U.S. Patent 5,716,987 assigned to Bristol-Myers Squibb, Prophylactic and therapeutic treatment of skin sensitization and irritation (February 1998).

70. Wille, J., Kydonieus, A., and Castellana, F., U.S. Patent 5,618,557 assigned to Bristol-Myers Squibb, Prophylactic treatment of allergic contact dermatitis (April 1997).

71. Wille, J., Kydonieus, A., and Castellana, F., World Patent Application WO 9,718,782 assigned to Bristol-Myers Squibb, Treatment with calcium channel blockers for drug induced hypersensitivity (May 1997).

72. Granstein, R. D. and Gallo, R. L., World Patent Application WO 9,009,792 assigned to General Hospital Corp., Topical application of amiloride or analogues thereof for treatment of inflammation (September 1990).

73. Grant, A. and Diezel, W., U.S. Patent 5,202,130 assigned to Johns Hopkins, Suppression of exzematous dermatitis by calcium transport inhibition (April 1993).

74. Sharpe, R. J., South African Patent ZA 9,006,583 assigned to Beth Israel Hospital, Treatment of cutaneous hypersensitivity with topical calcium channel blockers (September 1991).

75. Diezel, W., East German Patent DD 297,062 assigned to TKS Optimum, Magnesium salts as topical inflammation inhibitors of the skin (January 1992).

76. Hahn, G. S. and Theuson, D. O., World Patent Application WO 9,619,181 assigned to Cosmederm Technologies, Formulation and method for reducing skin irritation (June 1996).

77. De Lacharriere, O. and Breton, L., French Patent 2,740,341 assigned to L'Oreal, Use of metallic salts in the treatment of cutaneous pain and prevention of irritation (October 1996).

78. Modak, S. M. and Advani, B. H., U.S. Patent 5,708,023 assigned to Columbia University, Zinc gluconate gel compositions (January 1998).

79. Dwyer, D. S. and Esenther, K., U.S. Patent 5,489,441 assigned to Procept Inc., Method for suppressing immune response associated with psoriasis, contact dermatitis and diabetes mellitus (February 1996).

80. Missaen, J. et al., Ruthenium Red and compound 48/80 inhibit the smooth-muscle plasma membrane of pig stomach cells, *Biochem. Biophys. Acta,* 1023, 449, 1990.

81. Kapus, A. et al., Ruthenium Red inhibits mitochondrial Na^+ and K^+ uniports induced by magnesium removal., *J. Biol. Chem.*, 265, 18063, 1990.

82. Richie, J. M. and Greene, N. M., Local anesthetics, in Goodman and Gilman's *The Pharmacological Basis of Therapeutics*, 8th ed., Gilman, A.G. et al., Eds., McGraw-Hill, New York, 1993, 312.

83. Bernstein, J. E., U.S. Patent 4,997,853 assigned to Galenpharma, Method and compositions utilizing capsaicin as an external analgesic (March 1991).

84. Bannon, Y. B., Corish, J., Corrigan, O., Geoghegan, E., and Masterson, J., U.S. Patent 5,298,257 assigned to Elan Transdermal, Method for treatment of withdrawal symptoms associated with smoking cessation and preparations for use in said method (March 1994).

85. Patel, D. C. and Ebert, C. D., U.S. Patent 4,855,294 assigned to Theratech, Method for reducing skin irritation associated with drug/penetration enhancer compositions (August 1989).

86. Waali, E. E., U.S. Patent 4,663,151 to Research Corporation, Aluminum chlorhydrate as a prophylactic treatment for poison oak, poison ivy and poison sumac dermatitis (May 1987).

87. Cauwenbergh, G., U.S. Patent 5,476,853 to Janssen Pharmaceutica, Agent for use as an anti-irritant (December 1995).

88. De Lacharriere, O. and Breton L., World Patent Application WO 9,717,077 to L'Oreal, Topical composition containing capsazepine (May 1997).

89. Breton, L., European Patent Application EP 0,723,774A assigned to L'Oreal, Use of an antagonist of CGRP in a cosmetic, pharmaceutical or dermatological composition (January 1996).

90. Schmidt, R. J., U.S. Patent 5,578,300 assigned to U.C.C. Consultants, Treatment of allergic contact dermatitis (November 1996).

91. Wilder, M. S., World Patent Application WO 860,256 to Centerchem, A method for preventing or alleviating skin irritation using a formulation containing superoxide dismutase (May 1986).

92. Huber, W. and Saifer, M. G., In *Superoxide and Superoxide Dismutases*, Michelson, A. M. et al., Eds., Academic Press, New York, 1977, 517.

15 Glucocorticoids

Michel Cormier, James Matriano, and Alfred Amkraut

CONTENTS

I. INTRODUCTION

As outlined in the first chapter, many drugs of interest for transdermal delivery have the potential to elicit a local inflammatory response. In addition, a number of complex factors associated with the system itself can influence the biocompatibility of the therapeutic transdermal system. Whether the initial insult is attributable to irritation, sensitization, or a combination thereof, glucocorticoids (GCs) have had a long history in the treatment of inflammatory processes. However, the physiological actions of GCs are diverse and include regulation of carbohydrate and protein metabolism, as well as hormonal regulation. With respect to anti-inflammatory activity, GCs have been used both topically and systemically. Systemic administration of GCs is frequently used to suppress inflammatory responses. However, practical considerations make their use difficult or unacceptable for concomitant transdermal therapy and attempts to develop an inhibitory strategy using GCs should be limited to topical administration.

The use of topical GCs offers several advantages, including reduced dose requirement of GCs, increased local concentration by focused targeting, and lowered risks of side effects. Much of the information concerning characterization, mechanism of action, and use of topical steroids has previously been compiled.[1] Here we shall briefly summarize the salient points important to the use of GCs in prevention of local inflammatory reactions, concentrating on the inhibition of irritation and contact sensitization.

II. MECHANISM OF ACTION

Steroids act by combining with cytoplasmic receptors on target cells.[2] The GC receptor (GR) is a ubiquitous molecule that consists of three domains: steroid binding, DNA binding, and modulatory. Inactive GR is complexed with proteins such as heat shock protein 90 (HSP90), HSP70, and immunophilin. Following GC uptake by the cell, GC binds to the steroid binding domain of the inactive GR, a process that induces a conformational change, releasing proteins such as HSP70, HSP90, and immunophilin from GR. The GC–GR complex translocates into the nucleus where the complex binds to glucocorticoid-response elements (GREs) of DNA. The currently acknowledged GRE DNA consensus sequence is GGTACnnnTGTTCT, where n is any nucleotide.[3] The modulation domain of the GR regulates the degree of the steroid's effects on the transcription of target gene(s). The activated DNA binding domain acts either directly or in combination with other proteins as a transcription activation or repression factor, resulting in increased or decreased production of its target proteins, respectively.[4–6]

Inhibition of transcription of target genes profoundly inhibits inflammation. Such is the case with the transcription factor NF-κB, a heterodimer (p50 and p65) important in the regulation of cytokine gene transcription. Cytoplasmic NF-κB is inactivated by a complex of inhibitory proteins such as IκBα and IκBβ. GCs have been demonstrated to inhibit translocation of NF-κB by increasing the rate of synthesis of IκBα. The increased expression of IκBα maintains sequestration of NF-κB in the cytoplasm, thereby inhibiting the transcription of a number of cytokine genes.[5,7]

Included in the list of GC targets are phospholipase A_2, leukotrienes (arachidonic acid and its metabolites), Interleukins (IL-1, IL-2, IL-3, IL-4, IL-6), tumor necrosis factor alpha (TNF-α), interferon gamma (IFN-γ), granulocyte/monocyte colony stimulating factor (GM-CSF), histamine, acute phase reactants, intracellular adhesion molecule (ICAM-1), and endothelial leukocyte adhesion molecule (ELAM-1) also known as E-selectin.[3] Inhibition of IL-1 production by monocyte/macrophages results in diminished antigen-presenting capacity, thereby inhibiting T cell activation. Inhibition of IL-2 and IFN-γ directly prevents T cell proliferation, activation, and differentiation. Reduced expression of ICAM-1 and ELAM-1 on vascular endothelial cells inhibits T cell and neutrophil trafficking.[8]

The anti-inflammatory and immunosuppressive effects of GCs occur at multiple levels. Gene targets vary with cell type, and the specific mechanisms of GC action remain undetermined in many cases. The cell types regulated by GCs include lymphocytes, monocyte/macrophages, basophils, mast cells, and endothelial cells.[3] Systemic administration of GCs results in an increase of circulating neutrophils and in a concomitant decrease of most other leukocytes. Topical application of GCs has been shown to diminish antigen-presenting capacity of Langerhans cells[9–15] as well as T cell and mast cell number.[16]

Reports demonstrate that susceptibility to the effect of GCs varies among different species.[17,18] In some cases, these differences have been linked to differences in the binding affinity of the GC to the GR. A notable example is the guinea pig, in which high levels of circulating hydrocortisone (HC) and a low GR affinity for GCs have been reported.[19] These findings indicate that caution will have to be exercised before extrapolating preclinical results to humans.

III. CONSIDERATIONS FOR GC INTERVENTION IN INFLAMMATION

Penetration of HC through the skin, although sufficient to treat mild inflammatory processes, is quite low. This type of therapy is not adequate for reduction of major skin inflammation. Permeation enhancers or an adequate vehicle have been used to increase HC effectiveness.[20] In addition, topical GCs with improved intrinsic potencies and higher skin permeability have been designed successfully. Increased potency has been accomplished by higher binding affinity of the GC to the GC receptor.[21] Higher skin permeability usually results from increasing the lipophilicity of the drug.[22] Other parameters such as binding to other proteins in skin and circulation may also affect the local or systemic persistence of GCs.

Because of glucocortocoids' extensive and diverse range of targets in the suppression of inflammatory processes, their clinical use for palliative treatment has been immense. Over the years, the pharmaceutical industry has developed a large number of GC derivatives. Although one would obviously want to use the most efficacious drug, the side effects of GCs, which parallel efficacy, can be severe, limiting their use. The main adverse systemic side effect is the inhibition of the pituitary–adrenal axis. This inhibition can become significant even in topical use when larger areas are treated.[23] GCs can significantly inhibit the immune system both locally and systemically, causing increased susceptibility to infection, particularly in otherwise immunosuppressed individuals. A potentially major local side effect of topical steroid application is thinning of the skin. This side effect usually appears after long-term application of steroids on the same site.[24,25] In practice, this side effect is not likely to be observed if the application site of the steroid is rotated (i.e., moved from one skin site to another). Finally, a troublesome side effect of transdermal GC delivery is the potential to develop contact sensitivity to the steroid. Although sensitization to GCs is rare, many reports have established its occurrence and severity.[26–31] Nevertheless, published information suggests that, in most documented cases, a predisposed terrain such as atopic dermatitis or a history of long-term topical steroid application on skin lesions such as psoriasis may favor the development of an immune response against the steroid.

Little use, if any, has been made of GCs to prevent skin reactions resulting from transdermal delivery. The reactions that are of most interest in the context of this monograph are drug- or excipient-induced irritation or sensitization. It is important to distinguish between these two types of inflammation because of the differences in the kinetic of appearance of the response.

IV. GC EFFECTS ON IRRITATION

Nonpharmacological irritation is caused by the caustic effect of an agent on skin components, most important, those of the epidermis or the papillary dermis. Apparently, irritation is linked to the cytotoxicity of the drug being delivered through the skin.[32] Damage to keratinocytes and other cellular components of the epidermis results in the release of inflammatory mediators, principally the products of arachidonic acid activation cascade (see Chapter 11). In addition, TNF-α and IL-1 are thought to be among the chief mediators of inflammation. IL-1α abounds in keratinocytes, whereas IL-1β is produced by Langerhans cells. Release of inflammatory mediators may also result from pharmacological activity of the drug. Drugs that can trigger this release include prostaglandins, neuropeptides, and vasodilators.[33–34]

Another mechanism of drug-induced irritation is degranulation of mast cells, possibly caused by a number of pharmacologic agents such as opiates.[35] Mast cells are located in the papillary dermis. Their granules contain histamine as well as other inflammation mediators. Mast cell degranulation also results from the action of TNF, IL-1, or neuropeptides. In vitro studies have demonstrated that mast cell degranulation can be inhibited by HC and other GCs; this inhibition is observed only at high concentrations of GCs.[36] Although the reported tissue concentrations cannot be achieved in peripheral tissues during systemic GC delivery, such concentrations are achieved during transdermal delivery of HC.[37] Unfortunately, in vivo demonstration of this effect in humans seems to be lacking. The mechanism of inhibition of mast cell degranulation by GCs may result from the increased stability of the cell plasma membrane by GC insertion into the lipid bilayer.

Although pretreating a skin site with GCs before application of an irritant may be effective, GC coadministered with an irritant may fail to have an effect. The stratum corneum acts as a reservoir for steroids and a long lag time exists between an application and the effective penetration of the steroid through this barrier.[38] As a result, permeation of GCs through the skin can trail diffusion of the irritant.

Furthermore, development of an effect on transcription and consequent decrease or increase in concentrations of affected proteins may lag the start of the irritant's caustic effect. Therefore, absence of pretreatment with the GC before initiating drug transdermal delivery may result in suboptimal anti-irritant effect of the GC. When developing a strategy of pretreatment or coformulation of GCs with a transdermal system, a comprehensive understanding includes knowledge of drug kinetics and GC permeation into the skin, formulation compatibility, and compliance. Moreover, because potency among GCs is related to their vasoconstrictive properties, potential changes in the pharmacokinetic or pharmacodynamic properties of transdermally delivered therapeutic drug(s) can be substantial.[39] As expected, many contradictory reports regarding the effect of steroids on irritation exist, probably as a result of these considerations.[40–44] In addition, efficacy of the GC probably will depend on the severity of the inflammation response.

To evaluate the effect of HC codelivery on drug-induced skin irritation, we studied the coadministration by electrically assisted delivery systems of HC with the mild irritant metoclopramide

HCl (MCP).[45] MCP is an antiemetic prescription drug. It is a water-soluble drug salt with cationic properties. Transport of MCP and HC can be accomplished using custom-built iontophoretic devices described as electrotransport (ET) delivery systems. While most of MCP transport is accomplished via iontophoresis (i.e., migration of ionized drug molecules in an electric field), HC transport is mainly the result of electroosmosis (i.e., migration of non-ionized molecules in an electric field). Electrotransport through the skin occurs chiefly through aqueous pathways (i.e., sweat glands and hair follicles). As a result, the stratum corneum, which accounts for most of the reservoir effect observed during the transdermal delivery of steroids, is bypassed during ET, resulting in a reduced transport lag time of HC.

The ET system comprised a silver anode (donor) reservoir gel containing a 10% aqueous solution of MCP and 0.5% HC. The electrodes were connected to a DC power source that supplied a constant level of electric current of 100 $\mu A/cm^2$.

A randomized crossover study was performed on seven Caucasian male volunteers. The study protocol was approved by the Medical Review Board at Alza. Informed, written consent was obtained from each subject. Each subject wore two electrotransport systems, one on each upper arm for 4 h. During the first week, four subjects wore two systems containing MCP and four subjects wore two systems containing MCP plus HC in the anode compartments. One week later, each subject repeated the procedure with the alternate type of metoclopramide system.

Skin sites were evaluated for irritation (a*) using a Minolta Croma Meter at 1, 4, 24, and 48 h following system removal. An a* value of 1 to 2 represents a slight redness or erythema, an a* value of 3.5 to 4.5 represents a moderate redness or erythema, and an a* value above 7 represents severe redness or erythema. Skin sites were also evaluated visually at 0, 4, 24, and 48 h following system removal.

To measure MCP delivery and confirm that the addition of HC does not affect MCP transport, blood samples (10 ml) were taken from each patient immediately before application of the systems (time 0 h) and at 0.5, 1, 2, 3, 4, 4.5, 5, 6, 8, and 20 h after system application. Plasma concentrations of MCP were determined by high-performance liquid chromatography (HPLC). Results clearly demonstrated that the addition of HC into the MCP-containing drug reservoir of the electrotransport system did not significantly affect the delivery of MCP into the bloodstream (no differences in C_{max}, T_{max}, and AUC). In addition, in vitro studies through human cadaver skin demonstrated that in similar conditions, HC flux was about 2.75 $\mu g/(cm^2\ h)$.

Figure 1 illustrates a plot of skin irritation (a*) vs. time following system removal from the skin for the skin sites in contact with the anodic donor reservoirs containing MCP only, or MCP with HC. As demonstrated, the addition of HC to the anodic reservoirs of MCP-containing ET systems resulted in less skin irritation compared to systems containing no HC. A similar effect of HC on MCP-induced irritation was observed with HC concentration as low as 0.05%. Visual evaluation yielded identical results.

These results demonstrate that the beneficial effect of HC can be achieved by simultaneous delivery of steroid and drug without HC pretreatment.

V. GC EFFECTS ON CONTACT SENSITIZATION

An irritant requires no prior exposure to produce inflammation. In contrast, a major distinguishing feature of immunity is memory: an induction or sensitization phase (1 to 2 weeks) is required to generate an immune response to a given antigen. Typically, no visible skin response is observed during this period. Thereafter, each reexposure to the sensitizing chemical (i.e., antigen) elicits an inflammatory response. The details of contact sensitization mechanisms have been discussed elsewhere in this book.

The mediators of inflammation observed during an irritation response are often identical to those observed during a sensitization response. Indeed, they are inextricably linked to pathways critical to elicit inflammation. Many of these pathways are coincidentally GC targets, potentially making

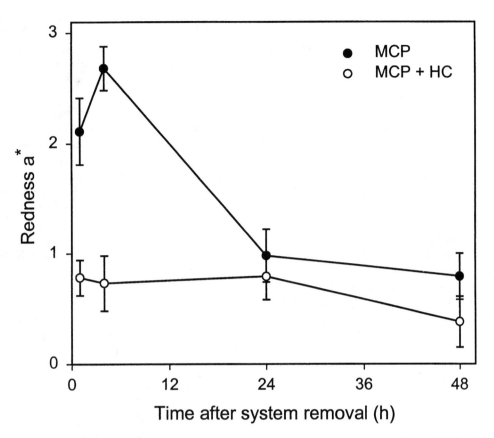

Figure 1   Skin erythema after 4 h electrotransport of metoclopramide (MCP) or MCP + 0.5% hydrocortisone (HC). Erythema was evaluated with the Minolta Chroma Meter at 1, 4, 24, and 48 h after removal of the ET systems. The measurement of skin erythema for these tests is given as a*, defined as the difference of the mean a* reading for the electrotransport-treated samples minus the mean a* reading for the untreated samples. Minolta measurements were made by taking the mean a* value of three readings at adjacent untreated sites and subtracting that value from the mean of three readings taken at the treated site.

GCs a broad-based anti-inflammatory agent. For example, with respect to inhibition of sensitization, GCs suppress key targets such as IL-2 production, and they inhibit antigen presentation.

The anti-inflammatory actions of GCs will obviously affect the efferent (elicitation) arm of the response (an inflammatory event). However, afferent (induction) inhibition is needed to prevent sensitization. Contact sensitization is believed to be initiated chiefly by presentation of the antigen on Langerhans cells. These cells migrate to the draining lymph node, where they encounter and activate specific T cells.[46]

Topical application of GCs has been demonstrated to reduce the number of Langerhans cells and alter antigen presenting cell function. After 10 to 14 days of treating guinea pig or human skin with topical GCs, Langerhans cells decrease significantly in number or disappear completely.[9,10] Toews et al.[47] showed that application of sensitizing compounds to sites with a decreased local density of Langerhans cells resulting from ultraviolet exposure led to anergy and eventual tolerance. This finding suggests that prevention of sensitization can occur by decreasing the density of Langerhans cells in the area of application. GCs trigger this decrease, but the decrease requires several days of treatment when sensitization could occur. GCs also have been shown to decrease cell surface Class II MHC expression.[11] Release of cytokines from the Langerhans cells, especially IL-1 and IL-6, is required for proper activation and expansion of T lymphocytes.[6,12,48] As indicated before, production and release of this cytokine in macrophages and monocytes is inhibited by GCs.

By pretreating skin with betamethasone and then applying a potent sensitizer, dinitrochlorobenzene, to the treated site, Burrows and Stoughton[49] demonstrated the efficacy of steroids in preventing sensitization in humans. Betamethasone was further applied twice daily for 14 days. This treatment blocked the development of the immune response in most subjects. However, the response to reexposure to dinitrochlorobenzene showed that subjects had not become tolerant to the drug.

Although transdermal delivery has been available for many years, only a few reports describe codelivery or pretreatment of a GC with a sensitizing drug in order to prevent sensitization to the drug.[39,50] Indeed, most reports show the effect of GCs on classic antigens such as poison oak or oxazolone.[51–54] This paucity of reports is probably the result of problems associated with coformulation of the agents and the effective codelivery of both agents. To demonstrate the effectiveness of this strategy, we studied the impact of codelivery of HC with the sensitizing agents benzoyl peroxide and chlorpheniramine (CP).[50] Sensitization to CP was achieved in female volunteers by repeatedly applying passive CP transdermal patches (with or without HC). Volunteers wore patches continuously on the same site for 3 weeks with a patch change every 2 to 3 days. A challenge with a CP patch (without HC) was performed 2 weeks after the last induction application to untreated skin sites. A similar protocol was used with benzoyl peroxide. HC flux through the skin was measured through isolated human epidermis and was found to be in the range 0.05 to 0.5 µg/(cm² h). Flux of CP was unaffected by the presence of HC. The results demonstrated that the incidence of sensitization toward CP was reduced from approximately 45 to 7.5% by codelivery of HC. A similar reduction of the sensitization to benzoyl peroxide was observed (Figure 2). A further reduction in the sensitization rate toward CP, without HC, was

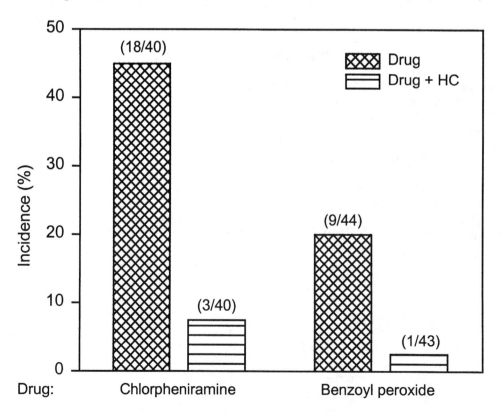

Figure 2   Incidence of sensitization toward chlorpheniramine and benzoyl peroxide in humans following nine applications on the same site of the respective drug. Induction systems contained the drugs chlorpheniramine maleate (8%) or benzoyl peroxide (5%) or the drug formulated with 2% hydrocortisone (HC). Challenge was performed with 8% chlorpheniramine maleate or 5% benzoyl peroxide.

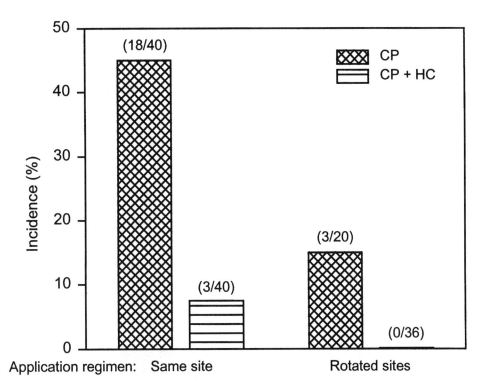

Figure 3   Incidence of sensitization toward chlorpheniramine in humans following nine applications on the same skin site or on different (rotated) sites. Systems contained 8% chlorpheniramine maleate (CP) or CP + 2% hydrocortisone (CP + HC). Challenge was performed with CP systems. The number in parentheses indicates the number of sensitized subjects over the total number of subjects.

achieved simply by rotating the application sites during the induction regimen. In this instance, different skin sites were exposed to CP patches without reexposure to any previously treated site. This scheme led to a reduction in the sensitization rate from 45% (18 of 40) to 15% (3 of 20). Moreover, under a rotating application regimen, codelivery with HC led to a further reduction in response from 7.5% (3 of 40) to 0% (0 of 36) (Figure 3). These 36 nonresponsive subjects underwent 12 additional applications of patches containing CP with HC under a rotating application regimen. Upon challenge with CP, no response could be elicited. Thereafter, an additional nine induction regimens with chlorpheniramine without HC were performed. Again, no response could be elicited with CP, suggesting that tolerance toward chlorpheniramine may have been achieved (Figure 4). Collectively, the inability to mount a sensitization response could be linked to the codelivery of HC during the induction phase.

The mechanism of tolerance, though not completely understood, frequently results from administering potentially antigenic substances in immune-privileged tissues. Classical experiments in contact sensitization have demonstrated this principle.[55] In addition, evidence indicates that tolerance may require antigen presence for prolonged maintenance,[56] a requirement that is accomplished during repeated transdermal therapy.

VI. CONCLUSION

GCs have been used for many years to suppress inflammation and immune responses, but their mechanism of action in suppressing contact sensitivity is still not entirely understood. As demonstrated in this book, a number of strategies are available to prevent or minimize skin reactions

Inductions	Challenge	Inductions	Challenge	Inductions	Challenge
⇩⇩⇩⇩⇩⇩⇩⇩⇩	3/20 (15%)				
⇕⇕⇕⇕⇕⇕⇕⇕⇕	0/36 (0%)	⇕⇕⇕⇕⇕⇕⇕⇕⇕⇕⇕⇕	0/36 (0%)	⇩⇩⇩⇩⇩⇩⇩⇩⇩	0/36 (0%)

Inductions:
⇩ Chlorpheniramine (8%)
⇕ Chlorpheniramine (8%) + hydrocortisone (2%)

Challenge: Chlorpheniramine (8%).

Figure 4 Incidence of sensitization toward chlorpheniramine in humans following nine applications on rotated sites. Induction and challenge were identical to Figure 3. Nonresponsive subjects exposed to CP + HC received 12 additional applications of CP + HC followed by a challenge with CP. Thereafter they received nine CP applications followed by a CP challenge. The numbers indicate the number of sensitized subjects over the total number of subjects. Percentages of sensitized individuals are given in parentheses.

occurring during the transdermal delivery of drugs. Due to the broad range of activity of GCs on the inflammatory processes, codelivery of GCs seems to be a preferred choice. The use of superpotent steroids may be limited due to the potential for local and systemic side effects. The use of HC may be a good alternative as the amount needed to produce inhibition is a small fraction of the endogenous production. In addition, local side effects such as skin thinning have not been observed with this steroid. Work is ongoing in our laboratory and elsewhere to develop this technology.

REFERENCES

1. Korting, H. C. and Maibach, H. I. (Eds). *Curr. Probl. Dermatol.*, 21, 1, 1993.
2. Ponec, M., Glucocorticoid receptors, *Curr. Probl. Dermatol.*, 21, 20, 1993.
3. Goodman and Gilman's *The Pharmacological Basis of Therapeutics*, 9th ed., McGraw-Hill, New York, 1996, 1465.
4. Corsini, E., Terzoli, A., Bruccoleri, A., Marinovich, M., and Galli, C. L., Induction of tumor necrosis factor-alpha in vivo by a skin irritant, tributyllin, through activation of transcription factors: its pharmacological modulation by anti-inflammatory drugs, *J. Invest. Dermatol.*, 108, 892, 1997.
5. Auphan, N., DiDonato, J. A., Rosette, C., Helmberg, A., and Karin, M., Immunosuppression by glucocorticoids: Inhibition by NF-κB activity through induction of IκB synthesis, *Science*, 270, 286, 1995.
6. Zanker, B., Walz, G., Wieder, K. J., and Strom, T. B., Evidence that glucocorticosteroids block expression of the human interleukin-6 gene by accessory cells, *Transplantation*, 49, 183, 1990.
7. Scheinman, R. I., Cogswell, P. C., Lofquist, A.K., and Baldwin, A. S., Role of transcriptional activation of IκBα in mediation of immunosuppression by glucocorticoids, Science, 270, 283, 1995.
8. Prens, E. P., Benne, K., Geursen-Reitsma, A. M., van Dijk, G., Benner, R., and van Joost, T. H., Effects of topically applied glucocorticosteroids on patch test responses and recruitment of inflammatory cells in allergic contact dermatitis, *Agents Actions*, 26, 125, 1989.
9. Belsito, D. V., Flotte, T. J., Lim, H. W., Baer, R.L., Thorbecke, G. J., and Gigli, I., Effect of glucocorticosteroids on epidermal Langerhans cells, *J. Exp. Med.*, 155, 291, 1982.
10. Berman, B., France, D. S., Martinelli, O. P., et al., Modulation of expression of epidermal Langerhans cell properties following in situ exposure to glucocorticosteroids, *J. Invest. Dermatol.*, 80, 168, 1983.
11. Furue, M., and Katz, S.I., Direct effects of glucocorticoids on epidermal Langerhans cells, *J. Invest. Dermatol.*, 92, 342, 1989.

12. Kitajima, T., Ariizumi, K., Bergstresser, P.R., and Takashima, A., A novel mechanism of glucocorti-coid-induced immune suppression: the inhibition of T cell-mediated terminal maturation of a murine dendritic cell line, *J. Clin. Invest.*, 98, 142, 1996.

13. Ashworth, J., Booker, J., and Breathnach, S. M., Effects of topical corticosteroid therapy on Langer-hans cell antigen presenting function in human skin, *Br. J. Dermatol.*, 118, 457, 1988.

14. Ashworth, J., Kahan, M.C., and Breathanach, S.M., Flow cytometrically-sorted residual HLA-DR + T6 + Langerhans cells in topical steroid-treated human skin express normal amounts of HLA-DR and CD1a/T6 antigens and exhibit normal alloantigen-presenting capacity, *J. Invest. Dermatol.*, 92, 258, 1989.

15. Mommaas, A.M., Influence of glucocorticoids on the epidermal Langerhans cell, *Curr. Probl. Der-matol.*, 21, 67, 1993.

16. Finotto, S., Mekori, Y. A., and Metcalfe, D. D., Glucocorticoids decrease tissue mast cell number by reducing the production of the c-kit ligand, stem cell factor, by resident cells, *J. Clin. Invest.*, 99, 1721, 1997.

17. Keightley, M. C., and Fuller, P. J., Cortisol resistance and the guinea pig glucocorticoid receptor, *Steroids*, 60, 87, 1995.

18. Klosterman, L. L., Murai, J. T., and Siiteri, P.K., Cortisol level, binding, and properties of corticos-teroid-binding globulin in the serum of primates, *Endocrinology*, 118, 424, 1986.

19. Keightley, M. C., and Fuller, P. J., Unique sequences in the guinea pig glucocorticoid receptor induce constitutive transactivation and decrease steroid sensitivity, *Mol. Endocrinol.*, 8, 431, 1994.

20. Barry, B. W., Southwell, D., and Woodford, R., Optimization of bioavailability of topical steroids: penetration enhancers under occlusion, *J. Invest. Dermatol.*, 82, 49, 1984.

21. Hogger, P. and Rohdewald, P., Binding kinetics of fluticasone propionate to the human glucocorticoid receptor, *Steroids*, 59, 597, 1994.

22. Ackermann, C., Flynn, G. L., and Smith, W. M., Ether-water partitioning and permeability through nude mouse skin in vitro. II. HC 21-n-alkyl esters, alkanols and hydrophilic compounds, *Int. J. Pharm.*, 36, 67, 1987.

23. Munro, D. D., The effect of percutaneously absorbed steroids on hypothalamic-pituitary-adrenal function after intensive use in in-patients, *Br. J. Dermatol.*, 94, 67, 1976

24. Lavker, R. M., Schechter, N. M., and Lazarus, G. S., Effects of topical glucocorticoids on human dermis, *Br. J. Dermatol.*, 115, 101, 1986.

25. Lubach, D., Bensmann, A., and Bornemann, U., Steroid-induced dermal atrophy, *Dermatologica*, 179, 67, 1989.

26. Lauerma, A. I. and Reitamo, S., Clinical Reviews. Contact allergy to glucocorticoids, *J. Am. Acad. Dermatol.*, 28, 618, 1993.

27. Rivara, G., Tomb, R. R., and Foussereau, J., Allergic contact dermatitis from topical glucocorticoids, *Contact Dermatitis*, 21, 83, 1989.

28. Dooms-Goossens, A., Meinardi, M. M. H. M., Bos, J. D., and Degreef, H., Contact allergy to glucocorticoids: the results of a two-centre study, *Br. J. Dermatol.*, 130, 42, 1994.

29. Belsito, D. V., Allergic contact dermatitis to topical glucocorticosteroids, *CUTIS*, 52, 291, 1993.

30. Whitmore, S. E., Delayed systemic allergic reactions to glucocorticoids, *Contact Dermatitis*, 32, 193, 1995.

31. Freeman, S., Corticosteroid allergy, *Contact Dermatitis*, 33, 240, 1995.

32. Mize, N. K., Johnson, J. A., Hansch, C., and Cormier, M., Quantitative structure-activity relationship and cytotoxicity, *Curr. Probl. Dermatol.*, 23, 224, 1995.

33. Armstrong, R. A., Marr, C., and Jones, R. L., Characterization of the EP-receptor mediating dilatation and potentiation of inflammation in rabbit skin, *Prostaglandins*, 49(4), 205, 1995.

34. Baluk, P., Neurogenic inflammation in skin and airways, *J. Invest. Dermatol. Symp. Proc.*, 2(1), 76, 1997.

35. Casale, T. B., Bowman, S., and Kaliner, M., Induction of human cutaneous mast cell degranulation by opiates and endogenous opioid peptides: evidence for opiate and nonopiate receptor participation, *J. Allergy Clin. Immunol.*, 73(6), 775, 1984.

36. Grosman, N. and Jensen, S. M., Influence of glucocorticoids on histamine release and [45]calcium uptake by isolated rat mast cells, *Agents Actions*, 14, 21, 1984.

37. Schalla, W. and Schaefer. H., Localization of compounds in different skin layers and its use as an indicator of percutaneous absorption, *Percutaneous Absorption: Mechanisms, Methodology, Drug Delivery*, Bronaugh, R. L. and Maibach, H. I., Eds., Marcel Dekker, New York, 1985, chap. 22.

38. Foreman, M. I. and Clanachan, I., Steroid diffusion and binding in human stratum corneum, *J. Chem. Soc.*, 80, 3439, 1984.

39. Ito, M. K. and O'Connor, D. T., Skin pretreatment and the use of transdermal clonidine, *Am. J. Med.*, 91, 42S, 1991.

40. van der Valk, P.G.M. and Maibach, H. I., Do topical glucocorticoids modulate skin irritation in human beings? Assessment by transepidermal water loss and visual scoring, *J. Am. Acad. Dermatol.*, 21, 519, 1989.

41. Ramsing, D. W. and Agner, T., Efficacy of topical glucocorticoids on irritant skin reactions, *Contact Dermatitis*, 32, 293, 1995.

42. Duteil, L., Queille, C., Poncet, M., Ortonne, J. P., and Czernielewski, J., Objective assessment of topical glucocorticoids and non-steroidal anti-inflammatory drugs in methyl-nicotinate-induced skin inflammation, *Clin. Exp. Dermatol.*, 15, 195, 1990.

43. Anderson, C. D. and Groth, O., Influence on the dermal cellular infiltrate of topical steroid applications and vehicles in guinea pig skin: normal skin, allergic and toxic reactions, *Contact Dermatitis*, 10, 193, 1984.

44. Wilson, D. E., Kaidbey, K., Boike, S. C., and Jorkaski, D. K., Use of topical corticosteroid pretreatment to reduce the incidence and severity of skin reactions associated with testosterone transdermal therapy, *Clin. Ther.*, 20, 299, 1998.

45. Ledger, P., Cormier, M., and Campbell, P., U.S. Patent 5,693,010, Reduction of skin irritation during electrotransport delivery, 1997.

46. Kripke, M. L., Munn, C. G., Jeevan, A., Tang, J.M., and Bucana, C., Evidence that cutaneous antigen-presenting cells migrate to regional lymph nodes during contact sensitization, *J. Immunol.*, 145, 2833, 1990.

47. Toews, G. B., Bergstresser, P. R., and Streilein, J. W., Epidermal Langerhans cell density determines whether contact hypersensitivity or unresponsiveness follows skin painting with DNFB, *J. Immunol.*, 124, 445, 1980.

48. Katz, S., The skin as an immunological organ: allergic contact dermatitis as a paradigm, *J. Dermatol.*, 20, 593, 1993.

49. Burrows, W. M. and Stoughton, R. B., Inhibition of induction of human contact sensitization by topical glucocorticosteroids, *Arch. Dermatol.*, 112, 175, 1976.

50. Amkraut, A. A., Jordan, W. P., and Taskovich, L., Effect of coadministration of corticosteroids on the development of contact sensitization, *J. Am. Acad. Dermatol.*, 35, 27, 1996.

51. Kepel, E., Rooks II, W. H., Rodolfo, M. S., Ferraresi, R. W., and Shott, L. D., Poison ivy/oak-induced delayed hypersensitivity in the guinea pig: inhibition with fluocinononide, *J. Invest. Dermatol.*, 62, 595, 1974.

52. Evans, D. P., Hossack, M., and Thompson, D. S., Inhibition of contact sensitivity in the mouse by topical application of glucocorticoids, *Br. J. Pharmacol.*, 43, 403, 1971.

53. Meurer, R., Opas, E. E., and Humes, J. L., Effects of cyclooxygenase and lipoxygenase inhibitors on inflammation associated with oxazolone-induced delayed hypersensitivity, *Biochemical Pharm.*, 37, 3511, 1988.

54. Rietschel, R. L., Irritant and allergic responses as influenced by triamcinolone in patch test materials, *Arch. Dermatol.*, 121, 68, 1985.

55. Macher, E. and Chase, M. W., Studies on the sensitization of animals with simple chemical compounds, *J. Exp. Med.*, 129, 103, 1969.

56. Ramsdell, F. and Fowlkes, B. J., Maintenance of in vivo tolerance by persistence of antigen, *Science*, 257, 1130, 1992.

16 Ion Channel Modulation of Contact Dermatitis

John J. Wille, Agis F. Kydonieus, and Richard S. Kalish

CONTENTS

I. INTRODUCTION

Ion channel modulators are an important class of therapeutic agents used in the treatment of various human chronic diseases.[1] For example, calcium ion channel blockers diltiazem, nifedipine, and verapamil; the sodium/hydrogen ion channel inhibitor, amiloride; and the potassium ion channel modulator and loop-diuretic drugs ethacrynic acid and bumetinide are effective cardiovascular drugs. Ion channel modulating agents that inhibit the $Kv1.3$ K^+ channels in T cells and agents that inhibit chloride ion channel in inflammatory cells are potential new agents for treatment of inflammatory diseases such as arthritis.[2] This chapter focuses on the role of ion channel modulators as potential therapeutic agents for treatment of contract dermatitis.

The current modality of treatment of contact dermatitis is limited to low and high potency topical glucocorticosteroids such as topical hydrocortisone and oral prednisone, respectively.[3] Recently, Ramsing and Agner reported that topical betamethasone-17 valerate had efficacy on irritant skin reaction in human patch test against sodium lauryl sulfate (SLS).[4] While topical hydrocortisone creams provide limited short-term benefit, the more potent glucocorticosteroids such as prednisone tend to have serious systemic and immunosuppressive side effects. Recently, favorable clinical results have been reported for the macrolide antibiotics, e.g., tacrolimus (FK 506).[5] The nonsteroidal anti-inflammatory drugs, NSAIDs, such as indomethacin, have little practical use as topical anti-inflammatory agents mainly because of their low potency coupled with poor skin penetration.[6] With growing evidence for involvement of free radicals and reactive oxygen species in the etiology of photodamaged skin, topical application of antioxidants holds promise as a future therapy against skin inflammation.[7] This may account for the recent report that *N*-acetyl-cysteine was effective in blocking contact hypersensitive reaction (CHR) in mice.[8] Nevertheless, the search for newer, more potent and safer immunomodulatory agents has led to examination of ion channel modulators.

Topical administration of many drugs results in adverse skin reactions including the development of contact allergic dermatitis.[9] Many potentially systemically acting drugs that otherwise are therapeutically beneficial and attain sufficient systemic doses when administered transdermally are prohibited from clinical use because they are either irritating or sensitizing when delivered via a transdermal patch.[10] For example, skin sensitiziation has been reported to occur in >20% of all patients receiving Catapres TTS® transdermal clonidine, an antihypertensive and antianginal drug.[11] A major limiting factor at present in the development of new transdermal drugs is their potential to cause adverse skin sensitization reactions. An approach drug manufacturers have pursued is to avoid use of potentially immunizing drugs by searching with computer-based QSAR programs designed to identify structural analogs lacking the immunogenicity of known skin-sensitizing congener drugs.[12,13]

Another approach to the problem of transdermal drug immunogenicity is to develop countersensitizers, i.e., topical agents that rapidly and reversibly modulate the skin immune system, when they are applied either before or together with the sensitizing drugs. In this regard, it was reported that coadministration of topical hydrocortisone prevented the development of skin sensitization reactions in patients receiving topically sensitizing doses of the antihistamine chlorpheniramine.[14] There have been prior reports that ion channel inhibitors such as amiloride, lanthanum, and diltiazem inhibit the sensitization phase of CHR.[15,16] Wille and co-workers also reported that ethacrynic acid abrogates sensitization of skin due to topical delivery of albuterol, chlorpheniramine, clonidine, and nadolol.[17]

This chapter reviews some salient findings indicating that diverse ion channel modulators abrogate CHR and irritant contact dermatitis in mouse models.

II. ION CHANNEL MODULATORS

A. EFFECT OF ION CHANNEL MODULATORS ON SKIN IRRITATION

Lanthanum and cerium ion-containing salts were proposed earlier in the patent literature as possible treatments for the symptoms of dermatitis, based primarily on data showing their inhibitory effects on ATPase activity.[18] Lanthanum ions are also well-known reversible competitive inhibitors and calcium ion antagonists for many physiologically relevant calcium binding proteins, including the regulatory subunits of mammalian calcium ion channel membrane proteins.[19,20] Although Diezel and colleagues reported that both lanthanides and diltiazem, an organic calcium ion channel blocker, inhibited the sensitization phase of CHR in mice, they did not report their effects on skin irritation.[16] Recently, L'Oreal scientists, DeLacharriere and Breton, have claimed salts of lanthanides as cosmetic ingredients in creams for treatment of skin irritation.[21]

Gallo and Granstein were the first to report that the sodium/ATPase ion channel inhibitor, amiloride, was effective in reducing UV-induced tissue swelling in mice.[15] Alza Corporation scientists have claimed ammonium salts and ionophores as agents altering cellular pH, to have ameliorating effects on skin irritation due to topically applied drugs.[22] They posit these effects as direct interference with the Na^+/H^+-ATPase ion pump. Finally, it has been reported that ruthenium red, an agent that interferes with mitochondrial calcium transport, inhibits contact dermatitis.[23]

B. EFFECT OF ION CHANNEL MODULATORS ON CONTACT HYPERSENSITIVITY

The inhibition of CHR by calcium channel antagonists, diltiazem in mice and verapamil in humans, has been reported.[16,24,25] The mechanism of inhibition has not been determined but may relate to the specific inhibitory effect of calcium channel blockers on cytokine-stimulated lymphocyte migration.[26] The latter authors showed that DSDZ 202-79, a dihydropyridine analog, but not a stereoisomer of the analog, which was inactive as a calcium channel antagonist, inhibited lymphocyte migration, implicating release of IL-1 α, IL-1 β, and IL-8 in the mechanism of cutaneous immunity.

Recently, Matsunaga et al. reported that skin exposed to haptens but not irritants induced IL-1 β mRNA, signifying a role for epidermal IL-1β in regulating hapten-induced cytokine signaling in the early events of CHR.[27] These results have been confirmed by Cumberbatch et al., who were able to block dendritic antigen-presenting cell migration to the local lymph nodes following antigenic stimulation by injection of monoclonal antibodies to IL-1β.[28]

The generality that ion channel modulators are also effective topical immunosuppressants was strengthened by studies of Gallo and Granstein showing that amiloride, a sodium–hydrogen channel antagonist, inhibited allergic contact dermatitis.[15] This notion was later challenged by Lindgren et al., who reported that several analogs of amiloride that lacked Na^+/H^+ ion channel inhibitory activity retained inhibitory activity against CHR.[29]

In an effort to resolve these conflicting reports, we undertook further studies to explore the inhibitory effects of two calcium channel antagonists, nifedipine and verapamil, on transdermal drug-induced CHR and additional supportive studies demonstrating that these calcium channel antagonists as well as the sodium–hydrogen ion channel modulator, amiloride, are effective in blocking the induction phase of CHR in mice.

Earlier studies established that a vitamin A hypervitaminosis-enhanced CBA/J mouse model was useful in demonstrating the sensitization potential of a number of weakly sensitizing drugs including nadolol, a beta-blocking cardiovascular drug.[30] This model was later employed to demonstrate that nifedipine and verapamil inhibit the induction phase of CHR in nadolol-sensitized CBA/J mice.[31] Nifedipine was found (Figure 1) to be a more potent inhibitor of CHR than verapamil (100% vs. 0 at 24 h postchallenge, 80% vs. 42% at 48 h postchallenge, and 100% vs. 60% at 72 h postchallenge). These results agree with the fact that nifedipine is a more potent calcium channel blocking drug than verapamil, i.e., daily dosage for nifedipine is 2 mg vs. 50 to 100 mg for verapamil. Also, it would be expected that nifedipine would have a greater flux and therefore be

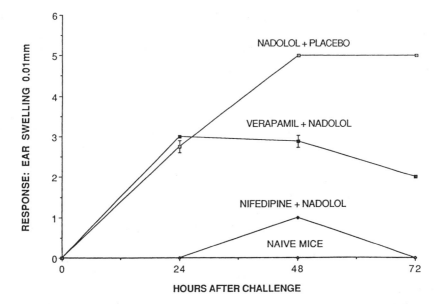

Figure 1   Abrogation of nadolol-induced contact hypersensitivity in CBA/J mice by calcium ion channel inhibitors. Mice (N = 10) were topically treated with either 0.5% nifedipine (nifedipine + nadolol, Δ-Δ), or 0.5% verapamil (verapamil + nadolol, ◯-◯) 1 day before each of three every-other-day topical nadolol (5% in vehicle) applications. Mice were challenged on the right ear with 1% nadolol 1 week after cessation of the last nadolol treatment. Ear thickness measurements were made 0, 24, 48, and 72 h after challenge. The left ear of each sensitized mouse was painted with vehicle only; it served as placebo control (nadolol + placebo, ·–·). Mice not sensitized with nadolol served as negative control (naive, □-□). (From Wille, J.J. et al., *Skin Pharm. Appl. Skin Physiol.*, 12: 15, 1999. With permission.)

more available transdermally than verapamil due to its smaller size (MW = 346.34) relative to verapamil (MW = 454.59).

In the same study, it was reported that both nifedipine and amiloride were effective inhibitors of the induction phase of dinitrochlorobenzene (DNCB)-induced CHR in mice. For example, a single application of nifedipine in a gel vehicle applied to the shaved abdomen of Balb/c mice 24 h prior to DNCB sensitization reduced the ear swelling response by an average of 80% relative to gel vehicle controls. Likewise, a single application of amiloride (1%) in a gel vehicle applied to the shaved abdomen of Balb/c mice 24 h prior to DNCB sensitization significantly reduced the ear swelling response by an average of 60% relative to vehicle control mice.

These studies confirm and extend the concept that interference with cutaneous ion channels inhibits the induction phase of CHR. The discrepant structure-activity for amiloride and its analogs requires further examination, and may reflect different sensitivities in relevant target cells used to assess ion channel activity vs. immune target cells regulating antigen processing and/or antigen presentation.

III. PREVENTION OF IRRITATION AND SENSITIZATION BY ETHACRYNIC ACID

Ethacrynic acid (ECA; Edecrin®) is a potent loop-diuretic drug often prescribed for the treatment of congestive heart failure.[32] It is still marketed in the U.S. but is now off-patent. Its chemical structure, formula weight, melting point, pKa, solubility in water and ethanol, and stability data are presented in Figure 2. Its diuretic activity is attributed to blockade of the sodium and potassium ion exchanger, resulting in the passive loss of potassium ions into the urine, and consequent failure of water uptake by tubule cells.[33] Part of the diuretic mechanism involves the covalent reaction of its chloride groups with sulfhydryl groups of proteins and enzymes such as carbonic anhydrase. A recent patent and literature search did not reveal any prior topical or dermatological applications. A patent was awarded to Bristol-Myers Squibb for prevention and treatment of irritant and allergic contact dermatitis.[34]

Wille et al. reported earlier that ECA in a gel vehicle prevented the induction phase of CHR in DNCB-sensitized Balb/c mice and in CBA/J mice sensitized with four different cutaneous drug sensitizers including albuterol, clonidine, chlorpheniramine, and nadolol.[17] Skin permeation studies showed no significant differences in flux rates of drug alone vs. drug in combination with ECA, eliminating the possibility that the expected null sensitization result was due to chemical interaction of ECA or a chemical complex between the drug and ECA that hindered transdermal delivery of the drug. Inhibition of nadolol-induced CHR required that ECA be applied to the skin site receiving the drug sensitizer delivered at least a few hours prior to sensitization. In addition, there was no significant difference in extent of inhibition of nadolol-sensitized CBA/J mice treated with ECA applied via an occluded gel vs. nonoccluded gel. Skin permeation studies also showed that the delivery of ECA was enhanced by an ethanol-containing gel relative to an aqueous gel formulation. These studies provided evidence that ECA is both a novel topical immunosuppressant and may permit the transdermal delivery of drugs that otherwise are safe but cause allergic skin reactions in patients that are sensitized by topical delivery of the drug.

In a recent study, Wille et al. reported that ECA was effective in inhibiting the elicitation phase of CHR. Balb/c mice were sensitized to DNCB on their bellies and challenged 5 days later on the ear with DNCB.[35] Positive control mice painted on the DNCB-challenged ear with a placebo gel vehicle, not containing ECA, developed significant ear swelling 24 h later. By contrast, the ear-swelling response was drastically reduced (>65%) in DNCB-sensitized mice that were treated with 1% ECA in gel vehicle 1 h after DNCB ear challenge. The ear swelling response was suppressed to the same extent by either 1% ECA or 1% hydrocortisone. In addition, it was shown that ECA was just as effective in suppressing the ear swelling response when applied 1 h after ear challenge in oxazolone-sensitized mice. Ethacrynic acid was reported to be very effective in preventing both the induction and elicitation phases of sensitization induced by the hair coloring oxidative dye,

ETHACRYNIC ACID

(2,3-dichloro-4 (2-methylene-1-oxobutyl)-phenoxyl acetic acid)

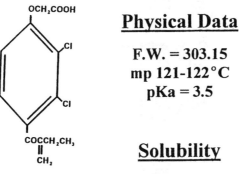

Physical Data

F.W. = 303.15
mp 121-122°C
pKa = 3.5

Solubility

Water 0.06%
Ethanol 66.0%

Stability

100% (21 Days at Room Temperature)

Figure 2 Physicochemical properties of ethacrynic acid: FW, formula weight; mp, melting point pKa, acid dissociation constant. Stability of ECA was determined from samples held for different lengths of time at pH 5 in an aqueous medium and withdrawn for HPLC analysis against authgentic ECA samples.

para-phenylenediamine (PPD). It suppressed induction of CHR by 43, 55, and 66% when assessed at 24, 48, and 72 h postchallenge, and totally inhibited the elicitation phase of PPD-induced CHR assessed at 24, 48, and 72 h postchallenge. These results indicate that ECA suppression is independent of the specific antigen used to immunize animals and acts generally to inhibit the efferent and well as the afferent arm of the skin immune system.

The good efficacy of ECA in inhibiting both the elicitation and induction phase of CHR prompted us to study its effect of skin irritation. A rapid and reliable mouse ear swelling test was developed that yielded quantitative assessment of irritant potency of a test substance. Preliminary experiments showed that the acetone vehicle alone causes no detectable ear swelling compared to untreated mouse ears. Irritant concentrations were chosen by first conducting a dose–response study to determine the lowest dose that produces significant ear swelling. Figure 3 presents data showing that 1% ECA applied to irritant-treated ears within 5 to 10 min after topical application significantly reduced ear swelling for a panel of six different irritants. It completely reduced the ear swelling due to 0.1% phorbol myristate acetate (PMA), 25% lactic acid (LA), and 1% trans-retinoic acid (tRA), and significantly reduced ear swelling due to 2% DNCB, 5% capsaicin (CA), and 2.5% arachidonic acid (AA). It was also reported that topical application of 1% ECA 2 h before topical application of 5% AA was also an effective treatment regime. The ear swelling response that was measured at peak swelling 2 h postchallenge with 5% AA was completely prevented, while ECA significantly reduced the ear swelling response due to topical ear application of 2% DNCB.

The anti-irritant activity of ECA was also compared with that of two topical NSAIDs, 1% ibuprofen or 1% indomethacin. Neither was as effective as ECA in preventing irritation produced by 5% AA alone, nor was topical 1% HC as effective as 1% ECA in reducing 5% AA-induced ear swelling.

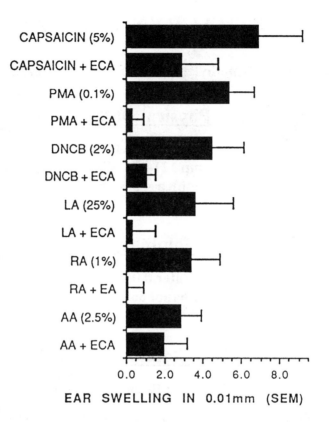

Figure 3   A. Histogram plot of data showing the difference in ear swelling with irritant alone vs. irritant plus ECA. Ears were treated first with irritants (a-f), and then 5 to 10 min later with 1% ECA. Irritants: (a) PMA (0.1%), (b) t-RA(1%), (c) DNCB (2%), (d) LA (25%), (e) CA (5%), and (f) AA (2.5%). B. Histogram plot of data showing the difference in ear swelling when mouse ears were pretreated with 1% ECA 2 h before topical application of irritants, 2% DNCB or 5% AA. (From Wille, J.J. et al., *Skin Pharm. Appl. Skin Physiol.*, 11: 282, 1998. With permission.)

Finally, ECA treatment was shown to prevent surfactant-induced cumulative skin irritation. ECA pretreatment was highly effective in preventing ear swelling due the surfactant, disodium laureth sulfonate (DSS), which was almost completely prevented by a 1-h pretreatment preceding each surfactant treatment. Although not as effective, topical ethacrynic acid significantly reduced, by 60%, the extent of ear swelling when presented simultaneously with 10% sodium lauryl sulfate (SLS). By contrast, posttreatment with 1% ECA had only a modest inhibitory effect on 10% SLS-induced irritation. Taken as a whole, the above results substantiate that ECA has broad-acting cutaneous anti-irritant activity.

IV. PREVENTION OF IRRITATION AND SENSITIZATION BY PHENOXYACETIC ACID METHYL ESTER (PAME)

The aim of another study was to develop a nondrug congener of ECA that is as potent an inhibitor of irritant and allergic contact dermatitis as ethacrynic acid.[36] Figure 4 is a computer-generated diagram of the stereochemical structures of PAME and ECA. PAME has the same phenoxyacetic acid backbone minus the chloride groups and methylene alkyl chain substituents and is the methyl ester of the phenoxyacetic acid. Unlike its chemical analog, it lacks topical diuretic activity. PAME-treated mice do not lose weight relative to vehicle-treated control mice. By contrast, ECA-treated mice lost $\geq 10\%$ body weight on average when treated topically for 4 consecutive days, but regained their original average body weight when the treatment was discontinued. In addition to losing body weight, chronic treatment of mouse skin with $\geq 1\%$ ECA results in red inflamed-looking skin. By contrast, PAME-treated mouse skin appeared normal.

The anti-irritant activity of PAME was assessed by a short-term mouse ear swelling test to quantitatively measure irritation that develops within 1 to 2 h after painting Balb/c mouse ears with an irritant. For every test irritant, preliminary dose ranging studies were conducted and the minimum concentration required to develop significant ear swelling employed as the positive control concentration. In a pretreat design, 1% PAME in vehicle was applied to the mouse ear 2 h earlier than a single application of 0.5% AA in vehicle to the same ear. In a posttreat design, 1% PAME in vehicle was applied 15 min after a single application of 0.5% AA. PAME completely prevented both pre- and posttreat AA-induced ear swelling response; PAME-treated ears were neither swollen nor red, indicating that the erythema associated with AA treatment was also inhibited. PAME also prevented ear swelling when applied 15 min after painting mouse ears with 1% trans-RA.

The efficacy of PAME was also tested on DNCB-induced irritation in mice. DNCB applied topically to mouse ear skin at a concentration of 2% was reported to be a skin irritant. The anti-irritant activity of PAME was compared with ECA, indomethacin (IND), and ibuprofen (IBU). Both PAME and ECA significantly reduced ear swelling, while both NSAIDs were without appreciable effect. PAME was also reported to inhibit irritation induced by topical application of PMA, a potent inflammatory agent and tumor promoter. By contrast, topical indomethacin was completely without effect.

Three experimental protocols were designed to test the ability of PAME to inhibit surfactant-induced irritation. In the first design, 1% PAME in gel vehicle was applied to mouse ears prior to twice-daily single applications of 15% DSS for 3 consecutive days; it reduced erythema and ear swelling by 58%. In the second design, 1% PAME in gel vehicle, applied to mouse ears simultaneously with 10% SLS in gel vehicle twice daily, 1 h apart, for 2 consecutive days, reduced ear swelling by 33%. In the third design, 1% PAME in gel vehicle, applied to mouse ears twice daily, 1 h apart, 5 min after each single application of 10% SLS, reduced ear swelling by 62%. The posttreatment protocol was equally as effective as the pretreatment protocol. Histological analysis performed on ear skin taken from the same mice used in the posttreatment protocol above showed that PAME completely reversed SLS-induced epidermal hyperproliferation and reduced dermal induration and leukocytic infiltration. By comparison, ECA treatment was less effective in reducing SLS-induced inflammation.

PAME was examined for its ability to inhibit the elicitation phase of contact hypersensitivity response. DNCB-sensitized mice treated 5 min after DNCB ear challenge with PAME (1%) exhibited a >60% reduction in ear swelling response. PAME was also effective in inhibiting the elicitation phase in oxazolone-sensitized mice. Topical application of PAME (1%) 5 min after ear challenge substantially reduced the ear swelling (84%).

PAME was also effective in inhibiting both the induction and elicitation phases of para-phenylene-diamine-induced contact hypersensitivity response. PAME (0.5%) was applied 1 day prior to each of the PPD applications to the shaved abdominal skin of CBA/J mice. It inhibited 70, 83, and 98% of the ear swelling response measured at 24, 48, and 72 h after challenge, respectively. PAME, applied 30 min prior to ear challenge in PPD-sensitized CBA/J mice, inhibited the elicitation phase by 80, 100, and 100% of the ear swelling response measured at 24, 48, and 72 h, respectively.[120]

V. SUMMARY AND CONCLUSIONS

Earlier studies provided evidence that ion channel antagonists interfere with CHR and have potential therapeutic activity for treatment of inflamed skin. These findings have now been confirmed and extended to include ethacrynic acid and phenoxyacetic acid methyl ester.[14–17,21–25,29,31,35] Both ethacrynic acid and PAME are effective and act as topical inhibitors of cutaneous irritation and

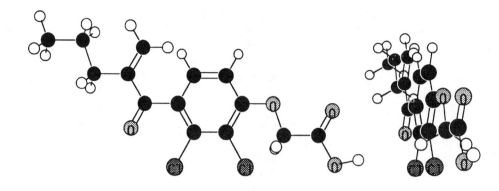

ECA

ECA

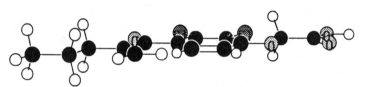

ECA molecule 0

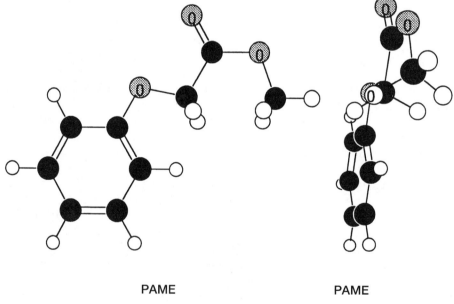

PAME

PAME

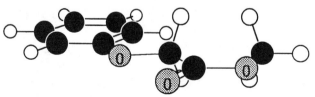

PAME molecule 0

Figure 4 Computer-generated stereomolecular structures of ECA (a) and PAME (b).

CHR. ECA and PAME appear to be active in suppressing both the induction and elicitation phases of CHR, indicating that they are useful in preventing and treating adverse skin reactions that occur upon single or repeated environmental exposure and afford protection in the transdermal delivery of an expanding repertoire of commercially important drugs that cause skin sensitization, e.g., antihypertensive (clondine), beta-blocker (nadolol), anti-asthmatic (albuterol), and antihistaminic (chlorpheniramine) drugs.

Currently, it is proposed that both irritation and sensitization are mediated by epidermally derived cytokines. For example, cytokine mRNAs upregulated by both irritants, allergens, and tolerogens during the early events of allergic contact dermatitis (ACD) include: TNF-α, IFN-γ, MIP-2, and GM-CSF, while class II MHC complex I-Aα, Il-1α, IL-1β, IFN-induced protein (IP)-10, and macrophage inflammatory protein (MIP)-2 mRNAs are specifically upregulated only after allergen painting.[37–40] Langerhans cells have also been shown to be the primary source of IL-1β, and MHC class II-Ig and MHC class I-Aα, while keratinocytes are a major source of TNF-α, IL-1α, IP-10, and MIP-2. TGF-β has an immunosuppressive effect on Langerhans cell cytokine production and on the CHR.[41] T cell-produced IL-4 and macrophage-produced IL-10 also have been reported to play a role in suppression of the elicitation phase of ACD.[42–46]

The mechanism by which topical treatment with a loop-diuretic drug suppresses both the induction and elicitation phase of contact hypersensitivity is not well understood. Loop diuretics interfere with the uptake of potassium in the mammalian loop of Henle through their action on the sodium/potassium ATPase.[1] These actions may be mediated by its inhibitory effect on potassium ion channels, but the actual cell target is unknown. Other ion channel modulators such as lanthanides appear to alter the Langerhans cell's ability to act as an antigen-presenting cell, and are reversible competitive inhibitors of Langerhans cell surface ATPase.[29] Although oubain (Na$^+$/K$^+$ ATPase inhibitor) and two other Ca^{2+}/Mg^{2+} ATPase inhibitors (ruthenium red and vanadate) failed to inhibit Langerhans cell ATPase, they may be potential inhibitors of CHR.[16] In agreement with this hypothesis, amiloride, a Na$^+$/K$^+$ ATPase inhibitor, is a potent inhibitor of CHR.[15] However, some analogs of amiloride with no ion channel activity retain immunosuppressive action.[29] These findings indicate the need for caution in overinterpreting ion channel activity correlations as causal agents of immune suppression.

ECA and PAME prevented cutaneous irritation to a wide range of irritants. The fact that ECA has less inhibitory effect on AA-induced irritation when administered a few minutes after arachidonic acid than when administered 1 h before AA may indicate that ECA has an upstream effect on AA metabolism. This agrees with data showing that ECA was superior to topical hydrocortisone in preventing AA-induced ear swelling and was better than ibuprofen and indomethacin, both of which interfere with the generation of AA metabolites. The inhibition of PMA-induced irritation by ECA and PAME suggests that they may interfere with ion channel activity associated with PKC-mediated signal transduction.

The broad spectrum activity of ECA and PAME against such diverse allergens and irritants as AA, DNCB, retinoic acid, lactic acid, and surfactants is not easily explained by any existing hypotheses. One possibility is that ECA interacts with ion channel lipoproteins in the cell membranes and blocks singlet oxygen generation, thereby preventing surface-activated protein kinases, AP-2 activation, and intercellular adhesion molecule-1(ICAM-1) gene expression, as part of a common irritant-provoked signal transduction cascade, in a manner similar to that proposed for UV-A radiation-induced skin irritation and immunosuppression.[47]

REFERENCES

1. Goodman and Gilman's *The Pharmacological Basis of Therapeutics*, 7th Edition. Goodman Gilman A, Goodman LS, Rall TW, Murad F, Eds., MacMillan, New York, 1985, 896–900.

2. Inflammation Research Association Meeting, New York Academy of Sciences, Ion channel modulation as a drug discovery target in inflammatory disease, New York, January 18, 1995.

3. Friedmann PS.: Pharmacological modulation of the skin immune system, in: *Skin Immune System,* Bos J, Ed., CRC Press, Boca Raton, FL, 1989, 462–467.

4. Ramsing DW, Agner T.: Efficacy of topical corticosteroids on irritant skin reactions. *Contact Dermatitis* 32: 293, 1995.

5. Ruzicka T, Bieber T, Schopf E, et al.: A short-term trial of tacrolimus (FK506) ointment for atopic dermatitis. *N.E.J.M.* 337: 816, 1997.

6. Bachmann H and Hofmann P.: Tenoxicam: a non-steroidal anti-inflammatory drug for topical application. *Pharmacol. Skin* 1: 256–257, 1987.

7. Darr D and Fridovich I.: Free radicals in cutaneous biology. *J. Invest. Dermatol.* 102: 671, 1994.

8. Hemelaar PJ, Biejersbergen van Henegouwen GMJ.: Protective effect of N-acetylcysteine on UVB induced immunosuppression by inhibition of the action of cis-urocanic acid. *Photochem. Photobiol.* 63: 322, 1996.

9. Fischer AA.: Contact dermatitis from topical medicaments. *Semin. Dermatol.* 1: 49, 1982.

10. *Textbook of Contact Dermatitis,* Rycroft R, Menne T, Frosch P, and Benezra C, Eds., Springer-Verlag, 1992, 540–653.

11. Maibach HI.: Clonidine: irritant and allergic contact dermatitis assays. *Contact Dermatitis* 12:192, 1985.

12. Enslin K et al.: Predictions of rabbit irritation severity by structure-activity relationships, in: *Irritant Contact dermatitis Syndrome,* Van der Valik P and Maibach HI, Eds., CRC Press, Boca Raton, FL, 1995.

13. Benezra C et al.: Molecular aspects of allergic contact dermatitis, in: *Textbook of Contact Dermatitis,* Rycrofty R, Menne T, Frosch P, and Benezra C, Eds., Springer-Verlag, New York, 1992, 105–119.

14. Amkraut A, Jordan W, and Taskovich L.: Effect of co-adminstration of corticosteroids on the development of contact sensitization. *J. Am. Acad. Dermatol.* 35: 27, 1996.

15. Gallo RL and Granstein RD.: Inhibition of allergic contact dermatitis and ultraviolet irradiation-induced tissue swelling in the mouse by amiloride. *Arch. Dermatol.* 125: 502, 1989.

16. Diezel W, Gruner S, Diaz LA, and Anhalt GJ.: Inhibition of cutaneous contact hypersensitivity by calcium transport inhibitors lanthanum and diltiazem, *J. Invest. Dermatol.* 93: 322, 1989.

17. Kalish RS, Wood JA, Wille, JJ, and Kydonieus A.: Prevention of contact hypersensitivity to topically applied drugs by ethacrynic acid: potential application to transdermal drug delivery. *J. Control Rel.* 48: 79, 1997.

18. Wolfgang, D.: East German Patent 297062. Magnesium salts as topical inflammation inhibitors for the skin (January 1992).

19. Holiday J and Spitzer N.: Calcium channels in the regulation of cell development and cellular interactions, in: *Calcium Channels,* Herwoitz L, Partridge L, and Leach I, Eds., CRC Press, Boca Raton, FL, 1991, 237.

20. Lee KS and Tsien RW.: Mechanism of calcium channel blockade by verapamil, D600, diltiazem, and nitredepine in single dialysed heart cells. *Nature* 302: 790, 1983.

21. Delacharriere O and Breton L.: Utilisation de sel de lanthanide, de tain, de zinc, de manganese, d'yttrium, de cobalt, de baryum, de strontium dans une composition pour la peau. Republique Francaise Institut National de la Propriete Indistrielle, Pub. No. 2, 740, 341.

22. Cormier JM, Ledger PW, and Amkraut A.: U.S. Patent 516074.: Reduction or prevention of skin irritation by drugs. Issued November 1992.

23. Dwyer DS and Esenther K. U.S. Patent 5489441: Method for suppressing immune response associated with psoriasis contact dermatitis and diabetes melitus. Issued February 1996.

24. Gruner S, Diezel W, Strunk D, Eckert R, Siems W, and Anhalt GJ.: Inhibition of Langerhans cell ATPase and contact sensitization by lanthanides-role of T-suppressor cells. *J. Invest. Dermatol.* 97: 478, 1991.

25. McFadden J, Bacon K, and Camp R.: Topically applied verapamil hydrochloride inhibits tuberculin-induced delayed-type hypersensitivity reactions in human skin. *J. Invest. Dermatol.* 99: 784, 1992.

26. Bacon K, Westwick J, and Camp RDR.: Potent and specific inhibition of IL-8, IL-1 alpha, and IL-1beta-induced in vitro lymphocyte migration by calcium channel antagonists. *Biochem. Biophys. Res. Commun.* 165: 349, 1989.

27. Matsunaga T, Katayama H, and Nishioka K.: Epidermal cytokine mRNA expression induced by hapten differs from that induced by primary irritants in human skin organ culture system. *J. Dermatol.* 25: 421, 1998.
28. Cumberbatch M, Dearman RJ, and Kimber I.: Langerhans cells require signals from both tumor necrosis factor-alpha and interleukin 1-beta for migration. *Immunology* 92: 388, 1997
29. Lindgren AM, Granstein RD, Hosoi J, and Gallo RL.: Structure-function relations in the inhibition of murine contact hypersensitivity by amiloride. *J. Invest. Dermatol.* 104: 38, 1995.
30. Kalish RS, Wood JA, Wille JJ, and Kydonieus A.: Sensitization of mice to topically applied drugs: albuterol, chlorpheniramine, clonidine, and nadolol. *Contact Dermatitis* 33: 407, 1995.
31. Wille JJ, Kydonieus A, and Kalish RS.: Several different ion channel modulators abrogate contact hypersensitivity in mice. *Skin Pharm. Skin Physiol.*, in press.
32. Physicians' Desk Reference, 50th ed., Medical Economics Co., Montvale, NJ, 1996.
33. Good and Gilman's *The Pharmacological Basis of Therapeutics*, 8th ed., Good Gilman A, Rall TW, Nies AS, and Taylor P, Eds., MacMillan, New York, 1993, 764–783.
34. Wille JJ et al.: Prophylactic and therapeutic treatment of skin sensitization and irritation. U.S. Patent 5,686,100. Issued November 11, 1997.
35. Wille JJ, Kydonieus A, and Kalish RS.: Inhibition of irritation and contact hypersensitivity by ethacrynic acid. *Skin Pharm. Skin Physiol.*, in press.
36. Wille JJ, Kydonieus A, and Kalish RS.: Inhibition of irritation and contact hypersensitivity by phenoxyacetic acid methyl ester. *Skin Pharm. Skin Physiol.*, in press.
37. Enk, AH and Katz, SJ.: Early molecular events in the induction phase of contact sensitivity. *Proc. Natl. Acad. Sci. U.S.A.* 89: 1398–1402, 1992.
38. Enk, AH, Angeloni, VL, Udey, MC, and Katz, SI.: An essential role for Langerhans cell-derived IL-1β in the initiation of primary immune responses in skin. *J. Immunol.* 150: 3698–3704, 1993.
39. Kutsch, CL, Norris, DA, and Arend, WP.: Tumor necrosis-α induces interleukin-1α and interleukin-1 receptor antagonist production by cultured human keratinocytes. *J. Invest. Dermatol.* 101: 79–85, 1993.
40. Groves, RW, Allen, MH, Ross, EL, Barker, JNWN, and MacDonald, DM.: Tumor necrosis factor alpha is proinflammatory in normal human skin and modulates cutaneous adhesion molecule expression. *Br. J. Dermatol.* 132: 345–352, 1995.
41. Epstein, SP, Baer, RL, Thorbecke, GJ, and Belsito, DV.: Immunosuppressive effects of transforming growth factor-β: inhibition of the induction of Ia antigen on Langerhans cells by cytokines and of the contact hypersensitivity response. *J. Invest. Dermatol.* 96: 873–837, 1991.
42. Rowe, A and Bunker, CB.: Interleukin-4 and the interleukin-4 receptor in allergic contact dermatitis. *Contact Dermatitis* 38: 36–39, 1998.
43. Asada, H, Linton, J, and Katz, SI.: Cytokine gene expression during the elicitation phase of contact sensitivity: regulation by endogenous *Il-4*. *J. Invest. Dermatol.* 108: 406–411, 1997.
44. Rivas, JM and Ullrich, SE.: Systemic suppression of delayed-type hypersensitivity by supernatants from UV-irradiated keratinocytes. *J. Immunol.* 149: 3865–3871, 1992.
45. Enk, AH, Angeloni, VL, Udey, MC, and Katz, SI.: Inhibition of Langerhans cell antigen-presenting function by Il-10. *J. Immunol.* 151: 2390–2398, 1993.
46. Fox, FE, Kubin M, Cassin M, Niu, Z, Hosoi J, Torii, J, Granstein, RD, Trinchieri G, and Rook AH.: Calcitonin gene-related peptide inhibits proliferation and antigen presentation by human peripheral blood mononuclear cells: effects of B7, interleukin 10, and interleukin 12. *J. Invest. Dermatol.* 108: 43–48, 1997.
47. Grether-Beck S, Olaizola-Horn S, Schmitt H, Grewe M, Jahnke A, Johnson JP, Brivada K, Sies H, and Krutman, J.: Activation of transcription factor AP-2 modulates UVA radiation- and singlet oxygen-induced expression of the human intercellular adhesion molecule 1 gene. *Proc. Natl. Acad. Sci. U.S.A.* 93:14586–91, 1996.

17 Mast Cell Degranulating Agents Modulate Skin Immune Responses

John J. Wille and Agis F. Kydonieus

CONTENTS

I. INTRODUCTION

A. BACKGROUND

Mast cells are important mediators of both nonspecific cutaneous inflammation and of the immunological functions associated with allergy and delayed type hypersensitivity (DTH) reactions.[1] Mast cells are a histiotype cell found in most soft tissues and organs of mammals and humans. They are recognized histologically by the presence of intracytoplasmic granules that stain with metachromatic dyes such as azure A and toluidine blue. Mast cells can be classified in two subtypes, connective tissue mast cells (CTMC) and mucosal mast cells (MMC). The former are found in the skin and serosal tissues, while the latter are predominately located in mucosal tissues (eye, nose, intragastral tissue). Besides differences in anatomical location, the two types differ in granule-staining properties, protease types, and ontogeny.[2] It is presumed that both arise from a common bone marrow-derived precursor. We are concerned here with CTMC found in skin. These are found abundantly in the upper papillary dermis in close proximity to capillaries and are seen frequently in close association with cutaneous nerves.

Cutaneous mast cells play an auxiliary function as part of the host's immediate line of defense by aiding in the detection and signaling of invading parasites, antigens, and allergens. Through release of mediators, they initiate a cascade of nonspecific inflammatory responses. For example, in response to skin injury they generate and directly secrete arachidonic acid metabolites prostaglandins (PGD_2, PGE_2, PGI_2), and leukotrienes (C_4, D_4, and E_4 and LKB_4).[3]

The main role of skin mast cells is to confront antigen/allergen attack via the skin's immunological surveillance system. In particular, mast cells are involved in the development of immediate or type I delayed-type hypersensitivity (DTH) and type II DTH or contact hypersensitivity reactions (CHR) of the skin.[1] This chapter is concerned with the role of mast cells in contact hypersensitivity. There is scant knowledge of mast cell involvement in CHR, and much of it deals with release of serotonin in rodents. Askenase and colleagues have shown that mast cell release of serotonin is critical in suppressor T cell formation, and in priming helper T cells to produce IgE-like molecules in lymphoid centers that are transported to the periphery where they bind and confer antigen-specific memory to cutaneous mast cells.[4]

The best evidence for a role of mast cells in CHR is the defective CHR observed in two strains of mast cell-deficient mice.[4] Askenase and co-workers have recently reviewed this and conflicting evidence for the dependence of CHR on mast cells, and have speculated that there may be other sources of mediators such as serotonin coming from platelets.[1] Recently, it was reported that UVB-induced immunosuppression of CHR is defective in W/W^v mast cell-deficient mice. Additional evidence for a mast cell dependence is the observation that DTH responses are preferentially elicited at cutaneous sites enriched in mast cells, and that such sites exhibit evidence of partial mast cell degranulation.[1]

The mechanism of mast cell degranulation has been primarily worked out in type I DHT responses, and it is presumed that similar events occur during the elicitation phase of CHR. In the former, mast cell degranulation occurs via a transmembrane signal that mobilizes IgE or IgE-like receptor cross-linking, leading ultimately to activation of granule exocytosis and release of mediators. These include vasoactive amines, proteolytic enzymes, and matrix proteoglycans. Among vasoactive mediators are histamine, serotonin, and platelet-activating factor, PAF.[1,5] Among proteolytic enzymes and proteins released are the neutral proteases, chymase and tryptase, eosinophil chemotactic factors, and granule matrix heparin sulfate proteoglycans.[5] Additional soluble mediators released include cytokines IL-3, IL-4, IL-5, IL-6, and GM-CSF.[6–8] Of particular interest to the subject of this chapter is the recent report that UV radiation results in mast cell release of tumor necrosis factor-alpha (TNF-α).[9,10]

There are a large number of nonimmunological stimuli or secretagogues that can cause mast cell degranulation. Examples include the neuropeptides such as substance P, somatostatin, neurotensin, and nerve growth factors; calcium ionophore; A 23187; dextran; morphine sulfate; chymotrypsin; tetradecanoylphorbol acetate; dimethyl sulfoxide; sulfur mustards, *Escherichia coli* fimbriae; exogenous type II phospholipase A_2; such physical factors as ultrasound, sunlight, heat, cold, and pressure; and physiological conditions such as skin injury, hypoxia, osmotic changes, and emotional stress.[11–19] Other, less well characterized agents include: tridecylresorcinolic acid, a sodium–potassium ATPase ion channel blocker, estradiol, clonidine, progesterone, and carbachol.[20–24]

B. Contact Hypersensitivity: The Achilles' Heel of Transdermal Drug Delivery

A major obstacle to the transdermal delivery of drugs is the development of allergic contact dermatitis (ACD). Delayed contact hypersensitivity responses are reported to occur for many topical medicaments surveyed by patch testing, including: benzocaine, chlorpheniramine, diphenhydramine, neomycin sulfate, penicillin, promazine, and sulfanilamide.[25] Therapeutic agents such as drugs also cause ACD when administered transdermally (e.g., clonidine) and this presents a significant problem.[26] In addition, most beta-blockers, antiasthmatics, and antihistamines are known sensitizing drugs. In general, ACD may be caused by varied and numerous agents, for example, metals (e.g., nickel), fragrances, chemicals, cosmetics, textiles, pesticides, pollen, and the like.[27]

Previous efforts to address the problem of ACD by prophylactically treating the skin to prevent the onset of the induction phase of ACD and/or to therapeutically prevent or reduce the adverse effects of the elicitation phase include the use of lanthanum citrate and diltazium hydrochloride, corticosteroids, verapamil hydrochloride, and the diuretic, amiloride.[28–31] Recently, Wille and co-workers reported that ethacrynic acid yielded significant prevention of contact sensitization to a wide variety of skin-sensitizing drugs, including albuterol, chlorpheniramine, clonidine, and nadolol.[32]

This chapter deals with experimental studies that define a critical connection between agents that cause mast cell degranulation and also inhibit CHR in mice. In particular, it focuses on *cis*-urocanic acid as it has an established history and linkage to events that mediate UVB-induced immunosuppression. It is hoped that the heuristic approach we have taken here will spur additional research to find more potent topical agents that specifically abrogate contact allergic dermatitis.

II. EFFECT OF *CIS*-UROCANIC ACID ON MAST CELL DEGRANULATION

A. Preparation of Purified *cis*-Urocanic Acid and Its Permeation through Excised Skin

A central question with regard to the effect of urocanic acid on mast cells and, for that matter, with other targets is whether the effects seen are specific to the cis isomer or to some indeterminate mixture of the trans and cis isomers. For this reason, we prepared purified *cis*-urocanic acid (C-UA). This was accomplished by exposure of a saturated solution of *trans*-urocanic acid (T-UA) to 313 nm of UV light, which yielded an equilibrium ratio of 70:30 of cis/trans isomers. C-UA was further purified by Dowex-1 X8 ion exchange chromatography and by high pressure liquid chromatography of the pooled chromatographic eluates. Figure 1 presents chromatographic profiles of purified C-UA. NMR studies confirmed that the material was >99% the cis isomer. The solubility of purified C-UA was determined to be 25 mg/ml in water, while the solubility of the trans isomer was only 1.1. mg/ml in water at 20°C. This differs from the reported value of 1 to 2 mg/ml for the cis isomer.[33] The implications of higher water solubility of the cis isomer relative to the trans isomer suggest a greater diffusibility and transport into the dermis following UVB irradiation, where we believe it has greater access to dermal mast cells.

Another question we addressed was the permeation of purified C-UA through both mouse and human skin. Figure 2 summarizes data showing a roughly parabolic relationship between the observed flux ($\mu g/cm^2/h$) and concentration of the topically applied dose of C-UA in vehicle for both mouse and human skin. As expected, mouse skin with a thinner *stratum corneum* than human skin was two to three times more permeable than human skin with its thicker *stratum corneum* over the concentration range tested. It was also shown that percutaneous absorption of C-UA, formulated in an ethanolic gel vehicle (75% ethanol in 2.5% HPMC), enhances C-UA permeation relative to a water vehicle. The importance of these studies rests in future use of C-UA in transdermal

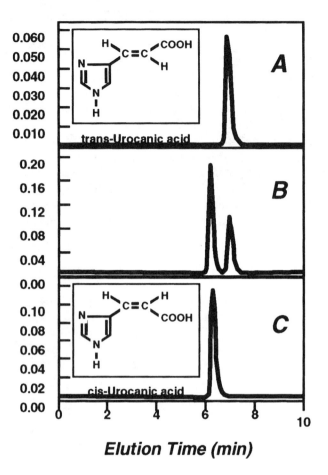

Elution Time (min)

Figure 1   HPLC analysis of solutions containing: (A) all *trans* (E)- urocanic acid (T-UA) in water, (B) a 70:30 mixture of *cis*-urocanic acid (C-UA)/T-UA obtained after equilibrium (30 h) of the photoisomerization reaction, and (C) chromatographically purified C-UA. Ordinate: relative absorbance units. Abscissa: elution time (min). Chemical structures of T-UA and C-UA are depicted in the inserts. (From Wille JJ et al.: *Skin Pharm Appl Skin Physiol*, 12: 20, 1999. With permission.)

delivery systems, where sustained delivery is required at levels that target dermal mast cell degranulation-induced immunosuppression of CHR. The C-UA concentrations in vehicles that accomplish these goals correspond to skin permeation flux rates in the range of 10 to 50 μg/cm^2 /h.

B. Mast Cell Degranulation Induced by Topical *cis*-Urocanic Acid

1. C-UA but Not T-UA Depletes Mast Cell Chymase

Human skin organ cultures were prepared as previously described and the skin explants exposed on the dermal side to solutions containing C-UA in culture media. C-UA–induced mast cell degranulation was detected immunocytochemically by depletion of human mast cell-specific chymase enzyme, a marker enzyme of mast cells.[34] Figure 3 shows that as little as 1 μg/ml of C-UA was able to significantly reduce the chymase content of mast cells by greater than 75% over untreated controls (88 ± 12 positive mast cells per mm^2) as detected by immunocytological reduction in chymase-specific staining. This degranulating effect of C-UA was even more potent than 5 mM morphine sulfate (37 ± 15, positive mast cell per mm^2). In a series of further skin organ culture experiments, it was shown that it required more than five times the dose of T-UA to achieve an equivalent amount of chymase release.

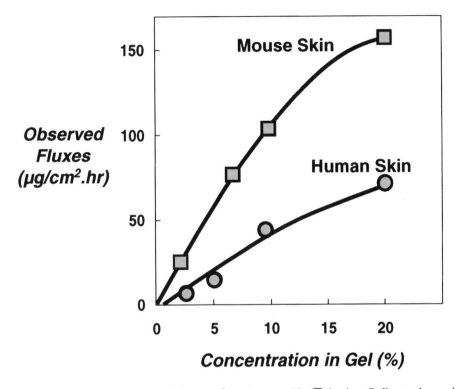

Figure 2   Permeation of C-UA through human (●) and mouse skin (■) in vitro. Ordinate: observed fluxes; abscissa: concentration of C-UA in HPMC gel. (From Wille JJ et al.: *Skin Pharm Appl Skin Physiol*, 12: 21, 1999. With permission.)

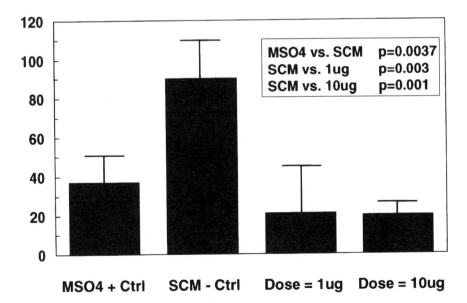

Figure 3   Depletion of mast cell-specific chymase by C-UA in human skin organ culture. Positive control, 5 mM morphine sulfate (MSO_4 + ctrl); negative control, skin culture medium (SCM); C-UA treatment (dose = 1 µg/ml): C-UA treatment (dose = 10 µg/ml). Ordinate: chymase-positive mast cells per microscopic field. The oval box encloses the p values calculated from ANOVA two-way comparisons as shown. (From Wille JJ: *Skin Pharm Appl Skin Physiol*, 12: 22, 1999. With permission.)

2. C-UA but Not T-UA Induces E-Selectin on Target Endothelial Cells

Previous studies indicated that E-selectin, a cell adhesion protein, is expressed on dermal endothelial cells following UVB irradiation and after exposure to mast cell-derived TNF-α.[34] Endothelial cell membranes expressing E-selectin aid in leukocyte extravasation by binding ligand present on the surface of leukocytes. Regulation of the induction of these adhesion proteins is therefore of importance in leukocyte trafficking during the process of skin inflammation. The results of neonatal foreskin organ culture experiments to which either the cis or trans isomers of urocanic acid were added are presented in Figure 4. E-selectin expression was significantly greater 6 h after C-UA treatment than after T-UA treatment for all doses examined (10, 75, and 200 μg/ml), and was equivalent to the level of expression seen for the positive control (5 ng/ml of TNF-α).

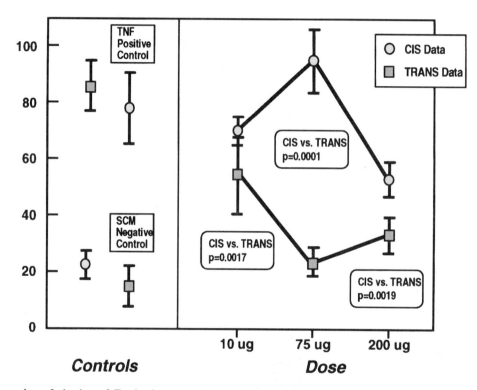

Figure 4   Induction of E-selectin expression by C-UA vs. T-UA. Controls (left panel: two sets were performed as standards for the C-UA and T-UA experiments): positive controls, 100 ng/ml of TNF-α; negative control (skin culture medium, SCM). Dose (right panel): C-UA and T-UA were added at 10, 75, and 200 μg/ml to the culture medium of the human skin organ cultures. Ordinate: number of positive microvessel profiles per mm². Oval boxes enclose the probability values, p, for two-way ANOVA test. (From Wille JJ: *Skin Pharm Appl Skin Physiol*, 12: 22, 1999. With permission.)

3. Other Immunomodulatory Agents Affect Cutaneous Mast Cells

a. Hydrocortisone

Hydrocortisone is perhaps the most widely prescribed and most common over-the-counter drug used for effective treatment of the symptoms of contact allergy.[35] In contrast, antihistamines that are effective in type I immediate-type hypersensitivity reactions are notoriously ineffective in this regard, i.e., allergic patch test results are unaffected in patients receiving routine dose regimens of antihistamine vs. patients not receiving any antihistamines. The mechanism of glucocorticosteroid suppression of contact dermatitis is not yet fully understood and appears to involve multiple targets, including lymphocytes, monocyte/macrophages, and epidermal Langerhans cells.[36,37] Recent reports indicate that prolonged treatment of human skin with glucocorticosteroids such as hydrocortisone deplete the skin of mast cells.[38,39] There are even suggestions that chronic steroid treatment of human skin may desensitize skin making it unresponsive to drug-induced sensitization.[40]

b. Cyclosporins

Cyclosporin A (CsA) is now widely used in the treatment of graft rejection and has been tested for its effects on cutaneous immunity.[41] Cyclosporin A(CsA) acts primarily on T lymphocytes, and inhibits the production of IL-2 and interferon-γ by T cells, and it reduces the expression of HLA-DR antigens on stimulated cells.[42–45] Marone et al. reported that CsA inhibited IgE- and non-IgE-mediated release of histamine and leukotriene C from human lung mast cells.[46] These effects of CsA are presumably due to a direct interaction of this lipophilic drug with cell membranes, that inhibits granule exocytosis as reported for cytolytic T lymphocytes and rat basophilic leukemic cells, as well as human peripheral blood basophils.[47–49] In another study, CsA inhibited the release of histamine and *de novo* synthesis of Prostaglandin D_2 from human skin mast cells challenged with anti-IgE antibody, but had no effect on histamine release of mast cells challenged with either A23187 or substance P.[50] CsH, an analog that does not bind to cyclophilin, was unable to inhibit anti-IgE–induced mast cell degranulation, indicating that CsA mediates its effect via the cyclophilin pathway. The inhibitory effect of CsA on the immunologic activation of human cutaneous mast cells is limited to IgE-mediated release of inflammatory cytokines that play a role in immune reactions.[6] As such, CsA is expected to be most effective in preventing contact allergic responses. By contrast, it has not been effective in blocking the elicitation step of allergic contact dermatitis.[51] The reason for this is unknown, but failure to block the elicitation phase of CHR could be explained if CsA has no effect on TNF-α release, as suggested by its failure to inhibit non-IgE–induced degranulation.

III. EFFECT OF *CIS*-UROCANIC ACID ON SKIN IMMUNE SYSTEM

There are still many questions that remain unanswered. What is the source of TNF-α generated by UVB and C-UA? Are Langerhans cells the major target of C-UA–induced mast cell degranulation? If not, what other cell targets are involved? What are the alterations in Langerhans cells induced by mast cell mediators that render them less immunogenic? Are the changes induced by mast cell mediators that alter Langerhans cell antigen presentation the same as those that result in systemic immune tolerance?

A. CELLULAR TARGETS

1. Keratinocytes

Although keratinocytes are known to produce many immunologically active cytokines, Ullrich and co-workers reported that C-UA had no direct effect on the secretion of TNF-α nor on the immunosuppressive cytokines IL-4 or IL-10.[52] Neither C-UA nor T-UA is toxic to either dermal fibroblasts or normal human keratinocytes as assessed by in vitro cytotoxicity assays at concentrations below 1.5 mg/ml, nor did C-UA elicit PGE_2 release (Wille et al., unpublished). Other possibilities include release of TNF-α from mast cells that stimulate keratinocyte CSF-1 or inhibit keratinocyte IL-7, both of which could interfere with dendritic cell maturation (see Ullrich, Chapter 20 in this book).

2. Langerhans Cells

C-UA has been shown to mimic many of the deleterious morphological and biochemical effects induced by UV irradiation on Langerhans cells, including loss of dendrites, cytoskeletal modifications, and changes in their rate of migration to draining lymph nodes.[53–55] There is uncertainty as to how such alterations result in immunosuppression. The above deleterious effects of UVB and C-UA can be reversed by antibody to C-UA.[56] TNF-α may upregulate Langerhans cell IL-4 and IL-10 and increase their immunosuppressive potential and ability to anergize T cells by ablation of their B7 costimulatory signals. In addition, TNF-α induces laminin surface receptors on intraepidermal Langerhans cells, which may either slow down or speed up their transit from the epidermis to the lymph nodes.[57] IL-4 secretion by Langerhans cells may attract monocytes, which secrete IL-10, leading to deranged costimulatory B7 expression on Langerhans cells and interfere with Th1 activation through apoptosis induction, and at the same time favor the activation of Th2 cells and the production of IL-10 required for the induction of immune tolerance.[58]

B. Immunosuppression and Tolerance

1. Inhibition by C-UA of Contact Hypersensitivity

Previous work reported that C-UA inhibited both induction and elicitation phases of the contact hypersensitivity response in mice, but had no effect on irritation or immediate-type allergic response.[59] Wille et al., using highly purified C-UA, have confirmed and extended these results, but were unable to confirm an effect on elicitation.[60]

Earlier, action spectra data for CHR that showed a similarity to the absorption spectra of DNA damage and to the absorption spectrum of C-UA prompted De Fabo and Noonan to speculate C-UA mediates UVB-induced CHR suppression.[61] Reeves et al. have reported that there is a lack of correlation between suppression of contact hypersensitivity by UV radiation and photosensitization of epidermal urocanic (UA) acid in hairless mice.[62] Later, Morison and Kelly found no correlation between skin content of UA and extent of UVB-induced immunosuppression.[63] However, their experiments are open to other interpretations, since their manipulations to achieve different urocanic acid levels were either immunosuppressive by themselves (hair plucking) or indirectly led to mast cell degranulation and release of immunosuppressive cytokines. C-UA has been implicated in a wide variety of immune functions including suppression of CHR, induction of a serum suppressor factor, inhibition of epidermal cell cytokine IL-1, defective dendritic cell antigen presentation, prolongation of murine skin allograft survival, and regulation of tumor antigen presentation.[64–73]

Histamine, histamine receptors, and prostaglandin E_2, all mast cell mediators, affect C-UA–induced immunosuppression.[74–77] For example, C-UA but not T-UA downregulates histamine-induced cyclic AMP production by dermal fibroblasts.[78] The effect of C-UA on histamine metabolism is probably indirect, as urocanic acid isomers failed to compete with radiolabeled histamine for rat brain H1, H2, or H3 receptors.[79] Interestingly, they found that C-UA displayed a weak interaction with the GABA (gamma-aminobutyric acid) receptor. The significance of this is unknown as the presence of GABA receptors in skin has not yet been reported. A role for antioxidants in immunosuppresion has also been investigated. N-acetylcysteine, an antioxidant, reverses C-UA–induced immunosuppression, implicating C-UA in free radical formation and, perhaps, may instigate activation of AP-2 nuclear transcription factor, which is involved in UV immunosuppression, via lipid peroxidation of cell membranes.[80,81]

Perhaps the most compelling evidence that C-UA mediates UVB-induced immunosuppression is evidence that dermal injection of an antibody to TNF-α reversed the immunosuppressive effects of both UVB and C-UA, suggesting that TNF-α released locally in the area of Langerhans cells is responsible for the cascade of events mediating immunosuppression.[82] Further support for a relationship between C-UA–mediated immunosuppression comes from work by Moodycliff and co-workers[83,84] and El-Ghorr and Norval,[56] who reported that a monoclonal antibody to C-UA has a differential effect on reversal of UVB-induced immunnosuppression of DHT responses. The latter authors also report that the C-UA antibody did not prevent the accumulation of dendritic cells into local lymph nodes. Recently, Yamazaki et al. have shown that TNF-α, RANTES, and MCP-1 are potent chemotactic attractants for Langerhans cells and may influence their migration from the epidermis to regional lymph nodes during contact sensitization.[85] Further, Jakob and Udey reported that both IL-1 and TNF-α aid in the emigration of Langerhans cell by reducing E-cadherin interaction of Langerhans cells to epidermal keratinocytes.[86] Experiments using anti-IL-1β antibody administered systemically prior to skin sensitization abolished Langerhans cell accumulation in the draining lymph nodes and also inhibited TNF-α–induced migration and dendritic cell accumulation.[87] Interestingly, Price et al. have reported that antibody to alpha 6 integrin (laminin) but not an anti-alpha 4 integrin (fibronectin) blocks Langerhans emigration and dendritic cell accumulation during the induction phase of contact sensitization.[88]

The possibility that the immunosuppressive effects of both C-UA and UVB is mediated by DNA damage is supported by studies showing reversal of both immunosuppression and pyrimidine dimer formation in skin exposed to liposome-mediated DNA repair enzymes and by UVA radiation reversal of both C-UA and UVB-induced immunosuppression.[89,90]

Since UV-induced DNA damage in keratinocytes mediates IL-6 mRNA and cytokine release, there may be a common pathway underlying cytokine regulation of immunosuppression and its reversal by countervailing cytokines.[91]

Cytokine-driven skin immune regulatory processes also appear to underlie the earlier discovery that alpha 6 integrin is expressed on epidermal Langerhans cells exposed to TNF-α, and supports the hypothesis that Langerhans cell migration is orchestrated by a cascade of cytokines. We propose that exposure of Langerhans cells to mast cell-derived TNF-α, prior to induction of sensitization, may interrupt the normal sequence of steps required for Langerhans cell maturation.

The remainder of this chapter attempts to address these questions and to offer some plausible scenarios that accommodate both established facts and general knowledge. Our results show that C-UA is a potent mast cell degranulating agent, and that the TNF-α is released in sufficient quantities to initiate dermal events involved in the cascade of inflammation Our in vivo murine sensitization studies establish that administration of C-UA during the induction phase downregulates CHR. Further, we have shown that other agents that promote mast cell degranulation also suppress CHR. These results suggest that temporally inappropriate induction of the mast cell degranulation during the initiation phase of ACD may interfere with downstream events associated with full expression of the CHR upon elicitation.

2. C-UA Inhibits the Induction Phase of Contact Sensitivity

Table 1 presents data showing that purified C-UA, incorporated into vehicle (2.5% HPMC in 75% ethanol) and applied 24 h prior to 2,4-dinitrochlorobenzene (DNCB) sensitization, was effective in preventing ear swelling in mice. The extent of suppression observed 24 h postchallenge was greater than 70% and was still evident when measured 72 h postchallenge. There were no signs of local irritation or inflammation associated with prolonged skin contact with concentrations of C-UA below 20% in HPMC gel. In an attempt to achieve total abrogation of the ear swelling response, mice were pretreated prior to DNCB sensitization with increasing doses of purified C-UA. Nearly complete (>85%) elimination of the sensitization response can be attained at or above 10% C-UA, and a dose response for prevention was established.

A further question we addressed experimentally was the requirement for 24 h pretreatment with the mast cell degranulating agent, C-UA. In separate studies, codelivery of C-UA and DNCB was compared to 24-h pretreatment prior to DNCB sensitization. Codelivery was found to be minimally effective relative to 24-h pretreatment.

3. Other Mast Cell Degranulating Agents Suppress CHR

The question arose whether other mast cell degranulating agents also act as to suppress CHR. We found that chloroquine applied topically at 1% chloroquine in 2.5 HPMC gel vehicle significantly inhibited the ear swelling response (>40%), using the 24-h pretreatment protocol. Capsaicin, another

TABLE 1
Inhibition of Contact Sensitivity by *cis*-Urocanic Acid

Treatment (in hours)	Ear Swelling (mm × 10^2)	Percent (%) Suppression[a]
None (HMPC gel)		
24	0	
72	0	
DNCB (100 µg)		
24	8.9	—
72	7.2	—
Cis-Urocanic Acid (1%) + DNCB (100 µg)		
24	2.6	71
72	4.8	33
Cis-Urocanic Acid (5%) + DNCB (100 µg)		
24	1.8	80
72	3.0	59

[a] The data were analyzed for significance by Student t test. The p-values between the following pairs were (a) $p < 0.01$ for 1%C-UA—24 h vs. DNCB—24 h, (b) $p \leq 0.05$ for 1% C-UA—48 h vs. DNCB—48 h, (c) $p < 0.01$ for 5% C-UA—24 h vs. DNCB—24 h, (d) $p \leq 0.05$ for 5% C-UA—48 h vs. DNCB—48 h.

mast cell secretagogue, inhibited DNCB sensitization (>30%) when applied topically at 1% in the 2.5% HPMC gel vehicle, using the 24-h pretreatment protocol. Although the reduction in CHR is small, no effort was made to optimize the secretagogue's dosage.

It has already been established that UV-irradiation at doses (1 to 3 MED) that suppress contact hypersensitivity are highly effective at degranulating mast cells in the neonatal foreskin organ culture model.[9] Release of TNF-α into the medium was confirmed by the human skin organ culture assay that permits detection of inducible E-selectin expression on the dermal microvasculature. Induction had kinetics similar to other mast cell secretagogues (e.g., substance P).

4. C-UA Induces Immune Tolerance

A state of immune unresponsiveness also known as "immune tolerance" was shown to exist in mice which had been treated with only one application of C-UA, to the shaved abdomen, but were resensitized 2 weeks later on their shaved backs and subsequently 5 days later rechallenged on their left ears. Figure 5 presents data showing that one-time pretreatment with either a 1 or 5% C-UA gel induced greater than 50% suppression relative to naive mice receiving their first sensitization on the shaved backs at the same time. The figure also presents data showing that the level of immune tolerance (unresponsiveness) achieved in the absence of a second pretreatment is about half of that achieved by a single C-UA application in the same animal.

5. Cromolyn Promotes Contact Sensitization

Sodium cromolyn is a drug that stabilizes mast cell membranes (*Physicans' Desk Reference*) and has been used clinically to treat type 1 immediate-type allergic reactions. It might be expected to be effective in suppressing the elicitation phase of CHR. We hypothesized that if countersensitizers act via induction of mast cell degranulation, an agent such as sodium cromolyn that stabilizes mast cell membranes would not suppress contact hypersensitivity, and might even enhance contact sensitization. In a murine contact sensitization model, we used a water-soluble chemical sensitizer, trinitrobenzene sulfonate, TNBS, to sensitize mice. Cromoyln

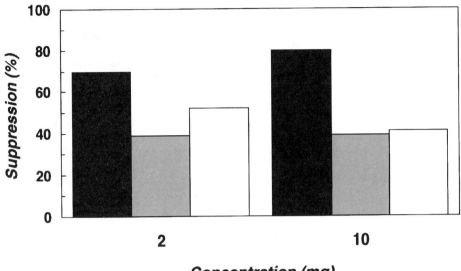

Figure 5 Induction of immune suppression and immune tolerance by *cis*-urocanic acid. Balb/c mice (8 per group)) received a single application of C-UA prior to primary site sensitization with DNCB and displayed immune suppression at 24 h (■) and 48 h (hatched bar) post ear challenge; these same mice were then resensitized 2 to 3 weeks later with 1% DNCB at a second skin site, and subsequently rechallenged 5 days later. The resensitization data (□) show there is a significant reduction in ear swelling relative to control mice that did not receive C-UA treatment during primary site sensitization. (From Wille JJ et al.: *Skin Pharm Appl Skin Physiol*, 12: 25, 1999. With permission.)

was injected intradermally 1-h before TNBS sensitization. These results showed that cromolyn treatment enhanced ear swelling response over the positive control at both 24 and 48 h postchallenge.

IV. SUMMARY AND CONCLUSIONS

The search for effective inhibitors of transdermal drug-induced contact sensitization was directed to dermal mast cell degranulating agents (MCDAs). Human skin organ cultures were employed to test whether C-UA and other potential MCDAs cause mast cell degranulation. These were then each tested for their ability to inhibit the initiation phase of the contact hypersensitivity reaction (CHR). C-UA, at 1 μg/ml, significantly depleted mast cell chymase, whereas T-UA was relatively ineffective. C-UA also induced local effects of liberated mast cell TNF-α, as detected by E-selectin expression on the microvascular dermal endothelium. C-UA significantly reduced (>80%) the ear swelling response in Balb/c mice, when applied 24 h prior to application of a sensitizing amount of dinitrochlorobenzene (DNCB), and induced a prolonged (>3 weeks) state of immune tolerance (>40%). Similar immunosuppressive effects were observed with chloroquine and capsaicin. Pretreatment with cromolyn, a mast cell membrane stabilizer, was unable to inhibit DNCB-induced CHR. It is suggested that one mechanism for UVB-induced immunosuppression is the production of C-UA, which degranulates mast cells, producing local TNF-α effects during the initiation phase of CHR. TNF-α, and possibly other mast cell mediators, may interfere with downstream events associated with accessory cell function. Mast cell degranulating agents may be a new class of topical immunosuppressants, i.e., countersensitizers, whose administration might permit the transdermal delivery of drugs which otherwise cannot now be so delivered because of their known sensitizing potential.

REFERENCES

1. Van Loveren H, Teppema JS, and Askenase PW.: Skin Mast Cells, in: *The Skin Immune System*, Bos, J (Ed.), 1990, 172.
2. Kirshenbaum AS, Kessler SW, Goff JP, and Metcalfe DD.: Demonstration of the origin of human mast cells from CD34+ bone marrow progenitor cells, *J Immunol*, 146: 1410, 1991.
3. Metzger H, Alcaraz G, Hohman R, Kinet JP, Pribluda R, and Quatro R.: The receptor with high affinity for immunoglobulin E, *Annu Rev Immunol*, 4: 419, 1986.
4. Askenase PW, Van Loveren H, Kopf, SK, Ron Y, et al.: Defective elicitation of delayed-type hypersensitivity in W/Wv and Sl/Slv mast cell -deficient mice. *J Immunol*, 31: 2687, 1983.
5. Ishizaka T and Ishizaka K.: Activation of mast cells for mediator release through IgE receptors. *Prog Allergy*, 34: 188, 1984.
6. Plaut M, Pierce JH, Watson CJ, Hanlery-Hyde J, Nordan RP, and Paul WE.: Mast cell lines produce lymphokines in response to cross-linkage of Fc ε RI or to calcium ionophores. *Nature*, 339: 64, 1989.
7. Wodner-Filipowicz A, Heusser CH, and Morini C.: Production of the hemopoietic growth factors GM-CSF and interleukin-3 by mast cells in response to IgE receptor mediated activation. *Nature*, 39: 150, 1989.
8. Burd PR, Rogers HW, Gordon JR, Martin CA, Jayaraman S, Wilson SD, Dvorak AM, Gali SJ, and Dorf ME.: Interleulin-3 dependent and independent mast cells stimulated with IgE and antigen express multiple cytokines. *J Exp Med*, 70: 245, 1989.
9. Lavker RM, Kaminer MS, and Murphy GF.: Mast cell degranulation results in endothelial activation after acute exposure of human skin to UV irradiation, in: Marks and Plewig (Eds.), *Environmental Threat to the Skin*, Martin Dunitz, London, 1992, 125.
10. Walsh LJ, Trinchieri G, Waldorf HA, Whitaker D, and Murphy GF.: Human dermal mast cells contain and release tumor necrosis factor-α, which induces endothelial leukocyte adhesion molecule-1. *Proc Natl Acad Sci USA*, 8: 4220, 1991.
11. Shahanan F, Danburg JA, Fox J, et al.: Mast cell heterogeneity effects of neurogenic peptides on histamine release, *J Immunol*, 135: 133, 1985.
12. Ali H, Leung KBP, Pearce FL, Hayes MA, and Foreman JC.: Comparison of histamine releasing action of substance P on mast cells and basophils from different species and tissues. *Int Arch Allergy Appl Immunol*, 79: 413, 1986.
13. Bruni A, Bigon E, Boarato E, Mietto L, et al.: Interaction between nerve growth factor and lysophosphatidylserine on rat peritoneal mast cells. *FEBS Lett*, 138: 190, 1982.
14. Friedman MM and Kaliner MA.: Human mast cells and asthma. *Am Rev Respir Dis*, 135: 1157, 1987.
15. Taki M and Endo K.: Effect of potent selective protein kinase C inhibitor on histamine release from rat mast cells. *J Pharm Sci*, 82: 209, 1983.
16. Frosch DJ, Duncan S, and Kligman AM.: DMSO is a mast cell degranulator. *Br J Dermatol*, 102: 263, 1980.
17. Riimaru T, Nakamura M, Yano T, et al.: Mediators, initiating the inflammatory response, released in organ culture by full-thickness human skin explants exposed to the irritant, sulfur mustard, *J Invest Dermatol*, 96: 888, 1991.
18. Malavlya A, Ross E, Jakschik BA, and Abraham SN.: Mast cell degranulation induced by type 1 fimbriated *Escherichia coli* in mice, *J Clin Invest*, 93: 1645, 1994.
19. Urakami M, Hara N, Kudo I, and Inoue K.: Triggering of degranulation in Mast cells by exogenous type II phospholipase A2. *J Immunol*, 151: 5675, 1993.
20. Shoji N, Umeyama A, Takemoto T, Kobayoshi, N, and Okizumi Y.: Mast cell degraulation by Na+-K+-ATPase ion channel blocker, tridecylresorcylic acid-(TRA). *J Nat Products*, 47: 530, 1984.
21. Vliagoftis H, Dimitriadou V, Roznicicki JJ, Corrreial I, Raam S, and Theoharides TC.: Estradiol augments while tamoxafin inhibits rat mast cell secretion, *Int Arch Allergy Immunol*, 98: 398, 1992.
22. Marathius K, Lambracht-Hall M, Savala J, and Theoharides TC.: Endogenous regulation of rat brain mast cell serotonin release. *Int Arch Allergy Immunol*, 95: 332, 1991.
23. Vliagoftis H, Dimitriadou V, and Theoharides TC.: Progesterone triggers selective mast cell secretion of 5-hydroxytryptamine. *Int. Arch Allergy Immunol*, 93: 113, 1990.
24. Dimitriadou V, Lambrecht-Hall M, Reichler J, and Theoharides TC.: Histochemical and ultrastructural characterization of rat brain perivascular mast cells stimulated with compound 48/80 and carbochol. *Neuroscience*, 39: 209, 1990.

25. Fischer AA.: Contact dermatitis from topical medicaments. *Semin. Dermatol.,*1: 49, 1982.

26. Maibach HI.: Clonidine: irritant and contact dermatitis assays. *Contact Dermatol*, 12: 192, 1985.

27. *Fisher's Contact Dermatitis*, 4th Edition, Reitchel RL, Fowler JE(eds), Williams & Wilkins, Baltimore, MD, pp.1, 1995.

28. Diezel W, Gruner S, Diaz LA, and Anhalt GJ.: Inhibition of cutaneous contact hypersensitivity by calcium transport inhibitors lanthanum and diltiazem. *J Invest Dermatol*, 93: 322, 1989.

29. Amkraut A, Jordan W, and Taskovich L.: Effect of co-administration of corticosteroids on the development of contact sensitization. *J Am Acad Dermatol*, 35: 27, 1996.

30. McFadden J, Bacon K, and Camp, R.: Topically applied verapamil hydrochloride inhibits tuberculin-induced delayed-type hypersensitivity reactions in human skin. *J Invest Dermatol*, 99: 784, 1992.

31. Gallo RL and Granstein RD.: Inhibition of allergic contact dermatitis and ultraviolet irradiation-induced tissue swelling in the mouse by amiloride. *Arch Dermatol,* 125: 502, 1989.

32. Kalish RS, Wood JA, Kydonieus A, and Wille JJ.: Prevention of contact hypersensitivity to topically applied drugs by ethacrynic acid: potential application to transdermal drug delivery. *J Control Rel,* 48: 79, 1997.

33. CTFA Final Report on the Safety Assessment of Urocanic Acid. *J Am College of Toxicol*, 14: 388, 1995.

34. Klein LM, Lavker RM, Matis WL, and Murphy GF.: Degranulation of human mast cells induces an endothelial antigen central to leukocyte adhesion. *Proc Natl Acad Sci USA,* 86: 8972, 1989.

35. Freidmann PS, Pharmacological modulation of the skin immune system, in: JD Bos (ed). *Skin Immune System,* CRC Press, Boca Raton, FL, 1989, 461–483.

36. Snyder DS and Unanue ER.: Corticosteroids inhibit murine macrophage Ia expression and interleukin 1 production. *J Immunol*, 129: 1803, 1982.

37. Furue M and Katz SI, Direct effects of glucocorticosteroids on epidermal Langerhans cells. *J Invest Dermatol,* 92: 342, 1989.

38. Lavker RM, Schechter NM, and Lazarus GS.: Effects of topical corticosteroids on human dermis. *Br J Dermatol*, 115 (Suppl 31): 101, 1986.

39. Stahle M and Hagermark O.: Effects of topically applied clobetasol-17 propionate on histamine release in human skin. *Acta Dermatol Venerol*, 64: 239, 1984.

40. Burrows WM and Stoughton RB.: Inhibition of human contact sensitization by topical glucocorticosteroids. *Arch Dermatol,* 112: 175, 1976.

41. Shevach EM.: The effects of cyclosporin A on the immune system. *Annu Rev Immunol*, 3: 397, 1985.

42. Britton S and Palacios R.: Cyclosporin A. Usefulness, risks and mechanism of action. *Immunol Rev,* 65: 5, 1982.

43. Bunjes D, Hardt C, Rollinghoff M, and Wagner H.: Cyclosporin A mediates immunosuppression of primary cytotoxic T-cell responses by impairing the release of interleukin-1 and interleukin-2. *Eur J Immunol,* 11: 657, 1981.

44. Reem GH, Cook IA, and Vilcek J.: Gamma-interferon synthesis by human thymocytes and T lymphocytes is inhibited by cyclosporin A. *Science*, 221: 63, 1983.

45. Lillehof HS, Malek TR, and Shevach EM.: Differential effect of cyclosporin A on the expression of T and B lymphocyte activation antigens. *J Immunol*, 133: 244, 1984.

46. Marone G, Treiggiani M, Cirillo R, Giacummo A, et al.: Cyclosporin A inhibits the release of histamine and peptide leukotriene C from human lung mast cells. *La Ricerca Clin Lab*, 18: 53, 1988.

47. Kahan BD.: Cyclosporin: the agent and its actions. *Transplant Proc,* 17(Suppl 1): 5, 1985.

48. Trenn G, Taffs R, Hohman RJ, Kincaid R, Shevach EM, and Sitkovsky M.: Biochemical characterization of the inhibitory effect of CsA on cytolytic T lymphocyte effector functions. *J Immunol*, 142: 3796, 1989.

49. Hultsch T, Rodriguez JL, Kaliner MA, and Hohman RJ.: Cyclosporin A inhibits degranulation of rat basophilic leukemia cells and human basophils. *J Immunol*, 144: 2659, 1990.

50. Trigiani M, Cirillo R, Lichtenstain LM, and Marone G.: Inhibition of histamine and prostaglandin D2 release from human lung mast cells by ciclosporin A. *Int Arch Immunol*, 88: 253, 1989.

51. Borel JF, Feurer C, Magnee C, Stahelin H.: Effects of the new anti–lymphocyte peptide Cyclosporin A in animals, *Immunology*, 32: 1017, 1977.

52. Yarosh DB, Alas L, Kibital AL, and Ullrich SE.: Urocanic acid, immunosuppressive cytokines, and the induction of human immunodeficiency virus. *Photodermatol Photoimmunol Photomed*, 9: 127, 1992.

53. Kurimoto I and Streilein JW.: Deleterious effects of cis-urocanic acid and UVB radiation on Langerhans cells and on the induction of contact hypersensitivity are mediated by tumor necrosis factor-α. *J Invest Dermatol*, 99: 69s, 1992.

54. Bacci, S., Nakamura, T., and Streilein, J.W., Failed antigen presentation after UVB radiation correlates with modification of Langerhans cells cytoskeleton, *J Invest Dermatol*, 107: 838, 1996.

55. Moodycliffe AM, Kimber I, and Norval M.: The effect of ultraviolet B irradiation and urocanic acid isomers on dendritic cell migration. *Immunology*, 77: 394, 1992.

56. El-Ghorr, A.A. and Norval, M., A monoclonal antibody to *cis*-urocanic acid prevents the UV-induced changes in Langerhans cells and DTH responses in mice, although not preventing dendritic cell accumulation in lymph nodes draining the site of irradiation and contact hypersensitivity responses, *J Invest Dermatol*, 105: 264, 1994.

57. Iofredda MD, Whittaker D, and Murphy GF.: Mast cell degranulation upregulates $\alpha 6$ integrins on epidermal Langerhans cells. *J Invest Dermatol*, 101: 749, 1993.

58. Lambert RW and Granstein RD.: Neuropeptides and Langerhans cells. *Exp Dermatol*, 7: 73, 1998.

59. Laerma AI and Maibach HI.: Topical *cis*-urocanic acid suppresses both induction and elicitation of contact hypersensitivity in Balb/c mice. *Acta Derm Venereol (Stockh)*, 77: 272, 1995.

60. Wille JJ and Kydonieus A.: Transdermal treatment with mast cell degranulating agents for drug induced hypersensitivity. PCT EP 612525., February 1993.

61. De Fabo EC and Noonan FP.: Mechanism of immune suppression by ultraviolet irradiation in vivo. *J Exp Med*, 157: 84, 1983.

62. Reeve VE, Boehm-Wilcox C, Bosnic M, Cope R, and Ley RD.: Lack of correlation between supresion of contact hypersensitivity by UV radiation and photosensitization of epidermal urocanic acid in hairless mice. *Photochem Photobiol*, 60: 268, 1994.

63. Morison WL and Kelley SP.: Urocanic acid may not be the photoreceptor for UV-induced suppression of contact hypersensitivity. *Photodermatology*, 3: 98, 1986.

64. Ross JA, Howie SEM, Norval M, Maingay P, and Simpson TJ.: Ultraviolet irradiated urocanic acid suppresses delayed-type hypersensitivity to Herpes simplex virus in mice. *J Invest Dermatol*, 87: 630, 1986.

65. Ross JA, Howie SEM, Norval M, and Maingay J.: Two phenotypically distinct cells are involved in UV-irradiated urocanic acid-induced suppression of the efferent DTH response to HSV-1 in vivo, *J Invest Dermatol*, 89: 230, 1987.

66. Norval M, Simpson TJ, Bardshiri E, and Howie, SEM.: Urocanic acid analogues and the suppression of the delayed type hypersensitivity response to Herpes simplex virus. *Photochem Photobiol*, 9: 633, 1989.

67. Ross JA, Howie SEM, Norval M, and Miangay J.: Systemic administration of urocanic acid generates suppression of the delayed type hypersensitivity response to herpes simplex virus in a murine model of infection. *Photodermatology*, 5: 9, 1988.

68. Ross JA, Howie SEM, Norval M, and Maingay JP.: Induction of suppression of delayed type hypersensitivity to Herpes simplex virus by epidermal cells exposed to UV-irradiated urocanic acid in vivo. *Viral Immunol*, 1: 191, 1988.

69. Harriot-Smith TG and Halliday WJ.: Suppression of contact hypersensitivity by short-term ultraviolet irradiation:II. The role of cis-urocanic acid. *Clin Exp Immunol*, 72: 174, 1988.

70. Rasanen L, Jansen CT, Reunala T, and Morrison H.: Stereospecific inhibition of human epidermal cell interleukin-1 secretion and HLA-DR expression by cis-urocanic acid. *Photodermatology*, 4: 182, 1987.

71. Noonan FP, De Fabo EC, and Morrison H.: Cis urocanic acid, a product formed by ultraviolet B irradiation of the skin, initiates an antigen presentation defect in splenic dendritic cells in vivo. *J. Invest Dermatol*, 90: 92, 1988.

72. Gruner S, Oesterwitz H, Stoppe H, Henke W, Eckert R, and Sonnischsen N.: Cis-urocanic acid as a mediator of ultraviolet light-induced immunosuppression. *Semin Hematol*, 1: 102, 1992.

73. Beissert S, Mohammad T, Torri H, Lonati A, Yan Z, Morrison H, and Granstein, R.D.: Regulation of tumor antigen presentation by urocanic acid. *J Immunol*, 169: 92, 1997

74. Norval M, Gilmour JW, and Simpson TJ.: The effect of histamine receptor antagonists on immunosuppression induced by the cis-isomer of urocanic acid. *Photodermatol Photoimmunol Photomed*, 7: 243, 1990.

75. Hart P.H, Jaksic A, Swift G, Norval M, El-Ghorr ASA, and Finlay-Jones JJ.: Histamine involvement in UVB- and cis-urocanic acid-induced systemic suppression of contact hypersensitivity responses. *Immunology*, 91: 601, 1997.

76. Reeve VE, Bosnic M, and Rozinova E.: Carnosine (β-alanylhistidine) protects from the suppression of contact hypersensitivity by ultraviolet B(280-320 nm) radiation or by cis-urocanic acid. *Immunology*, 78: 99, 1993.

77. Hart PH, Jones CA, Jones KL, Watson CJ, Santucci I, Spencer LK, and Finlay-Jones, JJ.: Cis urocanic acid stimulates human peripheral blood monocyte prostaglandin E2 production and suppresses indirectly tumor necrosis factor-α. *J Immunol*, 150: 4514, 1993.

78. Palaszynski EW, Noonan FP, and De Fabo EC.: Cis-urocanic acid down-regulates the induction of adenosine 3′, 5′-cyclic monophosphate by either trans-urocanic acid or histamine in human dermal fibroblasts. *Photochem Photobiol,* 55: 165, 1992.

79. Laihia JK, Attila M, Neuvonen K, et al.: Urocanic acid binds to GABA but not to histamine (H1, H2 or H3) receptors. *J Invest Dermatol*, 11: 705–706, 1998.

80. Hemelaar PJ, Beijersbergen van Henegouwen GMJ.: The protective effect of N-acetylcsteine on UVB induced immunosuppression by inhibition of the action of cis-urocanic acid. *Photochem Photobiol,* 63: 322, 1996.

81. Krutmann J.: Ultraviolet A radiation induced immunomodulation: molecular and photobiological mechanism. *Eur J Dermato,* 8: 200, 1998.

82. Kurimoto I and Streilein JW.: cis-Urocanic acid suppression of contact hypersensitivity induction is mediated via tumor necrosis factor-α. *J Immunol*, 148: 3072, 1992.

83. Moodycliffe AM, Norval M, Kimber I, and Simpson TJ.: Characterization of a monoclonal antibody to cis-urocanic acid in the serum of irradiation mice by immunoassay, *Immunology,* 79: 667, 1993.

84. Moodycliffe AM, Bucana CD, Kripke ML, Norval M, and Ullrich SE.: Differential effects of a monoclonal antibody to cis-urocanic acid on the suppression of delayed and contact hypersensitivity following ultraviolet irradiation, *J Immunol,* 157: 2891, 1996.

85. Yamazaki S, Yokezeki H, Sahoh T, Katayama I, and Nishioka K.: TNF-α, RANTES, and MCP 1 are major chemoattractants of murine Langerhans cells to the regional lymph nodes. *Exp Dermatol*, 7: 35, 1998.

86. Jakob T and Udey MC.: Regulation of E-cadherin-mediated adhesion in Langerhan cell-like dendritic cells by inflammatory mediators that mobilize Langerhans cell in vivo. *J Immunol*, 160: 4067, 1998.

87. Cumberbatch M, Dearman RJ, and Kimber I.: Langerhans cells require signals from both tumor necrosis factor-alpha and interleukin-1 beta for migration. *Immunology,* 92: 388, 1997.

88. Price AA, Cumberbatch M, Kimber I, and Ager A.: Alpha 6 integrins are required for Langerhans cell migration from the epidermis. *J Exp Med,* 186: 1725, 1997.

89. Reeve VE, Bosnic M, et al.: Ultraviolet A radiation (320–400 nm) protects hairless mice from immunosuppression induced by ultraviolet B radiation (280–320 nm) or cis-urocanic acid. *Int Arch Allergy Immunol,* 115: 316, 1998.

90. Yarosh DB and Kripke ML.: DNA repair and cytokines in anti-mutagensis and anticarcinogenesis. *Mutation Res,* 350: 255, 1996.

91. Petit-Frere C, Clingen PH, Grewe M, Krutman J, Roza L, Arlett CF, and Green MHL.: Induction of interleukin-6 production by ultraviolet radiation in normal human epidermal keratinocytes and in a human keratinocyte line is mediated by DNA damage. *J Invest Dermatol,* 111: 354, 1998.

18 Modulation of Neurogenic Inflammation by Strontium

Gary S. Hahn

CONTENTS

I. INTRODUCTION

When the skin is exposed to irritating chemicals found in the environment or in many topical products, rapid-onset sensory irritation characterized by stinging, burning, and itching may occur. These sensations may be present without any visible changes in the skin's appearance, or may be accompanied by erythema with or without edema.[40] The fact that nerves in the skin could cause dermal erythema was first described by Bayliss, who demonstrated that electrical stimulation of the spinal cord could produce vasodilatation in the skin.[2] The ability of nerves to mediate dermal inflammation in response to irritating chemical exposure was first described by Bruce, who found that the inflammatory response of the skin to mustard oil was diminished when the sensory nerves innervating the application site were damaged.[5] Bruce termed this response the "axon reflex" to indicate that nerves actively contribute to inflammation in chemically induced skin damage. Later studies by Thomas Lewis on chemically induced skin irritation further strengthened the role of skin nerves in irritant reactions through the skin's "triple response" of localized erythema, edema, and an erythematous flare that may extend for several centimeters around the site of chemical application or physical trauma.[21,22] This "triple response of Lewis" can occur after exposure to insect bites, localized pressure (e.g., firm rubbing of the skin with a pointed object), direct electrical stimulation of the skin, and by many chemically and biologically unrelated substances such as histamine, neuropeptides (e.g., substance P), and many acidic and basic chemicals found in cosmetics, personal care products, pharmaceuticals, and during occupational exposure. Lewis suggested that activation of sensory nerves from injurious skin exposure resulted in signals sent to the spinal cord and, ultimately, the brain where irritant sensations reach conscious awareness. Lewis also hypothesized a novel pathway for nerve conduction that was counterintuitive. He proposed that the flare and inflammation of the triple response occurred when irritant-stimulated nerves sent a retrograde (backward) conduction of nerve impulses from the spinal cord to the site of injury, causing a local inflammatory reaction at the site of stimulation. This process, now confirmed, is called "neurogenic inflammation."[27]

II. NEUROGENIC INFLAMMATION

It is known that the skin contains distinct nerves that convey sensations of touch, vibration, position sense, and temperature.[24] Nerves that transmit the sharp, highly localized pain of a pin prick or paper cut (A delta fibers) are thin (1 to 5 µm in diameter), slowly conducting (5 to 30 m/s) compared to the most rapidly conducting nerves (80 to 120 m/s), and are thinly myelinated. In contrast, stinging, burning, itching, and poorly localized burning pain are transmitted by a subset of type C fibers that are thinner (0.2 to 1.5 µm in diameter), slowly conducting (0.5 to 2 m/s), unmyelinated, and chemically sensitive. Also called "nociceptors" (from the Latin *nocere*, to injure), these neurons are exquisitely sensitive to slight, transient changes in their biochemical milieu. Chemically sensitive nociceptors are also sensitive to certain forms of mechanical stimulation (e.g., wool) and elevated temperatures, and are thus termed "polymodal nociceptors." Type C nociceptors are present throughout the dermis and extend to the outermost layer of the viable epidermis, thus acting as one of the skin's earliest warning systems.[19] When their chemical environment is altered by slight changes in pH, or by chemical irritants, nociceptors depolarize, synapse in the dorsal root ganglion (DRG) of the spinal cord, and continue via neurons in the lateral spinothalamic tract to the brain, where their annoying aspects are fully appreciated. If the magnitude of the irritant stimulus is sufficiently high, interneurons in the DRG or local conduction of depolarizing signals within the terminal arborization of a single nerve fiber send a retrograde depolarization signal down the activated fiber that triggers the exocytosis of inflammatory mediators at the site of the irritant stimulus.[1,39] The principal mediators in humans include substance P, calcitonin gene-related peptide (CGRP), and neurokinin-A (a member of the substance P family). Substance P binds to stereospecific receptors on postcapillary venule endothelial cells, causing vasodilation (erythema) and extravasation (edema), and to substance P-specific receptors on neutrophils, macrophages, monocytes, and lymphocytes, causing chemotaxis and cellular activation. Additionally, substance P binds to nonstereospecific receptors on mast cells, causing them to degranulate and release histamine and other vasoactive inflammatory mediators. Histamine, in turn, binds to H1 histamine receptors on vascular endothelial cells, increasing extravasation, and to H1 receptors on a recently identified subset of type C neurons that appear to be itch specific.[36] CGRP binds to specific receptors on vascular endothelial cells and causes vasodilation without extravasation. Neurokinin-A does not activate mast cells, but does mimic substance P in causing extravasation and edema.

It is notable that the neurogenic inflammatory response ultimately activates the same immune system cells that participate in immediate, type 1 hypersensitivity, triggered by the IgE antibody and in the delayed, type 4 hypersensitivity, triggered by lymphocytes, but the activation of the response is neurally triggered. For this reason, the histological appearance of the reactions is very similar and may be indistinguishable when the response is chronic and causes the preeczematous condition cumulative irritant dermatitis that is responsible for considerable occupational disability.[3,42]

III. THE NEUROGENIC INFLAMMATION SYNDROME IS A CONTINUUM OF RESPONSES

To understand the clinical manifestations of the neurogenic inflammatory response, it is important to appreciate that it may occur in "quantum steps," depending on the nature and intensity of the irritating triggering process. Many chemicals activate only the afferent limb of the response that is perceived as stinging, burning, and/or itching without coexisting erythema and edema characteristic of the entire neurogenic reaction. These types of sensory irritation-only reactions are frequently experienced by people with sensitive skin upon exposure to many cosmetics and personal care products and may be reproducibly produced by applying acidic formulations of alpha-hydroxy acids (AHAs) to the faces of human subjects.[9] When the magnitude of the irritant stimulus is increased to a sufficient level, for example, by increasing the concentration of AHA in a facial challenge and/or by lowering its pH, transient erythema will accompany the sensory irritation reaction. At yet higher AHA concentrations used in chemical peels, edema may accompany the sensory irritation and erythema.[4]

IV. INHIBITORS OF NEUROGENIC INFLAMMATION IN CLINICAL USE

Several classes of substances are used to suppress type C nerve activation responsible for the purely sensory irritation reaction induced by chemical irritants or by exposure to irritating physical, disease, or environmental processes. Local anesthetics like lidocaine or procaine (Novocaine™) suppress the ability of neurons to depolarize and propagate an action potential necessary for nerve conduction by blocking sodium ion channels. Due to their nonspecific interaction with sodium channels in all classes of nerves, however, local anesthetics block not only irritant sensations but also tactile sensations, which causes numbness and other side effects.[34] Type C neurons also have stereospecific receptors for capsaicin, the ingredient in hot chili peppers responsible for their hot, burning qualities. When capsaicin binds to its receptor, the receptor opens an integral ion channel that allows sodium and calcium to enter the neuron, causing depolarization and transmission of an irritant signal.[7] When capsaicin is applied to the skin, it induces a potent burning sensation that can be accompanied by both erythema and edema. After repeated application of capsaicin, the neurons become desensitized, resulting in reduced sensitivity to subsequent irritant stimuli. This antinociceptive property of capsaicin has led to its use in topical analgesic products to reduce irritation from a variety of conditions.[6] The initial burning sensation caused by capsaicin has precluded its use in other than therapeutic products in which the initial discomfort is outweighed by its ultimate long-term benefit.

Many selective and nonselective inhibitors of specific mediators of the inflammatory component of neurogenic inflammation have been used to reduce itching or inflammation. Topical antihistamines block the H1 histamine receptor on type C nerves and in capillaries and have the well-known ability to reduce itching and edema caused by histamine release, but they do not reduce irritation caused by other mediators. Glucocorticoids are a mainstay for anti-inflammatory therapy and inhibit neurogenic inflammation. Antagonists of substance P, CGRP, and neurokinin-A have been tested with variable success in many animal and human conditions, but none have achieved clinical utility.[10,23] Many conventional anti-inflammatory agents can broadly inhibit neurogenic inflammatory reactions, but none can inhibit the initial and frequently rapid sensory irritation component that is often the most bothersome.

Since a safe compound capable of blocking sensory irritation and inflammation would provide considerable benefit, we sought to identify compounds that could effectively block sensory irritant reactions. Simple water-soluble strontium salts have proved to be potent and selective inhibitors of chemically induced sensory irritation and neurogenic inflammation in humans and do not produce numbness or loss of other tactile sensations.

V. STRONTIUM INHIBITS SENSORY IRRITATION AND NEUROGENIC INFLAMMATION

A. CLINICAL EVALUATION OF SENSORY IRRITATION

Since the first step in the cascade of responses that lead to the fully developed neurogenic inflammation syndrome is sensory irritation, strontium salts were first evaluated in sensory irritation models. All clinical studies were conducted according to double-blind, vehicle-controlled, random treatment assignment protocols in which each subject served as her own control. Test subjects were healthy women, aged 18 to 65, who self-reported a history of "sensitive skin" and were sensitive to lactic acid facial challenge. Treated skin sites were first washed with Ivory™ bar soap, followed by sequential application of test materials and sensory irritation evaluation. Statistical analysis of the mean sensory irritation differences between vehicle and strontium-treated groups was conducted using the Wilcoxon Signed Ranks Test for paired comparisons. All subjects provided informed consent and all protocols were reviewed by a safety committee.

B. SENSORY IRRITATION SCALE

Each minute for 10 to 60 min, depending on the study, subjects reported the magnitude of sensory irritation (stinging + burning + itching) according to the following scale:

0 = none		
1 = slight	Transient, barely perceptible irritation	
	Doesn't bother them	
2 = mild	Definite and continuous irritation	
	Bothers them	
3 = moderate	Distinctly uncomfortable irritation	
	Bothers them and interferes with concentration	
4 = severe	Continuous, intensely uncomfortable irritation	
	Intolerable and would interfere with daily routine	

C. ACIDIC IRRITANTS

1. Lactic Acid (7.5%, pH = 1.9) Sensory Irritation on the Face

Acidic formulations of alpha-hydroxy acids like lactic acid and glycolic acid have gained popularity in cosmetics because of their ability to exfoliate the skin and reduce some of the visible signs of aging.[38] Either lactic acid alone (7.5% in 10% ethanol/water vehicle, pH = 1.9), or an identical vehicle at the same pH containing various concentrations of strontium nitrate or strontium chloride was applied (0.1 g) to cheek sites, using cotton swabs (6 swipes) extending from the nasolabial fold to the outer cheek. Test materials were applied to the right or left side of subjects' faces sequentially, followed by sensory irritation assessment on each side for 10 min. A typical time–response curve for lactic acid (7.5%, pH = 1.9) on the face is presented in Figure 1. When the areas under both irritation curves is compared, strontium nitrate inhibited sensory irritation by 74% ($p < 0.01$). Both strontium nitrate and strontium chloride produced dose-dependent inhibition of sensory irritation when mixed with lactic acid Table 1.[15,16] In separate studies, the local anesthetic lidocaine (4%) was used as a positive control. When applied at the same time as the lactic acid, lidocaine did not produce significant inhibition (<10%), presumably since it requires time to be absorbed. When lidocaine (4%) was applied 5 min prior to the lactic acid, lidocaine inhibited by 51% ($p < 0.05$, n = 10). To determine whether the strontium cation was necessary for the observed anti-irritant activity, sodium chloride (250 mM) and sodium nitrate (250 mM) were mixed with the

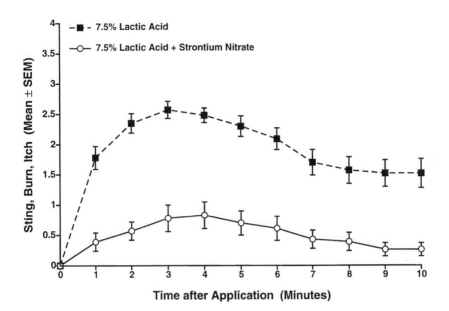

Time after Application (Minutes)

Figure 1   Lactic acid alone (closed squares) or with strontium nitrate (250 mM) was applied to the faces of 23 subjects and sensory irritation was assessed every minute for 10 min. (See text for scale.) Each data point represents the mean ± SEM irritation at each minute for all subjects. Total cumulative irritation (area under the curve) was inhibited by 68% ($p < 0.01$).

TABLE 1
Inhibition of Sensory Irritation Scores from 7.5% Lactic Acid (pH = 1.9)

Strontium Salt (mM)	Strontium Chloride[a]		Strontium Nitrate[a]	
	Inhibition[b]		Inhibition	
	% ± SEM	(# subjects, p)	% ± SEM	(# subjects, p)
500	75 ± 7	(n = 16, p < 0.005)	68 ± 6	(n = 24, p < 0.01)
250	65 ± 12	(n = 17, p < 0.01)	74 ± 7	(n = 23, p < 0.01)
125	64 ± 5	(n = 15, p < 0.01)	42 ± 14	(n = 15, p < 0.01)
63	30 ± 6	(n = 8, p < 0.01)	34 ± 8	(n = 16, p < 0.01)

[a] Strontium nitrate or strontium chloride hexahydrate was either mixed with the lactic acid vehicle (7.5%, pH = 1.9, 10% ethanol/water).

[b] The total cumulative irritation in each study (scores of 1 + 2 + 3 + 4) for the lactic acid-treated side of the face was compared to the lactic acid + strontium-treated side of the face (areas under the curves) and irritation inhibition was calculated as a percent difference.

---

lactic acid and compared to strontium nitrate (250 mM) or strontium chloride (250 mM). In both instances, sodium nitrate or sodium chloride produced insignificant (<15%, NS) inhibition of sensory irritation, proving that the nitrate or chloride anions did not produce the observed anti-irritant activity.

Pretreatment with either strontium nitrate or strontium chloride from 1 to 15 min prior to the same lactic acid facial challenge produced a similar level of sensory irritation inhibition. Substantial anti-irritancy was also observed when strontium nitrate was applied several minutes after lactic acid was applied.

2. Glycolic Acid (6%, pH = 3.0) Sensory Irritation on the Face

The anti-irritant activity of strontium salts is also evident for less acidic AHA irritants similar to what could be used in over-the-counter cosmetic products. When glycolic acid (6% in 10% ethanol/water, pH = 3.0) with or without 250 mM strontium nitrate was applied to the faces of 94 subjects, the cumulative irritation inhibition by the strontium-containing solutions was 68% ($p < .01$) (Table 2). The incidence of each of the four scores of the glycolic acid only vs. the glycolic acid + strontium was (Score 4: 19 vs. 0 = 100% inhibition; Score 3: 96 vs. 16 = 83% inhibition; Score 2: 243 vs. 60 = 75% inhibition; Score 1: 338 vs. 215 = 36% inhibition; Score 0: 338 vs. 743 = 120% increase).

TABLE 2
Inhibition of Sensory Irritation Scores by Strontium Nitrate

	Irritation Score	% Inhibition of Sensory Irritation Scores[a]			
		Glycolic Acid (6%, pH = 3.0)	Glycolic Acid (70%, pH = 0.6)	Ascorbic Acid (30%, pH = 1.7)	Thioglycolate Depilatory (4%, pH = 12)
Subjects (#)		94	19	20	23
Total scores (#)		1034	209	110	506
None	(0)	−120[b]	−381	−260	−65
Slight	(1)	36	−6	63	40
Mild	(2)	75	43	91	76
Moderate	(3)	83	92	100	71
Severe	(4)	100	100	100	—

[a] Sensory irritation was induced by glycolic acid (70%, pH = 0.6) application to arms, glycolic acid (6%, pH = 3.0) application to the face, ascorbic acid (30%, pH = 1.7) application to the face; calcium thioglycolate (4%, pH = 12) depilatory application to the legs. For each study, the incidence of each of the four sensory irritation scores (0–4) for the irritant alone and the irritant plus strontium nitrate treatment was compared. Each number represents the percent inhibition of each irritation score incidence induced by strontium nitrate.

[b] Negative inhibition values represent an increase in the score incidence.

3. Glycolic Acid (70%, pH = 0.6) Sensory Irritation on the Arms

Nineteen subjects were treated with 70% glycolic acid (pH = 0.6) with or without strontium nitrate (20% [945 mM]) on 2″ × 4″ rectangular sites on the right or left midvolar forearm and sensory irritation was evaluated every minute for 10 min, followed by neutralization with sodium bicarbonate. Within seconds after glycolic acid application (time 0 in Figure 2), sensory irritation differences were apparent between the two groups (mean ± SEM = 0.53 ± 0.16 for glycolic only vs. 0.16 ± 0.09 for glycolic + strontium), indicating that strontium had an immediate onset of action. Sensory irritation peaked at minute 4 (2.53) and remained at a plateau (range = 2.32 to 2.68) for the remainder of the study. In contrast, irritation on the strontium-containing sites ranged from 0.63 at minute 4 and stayed within the range of 0.63 to 0.79 for the rest of the study. Strontium inhibited cumulative irritation by 75% ($p < 0.005$). The data in Table 2 present the percent inhibition of each of the four sensory irritation scores induced by strontium nitrate. During the study, the 19 subjects reported 209 irritation scores. The incidence of each of the four scores of the glycolic acid only vs. the glycolic acid + strontium was (Score 4: 41 vs. 0 = 100% inhibition; Score 3: 50 vs. 4 = 92% inhibition; Score 2: 44 vs. 25 = 43% inhibition; Score 1: 47 vs. 50 = 6% increase; Score 0: 27 vs. 130 = 381% increase). In other studies, measurement of skin turnover using the dansyl chloride technique[18] demonstrated that strontium nitrate did not affect the stimulatory effect of glycolic acid on skin turnover.

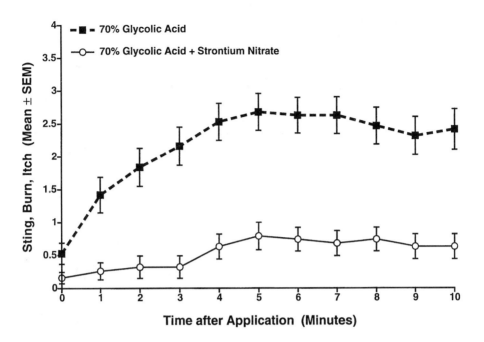

Figure 2   Glycolic acid (70%, pH = 0.6) only (closed squares) or with strontium nitrate (20%) (open circles) was applied to the forearms of 19 subjects and sensory irritation was measured every minute for 10 min. Each data point represents the mean ± SEM irritation at each minute for 19 subjects. Total cumulative irritation (areas under the curve) was inhibited by 75% ($p < 0.005$).

Clinical studies of a 70% glycolic acid (pH = 0.6) chemical peel solution with strontium nitrate applied to the whole face in over 150 human subjects demonstrated substantially reduced sensory irritation and erythema without reducing the expected benefits of the peel, as judged by clinical response or by histological analysis.[13,35]

4. Ascorbic Acid (30%, pH = 1.7) Sensory Irritation on the Face

Ascorbic acid has gained popularity as an ingredient used in "treatment cosmetics" for its antioxidant activity and ability to stimulate collagen synthesis.[9a] Since ascorbic acid is most stable and bioavailable in aqueous formulations at highly acidic pH (e.g., pH < 3), a 30% aqueous solution of ascorbic acid (pH = 1.7) was evaluated for sensory irritation with or without strontium nitrate (250 mM). After application to the face of 20 subjects, the cumulative irritation inhibition by the strontium-containing solutions was 84% ($p < 0.005$) (Table 2). The incidence of each of the four scores of the ascorbic acid only vs. the ascorbic acid + strontium was (Score 4: 1 vs. 0 = 100% inhibition; Score 3: 13 vs. 0 = 100% inhibition; Score 2: 23 vs. 2 = 91% inhibition; Score 1: 48 vs. 18 = 63% inhibition; Score 0: 25 vs. 90 = 260% increase).

5. Aluminum/Zirconium Salt Erythema on the Arms

Aluminum salts, with or without zirconium salts, are the only approved active ingredients of antiperspirants in the U.S. and frequently cause both sensory irritation and inflammation when used as directed.[29] Aluminum/zirconium salt solution (25%) with or without strontium nitrate (500 mM) or strontium chloride (500 mM) was applied to the arms of 29 subjects using occluded patches for 21 days and the magnitude of visible inflammation was evaluated every day. Inflammation was visually measured according to the following scale:

0 =   No evidence of erythema
1 =   Minimal erythema
2 =   Definite erythema
3 =   Erythema and papules

The data in Figure 3 demonstrate that both strontium nitrate (500 mM) or strontium chloride (500 mM) caused nearly complete inhibition of erythema development during the first week and substantially inhibited erythema during the second and third weeks. Total erythema caused by the aluminum/zirconium salts, calculated as the percent difference of the areas under the 21-day irritation curves, was reduced by 64% ($p < 0.0001$) by strontium nitrate and by 66% ($p < 0.0001$) by strontium chloride.

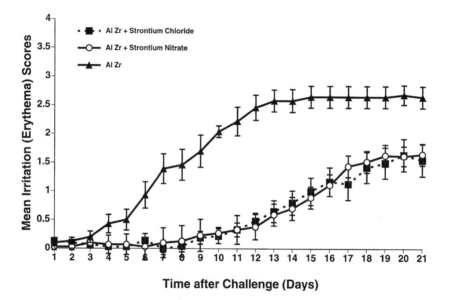

Figure 3   Strontium nitrate (500 mM, open circles) or strontium chloride (500 mM, closed squares) was mixed with the aluminum/zirconium salt solution each day when a new patch was applied. Each data point represents the mean ± SEM for 29 subjects. Total cumulative irritation (areas under the curve) was inhibited by 64% ($p < 0.0001$) for strontium nitrate and 66% for strontium chloride ($p < 0.0001$).

D. Basic Irritants — Calcium Thioglycolate Sensory Irritation on the Legs

Chemical depilatories are basic (pH = 9 to 12) and typically use calcium thioglycolate to dissolve hair keratin.[33] Twenty-three subjects shaved their legs with a safety razor to enhance irritation, then strontium nitrate pretreatment solution (10% w/v, in 10% ethanol/water) or vehicle was applied to 2″ × 4″ sites on the lateral portions of the legs. After 2 min, 5 g of depilatory lotion was applied to each leg followed by irritation evaluation every minute for 10 min. The data in Table 2 present the percent inhibition of each of the four sensory irritation scores induced by strontium nitrate. During the study, the 23 subjects reported 506 irritation scores. The incidence of each of the four scores of the depilatory vs. the depilatory + strontium was (Score 4: 0 vs. 0; Score 3: 7 vs. 2 = 71% inhibition; Score 2: 45 vs. 11 = 76% inhibition; Score 1: 88 vs. 53 = 40% inhibition; Score 0: 113 vs. 187 = 65% increase). Upon application of the depilatory, the mean sensory irritation score rose to approximately 1 during the first minute and remained at that level until minute 4, after which it declined to approximately 0.6 at the end of 10 min. Total irritation caused by the depilatory, calculated as the percent difference of the areas under the 20-min irritation curves, was reduced by 59% ($p < 0.01$).

E. Neutral Irritants (Histamine)

Histamine is contained in the preformed granules of mast cells and basophils and is released in response to many inflammatory stimuli, including substance P, during the neurogenic inflammatory process. It is a potent itch-producing chemical and directly activates type C nociceptors by binding to H1 histamine receptors in a pH-independent manner. Strontium nitrate (20%) in water or water alone was used to pretreat 4×6-cm sites on the volar forearms of 8 subjects 30 min and 5 min prior to intradermal injection of histamine (100 mcg in normal saline). Itch was assessed using a visual analog scale for 20 min. The mean itch magnitude each minute for all subjects was always less for the strontium-treated sites and reached statistical significance ($p < 0.05$) from minute 12 to the end of the study. The mean difference between the two groups continued to increase until it reached the maximum difference at 20 min, at which time itch was reduced 52% by strontium ($p < 0.05$).[43]

VI. STRONTIUM MECHANISM OF ACTION

Strontium salts can effectively suppress sensory irritation caused by chemically and biologically unrelated chemical irritants over a pH range of 0.6 to 12. Strontium's anti-irritant activity is not due to the nitrate or chloride anion alone, since sodium nitrate and sodium chloride were inactive at concentrations equimolar to active concentrations of strontium nitrate or strontium chloride. Strontium produces anti-irritation without reducing biological changes produced by exfoliative products containing alpha-hydroxy acids or beta-hydroxy acids, suggesting that its target site is intimately associated with the sensory nerves.

Water-soluble strontium salts have been reported to directly suppress neuronal depolarization when studied in animals.[14,37] Several mechanisms probably contribute to strontium's inhibitory activity. In vivo, strontium is a divalent ion with an ionic radius similar to the divalent calcium ion (1.13 vs. 0.99 Å, respectively).[31] Strontium also resembles calcium in its ability to traverse calcium-selective ion channels and trigger neurotransmitter release from nerve endings. In many systems, strontium is, however, less potent than calcium and thus can act as an inhibitor of calcium-dependent depolarization.[25,26,28,30,37] Strontium may act to block calcium dependent pathways which lead to neuronal depolarization. Neurons are also known to be sensitive to compounds that alter the electrostatic field surrounding their plasma membrane and ion channels.[17] Since strontium can alter the electrostatic field of ion channels and reduce ion permeation through them[11,32] strontium may suppress irritant-induced depolarization of unmyelinated sensory neurons. Strontium salts may also directly act on nonneuronal cells such as keratinocytes or immunoregulatory inflammatory cells. Recent reports demonstrate that strontium salts can suppress keratinocyte-derived TNF-α, IL-1α, and IL-6 in in vitro cultures.[8]

The fact that strontium can block irritation as intense as that produced by 70% unbuffered glycolic acid without causing numbness or other changes in cutaneous sensations suggests that strontium is exquisitely selective in its regulation of type C nociceptors (Figure 4). In contrast, local anesthetics like lidocaine or procaine not only block irritant sensations, but also block tactile sensations, producing numbness.[34] Recent studies support the concept that strontium is highly selective for only nociceptive subsets of sensory neurons since strontium nitrate (20%) applied to normal skin did not alter sensory thresholds for cold sensations, warmth sensations, or pain caused by cold or heat.[43]

VII. PRODUCT APPLICATIONS

Burning, stinging, and especially itching sensations are among the most troublesome symptoms that confront dermatologists. Given the paucity of agents that can rapidly and safely reduce sensory irritation, new and effective compounds are in great need. The rapid onset and anti-irritant potency of strontium salts suggests that they might have broad applications in topical products.

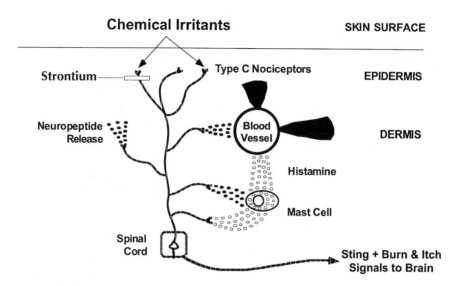

Figure 4 Chemical irritants activate unmyelinated type C nociceptors which trigger a wave of depolarization that synapses in the dorsal root ganglia (DRG) of the spinal cord, and is sensed as sting, burn, or itch. If the stimulation is of sufficient magnitude, interneurons in the DRG send a retrograde signal down the same C fibers which triggers the release of inflammatory substances including substance P, neurokinin A, calcitonin gene-related peptide (CGRP), and other mediators. These substances trigger vasodilation, and vascular permeability and activate inflammatory cells, including mast cells that, in turn, release another set of inflammatory mediators, including histamine, which further activate nociceptive sensory signals and inflammation.

A. COSMETICS AND PHARMACEUTICALS USED IN DERMATOLOGY

Both men and women typically use cosmetic products daily to beautify and protect the skin from environmental assault. Transient irritation from cosmetic products in the form of sensory irritation and/or erythema is frequent, especially when cosmetic "active ingredients" are used to reduce the appearance of fine lines and wrinkles. For people with "sensitive skin" due to inherently dry skin or other causes, the problem is compounded. Perhaps the most irritating products regulated as cosmetics in the U.S. are chemical peels used by dermatologists and aestheticians. Compounds regulated as over-the-counter drugs and prescription drugs also frequently have sensory irritation as a side effect that can reduce patient compliance and ultimately the therapeutic efficacy of the product. In addition to products intentionally applied to the skin, many workers are exposed to chemical irritants in the workplace that can result in considerable occupational disability.[3,20,44] Strontium salts, particularly strontium nitrate, have proven to be highly effective in reducing irritation and erythema from many irritating ingredients used in topical products and found in the workplace. The first strontium-containing cosmetic products will be available through physicians.

B. POTENTIAL FOR STRONTIUM USE IN OTHER ORGAN SYSTEMS

The neurogenic inflammation syndrome is believed to be pathogenically important in many irritating and inflammatory conditions, including irritant and allergic contact dermatitis, psoriasis, atopic dermatitis, ocular irritation and inflammation, allergic rhinitis, asthma, rheumatoid arthritis, inflammatory bowel disease, and other gastrointestinal disorders.[12] Topical application of strontium salts may act to reduce the initial stage of sensory irritation in these conditions and well as the later stage of frank inflammation.

Strontium salts represent a new class of selective inhibitors of sensory irritation and irritant contact dermatitis without local anesthetic side effects.

REFERENCES

1. Baluk P. Neurogenic inflammation in skin and airways. *J Invest Dermatol.* 1997; 2:76–81.
2. Bayliss WM. On the origin from the spinal cord of vasodilator fibres of the hind limb, and on the nature of these fibres. *J Physiol (London)* 1901; 26:173.
3. Björnberg A. Irritant Dermatitis. In: Maibach, HI, editor. *Occupational and Industrial Dermatology.* 2nd ed. Chicago: Year Book Medical Publishers; 1987. p. 15–21.
4. Brody HJ. *Chemical Peeling and Resurfacing.* 2nd ed. St. Louis, MO: Mosby; 1997. p. 73–108.
5. Bruce AN. Vasodilator axon reflexes. *Q J Physiol* 1913; 6:339.
6. Campbell E, Bevan S, Dray A. Clinical applications of capsaicin and its analogs. In: Wood J, editor. *Capsaicin in the Study of Pain.* New York: Academic Press; 1993. p. 255–272.
7. Caterina MJ, Schumacher MA, Tominaga M, Rosen TA, Levine JD, Julius D. The capsaicin receptor: a heat-activated ion channel in the pain pathway. *Nature* 1997; 389:816–824.
8. Celerier P, Richard A, Litoux P, Dreno B. Modulatory effects of selenium and strontium salts on keratinocyte-derived inflammatory cytokines. *Arch Dermatol Res* 1995; 287:680–682.
9. Christensen M, Kligman AM. An improved procedure for conducting lactic acid stinging tests on facial skin. *J Soc Cosmet Chem* 1996; 47:1–11.
9a. Colven RM, Pinnell SR. Topical vitamin C in aging. *Clin Dermatol* 1996; 14:227–234.
10. Donneren J, Amann R. The inhibition of neurogenic inflammation. *Gen Pharmacol* 1993; 24:519–529.
11. Elinder F, Medeja M, Arhem P. Surface charges of K+ : Effects of strontium on five cloned channels expressed on *Xenopus* oocytes. *J Gen Physiol* 1996; 108:325–332.
12. Geppetti P, Holzer P. *Neurogenic Inflammation.* Boca Raton FL: CRC Press; 1996. p. 1–324.
13. Greenway HT, Peterson C, Plis J, Cornell R, Hahn GS, Harper RA. Efficacy of a 70% glycolic acid peel product regimen containing the anti-irritant strontium nitrate (Abst) – Poster at American Academy of Dermatology — 1999. Manuscript to be submitted.
14. Gutentag H. The effect of strontium chloride on peripheral nerve in comparison to the action of "stabilizer" and "labilizer" compounds. *Penn Dent J* 1965; 68:37–43.
15. Hahn GS. Strontium is a potent and selective inhibitor of sensory irritation. *Dermatol Surg* 1999; 25: 1–6.
16. Hahn GS, Thueson DO. Inventors: Cosmederm Technologies, Inc., assignee. Formulations and Methods for Reducing Skin Irritation. U.S. Patent 5,716,625. February 10, 1998.
17. Hille B. *Ionic Channels of Excitable Membranes.* 2nd ed. Sunderland, MA: Sinauer Associates; 1992. p. 445–471.
18. Jansen LH, Hojyo-Tomoko MT, Kligman AM. Improved fluorescence staining technique for estimating turnover of human stratum corneum. *Br J Dermatol* 1973; 90:9–12.
19. Kennedy WR, Wendelschafer-Crabb G. The innervation of the human epidermis. *J Neurol Sci (Netherlands)* 1993; 115:184–190.
20. Lammintausta K, Maibach, HI, Wilson D. Mechanisms of Subject (Sensory) Irritation: Propensity to non-immunologic contact urticaria and objective irritation in stingers. *Dermatosen* 1988; 36:45–49.
21. Lewis T. *The Blood Vessels of the Human Skin and Their Responses.* London: Shaw; 1927.
22. Lewis T. Observations upon reactions of vessels in human skin to cold. *Heart* 1930; 15:177.
23. Longmore J, Hill RG, Hargreaves RJ. Neurokinin-receptor antagonists: pharmacological tools and therapeutic drugs. *Can J Physiol Pharmacol* 1997; 75:612–621.
24. Martin JH, Jessell TM. Modality Coding in the Somatic Sensory System. In: Kandel ER, Schwartz JH, Jessell TM, editors. *Principles of Neural Science.* 3rd ed. New York: Elsevier; 1991. p. 341.
25. Meiri U, Rahamimoff R. Activation of transmitter release by strontium and calcium ions at the neuromuscular junction. *J Physiol* 1971; 215:709–726.
26. Mellow AM, Perry BD, Silinsky EM. Effects of calcium and strontium in the process of acetylcholine release from motor nerve endings. *J Physiol* 1982; 328:547–562.
27. Meyer RA, Campbell JN, Raja SN. Peripheral neural mechanisms of nociception. In: Wall PD, Melzack R, editors. *Textbook of Pain.* 3rd ed. London: Churchill Livingstone; 1994. p. 13–44.
28. Miledi R. Strontium as a substitute for calcium in the process of transmitter release at the neuromuscular junction. *Nature* 1966; 212:1233–1234.
29. Mueller WH, Quatrale RP. Antiperspirants and Deodorants. In: deVavarre MG, editor. *The Chemistry and Manufacture of Cosmetics* Vol. 3. 2nd ed. Wheaton, IL: Allured Publishing; 1993. p. 205–228.

30. Nakazato Y, Onoda Y. Barium and strontium can substitute for calcium in noradrenaline output induced by excess potassium in the guinea pig. *J Physiol* 1980; 305:59–71.

31. Pauling L. *Nature of the Chemical Bond and Structure of Molecules and Crystals.* 3rd ed. Ithaca, NY: Cornell University Press; 1960. p. 644.

32. Reuveny E, Jan YN, Jan,YL. Contributions of a negatively charged residue in the hydrophobic domain of the IRK1 inwardly rectifying K+ channel to K+-selective permeation. *Biophys J* 1996; 70:754–761.

33. Rieger MM, Brechner S. Depilatories. In: deVavarre MG, editor. *The Chemistry and Manufacture of Cosmetics* Vol. 4. 2nd ed. Wheaton, IL: Allured Publishing; 1993. p. 1229–1273.

34. Ritchie JM, Greene, NM. Local Anesthetics. In: Gilman AG, Rall TW, Nies AS, Taylor P, editors. *The Pharmacological Basis of Therapeutics.* 8th ed. New York: McGraw-Hill; 1993. p. 311–331.

35. Rubin MG, Harper RA, Hahn GS. Strontium nitrate in 70% free glycolic acid peels significantly reduces erythema and sensory irritation. (Abstr) – Poster at American Academy of Dermatology — 1999. Manuscript to be submitted.

36. Schmelz M, Schmidt R, Bickel A, Handwerker HO, Torebjörk HE. *J Neurosci* 1997; 17:8003–8008.

37. Silinsky EM, Mellow, AM. The relationship between strontium and other divalent cations in the process of transmitter release from cholinergic nerve endings. In: Skoryna SC, editor. *Handbook of Stable Strontium.* New York: Plenum Press; 1981. p. 263–285.

38. Stiller MJ, Bartolone J, Stern R, Kollias N, Gillies R, Drake LA. Topical 8% glycolic acid and 8% L-lactic acid creams for the treatment of photodamaged skin. A double–blind vehicle-controlled clinical trial. *Arch Dermatol* 1996; 132:631–636.

39. Szolcsanyi J. Neurogenic Inflammation: Reevaluation of Axon Reflex Theory. In: Geppetti P, Holzer P, editors. *Neurogenic Inflammation.* New York; 1996. p. 33–42.

40. Tausk F, Christian E, Johansson O, Milgram S. Neurobiology of the Skin. In: Fitzpatrick TB, Eisen AZ, Wolff K, Freedberg IM, Austen KF, editors. *Dermatology in General Medicine* Vol 1. 4th ed. New York: McGraw-Hill; 1993. p. 396–403.

41. Weltfriend SI, Bason M, Lammintausta K, Maibach HI. Irritant dermatitis (Irritation). In: Marzulli FN, Maibach HI, editors. *Dermatotoxicology.* 5th ed. Washington, D.C.: Taylor & Francis; 1996. p. 87–118.

42. Willis CM. The histopathology of irritant contact dermatitis. In: Van der Valk PG, Maibach HI, editors. *The Irritant Contact Dermatitis Syndrome.* Boca Raton, FL: CRC Press; 1996. p. 291–303.

43. Zhai H, Hannon W, Harper RA, Hahn, GS, Alessandra P, Maibach, HI. Strontium nitrate decreased itch magnitude and duration without effecting thermal pain or sensation in experimentally-induced pruritis in man. Submitted 1998.

19 Skin Tolerability of Iontophoretic Treatment

Bret Berner and Donald R. Wilson

CONTENTS

I. INTRODUCTION

Iontophoresis or the application of electric current to the skin is used to deliver drugs topically or systemically[1-3] or to extract interstitial fluid for diagnostic analysis.[4-6] An iontophoretic product for delivery of lidocaine for topical anesthesia is currently available,[7] and a patient-controlled analgesia iontophoretic system for fentanyl is in phase III clinical trials.[2] A reverse iontophoretic noninvasive glucose monitoring device[4,5] is in advanced clinical trials.

Clinical iontophoretic application of lidocaine, dexamethasone, and pilocarpine for a brief duration has resulted in a minimal incidence and severity of adverse skin reactions.[8] However, the formulation, drug, and current density can substantially influence the amount of skin irritation and sensation. As with passive transdermal systems, in particular transdermal clonidine,[9] the acceptability of these skin reactions becomes a therapeutic risk–benefit assessment. A variety of adverse events involving skin reactions have been reported, including mild-to-severe irritation, rare cases of sensitization, burns, pettichiae, folliculitis, itching, and pain.[8]

While numerous reviews of iontophoretic delivery exist,[1-3] there is currently only one recent review by Ledger[8] of skin tolerability and iontophoresis. In the present review, the literature is surveyed to describe the skin reactions or sensations and the conditions under which they are most frequently observed. A description of these skin reactions including grading scales and the techniques found particularly useful by the authors are then discussed.

II. SENSATION AND PAIN

While a large body of clinical literature now indicates the safety of short-term iontophoresis of steroids and nonsteroidal antiinflammatory drugs,[8] a variety of unpleasant sensations have been described, ranging from tingling and itching[10] to perceived changes in local temperature[8] to pain.[11]

The classical studies of Molitor and Fernandez[12] describe a nearly inverse hyperbolic relationship between current density and electrode area for the maximum tolerable current density. Given this near hyperbolic relationship, the product, i.e., the maximum tolerated total current, should be nearly constant. However, recruitment of additional nerve fibers, variation in the density and depth of cutaneous innervation among body sites, and numerous other variables cause considerable deviation. Except for selected data, total current does not appear to explain the data any better than current density. Prausnitz[13] reviewed the literature and modeled the perception and pain thresholds for current and current density vs. electrode area. With power laws there is still considerable variation in the data. Moreover, the current increases with the electrode area with an exponent of 0.21 and 0.33 and the current density scales inversely with electrode area with exponents of –0.79 and –0.67 for perception and pain, respectively.

There is some agreement that a value of 0.5 mA/cm^2 is the approximate threshold of pain,[11] but depending on the electrode area, frequency, and duration, this threshold may be exceeded considerably. For a very short duration, larger current densities and currents may be well tolerated.[13]

Tingling and itching have been associated with the recruitment of C fibers that have their nerve endings in the epidermis underlying the stratum corneum.[14] There is some evidence that adroit formulation may alter this sensation,[13] but this may reflect better electrode contact and the resulting more even current densities.

III. DESCRIPTION OF IRRITATION

As with chemically, mechanically, and light-induced skin irritation, the severity of an irritant response within a given area of skin to electric current increases with exposure, i.e., both the magnitude and duration of the applied stimulus. The unit of electrical magnitude that best relates to skin irritation is current density. In principle, for a given formulation the relative proportions of voltage, current, resistance, and skin area may all change, but the level of induced skin irritation should remain the same, providing current density and duration are held constant. Duration is the time that the skin is exposed to the stimulus. In the case where the stimulus is a series of repeated pulses, duration is the sum of all the pulses. Within a range of current densities, irritation can be quite insensitive to duration over more than an order of magnitude.

Since skin irritation induced by iontophoresis is associated with electric current, the lesion may be termed an electrical burn according to common medical usage.[15] Since the word "burn" first connotes a lesion caused by contact with heat or fire, the term is unfortunately misleading. The skin irritation produced by the iontophoretic range of current densities is not a thermal burn caused by heat. As a thermoregulatory organ, human skin is a heat sink. Resting blood flow to the skin is about 0.25 $ml/cm^2/min$. When the skin is heated until maximally vasodilated, this flow may increase seven times to 1.75 $ml/cm^2/min$.[16] In practice, no increase above normal body temperature can be detected in the skin with either skin surface or infrared probes when applying iontophoretic current densities.

Skin irritation from iontophoresis compares best with chemical irritation and primary irritant dermatitis, and may in fact have a real chemical cause. Here again, "burn" cannot be avoided since severe primary irritation is also termed a chemical burn or dermatitis escharotica.[15] The necrosis depicting a third degree heat burn also characterizes a chemical burn. The terms "first-degree burn" or "erythema" and "second-degree burn" or "vesiculation" correspond, respectively, to conditions seen in mild and moderate primary irritant dermatitis, but are not used to describe chemical irritation.

Burns resulting from iontophoresis have been linked to excessive current density passing through the tissue, resulting from shunts or poor electrode contact or the electrode or a wire touching the body and to changes in pH. While pH changes do not account for these other cases of localized high current density and burns, Molitor and Fernandez[12,17] and later Schwarz et al.[11] did show relationships between burns and the basic and acidic pH that may be generated at certain electrode materials such as platinum. Selection of a different electrode material is often advisable for this reason.

Iontophoretic chemical irritation may occur when copper or platinum electrodes are used. In this case, hydroxyl (OH^-) groups are produced at the cathode, and hydrogen ions (H^+) are produced at the anode.[18] These, respectively, create basic and acidic irritation under the electrodes which may ultimately cause necrosis. At equal normality, the irritation response to a base will be stronger than to an acid. Scarring results when necrosis is produced. If the copper leads from iontophoretic electrodes accidentally contact the skin for a period of time, pH irritation will be demonstrated and necrosis may occur.

In clinical usage where the pH and current have been optimized, only transient erythema has been reported. This transient erythema typically lasts from less than 1 h to a day[19] and is not of any clinical significance.

When pH is controlled through the cautious selection of electrodes and electrolytes, excessive iontophoretic current densities may still produce skin irritation similar to that of soap. These conditions may occur at high current densities where there is substantial convective flow, as may be demonstrated by a potassium efflux from the skin associated with iontophoretic irritation.[20]

Under these conditions of moderate iontophoretic irritation, the erythema and edema across the skin site are rarely uniform. Instead, a peppering of palpable red spots occurs, and many spots have visible hairs emanating from their centers (i.e., folliculitis). Spots without hairs often fit the pattern where hair should be. Upon close inspection, many spots have small fluid vesicles raised above the skin surface. Air in the vesicles or loose scale on the surface may give them a whitish cap. The vesicles are filled with a yellowish serous exudate, and a small scab or eschar quickly forms if the vesicle ruptures, suggesting a high initial fibrinogen content. The scabs trigger local scaling around their periphery. Both scabs and scale cause the skin to feel rough during the recovery phase.

In the analogy between soap[21] and iontophoresis, both appear to have identified the same path of least resistance through the hair follicle to reach the dermis, and the density of the irritant stimulus appears to be strongest within the follicle. Beyond this, the similarity is unclear. Soaps may be envisioned to attack cell membranes, alter membrane potentials, and trigger the release of cytokines and vasoactive agents that initiate the irritation response. The mechanism by which iontophoretic current, devoid of heat and pH effects, causes irritation is less known. Nevertheless, an increased efflux of potassium, indicating potential disruption of membrane function, has been associated with iontophoretic irritation,[20] and prostaglandins have been determined after iontophoresis.[22] Histamine release has also been associated with iontophoretic irritation.[23] These similarities suggest that the analogy may also be physiologically correct.

In addition, iontophoretic current at sufficient current densities causes electroosmosis, a flow of water.[24] This may contribute to a physical electroosmotic effect that helps create interstitial edema and vesiculation. However, the suppression of vesicles and iontophoretic irritation by treatment with corticosteroids[25] supports a purely physiological, rather than a physical, mechanism.

In some individuals, the iontophoresis-induced spots are small and numerous, suggesting that sweat ducts have become the preferred electrical path. The conduction of electric current through sweat ducts is demonstrated in using iontophoresis to treat hyperhidrosis on the hands and feet.[26] Here, where hair is absent, vesiculation may occur, but it more closely resembles milliaria crystallina[18] of an active sweat gland producing sweat in a duct that is physically occluded by iontophoresis.[18] The vesicles of milliaria crystallina are formed above the basal membrane by sweat pressure and typically have little erythema or tissue edema and do not itch.

There is much intersubject variability in the way that iontophoretic irritation manifests itself, but there is always a strong similarity in the type of response shown by a given individual. Individuals usually show variability only in the intensity of a response, and their response may be more severe in the winter season. To illustrate extremes between subjects, one person may have reactions characterized by four or five rather large vesicular spots rising from a region of relatively normal skin. Here, the electric current appears to have selected just a few low resistance hair follicles and did not pass uniformly through the skin. Another person may demonstrate an even erythema and edema pattern, indicating a more uniform passage of current. An almost uniform or blotchy pattern may result when the reactions of small palpable spots blend together.

Some individuals mention that site irritation increases and itches during bathing or vigorous exercise. While skin reactions usually occur just in the electrode region, strong reactions often cause an erythemic and edematous flare that fades with distance from the site. If the electrode site is vesiculated, the vesicles are usually confined to the electrode region. High irritant responders fall into two general categories: (a) those who possess a maximum response soon after the iontophoretic electrodes are removed from the skin and (b) those who show a maximum response 2 to 3 days after electrode removal. Both vigorous exercisers who sweat profusely and those who rarely sweat at all may fall into the delayed maximum response category. Regardless of the time to reach a maximum response, once the peak occurs, itching disappears immediately, and the site progresses through the rapid recovery phase typical of irritant reactions. During the first week of recovery, most vesicles rupture to become scabs which trigger localized scaling; the remaining vesicles are slowly reabsorbed. Erythema and edema also began to clear. During the second week, residual erythema and edema usually clear completely. Any remaining scale and scabs usually slough away in the third week. A tan response may persist in some subjects for several months. No scarring occurs.

IV. EVALUATION OF IRRITATION IN ANIMALS AND IN MAN

The evaluation of irritation from iontophoretic devices is complicated by the multiple potential irritant sources: (a) iontophoresis, (b) chemical from the formulation, and (c) mechanical from the device. Separate studies need to be designed for each source.

Mechanical irritation can be determined from passive wear studies, i.e., no current, and from careful observation of the areas beyond the electrodes. Mechanical effects for devices can range from transient erythema that disappears within 1/2 hour to abrasions or blisters. Reducing these reactions is accomplished through adroit device design and passive wear studies. Edge effects and slippage of a tightly attached device can be the major sources of mechanical irritation of devices.

Chemical irritation can be addressed with both passive and placebo-controlled iontophoretic studies. Classical skin irritation testing of the formulation under passive conditions in rabbits[27] or in man[28] can provide information on the chemically induced irritation from a component in the formulation. However, skin irritation increases almost linearly with the flux of the irritant compound over the mild-to-moderate irritant response regime. Consequently, iontophoresis can enhance the flux and the ensuing reaction to an irritating agent well beyond that observed by passive delivery alone. To establish a no-effect level for a potential irritant, iontophoretic studies with and without that agent may be necessary. Observation of the placebo site should help separate irritation resulting from the agent from iontophoresis or other sources. Similarly, a balance of efficacious delivery and acceptable skin irritation may be achieved through a study of irritation under iontophoresis at different current densities. While in a passive study, the flux may be controlled through the concentration of the irritant, the current density most easily controls the flux in an iontophoretic study.

Iontophoretically induced irritation has been evaluated in rabbits[8] and in pigs.[29] In cases where the drug was the source of irritation or where at most transient erythema was produced in man, these animal models were reasonably predictive. However, in cases where moderate irritant responses with vesiculation to iontophoresis alone were produced in man, both the rabbit and pig models have given false negatives.

The evaluation in man of iontophoretic irritation follows the conventional approach of Draize with separate erythema and edema scores. These scores may then be combined to form a single primary irritant index[27] to categorize the severity of the irritant. For moderate irritants, additional features are scored, in particular, spots such as vesicles, scale, and tanning. The scale to score spots consists of the following:

s   The total number of spots
sv   Spots within the site containing vesicles, e.g., follicular vesicles, milliaria
        or spots with whitish scale on top
se   Spots with eschar, dried or wet scabs

These spots are particularly important to characterize from 48 h to 1 week after removal of the system.

During the recovery phase from irritation, the skin may develop a scaly surface. Scoring of this scaling may be done as follows:

Light   Fine, barely visible or sporadic
Moderate   Clearly noticeable and abundant
Severe   Large dense sheets; erythema is difficult to evaluate

During recovery, skin which is normally pigmented, e.g., olive skin tone, will often develop a tan response when stimulated by irritation, e.g., chemical, friction, or ultraviolet radiation. This tanning response should be noted.

V. SENSITIZATION

Contact allergy or sensitization connotes the immune response to repeated exposure to the sensitizing agent. Sensitization may result from passive administration, but in principle, iontophoresis could increase the incidence of sensitization. The incidence of sensitization is typically higher when the irritant is applied under irritant conditions.[30] When iontophoretic irritation occurs, the incidence of sensitization could increase. Moreover, weak sensitizers, such as nicotine, may exhibit a dose response, and the enhanced iontophoretic delivery could result in increased sensitization. There are, however, surprisingly few cases of skin sensitization during iontophoresis in the literature.[8] This may be a tribute to the limited selection of agents and the use of nonirritating conditions for clinical iontophoresis.

Evaluation of contact allergy for transdermal and iontophoretic delivery is best conducted by a modified Buehler test.[30] The formulation should be evaluated both passively and under iontophoretic delivery. Typical paradigms involve an induction phase consisting of application three times weekly for 3 weeks, followed by a 2-week rest period and a challenge phase. A positive response should be followed by a rechallenge. These challenge phases may involve only passive delivery to help separate irritant and sensitization responses. Iontophoretic delivery in the challenge phases should only be used to deliver the agent and should certainly be used under non-irritating conditions. This paradigm can be applied to guinea pigs and to man with the caveat that the investigators have observed a false positive in guinea pigs.

The duration of the induction phase may need to be lengthened. Clonidine was a false negative in guinea pigs and in man using the standard 2- to 3-week induction phase, and an induction phase of 4 to 12 weeks has been shown to be more predictive for transdermal delivery.[31] This may also be true for iontophoretic delivery.

VI. CONCLUSIONS

The skin tolerability of clinical iontophoresis has been quite acceptable. Irritant reactions may be studied with minor additions to the existing paradigms. Some caution should be used with regard to the predictive power of animal models for irritation and sensitization during iontophoresis.

REFERENCES

1. A. Banga and Y.W. Chien, Iontophoretic delivery of drugs: fundamentals, developments, and biomedical applications, *J. Controlled Rel.*, 7:1–24 (1988).
2. B. Berner and S.M. Dinh, *Electronically Controlled Drug Delivery*, CRC Press, Boca Raton, FL (1998).
3. J. Singh and K.S. Bhatia, Topical iontophoretic drug delivery: pathway, principles, factors, and skin irritation, *Med. Res. Rev.*, 16:285–329 (1996).
4. R. T. Kurnik, B. Berner, J. Tamada, and R.O. Potts, Design and simulation of a reverse iontophoretic glucose monitoring device, *J. Electrochem. Soc.*, 145:4119–4125 (1998).
5. J.A. Tamada, N.J.V. Bohannon, and R.O. Potts, Measurement of glucose in diabetic subjects using noninvasive transdermal extraction, *Nature Med.*, 1:1198–1201 (1995).
6. G. Rao, P. Glikfeld, R.H. Guy, Reverse iontophoresis: development of a noninvasive approach for glucose monitoring, *Pharm. Res.*, 10:1751–1755 (1993).
7. L. Zeltzer, M. Regalado, L.S. Nichter, D. Barton, S. Jennings, and L. Pitt, Iontophoresis versus subcutaneous injection: a comparison of two methods of local anesthesia delivery in children, *Pain*, 44:73–78 (1991).
8. P.W. Ledger, Skin biological issues in electrically enhanced transdermal delivery, *Adv. Drug Delivery Rev.*, 9:289–307 (1992).
9. M.R. Holdiness, A review of contact dermatitis associated with transdermal therapeutic systems, *Contact Dermatitis*, 20:3–9 (1989).
10. D.L. Kellog, J.M. Johnson, and W.A. Kosiba, Selective abolition of adrenergic vasoconstrictor responses in skin by local iontophoresis of bretylium, *Am. J. Physiol.*, 257: H1599–H1606 (1989).
11. V. Schwarz, C.H. Sutcliffe, and P.P. Style, Some hazards of the sweat test, *Arch. Dis. Childhood*, 43:695–701 (1968).
12. H. Molitor and L. Fernandez, Studies on iontophoresis: experimental studies on the causes and prevention of iontophoretic burns, *Am. J. Med. Sci.* 198:778–785 (1939).
13. M.R. Prausnitz, The effects of pulsed electrical protocols on skin damage, sensation, and pain, *Proc. Intern. Symp. Control. Rel. Bioact. Mater.*, 24:25–26 (1997).
14. R. Myyra, M. Dalpra, and J. Globerson, Electrical erythema?, *Anesthesiology,* 69:440.
15. *Dorland's Illustrated Medical Dictionary*, W. B. Saunders, Philadelphia, PA, 26th ed., p. 197 (1985).
16. A. C. Guyton, *Textbook of Medical Physiology*, WB Saunders, Philadelphia, p. 379 (1976).
17. H. Molitor, Pharmacologic aspects of drug administration by ion-transfer, *Merck Rep.*, 22–29 (1943).
18. K. Grice, H. Sattar, and H. Baker, Treatment of idiopathic hyperhidrosis with iontophoresis of tap water and poldine methosulphate, *Br. J. Derm.*, 86:72–78 (1972).
19. E. Camel, M. O'Connell, B. Sage, M. Gross, and H.I. Maibach, The effect of saline iontophoresis on skin integrity in human volunteers, *Fundam. App. Toxicol.*, 32:168–178 (1996).
20. M.J.N. Cormier, P.W. Ledger, J. Johnson, J.B. Phipps, and S. Chao, Reduction of skin irritation and resistance during electrotransport, U.S. Patent 5,624,415 (1997).
21. R.H. Bruner, Pathological processes of skin damage related to toxicant exposure, in D. W. Hobson (Ed.), *Dermal and Ocular Toxicology Fundamentals and Methods*, CRC Press, Boca Raton, FL, pp. 73–109 (1991).
22. N.K. Mize, M. Buttery, P. Daddona, P. Morales, and M. Cormier, Reverse iontophoresis: monitoring prostaglandin E2 associated with cutaneous inflammation in vivo, *Exp. Dermatol.*, 6: 298–302 (1997).
23. P. Leung and H. Chai, Localized urticaria induced by direct electric current stimulation, *Ann. Allergy*, 43:291–292 (1979).
24. L.P. Gangarosa, A. Ozawa, M. Ohkido, Y. Shimonura, and J.M. Hill, Iontophoresis for enhancing penetration of dermatologic and antiviral drugs, *J. Dermatol.*, 22:865–875 (1995).
25. P.W. Ledger, M.J.N. Cormier, and P.S. Campbell, Reduction of skin transport during electrotransport delivery, U.S. Patent 5,693,010 (1997).
26. F. Levit, Simple device for treatment of hyperhidrosis by iontophoresis. *Arch Dermatol.*, 98:505–507 (1968).
27. J.H. Draize, G. Woodard, and H.O. Calvery, Methods for the study of irritation and toxicity of substances applied topically to the skin and muscous membranes, *J. Pharmacol. Exp. Ther.*, 82:377–390 (1944).

28. C.G.T. Mathias, Clincial and experimental aspects of cutaneous irritation, in F.N. Marzulli and H.I. Maibach (Eds.), *Dermatotoxicology*, 2nd ed., Hemisphere Publishing, New York, pp. 167–183 (1983).

29. N.A. Monteiro-Rivere, Altered epidermal morphology secondary to lidocaine iontophoresis: *in vivo* and *in vitro* studies in porcine skin, *Fund. Appl. Toxicol.*, 15:174–185 (1990).

30. F.N. Marzulli and H.I. Maibach, Contact allergy: predictive testing in human, in F.N. Marzulli and H.I. Maibach (Eds.) *Dermatotoxicology*, 2nd ed., Hemisphere Publishing, New York, pp. 279–299 (1983).

31. B. Berner and A. F. Kydonieus, Novel drug delivery systems, in P.G. Welling, A. Banakar, and L. Lasagna (Eds.), *The Drug Development Process*, Marcel Dekker, New York, pp. 169–201 (1996).

20 The Effects of Ultraviolet Radiation on the Immune Response

Stephen E. Ullrich

CONTENTS

I. INTRODUCTION

Exposing the skin to the ultraviolet (UV) radiation present in sunlight has a number of effects. Some are positive, such as the stimulation of vitamin D synthesis, and some are negative, such as the induction of skin cancer. In addition, UVB (280 to 320 nm) radiation is immune suppressive, and studies with experimental animals and biopsy-proven skin cancer patients have provided strong evidence to suggest that the suppressive effect of UVB radiation on the immune system is a major risk factor for skin cancer induction.[1,2] Because skin cancer is the most prevalent form of human neoplasm (approximately one third of all newly diagnosed cancers are skin cancers), it is important to determine how UVB irradiation of the skin activates immune-suppressive pathways (Figure 1). This chapter reviews the mechanisms involved in inducing immune suppression by UVB exposure.

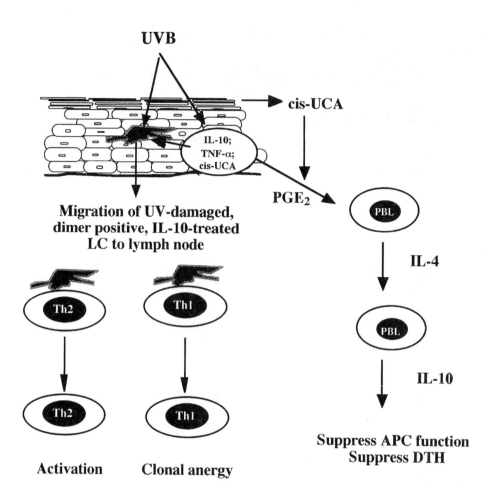

Figure 1   Suggested pathways involved in UVB-induced immune suppression. See text for details. (From Kimber, I. and Selgrade, M.K., Eds., *T Lymphocyte Subpopulations in Immunotoxicology*, John Wiley & Sons, New York, 1998. With permission.)

II. TARGETS OF UVB RADIATION WITHIN THE SKIN

A. CELLULAR TARGETS

1. Langerhans Cells

Staining epidermal sheets with ATPase or monoclonal anti-Ia antibody reveals a dendritic cell network that functions as the first line of defense against invading microorganisms and other environmental insults. Upon encountering antigen, the epidermal Langerhans cell takes up the antigen (or hapten in the case of a contact allergen), migrates to the draining lymph nodes, and initiates an immune response by presenting the antigen to T cells. Data to support this sequence of events in vivo came from studies by Kripke and colleagues.[1] Mice were sensitized with a fluorescent contact allergen, fluorescein isothycyanate (FITC), and 18 h later the FITC+ cells were recovered from the draining lymph nodes. The antigen-presenting cell capability of these hapten-positive cells was determined by measuring the induction of contact hypersensitivity (CHS) when the dendritic cells were injected into normal mice. The cells that presented the antigen were dendritic in morphology, Ia+, Birbeck granule+, and radioresistant.[3,4] In addition, these cells were able to stimulate the proliferation of FITC-specific T cell lines.[5] These findings confirm that epidermal Langerhans cells that encounter antigen in the skin do indeed migrate to the draining lymph node where they initiate an immune response. (For a more complete discussion of Langerhans cell function, see Chapter 8.)

That UVB-irradiation of the skin may affect Langerhans cell function and modulate the immune response was first proposed by Toews and colleagues.[6] Exposing mice to relatively low doses of UVB radiation altered both the morphology and function of epidermal Langerhans cells. Not only was the dendritic network of Ia+, ATPase+ cells destroyed after UVB irradiation, but sensitization through the Langerhans cell-depleted skin failed to induce contact sensitization. Perhaps the most interesting result presented in this study was the observation that when mice that were originally sensitized through UVB-irradiated skin were immunized a second time with the same hapten applied to nonirradiated skin, they failed to respond. This suggests the induction of immune tolerance by UVB exposure. The subsequent discovery that UVB exposure induced hapten-specific splenic suppressor T cells further supported the hypothesis that UVB irradiation of the skin sends a tolerance-inducing signal to the immune system.[7]

Formal proof that Langerhans cells were indeed the targets of UVB radiation came from the experiments performed by Cruz and colleagues. Langerhans cell populations were identified and purified from the skin by fluorescent activated cell sorting (FACS). These cells were then irradiated with UVB, conjugated with hapten, and used as a dendritic cell vaccine. Because injecting UVB-irradiated cells suppressed CHS, and because the animals were rendered tolerant to subsequent sensitization with the same hapten, these data indicate that Langerhans cells within the skin are one target of UVB radiation.[8,9]

2. Keratinocytes

Keratinocytes are the most abundant cell type within the epidermis, and the highly regulated growth and differentiation of keratinocytes provides for the essential barrier function of the skin.[10] Keratinocytes can also influence immune function by secreting biological response modifiers and/or cytokines. Resting keratinocytes secrete relatively few cytokines, but upon activation by external stimuli such as tumor promoters or UVB light, keratinocytes release a wide variety of cytokines, growth factors, and biological response modifiers.[11] Some of these have been shown to play an important role in the immune suppression induced by UVB radiation, including prostaglandin E_2 (PGE_2),[12] tumor necrosis factor alpha (TNF-α),[13] alpha-melanocyte stimulating hormone (α-MSH),[14] and interleukin (IL)-10.[15] Because most of these cytokines have UV-responsive transcriptional control sequences in the 5′ noncoding promoter region of the gene (i.e., NF-$\kappa\beta$ and AP-1), it is generally believed that activation of these sites by UVB irradiation explains the increase in cytokine production.

Alternatively, data generated by others indicate that inhibiting the production of keratinocyte-derived growth factors by UVB radiation may contribute to immune suppression. Interleukin-7 is a growth factor for dendritic T epidermal cells and colony-stimulating factor-1 (CSF-1) is a growth factor for Langerhans cells. Following UVB radiation the secretion of IL-7 and CSF-1 by keratinocytes is suppressed.[16,17] Similarly, IL-15, which is a non-T cell-derived cytokine that binds to the α and β chains of the T cell receptor and promotes the activation of T cells, is constitutively produced by keratinocytes.[18,19] Production of IL-15 is suppressed following UVB exposure.[19] Blauvelt et al. suggest that removing IL-15 from the epidermal cytokine milieu may contribute to the suppression of T cell-mediated immune reactions by UVB radiation.[19]

Recently, Aragane et al.[20] investigated the mechanism through which UVB exposure inhibits cytokine production. Interferon-gamma (IFN-γ) activates an IFN-stimulated response element (ISRE) located in promoter region of the IL-7 gene, and activating ISRE initiates IL-7 secretion. Aragane and colleagues isolated nuclear extracts from IFN-γ–treated keratinocytes that were or were not exposed to UVB radiation and examined binding of interferon regulatory factor-1 (IFR-1) to

ISRE using electrophoretic mobility shift assays. When extracts were isolated from IFN-γ–treated nonirradiated keratinocytes, gel-shift assays demonstrated binding of IFR-1 to ISRE. But when the nuclear extracts were recovered from IFN-γ–treated, UVB-irradiated cells, binding of IFR-1 to ISRE was suppressed. Northern blot analysis confirmed these findings by indicating suppression of IFR-1 mRNA production.

The mechanism may include suppressing the activation of the signal tranducer and activator of transcription (STAT)-1 by UVB radiation. Interferon binding to its receptor causes dimerization of the receptor which allows the receptor-associated Janus kinases (Jak)-1 and 2 to come in close proximity, phosphorylate each other, and activate kinase activity. Jak 1 and 2 then phosphorylate STAT-1, which causes it to form a homodimer that translocates to the nuclease and activates IFN-γ responsive genes by binding to the IFN-γ–activated sequences (GAS) found in the promoter region of the gene. Aragane et al. reported that UVB irradiation of cells prevents phosphorylation of STAT-1.[21] This would interfere with the dimerization and translocation of this protein to the nucleus, thus preventing STAT-1 binding to the GAS element and thereby suppressing IL-7 production.

From these types of observations it is now becoming clear that UVB exposure by either promoting the release of immune suppressive cytokines by keratinocytes or by suppressing the release of critical keratinocyte-derived growth factors can negatively influence immune function. Of course the molecular mechanisms involved in the differential suppression of the expression of IFR-1 mRNA and the enhanced expression of others (i.e., IL-10 mRNA)[15] in UVB-irradiated keratinocytes remain to be seen.

3. Nerve Cell Endings

Immunologists and neurologists have long recognized the close association between the two systems they study. We know, for example that stress and anxiety can adversely affect immune function. Increasing evidence is accumulating to suggest that UVB exposure may downregulate cutaneous immunity by inducing nerve cells within the skin to release immune modulatory substances. One example is calcitonin gene-related peptide (CGRP). Hosoi et al. found that epidermal nerve cell fibers are rich in CGRP and are intimately associated with epidermal Langerhans cells. Furthermore, CGRP was found to inhibit Langerhans cell antigen-presenting cell function, and the elicitation of a delayed-type hypersensitivity (DTH) reaction.[22] Following UVB irradiation of the skin, CGRP production increases, and treating UVB irradiated rats and mice with a CGRP receptor antagonist interferes with UVB-induced vasodilatation and UVB-induced immune suppression. Similar to the effects of UVB irradiation, topical application of CGRP depletes Ia+ epidermal Langerhans cells.[23,24] Recently, Niizeki et al. confirmed that UVB-induced immune suppression is blocked by CGRP receptor antagonists and further demonstrated that these antagonists blocked the UVB-induced depletion of Langerhans cells from the skin. In addition, they suggest that CGRP mediates its suppressive effects through TNF-α, because treating mice with CGRP plus neutralizing anti-TNF-α antibody blocked both the induction of immune suppression and depletion of epidermal Langerhans cells.[25] These studies clearly indicate that nerve cells are another cellular target for UVB radiation within the skin and that irradiation of nerve cell endings induces them to produce and release immune modulatory substances.

B. Molecular Targets In Skin Cells

1. DNA

The formation of pyrimidine dimers and 6-4 photoproducts at dipyrimidine sites in irradiated DNA is a characteristic response to UVB exposure. In nonmelanoma UVB-induced skin cancers, UVB-induced signature mutations in the *p53* tumor suppressor gene have been shown to be a key component in the disease pathway leading to cancer induction.[26–28] A considerable amount of evidence is accumulating to suggest that the induction of pyrimidine dimers by UVB radiation is also the initiating event in the activation of immune suppressive pathways. In a series of studies,[27–35] Kripke and colleagues demonstrated that reversal or repair of pyrimidine dimer formation blocks the induction of immune suppression.

In the first set of experiments, marsupials were exposed to UVB radiation and then exposed to visible light, and the effect this had on the generation of immune suppression was noted. Marsupials (*Monodelphis domestica*) were used because they possess a light-activated DNA repair enzyme. The photoreactivating repair enzyme forms a complex with the pyrimidine dimer and upon the absorption of energy provided by visible light splits the dimer, thus restoring the DNA to the native conformation and maintaining the fidelity of DNA replication. The photoreactivating enzyme is highly specific for pyrimidine dimers, and studies by others have shown that shining visible light on the marsupials after, but not before, UVB irradiation will activate dimer repair and prevent the induction of skin and eye tumors in UVB-irradiated animals.[29,30] Kripke and co-workers found that treating *Monodelphis domestica* with UVB light suppressed the induction of CHS. Treating the UVB-irradiated animals with visible light after, but not before, UVB exposure activated the photoreactivating enzyme which repaired pyrimidine dimer formation (85% suppression of dimer formation in the skin), and prevented the induction of immune suppression.[31]

Because there are fundamental differences in the nature of the immune response generated in placental mammals and marsupials, concerns were raised as to whether the data generated in the above mentioned study could be due to some unknown artifact. To address this concern, a second series of experiments were initiated in which a DNA repair enzyme, T4N5 bacteriophage endonuclease, was introduced into the skin of UVB-irradiated mice through the use of liposomes. These multilameller lipid vessels penetrate the cells of the epidermis, where they are destabilized by the acidic pH, thus delivering their contents intracellularly. Electron microscopic examination of murine skin treated with these liposomes documented delivery of T4N5 into the cytoplasm and nucleus of both keratinocytes and Langerhans cells.[32] When T4N5-containing liposomes were applied to the skin of UVB-irradiated mice, the number of cyclobutane pyrimidine dimers found in the skin was decreased and the induction of immune suppression was blocked. Control liposomes containing a heat-inactivated enzyme preparation did not reverse the induction of immune suppression. Furthermore, no suppressor cell activity was found in the spleens of UVB-irradiated mice that were treated with the T4N5-containing liposomes.[33] These data confirm those of the previous study and suggest that the UVB-induced pyrimidine dimer formation is indeed the initiating event in UVB-induced immune suppression and the induction of the antigen-specific suppressor T cells.

As mentioned above, cellular targets of UVB radiation within the skin include Langerhans cells and keratinocytes. Does pyrimidine dimer formation cause the UVB-induced inhibition of Langerhans cell antigen-presenting cell function and increased cytokine secretion? The role of DNA damage in the UVB-induced suppression of cutaneous antigen-presenting cell function was determined by observing the effect that T4N5-containing liposomes had on dendritic cell function. Using a monoclonal antibody specific for pyrimidine dimers, Vink et al. found that dimer-positive cells could be found in the epidermis, dermis, and draining lymph nodes of UVB-irradiated mice. A surprising result was that the dimer-positive cells persisted, particularly in the dermis, for at least 4 days after UVB exposure. When the mice were painted with the fluorescent hapten FITC, Ia+, FITC+, pyrimidine dimer+ cells (presumably migrating Langerhans cells) were found in the draining lymph nodes, and these cells exhibited reduced antigen-presenting activity when compared to dimer negative cells isolated from nonirradiated FITC-painted mice. Applying T4N5-containing liposomes to the skin of the UVB-irradiated mice both reduced the number of pyrimidine dimer+ cells found in the draining lymph nodes and blocked the impairment of antigen presentation. As before, applying liposomes containing the heat-inactivated enzyme preparation to the skin of UVB-irradiated mice had no effect on the number of dimer-positive cells found in the draining lymph node, nor did it reverse defective antigen presentation.[34]

Although it is reasonable to assume that the migrating FITC+, Ia+, dimer+ cells in the above-mentioned studies are UVB-damaged Langerhans cells, the identity of the UVB-damaged target cell was the focus of a subsequent study. Because DNA damage also plays a role in the production of cytokines by UVB-irradiated keratinocytes,[35] and because UVB-induced cytokines can influence antigen presentation by epidermal Langerhans cells,[36] it was not clear if applying T4N5-containing liposomes to the skin of UVB-irradiated mice directly affected Langerhans cell function or had an indirect effect and inhibited suppressive cytokine production by keratinocytes. To directly address this question, FITC+, dimer+, dendritic cells were purified by metrizamid gradients from the draining lymph nodes of UVB-irradiated mice and incubated in the dark with liposomes containing the photoreactivating enzyme. The dendritic cells were then exposed to visible light and their antigen-presenting cell function analyzed. Photoreactivation reduced the number of pyrimidine dimers present and totally restored antigen-presenting cell function. In addition, repair of pyrimidine dimer formation in vitro blocked T suppressor cell induction. Giving the photoreactivating light before liposome treatment did not reduce dimer formation nor restore immune function.[37] These two studies strongly suggest that UVB-induced DNA damage to cutaneous Langerhans cells initiates the well-described impairment of antigen-presenting cell function. Moreover, they imply that the UVB-induced suppression of antigen-presenting cell activity does not appear to be secondary to cytokine production, but a direct affect of UVB radiation on the DNA of Langerhans cells.

The use of T4N5-containing liposomes has also been instrumental in understanding the role of DNA damage in the production of immune modulatory cytokines by UVB-irradiated keratinocytes. Keratinocyte cultures or mouse skin was exposed to UVB radiation and then treated with T4N5-containing liposomes. Production of IL-10, both in vivo and in vitro, was significantly suppressed by T4N5-containing liposomes, but not by liposomes containing heat-inactivated enzyme.[35] In addition, treating UVB-irradiated keratinocytes cultures with T4N5-containing liposomes blocked the ability of supernatants from these cells to activate immune suppression in vivo, an activity previously attributed to keratinocyte-derived IL-10.[15,38]

Repairing UVB-induced pyrimidine dimer formation therefore prevents the induction of UVB-induced immune suppression, blocks the activation of the antigen-specific suppressor T cells, interferes with the UVB-induced impairment of antigen-presenting cell function, and suppresses the production of cytokines by UVB-damaged keratinocytes. This implies that UVB-induced DNA damage, primarily pyrimidine dimer formation, initiates UVB-induced immune suppression.

2. Urocanic Acid

In 1983, De Fabo and Noonan reported that the action spectra for UVB-induced suppression of CHS, UVB-induced DNA damage, and the isomerization of urocanic acid were very similar. Urocanic acid, a deamination production of histidine, is abundant in the outermost layers of the skin where it can be found as a trans isomer. Upon UVB-irradiation, *trans*-urocanic acid is isomerized into the cis form. Based on their inability to induce immune suppression when the stratum corneum of mice was removed by tape stripping immediately prior to UVB-irradiation, De Fabo and Noonan suggested the molecular target for UVB-induced immune suppression is located superficially, indicating a role for urocanic acid.[39] Since that initial observation, data reported by a number of different laboratories have demonstrated that *cis*-urocanic acid is immune suppressive. For example, *cis*-urocanic acid is found in the serum of UVB-irradiated mice.[40] Moreover, when Ross et al. injected cis-urocanic acid into mice, they were able to mimic the UVB-induced suppression of DTH to herpes simplex virus and induce splenic antigen-specific suppressor T cells.[41–43] Intravenous injection of *cis*-urocanic acid caused systemic impairment of antigen-presenting cell function, similar to what is observed following UV exposure.[44] Also topical application of *cis*-urocanic acid or intracutaneous injection altered Langerhans cells morphology and suppressed their antigen-presenting cell function.[45,46] The ability of UV radiation, *cis*-urocanic acid, and TNF-α to alter Langerhans cells morphology has been associated with a disruption of cytoskeletal organization.[47]

Little is known about the molecular mechanism(s) by which *cis*-urocanic acid initiates immune suppression. Because the immune suppressive effects of *cis*-urocanic acid can be blocked by antioxidants, some suggest free radical formation may be involved.[48] Palaszynski et al. reported that treating cultured fibroblast cell lines with *trans*-urocanic acid or histamine activates adenyl cyclase activity and causes increased production of adenosine 3′, 5′-cyclic monophosphate (cAMP). When *cis*-urocanic acid was added to the cells, cAMP production was suppressed. Because cAMP activity modulates cytokine production, the authors suggest that modulation of this important second messenger by *cis*-urocanic acid may modulate cytokine production by dermal fibroblasts which could alter immune function.[49] Whether *cis*-urocanic acid suppression of cAMP production is involved in the increased production of TNF-α by *cis*-urocanic acid-treated Langerhans cells as described by Kurimoto and Streilein[45] remains to be seen. In one other study, however, no increased production of immune-suppressive cytokines by *cis*-urocanic acid-treated keratinocytes was noted,[50] so it is not clear if modulation of cAMP production by *cis*-urocanic acid actually leads to a modulation of cytokine levels as suggested by Palaszynski et al.

Contrary to the above-mentioned studies, a number of laboratories report that they were unable to find a correlation between in vivo isomerization of urocanic acid and photoimmune suppression. Gibbs et al. noted differences in the in vivo action spectrum for isomerization of urocanic acid and UVB-induced immune suppression of CHS.[51] In particular, wavelengths in the UVA-II (320 to 400 nm) region of the solar spectrum that were very efficient at converting *trans*-urocanic acid to *cis*-urocanic acid were not immunosuppressive. Similarly, Reeve et al. found no correlation between isomerization of urocanic acid and the induction of immune suppression by UVB radiation.[52] In addition, when a *cis*-urocanic acid-specific monoclonal antibody was injected into UV-irradiated mice, two different groups found that while it blocked the UVB-induced suppression of DTH, it had no effect on UV-induced suppression of CHS,[53,54] and in a third study, only partial restoration (50 to 60%) of CHS in UV-irradiated mice injected with anti–*cis*-urocanic acid monoclonal antibody was reported.[55] Taken together, these findings suggest that while *trans*-urocanic acid serves as an important receptor within the skin for UV radiation and UV-induced immune suppression, the photoisomerization and production of *cis*-urocanic acid can account for some but not all of the suppressive effects of UV radiation on the immune system.

3. Membrane Lipid Peroxidation and Free Radical Formation

Irradiating cells with UV perturbs the function of a variety of molecules. In addition to inducing DNA damage and causing the isomerization of urocanic acid, alterations in the cellular redox equilibrium leading to free radical formation and membrane lipid peroxidation is another example of the ability of UV radiation to modulate the function of cellular macromolecules. Although we have recognized for years that UV irradiation of cells activates a variety of regulatory proteins as part of the response to UV-induced stress, some studies have suggested that UV-induced free radical formation may also contribute to the induction of immune suppression. For example, antioxidant treatment blocks the inhibition of antigen presentation by UVB,[56] abrogates UV-induced suppression of CHS,[57] and interferes with the induction of tolerance.[58]

It is generally assumed that the activation of transcriptional control sequences, such as AP-1 and NF-κβ by UVB radiation explains increased cytokine secretion. Data from a number of laboratories suggest that UV-induced free radical formation maybe the mechanism involved. Within minutes after UVC (254 nm) exposure, the Src tyrosine kinase which is normally found at the inner surface of the plasma membrane and participates in signal transduction is activated. This leads to a cascade of events that results in activation of Ha-Ras, Raf-1, c-jun amino-terminal protein kinase (JNK) and ultimately phosphorylation of positive regulatory sites in the activation domain of c-jun leading to the activation of AP-1. Addition of free radical scavengers (*N*-acetylcysteine; NAC) to the UVC-irradiated cells blocks these intracellular signaling pathways and interferes with the activation of AP-1.[59,60] Furthermore, UVC-induced signal transduction was blocked when the cells were treated with compounds such as vanadate and low molar concentrations of Triton X-100, which are known to interfere with membrane organization, suggesting the target of UV radiation resides at or near the cell membrane.[60] Subsequent experiments confirmed that the same pathways were involved in the activation of NF-κβ following UVC-irradiation, a pathway that was also inhibited by NAC-treatment.[61]

To rule out a role for UVC-induced DNA damage in the activation of transcriptional control elements, Devary and colleagues enucleated HeLa cells and then exposed them to UVC radiation. Because they observed binding of NF-κβ and AP-1 to DNA, they concluded that the UV-response did not require a nuclear signal, but in all probability the signal is initiated at the cell membrane.[61]

Unfortunately, the methodology employed in the above-mentioned experiments raises some concerns. The UVC light used as the source of radiation is not environmentally relevant because all UVC radiation is removed from the biosphere by the ozone layer. The use of HeLa cells as targets is also problematic, because the skin is the major target of UV radiation in vivo. Results from two important studies, however, suggest that UVB exposure of keratinocytes can activate many of the intracellular signaling pathways described above. First, using cell-free cytosolic keratinocyte extracts, Simon et al. confirmed that the target of UVB radiation that induced NF-κβ activation was a cell membrane component.[62] Second, Tobin et al. also observed that exposing keratinocytes to UVB radiation activated NF-κβ and AP-1. Of particular interest in this study was the identification of a very early upstream event that led to NF-κβ activation. Tobin et al. describe ligand-independent recruitment of the intracellular signal transducer TRAF-2 to the membrane-bound TNF-receptor following UVB exposure. The association occurs within 5 min of UVB exposure and is not inhibited by anti-TNF antibodies, but is blocked by cotransfection of dominant-negative mutants of TRAF-2.[63]

That lipid peroxidation may actually be linked to controlling UVB-induced cytokine secretion and thus may have the potential to impact on immune responsiveness was suggested by data published by Simon et al. In this study, cells were genetically engineered to overexpress heat shock protein 70. These proteins are normally used by cells to increase their resistance to environmental insults such as UVB radiation. Overexpression of heat shock protein 70 not only increased cell viability following UVB exposure, but also markedly decreased the secretion of IL-6 following induction of oxidative stress or treatment with UV radiation.[64]

Because AP-1 and NF-κβ activation is an necessary step in cytokine secretion, data indicating that the activation of these signaling pathways by a UV-induced membrane-associated lipid peroxidation step, although preliminary, strongly suggest that membrane lipids serve as an additional molecular target of UV radiation within the cell. In addition, although it is clear that activation of AP-1 and NF-κβ can occur in the absence of a nuclear signal, one consequence of UVB-induced DNA damage is the induction of DNA repair enzymes that have kinase activity and regulate gene transcription.[65] So what is not clear at the present time is how cross-talk between these two signaling pathways in intact cells contributes to UV-induced cytokine production and the induction of immune suppression.

III. EFFECTS OF UVB EXPOSURE ON THE CUTANEOUS IMMUNE RESPONSE

Local immune suppression is a term often seen when reading the literature concerning UVB-induced immune suppression. This refers to the situation where the hapten is applied directly to UVB-irradiated skin. The net result is a suppressed CHS response, activation of hapten-specific suppressor T cells, and hapten-specific tolerance. Suppressing CHS by applying haptens directly to UVB-irradiated skin has been demonstrated in both experimental animals[6] and in UVB-irradiated human volunteers.[66]

As mentioned above, it is generally accepted that UVB-induced alterations in Langerhans cell function is responsible for UVB-induced local immune suppression. Most recent studies have focused on determining the mechanism by which UVB irradiation of the skin alters the antigen-presenting cell function of epidermal Langerhans cells. From these studies two pictures have emerged, one indicating that direct UVB damage to the Langerhans cells results in impairment of antigen-presenting cell function, and the other suggesting that biological response modifiers made locally by UVB-irradiated epidermal cells suppress Langerhans cell function. Although an argument has been made that direct damage to the Langerhans cells may play a more important role in the UVB-induced impairment of Langerhans cell function,[37] these two effects of UVB radiation on the cutaneous immune system are not mutually exclusive.

A. LANGERHANS CELLS

Two papers published by Simon et al. nicely illustrate how direct irradiation of Langerhans cells alters immune responsiveness. In these experiments, UVB-irradiated Langerhans cells were used to present antigen to T cell clones in vitro. Two different types of T cell clones were used: type 1 (Th1) and type 2 (Th2) cells. Type 1 cells are T cells that secrete IFN-γ but not IL-4 upon activation, are involved in inflammatory immune reaction, such as DTH and CHS, and provide help to B cells for the production of complement-fixing antibodies. Type 2 cells, on the other hand, secrete IL-4 but not IFN-γ upon activation, provide help for the production of non-complement-fixing antibodies (IgG1 and IgE in the mouse), and are involved in the immune reactions often associated with allergy.[67] Simon and co-workers found that although normal Langerhans cells presented antigen equally well to Th1 and Th2 cells, UVB-irradiated Langerhans cells, while perfectly capable of presenting antigen to Th2 cells, lost their ability to present antigen to Th1 cells. Perhaps more interesting was the observation that not only was antigen presentation to Th1 cells suppressed, but antigen presentation by UVB-irradiated Langerhans cells rendered the Th1 cells tolerant, since they were unable to respond to subsequent stimulation with the same antigen presented by normal Langerhans cells.[68,69]

The potential mechanisms involved in the UVB alteration of Langerhans cell function, especially differential antigen presentation to Th1 and Th2 clones, are not readily apparent. Because binding of costimulatory molecules (CD80 and CD86) to their ligand on the T cell (CD28) plays an essential role in the induction of T cell activation, and since engagement of the T cell receptor without proper costimulation leads to tolerance induction, the effect of UVB exposure on the expression of these molecules on Langerhans cells has received some attention. Weiss et al. found that the upregulation of both CD80 and CD86 that occurs when Langerhans cells were placed in tissue culture was blocked by prior UVB irradiation. Downregulation of these costimulatory molecules correlated with a UVB-induced inhibition of the ability of the epidermal Langerhans cells to serve as stimulator cells in an allogeneic epidermal mixed leukocyte reaction. When effective CD80/CD86–CD28 signaling was restored by adding exogenous anti-CD28 monoclonal antibody, T cell proliferation was restored. These data suggest that the suppressive effects of low dose UVB radiation on antigen-presenting cell function are due, in part, to an inhibition of costimulatory molecule expression.[70]

Others have suggested that the effect of UVB radiation on the modulation of Langerhans cells costimulatory molecule expression in vivo may be more complicated than that described above. Laihia and Jansen exposed human volunteers to solar simulated UV radiation and observed alterations in costimulatory molecule expression over a period of 72 h. They found a triphasic response — an immediate (2 to 6 h) downregulation of Langerhans cell number, followed by a delayed up-regulatory phase (12 to 24 h) in which both the number of Langerhans cells and the intensity of CD80 and CD86 expression increased dramatically. Finally a late phase response (48 to 72 h) characterized by an influx of DR+ monocytes was noted.[71] The difficulty of interpreting these data in regard to the mechanisms involved in UVB-induced suppression of CHS is that, as we noted above, UVB-irradiated, pyrimidine dimer+, hapten-conjugated Langerhans cells migrate from the epidermis and within 18 h can be found in the draining lymph nodes. Because these are the cells that activate immune suppression in vivo,[34,37] the contribution of Langerhans cells expressing high levels of CD80 and CD86 that appear in the skin 48 to 72 h later is not clear.

Another mechanism by which UVB exposure may alter Langerhans cell function is through the induction of programmed cell death. Using an epidermal-derived dendritic cell line that retains many features of resident Langerhans cells, Kitajima et al. examined its susceptibility to apoptosis induction. They found that irradiation of the dendritic cells with relatively low doses of UVB radiation (25 to 100 J/m^2) delivered a signal that by itself did not induce apoptosis, but rendered the cells more susceptible to apoptosis induction. Culturing the UVB-irradiated dendritic cells with lipopolysaccharide (LPS) or using them to present antigen to a Th1 cell line resulted in decreased cell viability, increased condensation of nuclear DNA, and the formation of DNA laddering. Apoptosis was not induced by UVB alone, nor were normal nonirradiated cells induced to undergo apoptosis when they were used as antigen-presenting cells or stimulated with LPS.[72] These results are particularly intriguing in light of the findings of Süss and Shortman, suggesting that two subpopulations of dendritic cells exist, one that activates T cells and another that induces T cells to undergo apoptosis.[73] Perhaps a subpopulation of Langerhans cells exists that is more resistant to the UVB-induced apoptosis, and perhaps this cell preferentially activates Th2 cells.

Biologic response modifiers produced by irradiated cells at the site of UVB exposure can also influence antigen presentation by Langerhans cells. We have already seen that CGRP produced by UVB-irradiated nerve cells can suppress Langerhans cell antigen presentation.[22] Similarly, *cis*-urocanic acid has been shown to suppress Langerhans cell antigen-presenting cell function.[45-47] Keratinocyte-derived IL-10 is yet another example of a biologically active factor produced at the site of UVB-irradiation that can alter the antigen-presenting cell function of Langerhans cells. Enk et al. treated normal Langerhans cells with recombinant IL-10 and studied the effect this had on antigen presentation. The effects they observed were almost identical to those described by Simon et al.[68,69] Langerhans cells pretreated with IL-10 were able to present antigen to Th2 cells, but were not able to present antigen to Th1 cells. Furthermore, antigen presentation by IL-10–treated Langerhans cells tolerized the Th1 cells.[36] Subsequent studies by others have confirmed that IL-10 interferes with Langerhans cells antigen presentation[74] and that treating Langerhans cells with IL-10 induces immune tolerance.[75] Indeed, Dai and Streilein report that injecting syngeneic mice with hapten-conjugated Langerhans cells, pretreated with *cis*-urocanic acid, TNF-α, IL-10, and α-MSH suppressed the induction of CHS, and all but α-MSH were found to induce tolerance.[75] Potential mechanisms may include the effect of these cytokines, especially IL-10 on costimulatory molecule expression,[76] or on Langerhans cell apoptosis.[77]

The relative role of UVB-induced keratinocyte-derived cytokines in the suppression of CHS and tolerance induction was recently addressed by Niizeki and Streilein.[78] Previous studies from this group clearly demonstrated a role for UVB-induced TNF-α in local suppression of CHS.[13] Equally compelling were data presented by the same group suggesting that different mechanisms are involved in tolerance induction and immune suppression, since injecting UVB-irradiated mice with anti-TNF-α monoclonal antibody did not block tolerance induction.[79,80] Niizeki and Streilein attempted to resolve these conflicting results by determining whether TNF-α and IL-10 contributed equally to immune suppression and/or tolerance induction. To determine the role of locally produced IL-10 on CHS, recombinant IL-10 was injected into the dermis, and then a hapten was applied to the epidermis directly above the site of cytokine injection. When the magnitude of CHS that developed in these mice was compared to the positive controls, no difference was noted, suggesting that intradermally injected IL-10 could not suppress CHS. These mice were then rested and 14 days later hapten was painted on a previously untreated site to determine if intradermal IL-10 injection induced immune tolerance. The IL-10–injected mice failed to respond to a second sensitization, indicating tolerance induction by intracutaneously injected IL-10. The relevance of this finding to UVB-induced immune suppression and tolerance induction was demonstrated in experiments where injecting anti–IL-10 into UVB-irradiated mice had no effect on the induction of immune suppression after primary sensitization, but totally blocked tolerance induction in the same mice that were resensitized 14 days later. Conversely, injecting anti-TNF-α into UVB-irradiated mice blocked the induction of immune suppression, but did not interfere with tolerance induction. Thus, these findings confirm different mechanisms are involved in the induction of immune suppression and immune tolerance and suggest a preferential role for TNF-α in UVB-induced local immune suppression of CHS and IL-10 in tolerance induction.

B. INFILTRATING MACROPHAGES

In addition to the effects of UVB radiation on epidermal Langerhans cells, an important contribution to immune suppression is made by macrophages that migrate into the epidermis following UVB exposure. Cooper and colleagues observed that a non-Langerhans cells macrophage-like cell (CD1a⁻, CD11b⁺) migrated into human epidermis 72 h after UVB exposure.[81,82] These cells were found to present antigen to CD4⁺ suppressor/inducer T cells that help activate CD8⁺ T cells that exhibit suppressor cell function.[83,84] Kang et al. found that these inflammatory macrophages secreted large amounts to IL-10. In fact, they found that the major IL-10 producing cell in the UVB-irradiated epidermis is the CD11b⁺ infiltrating macrophage and suggest that the secretion of this cytokine by the infiltrating macrophages may account for its suppressive effects.[85]

To determine the role of the infiltrating macrophage in the suppression of CHS and tolerance induction in vivo, experiments using UVB-irradiated mice were initiated. The situation observed in mice was very similar to that described in humans: immediately after UVB exposure one saw a depletion of epidermal Langerhans cells and 72 h later, an influx of inflammatory macrophages, monocytes, and neutrophils. Applying a hapten to the skin of the UVB-irradiated mice immediately after exposure resulted in suppression of CHS, but tolerance was not induced when the hapten was applied immediately after exposure. Tolerance was only observed when the hapten was applied 72 h after UVB exposure, indicating a temporal association between macrophage infiltration and tolerance induction.[86] Confirmation that the infiltrating macrophages were responsible for tolerance induction came in subsequent studies in which haptenated epidermal cells from UVB-irradiate mice were injected into normal syngeneic controls. When monoclonal antibody was used to remove the CD11b⁺ cells from the tolerizing epidermal cell suspension, tolerance induction was lost.[87] In addition, injecting UVB-irradiated mice with anti-CD11b monoclonal antibody prevented the migration of the CD11b⁺ cells into the UVB-damaged epidermis. In addition to blocking tolerance induction, anti-CD11b also partially restored the UVB-induced immune suppression of CHS. Hammerberg and colleagues noted that epidermal structure in UVB-irradiated anti-CD11b-treated mice was better preserved and the keratinocytes in the UVB-irradiated skin showed less damage. They suggest that in addition to inducing immune tolerance, CD11b⁺ macrophages may further contribute to UVB-induced immune suppression by serving to amplify UVB-induced keratinocyte damage.[87]

IV. SYSTEMIC EFFECTS OF UVB EXPOSURE

The term "UVB-induced systemic immune suppression" refers to a situation where the UVB is applied at one site, and the hapten or antigen is administered at a distant nonirradiated site. The net result is systemic impaired antigen-presenting cell function, a suppressed CHS/DTH reaction, and the induction of antigen-specific suppressor, CD3⁺, CD4⁺, CD8⁻, T cells.[88–91] Often this type of immune suppression is called "high dose suppression," because the doses of UVB required to induce immune suppression are generally higher than those used in the local model. However, the amount of UVB needed to suppress in the systemic model varies depending on the immune response examined and the antigen used. Systemic suppression of DTH to infectious agents has been noted with doses as low as 0.7 to 2.7 kJ/m², a dose range that is comparable to that required to induce local immune suppression.[6,66,92,93] Systemic immune suppression has been observed in both UV-irradiated experimental animals and UV-irradiated human volunteers.[94]

The principal mechanism by which UVB irradiation of the skin activates systemic immune suppression is through the release of immune modulatory cytokines and biological response modifiers by irradiated skin cells, including PGE$_2$, TNF-α, *cis*-urocanic acid, and IL-10, because neutralizing their production and/or activity has been shown to reverse UVB-induced systemic immune suppression.[12,15,53,95]

One mechanism through which UV-induced cytokines and biological response modifiers alter immune reactivity is by altering the function of antigen-presenting cells. For example, splenic adherent cells isolated from mice injected with *cis*-urocanic acid failed to present antigen to immunized T cells.[44] Similarly, UVB-induced IL-10 mediates its suppressive effects by altering splenic antigen-presenting cell function. In these experiments, splenic adherent cells were isolated from mice exposed to UVB radiation or injected with supernatants from UVB-irradiated keratinocyte cultures. Neither of these populations of adherent cells was capable of presenting antigen to Th1 clones or T cell hybridomas, and neutralizing the IL-10 found in the keratinocyte supernatant or injecting the UVB-irradiated mice with anti–IL-10 reversed the immune suppression. Perhaps more interesting was the situation observed when these same splenic adherent cells were used to present antigen to Th2 cells. In this case, cytokine production by the Th2 cells was greatly enhanced when the antigen was presented by splenic adherent cells isolated from UVB-irradiated mice. Because the enhancement of cytokine production by antigen-presenting cells from UVB-irradiated mice was reversed by injecting the irradiated animals with monoclonal anti–IL-10, it appears that one consequence of UVB-induced IL-10 production is suppressed presentation to Th1 cells with an concomitant enhancement of antigen presentation to Th2 cells.[38]

From these data it appears that similar immune deviations occur in both the local and systemic model of UVB-induced immune suppression, a modulation of antigen-presenting cell function that ultimately leads to suppressed antigen presentation to Th1 cells, while antigen presentation to Th2 cells remains intact. The first paper suggesting that UVB exposure differentially affects the activation of T cell subsets was published by Araneo et al.[96] In these experiments, cytokine secretion by lymph node cells recovered from antigen-immunized, UVB-irradiated, or nonirradiated controls was measured. When the lymph node cells were isolated from UVB-irradiated mice, a decrease in IFN-γ production with an increase in IL-4 was noted, suggesting a shift toward an immune response predominated by Th2 cells. Data from a number of subsequent studies have supported this idea. Results from two studies indicate that the suppressor cells found in the lymphoid organs of UV-irradiated mice appear to mediate their effects by secreting IL-4 and/or IL-10. Rivas and Ullrich performed suppressor cell transfer experiments in which spleen cells from UV-irradiated mice were injecting into normal syngeneic controls. Injecting the recipient mice with antibodies specific for IL-10 or IL-4, but not isotype-matched control antibodies, blocked the transfer of immune suppression.[95] In addition, Yagi and colleagues cloned suppressor T cells from the spleen of UVB-irradiated mice. Upon antigenic stimulation these cells secreted IL-4 and IL-10 but not IFN-γ, indicating that they are Th2 cells. These cells suppressed when transferred into normal mice, and their suppressive activity was reversed with monoclonal anti–IL-10.[97]

A study of the effects of UVB radiation on the immune response to *Borrelia burgdorferi* provides further support for the hypothesis that UVB exposure suppresses Th1 cell activation and permits the development of Th2 cells. As mentioned above, Th1 cells provide help for the production of complement-fixing antibodies and are the T cells responsible for inducting DTH. Brown et al. studied the modulation of immunity to *B. burgdorferi* by UV radiation and found that UVB exposure suppressed both the DTH reaction and the production of *Borrelia*-specific complement-fixing IgG2a and IgG2b. In addition, UVB exposure caused a slight but significant increase in the production of *Borrelia*-specific noncomplement fixing IgG1. The immune suppressive effects of UVB radiation were reversed by injecting the irradiated mice with monoclonal anti–IL-10.[98]

One of the important signals that drive uncommitted T cell precursors down the Th1 pathway is IL-12.[99,100] The primary activation/differentiation of Th2 cells in vivo is also suppressed by IL-12.[101,102] Based on these findings, Schmitt et al. tested the hypothesis that IL-12 could interfere with UVB-induced immune suppression.[103] Injecting recombinant IL-12 into UVB-irradiated mice 4 h after irradiation but before antigenic stimulation blocked the induction of immune suppression. Reversal of immune suppression was observed regardless of whether CHS or classic DTH was used as the immunological end point. Associated with this block in UV-induced immune suppression was an abrogation of suppressor T cell induction. No immune suppression was noted when spleen cells from UVB-irradiated IL-12–injected mice were transferred into normal syngeneic recipients, whereas transfer of spleen cells from UVB-irradiated vehicle-treated donors into recipient mice shut down the induction of CHS in the recipient mice. In addition, the effect IL-12 injection had on the activity of preformed suppressor T cells was measured. In these experiments recipient mice were first injected with spleen cells from UVB-irradiated mice and then injected with IL-12 or the vehicle. Whereas the suppressor T cells interfered with the induction of an immune response in the vehicle-treated controls, as expected, injecting IL-12 into mice that received the UVB-induced suppressor cells interfered with immune suppression. Injecting IL-12 into control mice that received spleen cells from nonirradiated hapten-sensitized donors did not potentiate the immune response, suggesting that IL-12 administration was actually suppressing the activity of the UVB-induced suppressor cells and not simply enhancing the function of effector cells in these mice.[103]

Three subsequent reports confirmed that IL-12 administration overcomes UVB-induced immune suppression. Of particular interest in these studies was the observation the IL-12 administration could also reverse UVB-mediated tolerance induction.[104,105] Moreover, Schwarz et al.[106] recently provided evidence to suggest that the UV-induced suppressor cells that mediate hapten-specific immune tolerance in the local system are CD8+ cells and that IL-12 administration blocks their suppressive activity. Although different models of immune suppression were used, it is interesting to note that Schmitt et al. and Schwarz et al. both arrived at the same conclusion: IL-12 interferes with immune suppression by blocking the activity of suppressor T cells, rather than enhancing the function of helper T cells. Because of the essential role that IL-12 plays in the activation of Th1 cells, and since it has been reported that IL-12 can overcome the activation, differentiation, and cytokine secretion by Th2 cells,[107] the data indicating that IL-12 administration blocks UVB-induced immune suppression and breaks tolerance induction by suppressing the function of UVB-induced suppressor T cells provide further support for the hypothesis that UVB exposure shifts the immune response to one favored by Th2 cells.

Much of the work from my own laboratory has focused on the role of UVB-induced IL-10 in the generation of immune suppression. Although it is clear that IL-10 can influence Th1 cell activation by altering antigen presentation and suppressing IFN-γ secretion,[108] the major signal for the development of a Th2 response is IL-4.[109] Because of the critical nature of IL-4 in the development of Th2 cells, and since much of the available evidence suggests Th2 cells are involved in UVB-induced immune suppression, we decided to determine whether IL-4 plays a role in UVB-induced immune suppression. We initiated these experiments by asking if monoclonal anti–IL-4 could interfere with UVB-induced immune suppression. The protocol was similar to before: mice were injected with monoclonal anti–IL-4 within 4 h of UVB irradiation, and the effect this treatment had on UVB-induced suppression of DTH was measured. Monoclonal anti–IL-4 totally blocked the induction of immune suppression when compared to the response found in mice exposed to UVB and injected with isotype-matched antibody. When we looked in the serum of the irradiated mice, we found a dose-dependent induction of IL-4 following UVB exposure. However, we found no evidence supporting keratinocyte production of IL-4, since exposing keratinocyte cultures to UVB radiation did not cause the release of protein. Instead, we suggest that keratinocyte-derived PGE_2 causes the induction of serum IL-4 since treating the UVB-irradiated mice with a selective cyclooxygenase-2 inhibitor blocked serum IL-4 production.[110]

We were puzzled, however, by a result generated in the monoclonal antibody-blocking studies. As a control for these experiments, monoclonal anti–IL-10 was included because we previously demonstrated that this antibody effectively blocks UVB-induced systemic immune suppression. Because we knew that IL-4 and IL-10 are both found in the serum of UV-irradiated mice, why is it that when we neutralize the IL-4 with a specific monoclonal antibody the remaining IL-10 does not suppress DTH? One way to resolve this dilemma was to propose that UVB irradiation induces a cascade of events. Keratinocyte-derived PGE_2 enters the circulation where it induces serum IL-

4, and the IL-4 then causes the release of IL-10. Two pieces of evidence support this idea. First, injecting UVB-irradiated mice with monoclonal anti–IL-4 blocks the appearance of serum IL-10. Second, injecting normal mice with PGE_2 resulted in serum IL-4 and IL-10 production. We propose therefore that UVB exposure activates a cytokine cascade ($PGE_2 \rightarrow$ IL-4 $\rightarrow$ IL-10) that ultimately results in systemic immune suppression.[110]

While these experiments were in progress, Norval and El-Ghorr published additional data indicating an important role for IL-4 in the UVB-induced suppression. In these experiments IL-4–deficient mice were exposed to UVB radiation and immunized with herpes simplex virus or a contact allergen. Although CHS was suppressed in both the wild-type and the IL-4–deficient mice, DTH was not suppressed in the UVB-irradiated IL-4–deficient mice.[111] These results, in combination with our own, clearly indicate an important role for IL-4 in UVB-induced systemic immune suppression. Furthermore, these findings confirm previously published data indicating that different cytokines regulate DTH and CHS in the UVB-irradiated host.[95]

V. SUMMARY AND CONCLUSIONS

The UVB radiation present in sunlight is the primary cause of skin cancer induction, the most common form of human neoplasm. In addition, UVB radiation is immune suppressive and the immune suppression induced by UVB radiation has been identified as a major risk factor for skin cancer induction. Photocarcinogenesis involves the formation of DNA photoproducts, UVB-induced mutations of protooncogenes and tumor suppressor genes, and UVB-induced free radical formation (reviewed by Black et al.).[112] As we have seen here, many of the same signals are involved in the induction of immune suppression by UVB exposure. UVB-induced DNA damage, free radical formation, and the formation of unique photoproducts in the skin have all been shown to contribute to a cascade of events that ultimately leads to immune suppression, formation of suppressor T cells, and tolerance induction. Some of the steps in this cascade are presented schematically in Figure 1. UVB irradiation of the skin directly alters the function of epidermal Langerhans cells, so that when they migrate to the draining lymph nodes, Th1 cells are induced to undergo clonal anergy, whereas Th2 cell activation proceeds.[68,69] Similarly treating Langerhans cells with UVB-induced keratinocyte-derived cytokines (IL-10 and TNF-α) also interferes with epidermal Langerhans cell function,[45] and when IL-10–treated Langerhans cells are used to present antigen to T cell clones, Th1 cells are anergized, whereas Th2 cell activation proceeds normally.[36] Compelling evidence has been published suggesting that the molecular event initiating these changes in Langerhans cell function is UVB-induced pyrimidine dimer formation, since repairing pyrimidine dimer formation restores the antigen-presenting cell capacity of Langerhans cells and interferes with IL-10 and TNF-α secretion by UVB-irradiated keratinocytes.[34,35,37,113] The role of free radicals in this scheme cannot be ignored since others have shown that free radical scavengers will overcome the UVB-induced impairment of Langerhans cell antigen presentation and reverses cytokine production by UVB-irradiated keratinocytes.[56,64] Similarly, the contribution of infiltrating macrophages to immune suppression and tolerance induction must be considered.[85]

UVB exposure also suppresses the immune response to haptens and/or antigens applied or injected at a distant nonirradiated site. The release of cytokines and biologic response modifiers by UVB-irradiated keratinocytes appears to be the driving force behind the induction of systemic immune suppression. We found that UV-irradiated keratinocytes release IL-10, and that serum IL-10 is involved in UVB-induced systemic immune suppression.[15,95] While it does appear that keratinocyte-derived IL-10 is working locally to suppress Langerhans cell function, it does not appear that keratinocyte-derived IL-10 is involved in systemic immune suppression. Instead, we propose that PGE_2 released by UVB-irradiated keratinocytes activates a cytokine cascade involving at least IL-4 and IL-10 and ultimately suppresses DTH.[110] The cellular source of the IL-4 and IL-10 found in the serum of UVB-irradiated mice is not known; we suggest mast cells, peripheral blood monocytes, and T cells may all be involved. In addition, we suggest that *cis*-urocanic acid, by virtue of its ability to induce blood monocytes to secrete PGE_2,[114] may contribute to this cytokine cascade. This may help to explain why different experimental approaches, such as blocking PGE_2 production by indomethacin,[12] monoclonal anti–*cis*-urocanic acid antibody,[54] anti–IL-10,[15] and anti–IL-4,[110] have all been used to successfully block UVB-induced systemic immune suppression. We suggest that the ultimate result of this cytokine cascade is an alteration of systemic antigen presentation leading to a preferential suppression of Th1 cell activation and suppression of inflammatory immune reactions.

Acknowledgments: The work performed in my laboratory was supported by grants from the National Cancer Institute (CA-75575) and the National Institutes of Environmental Health Sciences (ES-07327).

REFERENCES

1. Kripke, M. L., Ultraviolet radiation and immunity: something new under the sun — Presidential address, *Cancer Res.,* 54:6102, 1994.
2. Streilein, J. W., Taylor, J. R., Vincek, V., Kurimoto, I., Shimizu, T., Tie, C., Colomb, C., Immune surveillance and sunlight induced skin cancer, *Immunol. Today,* 15:174, 1994.
3. Kripke, M, L., Munn, C. G., Jeevan, A., Tang, J.-M., Bucana, C., Evidence that cutaneous antigen-presenting cells migrate to regional lymph nodes during contact sensitization, *J. Immunol.,* 145:2833, 1990.
4. Bucana, C., Munn, C. G., Song, M. J., Dunner, K., Kripke, M. L., Internalization of Ia molecules into Birbeck granule-like structures in murine dendritic cells, *J. Invest. Dermatol.,* 99:365, 1992.
5. Muller, H. K., Bucana, C. D., Kripke, M. L., Cox, P. A., Saijo, S., Strickland, F. M., UV-irradiation of murine skin alters cluster formation between lymph node dendritic cells and specific T lymphocytes, *Cell Immunol.,* 157:263, 1994.
6. Toews, G. B., Bergstresser, P. R., Streilein, J. W., Epidermal Langerhans cell density determines whether contact hypersensitivity or unresponsiveness follows skin painting with DNFB, *J. Immunol.,* 124:445, 1980.
7. Elmets, C. A., Bergstresser, P. R., Tigelaar, R. E., Wood, P. J., Streilein, J. W., Analysis of the mechanism of unresponsiveness produced by haptens painted on skin to low dose UV radiation, *J. Exp. Med.,* 158:781, 1983.
8. Cruz, P. D., Nixon-Fulton, J., Tigelaar, R. E., Bergstresser, P. R., Disparate effects of in vitro UVB irradiation in intravenous immunization with purified epidermal cell subpopulations for the induction of CHS, *J. Invest. Dermatol.,* 92:160, 1989.
9. Cruz, P. D., Tigelaar, R. E., Bergstresser, P. R., Langerhans cells that migrate to skin after intravenous infusion regulate the induction of contact hypersensitivity, *J. Immunol.,* 144:2486, 1990.
10. Roop, D., Defects in the barrier. *Science,* 267:474, 1995.
11. Schwarz, T., Urbanski, A., Luger, T. A., Ultraviolet light and epidermal cell-derived cytokines, *Epidermal Growth Factors and Cytokines,* Vol. 10. Luger, T. A., Schwarz, T., Eds., Marcel Dekker, New York, 1994, 303.
12. Chung, H.-T., Burnham, D. K., Robertson, B., Roberts, L. K., Daynes, R. A., Involvement of prostaglandins in the immune alterations caused by the exposure of mice to ultraviolet radiation, *J. Immunol.,* 137:2478, 1986.
13. Yoshikawa, T., Streilein, J. W., Tumor necrosis factor-alpha and ultraviolet light have similar effects on contact hypersensitivity in mice, *Regional Immuno.,* 3:139, 1990.
14. Grabbe, S., Bhardwaj, R. S., Mahnke, K., Simon, M. M., Schwarz, T., Luger, T. A., α-Melanocyte-stimulating hormone induces hapten-specific tolerance in mice, *J. Immunol.,* 156:473, 1996.
15. Rivas, J. M., Ullrich, S. E., Systemic suppression of DTH by supernatants from UV-irradiated keratinocytes: an essential role for interleukin 10, *J. Immunol.,* 149:3865, 1992.
16. Schuhmachers, G., Ariizumi, K., Kitajima, T., Edelbaum, D., Xu, S., Shadduck, R. K., Gilmour, G. L., Bergstresser, P. R., Takashima, A., UVB radiation interrupts cytokine-mediated support of an epidermal-derived dendritic cells line (XS52) by a dual mechanism, *J. Invest. Dermatol.,* 106:1023, 1996.

17. Takashima, A., Matsue, H., Bergstresser, P. R., Ariizumi, K., Interleukin-7-dependent interaction of dendritic epidermal T cells with keratinocytes, *J. Invest. Dermatol.*, 105 (Suppl.):50S, 1995.

18. Sorel, M., Cherel, M., Dremo, B., Bouyce, I., Guilbert, J., Dubois, S., Lebeau, B., Raher, S., Minvielle, S., Jacques, Y., Production of interleukin-15 by human keratinocytes, *Eur. J. Dermatol.*, 6:209, 1996.

19. Blauvelt, A., Asada, H., Klaus-Kovtum, V., Altman, D. J., Lucey, D. R., Katz, S. I., Interleukin-15 mRNA is expressed by human keratinocytes, Langerhans cells, and blood-derived dendritic cells and is downregulated by ultraviolet B radiation, *J. Invest. Dermatol.*, 106:1047, 1996.

20. Aragane, Y., Schwarz, A., Luger, T. A., Ariizumi, K., Takashima, A., Schwarz T., Ultraviolet light suppresses IFN-gamma-induced IL-7 gene expression in murine keratinocytes by interfering with IFN regulatory factors, *J. Immunol.*, 158: 5393, 1997.

21. Aragane, Y., Kulms, D., Luger, T. A., Schwarz, T., Down-regulation of interferon gamma-activated STAT1 by UV light, *Proc. Natl. Acad. Sci. U.S.A.*, 94:11490, 1997.

22. Hosoi, J., Murphy, G. F., Egan, C. L., Lerner, E. A., Grabbe, S., Asahina, A., Granstein, R. D., Regulation of Langerhans cell function by nerves containing calcitonin gene-related peptide, *Nature*, 363:159, 1993.

23. Benrath, J., Eschenfelder, C., Zimmerman, M., Gillardon, F., Calcitonin gene-related peptide, substance P and nitric oxide are involved in cutaneous inflammation following ultraviolet irradiation, *Eur. J. Pharmacol.*, 293:87, 1995.

24. Gillardon, F., Moll, I., Michel, S., Benrath, J., Weihe, E., Zimmerman, M., Calcitonin gene-related peptide and nitric oxide are involved in ultraviolet radiation-induced immunosuppression, *Eur. J. Pharmacol.*, 293:395, 1995.

25. Niizeki, H., Alard, P., Streilein, J. W., Calcitonin gene-related peptide is necessary for ultraviolet B-impaired induction of contact hypersensitivity, *J. Immunol.*, 159:5183, 1997.

26. Brash, D. E., Rudolf, J. A., Simon, J. A., Lin, A., McKenna, G. J., Baden, H. P., Halperin, A. J., Ponten, J., A role for sunlight in skin cancer: UV-induced p53 mutations in squamous cell carcinoma, *Proc. Natl. Acad. Sci. U.S.A.*, 88:10124, 1991.

27. Kanjilal, S., Strom, S. S., Clayman, G. L., Weber, R. S., El-Naggar, A. K., Kapur, V., Cummings, K. K., Hill, L. A., Spitz, M. R., Kripke, M. L., Ananthaswamy, H. N., p53 mutations in nonmelanoma skin cancer of the head and neck: molecular evidence for field cancerization, *Cancer Res.*, 55:3604, 1995.

28. Ananthaswamy, H. N., Loughlin, S. M., Cox, P., Evans, R. L., Ullrich, S. E., Kripke, M. L., Sunlight and skin cancer: inhibition of p53 mutations in UV-irradiated mouse skin by sunscreens, *Nature Medicine*, 3:510, 1997.

29. Ley, R. D., Photorepair of pyrimidine dimers in the epidermis of the marsupial *Monodelphis domestica*, *Proc. Natl. Acad. Sci. U.S.A.*, 82:2409, 1985.

30. Ley, R. D., Applegate, L. A., Fry, R. J., Sanchez, A. B., Photoreactivation of ultraviolet radiation-induced skin and eye tumors of *Monodelphis domestica*, *Cancer Res.*, 51:6539, 1991.

31. Applegate, L. A., Ley, R. D., Alcalay, J., Kripke, M. L., Identification of the molecular target for the suppression of contact hypersensitivity by UV radiation, *J. Exp. Med.*, 170:1117, 1989.

32. Yarosh, D., Bucana, C., Cox, P., Kibitel, J., Kripke, M. L., Localization of liposomes containing a DNA repair enzyme in murine skin, *J. Invest. Dermatol.*, 103:461, 1994.

33. Kripke, M. L., Cox, P. A., Alas, L. G., Yarosh, D. B., Pyrimidine dimers in DNA initiate systemic immunosuppression in UV-irradiated mice, *Proc. Natl. Acad. Sci. U.S.A.*, 89:7516, 1992.

34. Vink, A. A., Strickland, F. M., Bucana, C., Cox, P. A., Roza, L., Yarosh, D. B., Kripke, M. L., Localization of DNA damage and its role in altered antigen-presenting cell function in ultraviolet-irradiated mice, *J. Exp. Med.*, 183:1491, 1996.

35. Nishigori, C., Yarosh, D. B., Ullrich, S. E., Vink, A. A., Bucana, C. D., Roza, L., Kripke, M. L., Evidence that DNA damage triggers interleukin 10 cytokine production in UV-irradiated murine keratinocytes, *Proc. Natl. Acad. Sci. U.S.A.*, 93:10354, 1996.

36. Enk, A. H., Angeloni, V., Udey, M. C., Katz, S. I., Inhibition of Langerhans cell antigen-presenting function by IL-10: a role for IL-10 in induction of tolerance, *J. Immunol.*, 151:2390, 1993.

37. Vink, A. A., Moodycliffe, A. M., Shreedhar, V., Ullrich, S. E., Roza, L., Yarosh, D. B., Kripke, M. L., The inhibition of antigen-presenting activity of dendritic cells resulting from UV irradiation of murine skin is restored by in vitro photorepair of cyclobutane pyrimidine dimers, *Proc. Natl. Acad. Sci. U.S.A.*, 94:5255, 1997.

38. Ullrich, S. E., Mechanism involved in the systemic suppression of antigen-presenting cell function by UV irradiation: keratinocyte-derived IL-10 modulates antigen-presenting cell function of splenic adherent cells, *J. Immunol.*, 152:3410, 1994.

39. De Fabo, E. C., Noonan, F. P., Mechanism of immune suppression by ultraviolet irradiation in vivo. I. Evidence for the existence of a unique photoreceptor in skin and its role in photoimmunology, *J. Exp. Med.*, 157:84, 1983.

40. Moodycliffe, A. M., Norval, M., Kimber, I., Simpson, T. J., Characterization of a monoclonal antibody to cis-urocanic acid: detection of cis-urocanic acid in the serum of irradiated mice by immunoassay, *Immunology*, 79:667, 1993.

41. Ross, J. A., Howie, S. E. M., Norval, M., Maingay, J., Two phenotypically distinct T cells are involved in UV-irradiated urocanic acid-induced suppression of the efferent DTH response to HSV-1 in vivo, *J. Invest. Dermatol.*, 89:230, 1987.

42. Ross, J. A., Howie, S. E. M., Norval, M., Maingay, J., Simpson, T. J., Ultraviolet-irradiated urocanic acid suppresses delayed type hypersensitivity to herpes simplex virus in mice, *J. Invest. Dermatol.*, 87:630, 1986.

43. Ross, J. A,. Howie, S. E. M., Norval, M., Maingay, J., Systemic administration of urocanic acid generates suppression of the delayed type hypersensitivity response to herpes simplex virus in a murine model of infection, *Photodermatology*, 5:9, 1988.

44. Noonan, F. P., De Fabo, E. C., Morrison, H., Cis-urocanic acid, a product formed by UVB irradiation of the skin, initiates an antigen presentation defect in splenic cells in vivo, *J. Invest. Dermatol.*, 90:92, 1988.

45. Kurimoto, I., Streilein, J. W., Cis-urocanic acid suppression of contact hypersensitivity induction is mediated via tumor necrosis factor-α, *J. Immunol.*, 148:3072, 1992.

46. Beissert, S., Mohammad, T., Torri, H., Lonati, A., Yan, Z., Morrison, H., Granstein, R. D., Regulation of tumor antigen presentation by urocanic acid, *J. Immunol.*, 159:92, 1997.

47. Bacci, S., Nakamura, T., Streilein, J. W., Failed antigen presentation after UVB radiation correlates with modifications of Langerhans cells cytoskeleton, *J. Invest. Dermatol.*, 107:838, 1996.

48. Hemelaar, P. J., Beijersbergen van Henegouwen, G. M. J., The protective effect of N-acetylcysteine on UVB-induced immunosuppression by inhibition of the action of cis-urocanic acid, *Photochem. Photobiol.*, 63:322, 1996.

49. Palaszynski, E. W., Noonan, F. P., De Fabo, E. C., cis-urocanic acid down-regulates the induction of adenosine 3',5'-cyclic monophosphate by either trans-urocanic acid or histamine in human dermal fibroblasts in vitro, *Photochem. Photobiol.*, 55:165, 1992.

50. Yarosh, D. B., Alas, L., Kibitel, A. L., Ullrich, S. E., Urocanic acid, immunosuppressive cytokines, and the induction of human immunodeficiency virus, *Photodermatol. Photoimmunol. Phototmed.*, 9:127, 1992.

51. Gibbs, N. K., Norval, M., Traynor, N. A., Wolf, M., Johnson, B. E., Crosby, J., Action spectra for the trans to cis photoisomerisation of urocanic acid in vitro and in mouse skin, *Photochem. Photobiol.*, 57:584, 1993.

52. Reeve, V. E., Boehm-Wilcox, C., Bosnic, M., Cope, R., Ley, R. D., Lack of correlation between suppression of contact hypersensitivity by UV radiation and photosensitization of epidermal urocanic acid in the hairless mouse, *Photochem. Photobiol.*, 60:268, 1994.

53. El-Ghorr, A. A., Norval, M., A monoclonal antibody to *cis*-urocanic acid prevents the UV-induced changes in Langerhans cells and DTH responses in mice, although not preventing dendritic cell accumulation in lymph nodes draining the site of irradiation and contact hypersensitivity responses, *J. Invest. Dermatol.*, 105:264, 1995.

54. Moodycliffe, A. M., Bucana, C. D., Kripke, M. L., Norval, M., Ullrich, S. E., Differential effects of a monoclonal antibody to cis-urocanic acid on the suppression of delayed and contact hypersensitivity following ultraviolet irradiation, *J. Immunol.*, 157:2891, 1996.

55. Hart, P. H., Jaksic, A., Swift, G., Norval, M., El-Ghorr, A. A., Finlay-Jones, J. J., Histamine involvement in UVB-and cis-urocanic acid-induced systemic suppression of contact hypersensitivity responses, *Immunology*, 91:601, 1997.

56. Caceres-Dittmar, C., Ariizumi, K., Xu, S., Tapia, F. J., Bergstresser, P. R., Takashima, A., Hydrogen peroxide mediates UV-induced impairment of antigen presentation in a murine epidermal-derived dendritic cell line, *Photochem. Photobiol.*, 62:176, 1995.

57. van den Broeke, L. T., Beijersbergen van Henegouwen, G. M., Topically applied N-acetylcysteine as a protector against UVB-induced systemic immunosuppression, *J. Photochem. Photobiol. B:Biol.*, 27:61, 1995.

58. Nakamura, T., Pinnell, S. R., Darr, D., Kurimoto, I., Itami, S., Yoshikawa, K., Streilein, J. W., Vitamin C abrogates the deleterious effect of UVB radiation on cutaneous immunity by a mechanism that does not depend on TNF-α, *J. Invest. Dermatol.*, 109:20, 1997.

59. Devary, Y., Gottlieb, R. A., Smeal, T., Karin, M., The mammalian ultraviolet response is triggered by activation of Src tyrosine kinases, *Cell*, 71:1081, 1992.

60. Adler, V., Schaffer, A., Kim, J., Dolan, L., Ronai, Z., UV irradiation and heat shock mediate JNK activation via alternative pathways, *J. Biol Chem*, 270:26071, 1995.

61. Devary, Y., Rosette, C., DiDonato, J. A., Karin, M., NF-κB activation by ultraviolet light is not dependent on a nuclear signal, *Science*, 261:1442, 1993.

62. Simon, M. M., Aragane, Y., Schwarz, A., Luger, T. A., Schwarz, T., UVB light induces a nuclear factor κB (NFκB) activity independently from chromosomal DNA damage in cell-free cytosolic extracts, *J. Invest. Dermatol.*, 102:422, 1994.

63. Tobin, D., van Hogerlinden, M., Toftgard, R., UVB-induced association of tumor necrosis factor (TNF) receptor 1 TNF receptor-associated factor-2 mediates activation of Rel proteins, *Proc. Natl. Acad. Sci. U.S.A.*, 95:565, 1998.

64. Simon, M. M., Reikerstorfer, A., Schwarz, A., Krone, C., Luger, T. A., Jäättelä, M., Schwarz, T., Heat shock protein 70 overexpression affects the response to ultraviolet light in murine fibroblasts: evidence for increased cell viability and suppression of cytokine release, *J. Clin. Invest.*, 95:926, 1995.

65. van Vuuren, A. J., Vermeulen, W., Ma, L., Weeda, G., Appeldoorn, E., Jaspers, N. G., van der Eb, A. J., Bootsma, D., Hoeijmakers, J. H., Humbert, S., Correction of xeroderma pigmentosum repair defect by basal transcription factor BTF2 (TFIIH), *EMBO J.*, 13:1645, 1994.

66. Cooper, K. D., Oberhelman, L., Hamilton, T. A., Baadsgaard, O., Terhune, M., Levee, G., Anderson, T., Koren, H., UV exposure reduces immunization rates and promotes tolerance to epicutaneous antigens in humans: relationship to dose, CD1a⁻DR⁺ epidermal macrophage induction, and Langerhans cell depletion, *Proc. Natl. Acad. Sci. U.S.A.*, 89:8497, 1992.

67. Mosmann, T. R., Sad, S., The expanding universe of T-cell subsets: Th1, Th2 and more, *Immunol. Today*, 17:138, 1996.

68. Simon, J. C., Tigelaar, R. E., Bergstresser, P. R., Edelbaum, D., Cruz, P. D., Ultraviolet B radiation converts Langerhans cells from immunogenic to tolerogenic antigen-presenting cells: induction of specific clonal anergy in CD4+ T helper 1 cells, *J. Immunol.*, 146:485, 1991.

69. Simon, J. C., Cruz, P. C., Bergstresser, P. R., Tigelaar, R. E., Low dose ultraviolet B-irradiated Langerhans cells preferentially activate CD4+ cells of the T helper 2 subset, *J. Immunol.*, 145:2087, 1990.

70. Weiss, J. C., Renkl, A. C., Denfeld, R. W., de Roche, R., Spitzlei, M., Schöpf, E., Simon, J. C., Low-dose UVB radiation perturbs the functional expression of B7.1 and B7.2 co-stimulatory molecules on human Langerhans cells, *Eur. J. Immunol.*, 25:2858, 1995.

71. Laihia, J. K., Jansen, C. T., Up-regulation of human epidermal Langerhans' cell B7-1 and B7-2 co-stimulatory molecules in vivo by solar-simulated irradiation, *Eur. J. Immunol.*, 27:984, 1997.

72. Kitajima, T., Ariizumi, K., Bergstresser, P. R., Takashima, A., Ultraviolet B radiation sensitizes a murine epidermal dendritic cell line (XS52) to undergo apoptosis upon antigen presentation to T cells, *J. Immunol.*, 157:3312, 1996.

73. Süss, G., Shortman, K., A subclass of dendritic cells kills CD4 T cells via Fas/Fas-ligand-induced apoptosis, *J. Exp. Med.*, 183:1789, 1996.

74. Beissert, S., Hosoi, J., Grabbe, S., Asahina, A., Granstein, R. D., IL-10 inhibits tumor antigen presentation by epidermal antigen-presenting cells, *J. Immunol.*, 154:1280, 1995.

75. Dai, R., Streilein, J. W., Ultraviolet B-exposed and soluble factor-pre-incubated epidermal Langerhans cells fail to induce contact hypersensitivity and promote DNP-specific tolerance, *J. Invest. Dermatol.*, 108:721, 1997.

76. Chang, C.-H., Furue, M., Tamaki, K., B7-1 expression of Langerhans cells is up-regulated by proin-flammatory cytokines, and is down-regulated by interferon-γ or by interleukin-10, *Eur. J. Immunol.*, 25:394, 1995.

77. Ludewig, B., Graf, D., Gelderblom, H. R., Becker, Y., Korczek, R. A., Pauli, G., Spontaneous apoptosis of dendritic cells is efficiently inhibited by TRAP (CD40-ligand) and TNF-α, but strongly enhanced by interleukin-10, *Eur. J. Immunol.*, 25:1943, 1995.

78. Niizeki, H., Streilein, J. W., Hapten-specific tolerance induced by acute, low-dose ultraviolet B radiation of skin is mediated via interleukin-10, *J. Invest. Dermatol.*, 109:25, 1997.

79. Shimizu, T., Streilein, J. W., Evidence that ultraviolet B radiation induces tolerance and impairs induction of contact hypersensitivity by different mechanisms, *Immunology*, 82:140, 1994.

80. Shimizu, T., Streilein, J. W., Local and systemic consequences of acute low-dose ultraviolet B radiation are mediated by different immune regulatory mechanisms, *Eur. J. Immunol.*, 24:1765, 1994.

81. Cooper, K. D., Fox, P., Neises, G. R., Katz, S. I., Effects of UVR on human epidermal cell alloantigen presentation: initial depression of Langerhans cell dependent function is followed by the appearance of T6-DR+ cells that enhance epidermal alloantigen presentation, *J. Immunol.*, 134:129, 1985.

82. Cooper, K. D., Neises, G. R., Katz, S. I., Antigen-presenting OKM5+ melanophages appear in human epidermis after ultraviolet radiation, *J. Invest. Dermatol.*, 86:363, 1986.

83. Baadsgaard, O., Salvo, B., Mannie, A., Dass, B., Fox, D., Cooper, K. C., In vivo ultraviolet-exposed human epidermal cells activate T suppressor cell pathways that involve CD4+CD45RA+ suppressor-inducer T cells, *J. Immunol.*, 145:2854, 1990.

84. Baadsgaard, O., Fox, D. A., Cooper, K. D., Human epidermal cells from ultraviolet light-exposed skin preferentially activate autoreactive CD4+2H4+ suppressor-inducer lymphocytes and CD8+ suppressor/cytotoxic lymphocytes, *J. Immunol.*, 140:1738, 1988.

85. Kang, K., Hammerberg, C., Meunier, L., Cooper, K. D., CD11b+ macrophages that infiltrate human epidermis after in vivo Ultraviolet exposure potently produce IL-10 and represent the major secretory source of epidermal IL-10, *J. Immunol.*, 153:5256, 1994.

86. Cooper, K. D., Duraiswamy, N., Hammergerg, C., Allen, E., Kimbrough-Green, C., Dillon, W., Thomas, D., Neutrophils, differentiated macrophages, and monocytes/macrophage antigen presenting cells infiltrate murine epidermis after UV injury, *J. Invest. Dermatol.*, 101:155, 1993.

87. Hammerberg, C., Duraiswamy, N., Cooper, K. D., Active induction of unresponsiveness (tolerance) to DNFB by in vivo ultraviolet-exposed epidermal cells is dependent upon infiltrating class II MHC+ CD11b[bright] monocytic/macrophagic cells, *J. Immunol.*, 153:4914, 1994.

88. Fisher, M. S., Kripke, M. L., Systemic alteration induced in mice by ultraviolet light irradiation and its relationship to ultraviolet carcinogenesis, *Proc. Natl. Acad. Sci. U.S.A.*, 74:1688, 1977.

89. Greene, M. I., Sy, M. S., Kripke, M. L., Benacerraf, B., Impairment of antigen-presenting cell function by UV radiation, *Proc. Natl. Acad. Sci. U.S.A.*, 76:6591, 1979.

90. Noonan, F. P., Kripke, M. L., Pedersen, G. M., Greene, M. I., Suppression of contact hypersensitivity by UV radiation is associated with defective antigen presentation, *Immunology*, 43:527, 1981.

91. Ullrich, S. E., Suppression of the immune response to allogeneic histocompatibility antigen by a single exposure to UV radiation, *Transplantation*, 42:287, 1986.

92. Jeevan, A., Denkins, Y., Brown, E., Kripke, M. L., Effects of UV radiation on infectious diseases, in *Biological Effects of Light*, Holick, M. F., Ed., Walter de Gruyter & Co., New York, 1992, 83.

93. Jeevan, A., Kripke, M. L., Alteration of the immune response to *Mycobacterium bovis* BCG in mice exposed chronically to low dose UV radiation, *Cell. Immunol.*, 130:32, 1990.

94. Moyal, D., Courbière, C., Le Corre, Y., de Lacharrière, O., Hourseau, C., Immunosuppression induced by chronic solar-simulated irradiation in humans and its prevention by sunscreens, *Eur. J. Dermatol.*, 7:223, 1997.

95. Rivas, J. M., Ullrich, S. E., The role of IL-4, IL-10, and TNF-α in the immune suppression induced by ultraviolet radiation, *J. Leukoc. Biol.*, 56:769, 1994.

96. Araneo, B., Dowell, T., Moon, H. B., Daynes, R. A., Regulation of murine lymphocyte production in vivo. UV radiation exposure depresses IL-2 and enhances IL-4 production by T cells through an IL-1 dependent mechanism, *J. Immunol.*, 143:1737, 1989.

97. Yagi, H., Tokura, Y., Wakita, H., Furukawa, F., Takigawa, M., TCRVβ7+ Th2 cells mediate UVB-induced suppression of murine contact photosensitivity by releasing IL-10, *J. Immunol.*, 156:1824, 1996.

98. Brown, E. L., Rivas, J. M., Ullrich, S. E., Young, C. R., Norris, S. J., Kripke, M. L., Modulation of immunity to *Borrelia burgdorferi* by ultraviolet irradiation: differential effect on Th1 and Th2 type immune responses, *Eur. J. Immunol.*, 25:3017, 1995.

99. Hsieh, C.-S., Macatonia, S. E., Tripp, C. S., Wolf, S. F., O'Garra, A., Murphy, K. M., Development of Th1 CD4+ T cells through IL-12 produced by *Listeria*-induced macrophages, *Science*, 260:547, 1993.

100. Magram, J., Connaughton, S. E., Warrier, R. R., Carvajal, D. M., Wu, C.-Y., Ferrante, J., Stewart, C., Sarmiento, U., Faharty, D. A., Gately, M. K., IL-12-deficient mice are defective in IFN-γ production and type 1 cytokine responses, *Immunity*, 4:471, 1996.

101. Morris, S. C., Madden, K. B., Adamovicz, J. J., Gause, W. C., Hubbard, B. R., Gately, M. K., Finkelman, F. D., Effects of IL-12 on in vivo cytokine gene expression and Ig isotype selection, *J. Immunol.*, 152:1047, 1994.

102. McKnight, A. J., Zimmer, G. J., Fogelman, I., Wolf, S. F., Abbas, A. K., Effects of IL-12 on helper cell-dependent immune responses in vivo, *J. Immunol.*, 152:2172, 1994.

103. Schmitt, D. A., Owen-Schaub, L., Ullrich, S. E., Effect of IL-12 on immune suppression and suppressor cell induction by ultraviolet radiation, *J. Immunol.*, 154:5114, 1995.

104. Müller, G., Salonga, J., Germann, T., Schuler, G., Knopp, J., Enk, A. H., IL-12 as mediator and adjuvant for the induction of contact sensitivity in vivo, *J. Immunol.*, 155:466, 1995.

105. Schwarz, A., Grabbe, S., Aragane, Y., Sandkuhl, K., Riemann, H., Luger, T. A., Kubin, M., Trinchieri, G., Schwarz, T., Interleukin-12 prevents ultraviolet B-induced local immunosuppression and overcomes UVB-induced tolerance, *J. Invest. Dermatol.*, 106:1187, 1996.

106. Schwarz, A., Grabbe, S., Mahnke, K., Riemann, H., Luger, T. A., Wysocka, M., Trinchieri, G., Schwarz, T., Interleukin-12 breaks ultraviolet light induced immunosuppressison by affecting CD8+ rather than CD4+ T cells, *J. Invest. Dermatol.*, 110:272, 1998.

107. Marshall, J. D., Secrist, H., DeKruyff, R. H., Wolf, S. F., Umetsu, D. T., IL-12 inhibits the production of IL-4 and IL-10 in allergen specific human CD4+ T lymphocytes, *J. Immunol.*, 155:111, 1995.

108. Fiorentino, D. F., Zlotnik, A., Vieira, P., Mosmann, T. R., Howard, M., Moore, K. W., O'Garra, A., IL-10 acts on the antigen-presenting cell to inhibit cytokine production by Th1 cells, *J. Immunol.*, 146:3444, 1991.

109. Kopf, M., Le Gros, G., Bachmann, M., Lamers, M. C., Bluethmann, H., Kohler, G., Disruption of the murine IL-4 gene blocks Th2 cytokine responses, *Nature*, 362:245, 1993.

110. Shreedhar, V., Giese, T., Sung, V. W., Ullrich, S. E., A cytokine cascade including prostaglandin E_2, interleukin-4, and interleukin-10 is responsible for UV-induced systemic immune suppression, *J. Immunol.*, 160:000, 1998.

111. El-Ghorr, A. A., Norval, M., The role of interleukin-4 in ultraviolet B light-induced immunosuppression, *Immunology*, 92:26, 1997.

112. Black, H. J., deGruijl, F. R., Forbes, P. D., Cleaver, J. E., Ananthaswamy, H. N., De Fabo, E. C., Ullrich, S. E., Tyrrell, R. M., Photocarcinogenesis: an overview, *J. Photochem. Photobiol. B: Biology*, 40:29, 1997.

113. O'Conner, A., Nishigori, C., Yarosh, D., Alas, L., Kibitel, J., Burley, L., Cox, P., Bucana, C., Ullrich, S., Kripke, M., DNA double strand breaks in epidermal cells cause immune suppression in vivo and cytokine production in vitro, *J. Immunol.*, 157:271, 1996.

114. Hart, P. H., Jones, C. A., Jones, K. L., Watson, C. J., Santucci, I., Spencer, L. K., Finlay-Jones, J. J., cis-Urocanic acid stimulates human peripheral blood monocyte prostaglandin E-2 production and suppresses indirectly tumor necrosis factor-alpha levels, *J. Immunol.*, 150:4514, 1993.

115. Kripke, M. L., Ultraviolet radiation and immunity: something new under the sun — Presidential address, *Cancer Res.*, 54:6102, 1994.

21 Immune Tolerance and Its Potential to Control Skin Reactions

Richard S. Kalish

CONTENTS

I. WHAT IS IMMUNE TOLERANCE?

Tolerance, or "anergy," to an antigen means that there is no obvious immune response to that antigen. This is not equivalent to lack of recognition. There are mechanisms of peripheral tolerance that require active immune suppression. Nor is tolerance always the lack of immune response, as tolerance may sometimes indicate the immune response has shifted, so as not to result in the expected pathology. Tolerance is also defined by the observed end point. For example, transplantation tolerance is defined as lack of graft rejection. This may reflect the deviation of the immune response toward antibody production (e.g., Th2 response), deletion of the allo-reactive T cells, or active suppression of the allo-reactive T cells.

Allergic contact allergens, or haptens, can also induce tolerance. Simple nonresponsiveness to a contact allergen may mean lack of interaction with the immune system. To confirm the presence of tolerance, it is necessary to demonstrate lack of response with rechallenge following adequate sensitization.

Immune tolerance has considerable clinical significance. Lack of tolerance or loss of tolerance underlies most autoimmune conditions, and induction of tolerance to transplantation antigens is the ultimate goal of transplantation immunology. Induction of tolerance to contact allergens could potentially find application in the development of transdermal drug delivery devices for potentially sensitizing drugs. Since the focus of this book is the development of transdermal drug delivery devices, this review of immune tolerance will focus on T lymphocytes and allergic contact dermatitis.

II. WHAT ARE THE MECHANISMS OF TOLERANCE?

Mechanisms of tolerance induction parallel the development of the immune system. Tolerance to autoantigens is developed during T lymphocyte maturation in the thymus, by a process termed "central tolerance." The primary mechanism of central tolerance is apoptosis of autoreactive T cells, by a process known as clonal deletion. T cells in the thymus interact with self-peptides presented by autologous major histocompatibility antigens (MHC). Immature T cells in the thymus that recognize self-peptide/MHC with high affinity are deleted by apoptosis, whereas immature T cells that recognize self-peptide/MHC with low affinity receive a positive signal.[1,2]

Peripheral tolerance is induced once the T lymphocytes have left the thymus. Peripheral tolerance is the focus of this review, as it is most relevant to allergic contact allergens and design of transdermal drug delivery devices.

Induction of tolerance revolves around antigen presentation and T cell activation. T cell recognition of antigen, or hapten, in the absence of the appropriate complement of signals can induce that T cell to become tolerant. When the T cell next encounters the antigen, it will not respond with full activation. One means by which this form of tolerance can be induced is by blocking of costimulatory signals (Table 1). High dose antigen, or peptide, can induce tolerance through presentation of antigen by nonprofessional antigen-presenting cells, which lack the complete set of signals. Immune deviation induces a qualitative change in the immune response from a Th1 to a Th2 reaction. This results in diminished cell-mediated pathology, such as allergic contact dermatitis. Oral tolerance is one means by which immune deviation can be induced. Tolerance induction with ultraviolet light is unique to the skin, and relevant for allergic contact dermatitis.

TABLE 1
Mechanisms of Peripheral Tolerance of T Lymphocytes

Antigen presentation by nonprofessional antigen presenting cells
Inhibition of costimulation
Immune deviation (Th1 vs. Th2): IL-10, TGF-β
Oral tolerance
Peptides
Ultraviolet light

All the above mechanisms of peripheral tolerance induction have in common interference with antigen presentation and T cell recognition. These processes will be reviewed in detail below.

III. CD28/B7 COSTIMULATION OF T CELL ACTIVATION

Presentation of antigen to T lymphocytes involves the interactions of multiple adhesion molecules. T cell receptor occupancy alone is not sufficient to induce T cell proliferation. Recognition of antigen by CD4+ cells in the absence of costimulatory signals can induce tolerance.[3,4] The interaction of CD28 and B7-1 (CD80) or B7-2 (CD86) has been shown to deliver such an essential costimulatory signal to both human[5-8] and murine[9-12] CD4+ T cells. CD28 is a T cell antigen and B7 is an inducible antigen of antigen presenting cells and T cells.

B7-1 (CD80) and B7-2 (CD86) are members of the immunoglobulin superfamily, coded by linked genes on human chromosome 3q13-q26.[13] Both molecules interact with CD28 and CTLA4, and B7-1 binds both CD28 and CTLA4 at the same site.[14] However, there is evidence that B7-1 and B7-2 may induce different responses from T cells. Both molecules bind CD28 with similar avidities. However, B7-1 has a higher affinity for CTLA4 than B7-2.[15] There is evidence that CTLA4 has a negative effect on T cell proliferation.[16]

IV. BLOCKING OF COSTIMULATION CAN INDUCE TOLERANCE

Blocking the CD28/B7 interaction can induce tolerance of CD4+ cells, and alloantigen-specific CD8+ cells.[17–19] CD28 associates with the activated T cell receptor zeta chain, and apparently facilitates interactions of the zeta chain with the protein tyrosine kinase lck.[20] Tolerant CD4+ cells have a block in T cell activation prior to activation of the ERK-1, ERK-2 kinases, and ras.[21,22] This block in ras activation inhibits the transcription factor AP-1, preventing IL-2 production. The tolerant cells retain the ability to proliferate to IL-2 and produce interferon-γ. IL-2 treatment can overcome tolerance induced by blocking of B7 costimulation.[23] Blocking of costimulation also can tolerize human poison ivy (urushiol)-specific CD8+ T cells, which is of direct relevance to allergic contact dermatitis.[24]

CTLA4Ig is a recombinant molecule formed by fusion of the extracellular domain of CTLA4 and IgG.[25] It is capable of blocking the interaction of B7 with CD28 on human T cells. CD28-blocking reagents such as CTLA4Ig are of interest for possible use in immunotherapy.[26,27] Experimental applications of CTLA4Ig in mice have included prolongation of pancreatic transplant survival[28] and treatment of systemic lupus erythematosus.[29]

A pharmacologic alternative to blocking of CD28-mediated costimulation is the use of the phosphatidylinositol 3-kinase inhibitor, wortmannin. The phosphatidylinositol 3-kinase pathway mediates some of the costimulatory effects of CD28, and inhibition with wortmannin can induce tolerance.[30]

V. CD40 AND CD40 LIGAND (CD40L) HAVE A ROLE IN COSTIMULATION AND THE INDUCTION OF TOLERANCE

The interaction of CD40 on B cells, with the CD40 ligand (CD40L) on T cells, activates B cells and induces Ig class switching.[31] T cell CD40L also interacts with CD40 on antigen-presenting cells (APC) to induce both costimulatory activity[32] and IL-12 production.[33] This includes the induction of B7-1 (CD80) and B7-2 (CD86).[34] Blocking antibodies to CD40L inhibit the allogeneic mixed lymphocyte reaction and synergize with blocking of CD28 costimulation to induce tolerance to organ allografts.[35]

VI. TOLERANCE INDUCTION BY BLOCKING OTHER MOLECULES WITH A ROLE IN T CELL ACTIVATION: LFA-1/ICAM-1, HEAT-STABLE ANTIGEN (HSA), VLA-4

ICAM-1/LFA-1 interactions are essential for T cell adhesion to APC.[36] Although ICAM-1/LFA-1 mediates adhesion, and not costimulation,[37] blocking of ICAM-1 inhibits human alloantigen responses in vitro,[38] prolongs cardiac allograft survival, induces long-term allograft tolerance in mice,[39] and suppresses allergic contact dermatitis.[40] Interference with LFA-3/CD2 interactions can also induce tolerance to alloantigen.[41]

Heat-stable antigen (HSA: CD24) is an additional costimulatory molecule for presentation of antigen to CD4+ cells.[42–44] HSA is a small, extensively glycosylated protein which is attached to the cell membrane by a glycosyl-phosphatidyl-inositol anchor,[45] and is linked to tyrosine kinases.[46] HSA is expressed on accessory cells, B cells, Langerhans cells, and activated T cells,[47] but not on resting mature T cells. It is expressed very early by activated T cells, and expression is transient. Langerhans cell costimulation mediated by HSA preferentially stimulates Th1 CD4+ cells.[48] HSA-mediated costimulation may be cooperative with CD28.[49] HSA can be homophilic,[50] and it is proposed that induction of T cell HSA by CD28 is required prior to HSA-mediated costimulation. HSA costimulation has been investigated primarily in murine systems; there are little human data on HSA.

VII. ANTIGEN PRESENTATION BY NONPROFESSIONAL ANTIGEN PRESENTING CELLS

Professional antigen-presenting cells are those with a high constitutive level of expression of both antigen-presenting (e.g., HLA-DR), adhesion (e.g., ICAM-1, LFA-1), and costimulatory molecules (e.g., CD80/CD86, CD40). Dendritic antigen-presenting cells of the lymph node, spleen, peripheral blood, and skin, including epidermal Langerhans cells, meet this definition. These cells are able to process and present antigen to T cells with high efficiency, and seldom induce tolerance under natural conditions. Monocytes and macrophages are able to process and present antigens to T cells, but only after sufficient activation. Depending upon their level of activation and expression of relevant molecules, they have the potential to induce tolerance. Many additional cell types, including keratinocytes, fibroblasts, and endothelial cells, have the potential to express HLA-DR under sufficient stimulation by cytokines. These are nonprofessional antigen-presenting cells.

Presentation of antigen by nonprofessional APCs can result in tolerance, presumably because these cells lack the full set of antigen presentation and costimulation molecules.[51] Keratinocytes express HLA-DR when induced with interferon-γ.[52,53] Presentation of antigen or hapten by HLA-DR–expressing epithelial cells,[54] or keratinocytes,[55] may result in tolerance. It is possible by this means to induce tolerance in mice by the intravenous injection of hapten-treated keratinocytes or fixed spleen cells. Incomplete signaling by the T cell receptor following antigen presentation by a nonprofessional APC leads either to tolerance or apoptosis mediated by Fas/Fas ligand (CD95).[56]

Tolerance induction by nonprofessional APC is likely to follow either treatment with high doses of antigen, or manipulations to deplete professional APCs. High antigen doses can result in uptake and presentation by unstimulated macrophages. Ultraviolet exposure of the skin results in depletion of Langerhans cells, which may result in hapten presentation by nonprofessional APCs, and tolerance.

VIII. IMMUNE DEVIATION (TH1 VS. TH2)

T helper (inducer) CD4 lymphocytes are classified by the cytokines they produce into two subsets.[57,58] Th1 cells produce IL-2, interferon-γ, and GM-CSF, whereas Th2 cells produce IL-3, IL-4, and IL-5. Th1 cells are responsible for delayed hypersensitivity reactions and Th2 cells produce helper factors for production of antibodies, including IgE. Th2 cells also produce IL-10, which inhibits cytokine production by Th1 cells, favoring IgE production.[59,60] IL-10 inhibits T cell proliferation and induces anergy.[61,62] Switching T cell cytokine profile from Th1 to Th2 can alter the nature of the immune response and suppress immunopathology. This immune deviation results in a form of tolerance. The immune system still recognizes the antigen, but the immune response does not produce pathology.

Allergic contact dermatitis is inhibited by IL-10[63,64] and potentiated by antibody to IL-10.[65] Dendritic cells cultured with IL-10 are unable to properly upregulate costimulatory molecules, such as CD86, and can induce tolerance.[66] α-Melanocyte-stimulating hormone (α-MSH) both inhibits contact sensitivity of mice with topical application and induces tolerance by an IL-10–dependent mechanism.[67] IL-10 production by keratinocytes is one of several proposed mechanisms for UV light-induced suppression of contact sensitivity (see below). Immune deviation also has a role in the tolerance induced by oral exposure to antigen.

IX. ORAL IMMUNE TOLERANCE

Oral feeding of antigens, or haptens, can result in tolerance.[68,69,70] At least two mechanisms of oral tolerance are supported by the data. Low dose feeding induces immunosuppressive transforming growth factor-β (TGF-β) producing T cells, while high dose feeding may lead to clonal deletion.[71] The induction of TGF-β–producing cells is an example of immune deviation. Intestinal epithelial cells produce the immunosuppressive cytokine TGF-β, which may promote the development of oral tolerance.[72] The chemokine macrophage inflammatory protein (MIP)-1α may also mediate oral tolerance induction.[73] Oral tolerance is capable of ameliorating several experimentally induced autoimmune diseases, including experimental allergic encephalomyelitis, collagen, and adjuvant-induced arthritis, uveitis, and diabetes in the nonobese diabetic mouse.[74] Clinical trials of oral tolerance are underway for myelin basic protein in multiple sclerosis,[75] type II collagen in rheumatoid arthritis, S-antigen in uveitis, and insulin in type I diabetes.

X. PEPTIDE-INDUCED TOLERANCE

Peptides can be used to induce tolerance by at least two mechanisms. The first mechanism is the administration of large doses of peptide containing the T cell epitope of interest. The peptide is presented by nonprofessional APCs, or by APCs that have not been fully activated. This presentation of peptide in the absence of the full complement of co-stimulatory signals results in tolerance.[76,77] It is possible to induce tolerance of human T cells to house dust mite (Der pI) allergen by culture with allergen in the presence of nonprofessional APCs.[78] Administration of peptides containing T cell epitopes is capable of inducing tolerance to both the peptide epitopes, and the proteins containing those epitopes.[79]

The second mechanism for the induction of tolerance with peptides requires the design of peptide analogs of T cell epitopes with amino acid substitutions. These altered peptide ligands can induce incomplete T cell receptor signaling with resultant tolerance,[80,81] and TGF-β production.[82] This tolerance is mediated by incomplete T cell receptor signaling, which results in inadequate tyrosine phosphorylation of the CD3 zeta chain and lack of recruitment of ZAP-70.[83] Design of altered peptide ligands requires knowledge of the MHC and T cell receptor contact positions of the natural peptide.[84] Amino acid substitutions are made in the T cell receptor contact positions, such that the peptide retains high affinity for the MHC molecule, with reduced affinity for the T cell receptor.

XI. ULTRAVIOLET LIGHT-INDUCED IMMUNOSUPPRESSION AND TOLERANCE

Exposure to ultraviolet B light (UVB) is both immunosuppressive and able to induce tolerance.[85–87] Multiple mechanisms are involved, including depletion of Langerhans cells and recruitment of APCs which favor tolerance induction.[88,89] UVB also induces keratinocytes to produce IL-10, resulting in immunosuppression and immune deviation. In contrast, the Th1 cytokine IL-12 can reverse UVB-induced immunosuppression and tolerance.[90] Urocanic acid is one potential mediator of the immunosuppressive effects of UVB.[91] UVB induces *trans*-urocanic acid to isomerize to *cis*-urocanic acid. The *cis*-urocanic acid has immunosuppressive effects[92,93] that may be partly mediated by IL-10.[94] Potential targets for UVB which induce immunosuppression include cyclobutyl pyrimidine dimers, urocanic acid, and TNF-α induction by keratinocytes. Mechanisms of UVB-induced tolerance and immunosuppression, as well as urocanic acid, are discussed at length in separate chapters.

XII. SUMMATION AND APPLICATION OF TOLERANCE TO CONTACT DERMATITIS CAUSED BY TRANSDERMAL DRUG DELIVERY

Induction of tolerance revolves around antigen presentation and recognition by T cells. Blocking of costimulation, or presentation by nonprofessional APCs can result in inadequate costimulation. Lack of costimulation induces incomplete T cell activation, which can leave the T cell viable, but minimally responsive. Alternately, presentation of antigen can result in apoptosis and clonal deletion. Clonal deletion is the primary mechanism of development of self-tolerance in the thymus (central tolerance), as well as certain forms of peripheral tolerance, such as high dose oral feeding. Immune deviation reduces immunopathology by shifting the immune response from a Th1 to a Th2 response, or by favoring the production of immunosuppressive cytokines such as IL-10 or TGF-β. Practical applications of these findings include tolerance induction by UVB, oral feeding, altered peptide ligands, and blocking of costimulation with agents such as CTLA4Ig.

Development of allergic contact dermatitis to topical drugs is a major limitation in the development of transdermal drug delivery systems.[94–99] For this reason, it would be advantageous to develop technology that would either prevent sensitization or induce tolerance to topically applied drugs. There are multiple potential targets for induction of tolerance to contact allergens (Table 2). Urocanic acid is one obvious potential mediator, as are manipulations that induce IL-10 production in the skin. Mast cells are a source of both IL-4 and TNF-α, which favor immune deviation and alter Langerhans cell density, respectively. Mast cell-activating agents may in this manner alter the allergic contact response. If the allergen is a protein, altered peptide ligands may induce tolerance. Ion channel inhibitors may inhibit cell signaling and activation of T cells, or APCs, thereby inducing tolerance.[100–103] Finally, pharmacologic manipulations that deplete epidermal Langerhans cells or inhibit Langerhans cell function should result in skin hyporesponsiveness or tolerance. Topical steroids are known to do both,[104] and one obvious application of this knowledge is the inhibition of sensitization to topically applied drugs by treatment with topical corticosteroid.[105]

TABLE 2
Potential Targets for Induction of Tolerance to Contact Allergens

Induction of IL-10 production in skin
Inhibition of cell activation (ion channel inhibitors)
  T cells
  Langerhans cells
Depletion of Langerhans cells
Inhibition of Langerhans cell function
  Ion channel inhibitors
  Corticosteroids
Mast cell production of IL-4 and TNF-α
Urocanic acid

REFERENCES

1. Liu CP, Crawford F, Marrack P, Kappler J. T cell positive selection by a high density, low affinity ligand. *Proc Natl Acad Sci USA* 95:4522–4526, 1998.
2. Chen W, Sayegh MH, Khoury SJ. Mechanisms of acquired thymic tolerance in vivo: intrathymic injection of antigen induces apoptosis of thymocytes and peripheral T cell anergy. *J Immunol* 160:1504–1508, 1998.

3. Jenkins MK, Schwartz RH. Antigen presentation by chemically modified splenocytes induces antigen-specific T cell unresponsiveness in vitro and in vivo. *J Exp Med* 165:302–319, 1987.

4. Quill H, Schwartz RH. Stimulation of normal inducer T cell clones with antigen presented by purified Ia molecules in planar lipid membranes: specific induction of a long-lived state of proliferative nonresponsiveness. *J Immunol* 138:3704–3712, 1987.

5. Jenkins MK, Taylor PS, Norton SD, Urdahl KB. CD28 delivers a costimulatory signal involved in antigen-specific IL2 production by human T cells. *J Immunol* 147:2461–2466, 1991.

6. Young JW, Koulova L, Soergel SA, Clark EA, Steinman RM, Dupont B. The B7/BB1 antigen provides one of the several costimulatory signals for the activation of CD4+ T lymphocytes by human blood dendritic cells in vitro. *J Clin Invest* 90:229–237, 1992.

7. Gimm CD, Freeman GJ, Gribben JG, Sugita K, Freeman AS, Morimoto C, Nadler LM. B-cell surface antigen B7 provides a costimulatory signal that induced T cells to proliferate and secrete interleukin 2. *Proc Natl Acad Sci USA* 88:6575–6579, 1991.

8. Freeman GJ, Gribben JG, Boussiotis VA, Ng JW, Restivo VA, Lombard LA, Gray GS, Nadler LM. Cloning of B7-2: a CTLA-4 counter-receptor that costimulates human T cell proliferation. *Science* 262:909–911, 1993.

9. Harding FA, McArthur JG, Groos JA, Raulet DH, Allison JP. CD28-mediated signalling co-stimulates murine T cells and prevents induction of anergy in T-cell clones. *Nature* 356:607–609, 1992.

10. Gross JA, Callas E, Allison JP. Identification and distribution of the costimulatory receptor CD28 in the mouse. *J Immunol* 149:380–388, 1992.

11. Hathcock KS, Laszio G, Dickler HB, Bradshaw J, Linsley P, Hodes RJ. Identification of an alternative CTLA-4 ligand costimulatory for T cell activation. *Science* 262:905–907, 1993.

12. Freeman GJ, Borriello F, Hodes RJ, Reiser H, Hathcock KS, Laszlo G, McKnight AJ, Kim J, Du L, Lombard DB, Gray GS, Nadler LM, Sharpe AH. Uncovering of functional alternative CTLA-4 counter-receptor in B7-deficient mice. *Science* 262:907–909, 1993.

13. Fernandez-Ruiz E, Somoza C, Sanchez-Madrid F, Lanier LL. CD28/CTLA-4 ligands: the gene encoding CD86 (B70/B7.2) maps to the same region as CD80 (B7/B7.1) gene in human chromosome 3q13-q23. *Eur J Immunol* 25: 1453–6, 1995.

14. Guo Y, Wu Y, Zhao M, Kong XP, Liu Y. Mutational analysis and an alternatively spliced product of B7 defines its CD28/CTLA4-binding site on immunoglobulin C-like domain. *J Exp Med* 181:1345–55, 1995.

15. Linsley PS, Greene JL, Brady W, Bajorath J, Ledbetter JA, Peach R. Human B7-1 (CD80) and B7-2 (CD86) bind with similar avidities but distinct kinetics to CD28 and CTLA-4 receptors. *Immunity* 1:793–801, 1994.

16. Waterhouse P, Penniger JM, Timms E, Wakeham A, Shahinian A, Lee KP, Thompson CB, Griesser H, Mak TW. Lymphoproliferative disorders with early lethality in mice deficient in Ctla-4. *Science* 270:985–988, 1995.

17. Lu P, Wang YL, Linsley PS. Regulation of self-tolerance by CD80/CD86 interactions. *Curr Opinion Immunol* 9:858–862, 1997.

18. Tan P, Anasetti C, Hansen JA, Melrose J, Brunvand M, Bradshaw J, Ledbetter JA, Linsley PS. Induction of alloantigen-specific hyporesponsiveness in human T lymphocytes by blocking interaction of CD28 with its natural ligand B7/BB1. *J Exp Med* 177:165–173, 1993.

19. Gribben JG, Guinan EC, Boussiotis VA, Ke XY, Linsley L, Sieff C, Gray GS, Freeman GJ, Nadler LM. Complete blockade of B7 family-mediated costimulation is necessary to induce human alloantigen-specific anergy: a method to ameliorate graft-versus-host disease and extend the donor pool. *Blood* 87:4887–4893, 1996.

20. Boussiotis VA, Barber DL, Lee BJ, Gribben JG, Freeman GJ. Differential association of protein tyrosine kinases with the T cell receptor is linked to the induction of anergy and its prevention by B7 family-mediated costimulation. *J Exp Med* 184:365–376, 1996.

21. Li W, Whaley CD, Mondino A, Mueller DL. Blocked signal transduction to the ERK and JNK protein kinases in anergic CD4+ T cells. *Science* 271:1272–1276, 1996.

22. Fields PE, Gajewski TF, Fitch FW. Blocked ras activation in anergic CD4+ T cells. *Science* 271:1276–1278, 1996.

23. Yi-qun Z, Lorre K, de Boer M, Ceuppens JL. B7-blocking agents, alone or in combination with cyclosporin A, induce antigen-specific anergy of human memory T cells. *J Immunol* 158:4734–4740, 1997.

24. Kalish RS, Wood JA. Induction of hapten specific tolerance of human CD8+ urushiol (poison ivy) reactive T-cells. *J Invest Dermatol* 108:253–257, 1997.

25. Linsley PS, Brady W, Urnes M, Grosmaire L, Damle NK, Ledbetter JA. CTLA-4 is a second receptor for the B cell activation antigen B7. *J Exp Med* 174:561–569, 1991.

26. Schwartz RH. Costimulation of T lymphocytes: the role of CD28, CTLA-4, and B7/BB1 in interleukin-2 production and immunotherapy. *Cell* 71:1065–1068, 1992.

27. Wallace PM, Rodgers JN, Leytze GM, Johnson JS, Linsley PS. Induction and reversal of long-lived specific unresponsiveness to a T-dependent antigen following CTLA4Ig treatment. *J Immunol* 154:5885–5895, 1995.

28. Lenshow DH, Zeng Y, Thistlethwaite JR, Montag A, Brady W, Gibson MG, Linsley PS, Bluestone JA. Long-term survival of xenogeneic pancreatic islet grafts induced by CTLA4Ig. *Science* 257:789–792, 1992.

29. Finck BK, Linsley PS, Wofsy D. Treatment of murine lupus with CTLA4Ig. *Science* 265:1225–1227, 1994.

30. Taub DD, Murphy WJ, Asai O, Fenton RG, Peltz G, Key ML, Turcovski-Corrales S, Longo DL. Induction of alloantigen-specific T cell tolerance through the treatment of human T lymphocytes with wortmannin. *J Immunol* 158:2745–2755, 1997.

31. Bowen F, Haluskey J, Quill H. Altered CD40 ligand induction in tolerant T lymphocytes. *Eur J Immunol* 25:2830–4, 1995.

32. Wu Y, Xu J, Shinde S, Grewal I, Henderson T, Flavell RA, Liu Y. Rapid induction of a novel costimulatory activity on B cells by CD40 ligand. *Curr Biol* 5:1303–11, 1995.

33. Cella M, Scheidegger D, Palmer-Lehmann K, Lane P, Lanzavecchia A, Alber G. Ligation of CD40 on dendritic cells triggers production of high levels of interleukin-12 and enhances T cell stimulatory capacity: T-T help via APC activation. *J Exp Med* 184:747–52, 1996.

34. McLellan AD, Sorg RV, Williams LA, Hart DN. Human dendritic cells activate T lymphocytes via a CD40: CD40 ligand-dependent pathway. *Eur J Immunol* 26:1204–10, 1996.

35. Larsen CP, Elwood ET, Alexander DZ, Ritchie SC, Hendrix R, Tucker-Burden C, Cho HR, Aruffo A, Hollenbaugh D, Linsley PS, Winn KJ, Pearson TC. Long-term acceptance of skin and cardiac allografts after blocking CD40 and CD28 pathways. *Nature* 381:434–8, 1996.

36. Boyd AW, Wawryk SO, Burns GF, Fecondo JV. Intercellular adhesion molecule 1 (ICAM-1) has a central role in cell-cell contact-mediated immune mechanisms. *Proc Natl Acad Sci USA* 85:3095–3099, 1988.

37. Bachmann MF, McKall-Faienza K, Schmits R, Bouchard D, Beach J, Speiser DE, Mak TW, Ohashi PS. Distinct roles for LFA-1 and CD28 during activation of naive T cells: adhesion versus costimulation. *Immunity* 7:549–557, 1997.

38. Boussiotis VA, Freeman GJ, Gray G, Gribben J, Nadler LM. B7 but not intercellular adhesion molecule-1 costimulation prevents the induction of human alloantigen-specific tolerance. *J Exp Med* 178:1753–1763, 1993.

39. Isobe M, Yagita H, Okumura K, Ihara A. Specific acceptance of cardiac allograft after treatment with antibodies to ICAM-1 and LFA-1. *Science* 255:1125–1127, 1992.

40. Murayama M, Yasuda H, Nishimura Y, Asahi M. Suppression of mouse contact hypersensitivity after treatment with antibodies to leukocyte function-associated antigen-1 and intracellular adhesion molecules-1. *Arch Dermatol Res* 289:98–103, 1997.

41. Bohmig GA, Kovarik J, Holter W, Pohanka E, Zlabinger GJ. Specific down-regulation of proliferative T cell alloresponsiveness by interference with CD2/LFA-3 and LFA-1/ICAM-1 in vitro. *J Immunol* 152:3720–3728, 1994.

42. Liu Y, Jones B, Aruffo A, Sullivan KM, Linsley PS, Janeway CA. Heat-stable antigen is a costimulatory molecule for CD4 T cell growth. *J Exp Med* 175:437–445, 1992.

43. Hubbe M, Altevogt P. Heat-stable antigen/CD24 on mouse T lymphocytes: evidence for a costimulatory function. *Eur J Immunol* 24:731–737, 1994.

44. Hough MR, Rosten PM, Sexton TL, Kay R, Humphries RK. Mapping of CD24 and homologous sequences to multiple chromosomal loci. *Genomics* 22:154–61, 1994.

45. Kay R, Rosten PM, Humphries RK. CD24, a signal transducer modulating B cell activation responses, is a very short peptide with a glycosyl phosphatidylinositol membrane anchor. *J Immunol* 147:1412–1416, 1991.

46. Stefanova I, Horejsi V, Ansotegui IJ, Knapp W, Stockinger H. GPI-anchored cell-surface molecules complexed to protein tyrosine kinases. *Science* 254:1016–1019, 1991.

47. Salamone MC, Achino B, Fainboim L. Cytoplasmic expression of a CD24-related epitope in human PHA activated normal T lymphocytes. *Immunol Lett* 34:109–13, 1992.

48. Enk AH, Katz SI. Heat-stable antigen is an important costimulatory molecule on epidermal Langerhans' cells. *J Immunol* 152:3264–3270, 1994.

49. Liu Y, Jones B, Brady W, Janeway CA Jr, Linsley PS. Co-stimulation of murine CD4 T cell growth: cooperation between B7 and heat-stable antigen. *Eur J Immunol* 22:2855–2859, 1992.

50. Kadmon G, Eckert M, Sammar M, Schachner M, Altevogt P. Nectadrin, the heat-stable antigen, is a cell adhesion molecule. *J Cell Biol* 118:1245–1258, 1992.

51. Nickoloff BJ, Turka LA. Immunological functions of non-professional antigen-presenting cells: new insights from studies of T-cell interactions with keratinocytes. *Immunol Today* 15:464–469, 1994.

52. Basham TY, Nickoloff BJ, Merigan TC, Morhenn VB. Recombinant gamma interferon induces HLA-DR expression on cultured human keratinocytes. *J Invest Dermatol* 83:88–90, 1984.

53. Griffiths CEM, Voorhees JJ, Nickoloff BJ. Characterization of intercellular adhesion molecule-1 and HLA-DR expression in normal and inflamed skin: modulation by recombinant gamma interferon and tumor necrosis factor. *J Am Acad Dermatol* 20:617–629, 1989.

54. Marelli-Berg FM, Weetman A, Frasca L, Deacock SJ, Imami N, Lombardi G, Lechler RI. Antigen presentation by epithelial cells induces anergic immunoregulatory CD45RO+ T cells and deletion of CD45RA+ T cells. *J Immunol* 159:5853–5861, 1997.

55. Gaspari AA, Kenkins MK, Katz SI. Class II MHC-bearing keratinocytes induce antigen-specific unresponsiveness in hapten-specific TH1 clones. *J Immunol* 141:2216–2220, 1988.

56. Hargreaves RG, Borthwick NJ, Montani MS, Piccolella E, Carmichael P, Lechler RI, Akbar AN, Lombardi G. Dissociation of T cell anergy from apoptosis by blockade of Fas/Apo-1 (CD95) signaling. *J Immunol* 158:3099–3107, 1997.

57. Mosmann TR, Cherwinski H, Bond MW, Giedlin MA, Coffman RL. Two types of murine helper T cell clone I. Definition according to profiles of lymphokine activities and secreted proteins. *J Immunol* 136:2348–2357, 1986.

58. Street NE, Mosmann TR. Functional diversity of T lymphocytes due to secretion of different cytokine patterns. *FASEB J* 5:171–177, 1991.

59. Fiorentino DF, Bond MW, Mosmann TR. Two types of mouse T helper cell IV. Th2 clones secrete a factor that inhibits cytokine production by Th1 clones. *J Exp Med* 170:2081–2095, 1989.

60. Moore KW, Vieira P, Fiorentino DF, Trounstine ML, Khan TA, Mosmann TR. Homology of cytokine synthesis inhibitory factor (IL10) to the Epstein-Barr virus gene BCRF1. *Science* 248:1230–1233, 1990.

61. Groux H, Bigler M, de Vries JE, Roncarolo MG. Inhibitory and stimulatory effects of IL-10 on human CD8+ T cells. *J Immunol* 160:3188–3193, 1998.

62. Groux H, Bigler M, de Vries JE, Roncarolo MG. Interleukin-10 induces a long-term antigen-specific anergic state in human CD4+ T cells. *J Exp Med* 184:19–29, 1996.

63. Meng X, Sawamura D, Tamai K, Hanada K, Ishida H, Hashimoto I. Keratinocyte gene therapy for systemic diseases. Circulating interleukin 10 released from gene-transferred keratinocytes inhibits contact hypersensitivity at distant areas of the skin. *J Clin Invest* 101:1462–1467, 1998.

64. Berg DJ, Leach MW, Kuhn R, Rajewsky K, Muller W, Davidson NJ, Rennick D. Interleukin 10 but not interleukin 4 is a natural suppressant of cutaneous inflammatory responses. *J Exp Med* 182:99–108, 1995.

65. Maguire HC, Ketcha KA, Lattime EC. Neutralizing anti-IL-10 antibody upregulates the induction and elicitation of contact hypersensitivity. *J Interferon Cytokine Res* 17:763–768, 1997.

66. Steinbrink K, Wolfl M, Jonuleit H, Knop J, Enk AH. Induction of tolerance by IL-10-treated dendritic cells. *J Immunol* 159:4772–4780, 1997.

67. Grabbe S, Bhardwaj RS, Mahnke K, Simon MM, Schwarz T, Luger TA. alpha-Melanocyte-stimulating hormone induces hapten-specific tolerance in mice. *J Immunol* 156:473–478, 1996.

68. Weiner HL, Gonnella PA, Slavin A, Maron R. Oral tolerance: cytokine milieu in the gut and modulation of tolerance by cytokines. *Res Immunol* 148:528–533, 1997.

69. Inada S, Yoshino S, Haque MA, Ogata Y, Kohashi O. Clonal anergy is a potent mechanism of oral tolerance in the suppression of acute antigen-induced arthritis in rats by oral administration of the inducing antigen. *Cell Immunol* 175:67–75, 1997.

70. Karpus WJ, Kennedy KJ, Smith WS, Miller SD. Inhibition of relapsing experimental autoimmune encephalomyelitis in SJL mice by feeding the immunodominant PLP139-151 peptide. *J Neurosci Res* 45:410–423, 1996.

71. Whitacre CC, Gienapp IE, Meyer A, Cox KL, Javed N. Oral tolerance in experimental autoimmune encephalomyelitis. *Ann NY Acad Sci* 778:217–227, 1996.

72. Galliaerde V, Desvignes C, Peyron E, Kaiserlian D. Oral tolerance to haptens: intestinal epithelial cells from 2,4-dinitrochlorobenzene-fed mice inhibit hapten-specific T cell activation in vitro. *Eur J Immunol* 25:1385–1390, 1995.

73. Karpus WJ, Lukacs NW. The role of chemokines in oral tolerance. Abrogation of nonresponsiveness by treatment with antimonocyte chemotactic protein-1. *Ann NY Acad Sci* 778:133–144, 1996.

74. Weiner HL. Oral tolerance for the treatment of autoimmune diseases. *Ann Rev Med* 48:341–51, 1997.

75. Hafler DA, Kent SC, Pietrusewicz MJ, Khoury SJ, Weiner HL, Fukaura H. Oral administration of myelin induces antigen-specific TGF-beta 1 secreting T cells in patients with multiple sclerosis. *Ann NY Acad Sci* 835:120–31, 1997.

76. Grunow R, Frutig K, Pichler WJ. Anergy induction in human CD4+ T-cell clones by stimulation with soluble peptides does not require cell proliferation and is accompanied by elevated IL4 production. *Cell Immunol* 173:79–86, 1996.

77. Falb D, Briner TJ, Sunshine GH, Bourque CR, Luqman M, Gefter ML, Kamradt T. Peripheral tolerance in T cell receptor-transgenic mice: evidence for T cell anergy. *Eur J Immunol* 26:130–135, 1996.

78. Fasler S, Aversa G, Terr A, Thestrup-Pedersen K, de Vries JE, Yssel H. Peptide-induced anergy in allergen-specific human Th2 cells results in lack of cytokine production and B cell help for IgE synthesis. Reversal by IL-2, not by IL-4 or IL-13. *J Immunol* 155:4199–4206, 1995.

79. Hoyne GF, Jarnicki AG, Thomas WR, Lamb JR. Characterization of the specificity and duration of T cell tolerance to intranasally administered peptides in mice: a role for intramolecular epitope suppression. *Int Immunol* 9:1165–1173, 1997.

80. Ryan KR, Evavold BD. Persistence of peptide-induced CD4+ T cell anergy in vitro. *J Exp Med* 187:89–96, 1998.

81. Fairchild PJ. Altered peptide ligands: prospects for immune intervention in autoimmune disease. *Eur J Immunogenet* 24:155–167, 1997.

82. Tsitoura DC, Gelder CM, Kemeny DM, Lamb JR. Regulation of cytokine production by human Th0 cells following stimulation with peptide analogues: differential expression of TGF-beta in activation and anergy. *Immunology* 92:10–19, 1997.

83. Matsushita S, Nishimura Y. Partial activation of human T cells by peptide analogs on live APC: induction of clonal anergy associated with protein tyrosine dephosphorylation. *Hum Immunol* 53:73–80, 1997.

84. Colovai AI, Liu Z, Harris PE, Cortesini R, Suciu-Foca N. Allopeptide-specific T cell reactivity altered by peptide analogs. *J Immunol* 158:48–54, 1997.

85. Toews GB, Bergstresser PR, Streilein JW. Epidermal Langerhans cell density determines whether contact sensitivity or unresponsiveness follows skin painting with DNFB. *J Immunol* 124:445–453, 1980.

86. Yoshikawa T, Rae V, Bruins-Slot W, Van den Berg JW, Taylor JR, Streilein JW. Susceptibility to effects of UVB radiation on induction of contact hypersensitivity as a risk factor for skin cancer in humans. *J Invest Dermatol* 95:530–536, 1990.

87. Tie C, Golomb C, Taylor JR, Streilein JW. Suppressive and enhancing effects of ultraviolet B radiation on expression of contact hypersensitivity in man. *J Invest Dermatol* 104:18–22, 1995.

88. Stingl G, Gazze-Stingl LA, Aberer W, Wolff K. Antigen presentation by murine epidermal Langerhans cells and its alteration by ultraviolet B light. *J Immunol* 127:1707–1713, 1981.

89. Meunier L, Bata-Csorgo Z, Cooper KD. In human dermis, ultraviolet radiation induces expansion of a CD36+ CD11b+ CD1- macrophage subset by infiltration and proliferation; CD1+ Langerhans-like dendritic antigen-presenting cells are concomitantly depleted. *J Invest Dermatol* 105:782–788, 1995.

90. Schmitt DA, Owen-Schaub L, Ullrich SE. Effect of IL-12 on immune suppression and suppressor cell induction by ultraviolet radiation. *J Immunol* 154:5114–5120, 1995.

91. Kurimoto I, Streilein JW. Deleterious effects of cis-urocanic acid and UVB radiation on Langerhans cells and on induction of contact hypersensitivity are mediated by tumor necrosis factor-alpha. *J Invest Dermatol* 99:69S–70S, 1992.

92. Kondo S, Sauder DN, McKenzie RC, Fujisawa H, Shivji GM, El-Ghorr A, Norval M. The role of cis-urocanic acid in UVB-induced suppression of contact hypersensitivity. *Immunol Lett* 48:181–186, 1995.

93. Norval M, Gibbs NK, Gilmour J. The role of urocanic acid in UV-induced immunosuppression: recent advances (1992–1994). *Photochem Photobiol* 62:209–217, 1995.

94. Moodycliffe AM, Bucana CD, Kripke ML, Norval M, Ullrich SE. Differential effects of a monoclonal antibody to cis-urocanic acid on the suppression of delayed and contact hypersensitivity following ultraviolet irradiation. *J Immunol* 157:2891–2899, 1996.

95. Bircher AJ, Howald H, Rufli T. Adverse skin reactions to nicotine in a transdermal therapeutic system. *Contact Dermatitis* 25:230–236, 1991.

96. Erkkola R, Holma P, Jarvi T, Nummi S, Punnonen R, Raudaskoski T, Rehn K, Ryynanen M, Sipila P, Tunkelo E. Transdermal oestrogen replacement therapy in a Finnish population. *Maturitas* 13:275–281, 1991.

97. Sentrakul P, Chompootaweep S, Sintupak S, Tasanapradit P, Tunsaringkarn K, Dusitsin N. Adverse skin reactions to transdermal oestradiol in tropical climate. A comparative study of skin tolerance after using oestradiol patch and gel in Thai postmenopausal women. *Maturitas* 13:151–154, 1991.

98. Lueg MC, Herron J, Zellner S. Transdermal clonidine as an adjunct to sustained-release diltiazem in the treatment of mild-to-moderate hypertension. *Clin Ther* 13:471–481, 1991.

99. Robinson MK, Parsell KL, Breneman DL, Cruze CA. Evaluation of the primary skin irritation and allergic contact sensitization potential of transdermal triprolidine. *Fundam Appl Toxicol* 17:103–119, 1991.

100. Gallo RL, Granstein RD. Inhibition of allergic contact dermatitis and ultraviolet radiation-induced tissue swelling in the mouse by topical amiloride. *Arch Dermatol* 125:502–506, 1989.

101. Lindgren AM, Granstein RD, Hosoi J, Gallo RL. Structure-function relations in the inhibition of murine contact hypersensitivity by amiloride. *J Invest Dermatol* 104:38–41, 1995.

102. Diezel W, Gruner S, Diaz LA, Anhalt GJ. Inhibition of cutaneous contact hypersensitivity by calcium transport inhibitors lanthanum and diltiazem. *J Invest Dermatol* 93:322–326, 1989.

103. Kalish RS, Wood JA, Kydonieus A, Wille JJ. Prevention of contact hypersensitivity to topically applied drugs by ethacrynic acid: potential application to transdermal drug delivery. *J Controlled Rel* 48:79–87, 1997.

104. Ashworth J, Brooker J, Breathnach SM. Effects of topical corticosteroid therapy on Langerhans cells antigen presenting function in human skin. *Br J Dermatol* 118:457–470, 1988.

105. Amkraut A, Jordan W, Taskovich L. Effect of co-administration of corticosteroids on the development of contact sensitization *J Am Acad Dermatol* 35:27–31, 1996.

22 Future Prospects and Areas of Promising Research

J. Wayne Streilein and Sharmila Masli

CONTENTS

I. INTRODUCTION

The preceding chapters in this book offer testimony to the remarkable advances that have taken place in the field of immunodermatology over the past few decades. This is especially true in the areas of research concerning contact hypersensitivity (CH) and allergic contact dermatitis (ACD).

In this chapter we will attempt to address four questions concerning future prospects for research in this field:

1. What do we now know for sure? — a summary of incontrovertible, experimentally verified facts about CH and ACD.
2. What do we think we know? — recent observations that require further verification and amplification.
3. What areas do we need to learn more about? — major gaps in our current knowledge and understanding of CH and ACD.
4. What would we really like to know next? — knowledge that would help to avoid acquisition of CH and ACD, and/or strategies that would reverse sensitization once it had taken place.

II. WHAT DO WE NOW KNOW FOR SURE?

As scientists we can look with some pride at several seminal observations which have been securely and repeatedly made during the past 25 to 30 years.

1. Skin contains bone marrow-derived cells of the dendritic type (Langerhans cells are the prototype) which capture antigens, process them into immunogenic moieties, and carry this information to draining lymph nodes for the initial activation of naive, antigen-specific T lymphocytes.
2. Exposure of skin to ultraviolet light B results in dramatic changes within cutaneous cells. Among these changes, alterations of cutaneous antigen-presenting cells (APCs), on the one hand, impair the capacity of epicutaneously applied haptens to induce contact hypersensitivity, and, on the other hand, promote the development of immunological tolerance to the hapten in question.
3. Cutaneous APCs are functionally plastic, i.e., they are capable of acquiring different sets of properties that promote or prejudice hapten-specific T cell responses in any of several different directions — Th1, Th2, tolerance, anergy, etc.
4. Keratinocytes contain, or can be encouraged to produce, a wide array of accessory molecules (cytokines, chemokines, cell-adhesion molecules, cell surface signaling molecules) that turn out to be major determinants of the functional properties that cutaneous APC adopt during an immunizing event.
5. Molecules that have the property of being haptens capable of inducing an adaptive immune response usually display irritant properties, and these properties help to define the immunogenic potential of haptens.

We regard these discoveries to be of fundamental importance to our current understanding of CH and ACD, and we believe that these findings are almost universally accepted by scientists working in this field.

III. WHAT DO WE THINK WE KNOW?

In the past few years, many exciting experimental observations have been made in the field of cutaneous immunology and contact hypersensitivity. Some of these findings may be of surpassing importance, but many are controversial and have yet to be fully embraced by the entirety of the scientific community. Nonetheless, it is important to generate this list, since future prospects in research in this area will be heavily influenced by the veracity of these findings.

1. While all agree that CH and ACD are primarily T cell-mediated immune reactivities, evidence is growing rapidly that CD8+ T cells are more important than CD4+ T cells as effectors.[1,2]

2. For universal sensitizers, such as trinitrochlorobenzene, the cutaneous proteins to which these haptens become covalently attached are cleaved by APC into immunogenic fragments that are loaded onto class I and II MHC molecules. Moreover, the haptenic moiety plays a central role in the high affinity with which the peptide/MHC complex is bound by the T cell receptor.[3–5]

3. Cytokines and neuropeptides released from dermal mast cells and from termini of cutaneous C type nerve fibers, respectively, make a major contribution to the cutaneous microenvironment when haptens are applied epicutaneously.[6] Because APCs are functionally plastic and responsive to nuances of their microenvironment, these neuropeptides and cytokines dictate the functional properties of local APCs and the nature of the subsequent immune response of T cells to cutaneous antigens.

4. Polymorphisms at certain genetic loci determine whether exposure of the skin of a given individual to a hapten will lead to the acquisition of CH or not. Examples of loci with important polymorphisms that determine immune responsiveness to haptens include the locus encoding cytochrome P450 (CYP) isoenzyme 2C9 which catalyzes prohaptens into the reactive metabolite,[7] and the *Tnfa* locus where susceptibility alleles rob certain strains of mice of the ability to develop CH when DNFB is painted on UVR-exposed skin.[8–10]

5. The irritant properties of haptens, which were originally thought to be operative largely during CH induction, now appear to be very important in determining the intensity of CH expression when hapten is applied to skin of presensitized individuals.[11,12]

We suspect that more than one of these observations will spawn experiments that will lead to important new insights into the mechanism of CH induction and expression and the pathogenesis of ACD.

IV. WHAT AREAS DO WE NEED TO LEARN MORE ABOUT?

There are many gaps in our knowledge of CH and ACD. Despite the apparent enormity of what has already been learned, much more remains to be learned. The following issues beg for experimental attention and answers.

A. THE ROLE(S) OF DIRECT AND INDIRECT HAPTEN-RECOGNIZING T CELLS IN CONTACT HYPERSENSITIVITY

In certain ways, there are lessons learned from transplantation immunology that are relevant to contact hypersensitivity. It is now well established that two different sets of T cell receptor repertoires recognize transplantation antigens.[13] One set of T cells bears receptors that directly recognize and bind to class I or II alloantigens; this is called the "direct pathway of allorecognition." In the direct pathway of allorecognition, donor-derived antigen-presenting cells (passenger leukocytes) constitutively express class I and II alloantigens and serve as the primary APCs. MHC alloantigens on these cells are recognized by T cells that are present in the normal lymphocyte pool at a very high frequency (compared to T cells that recognize other antigens). Moreover, when cultured in vitro with MHC alloantigenic stimulators, direct alloreactive T cells proliferate and secrete cytokines in a manner usually thought to be characteristic of previously primed cells. This is the basis of the mixed lymphocyte reaction — which only measures the responses of T cells recognizing class I and II alloantigens. The only other T cell recognition system in which a similar high frequency of T cells exists in naive individuals is the hapten system. Since haptens are known to derivatize MHC molecules directly, haptenated self-MHC class I and II molecules resemble MHC alloantigens, and are recognized directly by T cells present in the periphery at a high clonal frequency. We presume that epicutaneous application of hapten activates hapten-specific T cells of the "direct pathway" type.

A different set of T cells bears receptors that recognize alloantigens not as intact proteins, but as peptides loaded onto self-class I or II MHC molecules; this is called the "indirect pathway of allorecognition." In this pathway, alloantigen-specific T cells in normal individuals are present in the peripheral lymphocyte pool at extremely low frequencies (typically <1/100,000 lymphocytes). T cells of this type from naive individuals fail to respond to processed alloantigens in the mixed lymphocyte reaction and only do so if they are retrieved from a donor previously sensitized to the alloantigens in question. Since epicutaneously applied haptens derivatize cutaneous proteins both promiscuously and extensively, it is undoubtedly true that hapten-specific T cells are also activated via the "direct pathway," i.e., T cells that recognize hapten-conjugated peptides processed from cutaneous (epidermal) proteins into small fragments that are loaded on to self-class I and II MHC molecules. In fact, cytotoxic T cells of this type have been amply described in the recent past.[14,15]

In transplantation of solid tissue allografts, T cells of the direct and indirect pathway types differ significantly in their ability to participate in the rejection process, although both prove to be capable in their own right of destroying a graft. Moreover, the susceptibilities of indirect and direct alloreactive T cells to immunosuppression and tolerance induction are also different. Reasoning by analogy, hapten-specific T cells activated through the direct and indirect pathways may also differ in their capacity to effect CH and ACD, as well as their susceptibility to regulation and immunosuppression. It is very important that we learn the extent to which direct and indirect pathway T cells participate in CH and ACD.

B. The Basis for Irritant as Opposed to Immunogenic Properties of Xenobiotics

The relationship between the irritant properties of reactive molecules (such as xenobiotics) and the capacity of these molecules to act as haptens remains obscure. In the recent past, immunologists have paid increasing attention to the interactions that take place between innate immunity and adaptive immunity.[16] The adaptive immune response is an acquired (learned) response in which T and B lymphocytes display unique capacities (1) to recognize foreign molecules (antigens) with receptors of extraordinary diversity and specificity, (2) to distinguish foreign antigens from self-antigens and irrelevant molecules with great accuracy, and (3) to respond to subsequent encounters with the same foreign antigens in an exaggerated and accelerated manner. By contrast, innate immunity is spontaneous and inherent, and utilizes NK cells, macrophages, neutrophils, complement components, etc. to respond to intrusions by microorganisms. Recognition structures on innate immune cells are much less diverse than the receptors for antigen on adaptive immune cells, and these recognition structures are triggered by patterns of molecular species (often repetitive, and often carbohydrates and glycolipids) expressed on invading organisms. Immunologists are gradually appreciating that the success of an adaptive immune response to any particular antigen or pathogen is predicated on the success of the innate immune system to detect and warn of the existence of the pathogen. The concept of "danger" derives from this realization,[17] and the utilization of adjuvants by experimental immunologists attests to the importance of innate immunity in eliciting an adaptive immune response.

While there seems to be general appreciation that irritant properties of xenobiotics are related to their potential immunogenicity, we know very little about whether and to what extent haptens activate the innate immune system.[18] One might postulate that a xenobiotic only passes the threshold to becoming a hapten with the capacity to induce CH when it is able to trigger the activation of cells and molecules of the innate immune system.

C. THE ROLE(S) OF ATYPICAL CLASS I-LIKE MOLECULES IN THE ANTIGEN-PRESENTING FUNCTION OF CUTANEOUS CELLS

The expression of CD1a on Langerhans cells has served since the early 1980s as a singular marker in experimental studies of cutaneous immunology in human beings. In the recent past, CD1 isoforms have emerged as essential elements in immune responses about which we are only beginning to learn the meaning. For example, glycolipids are known to be displayed on CD1d molecules that are expressed on dendritic cells, macrophages, and other cells of bone marrow origin.[19] Subsets of α/β as well as γ/δ T cells display T cell receptors for antigen (Tcr) that specifically recognize glycolipid-bearing CD1 molecules on APC.[20,21] Yet despite the knowledge that CD1 isoforms are expressed on cutaneous APC, the role of γ/δ T cells in CH and ACD remains virtually unexplored. Of course, the discovery of dendritic epidermal T cells in mice more than a decade ago surprised and delighted immunologists.[22,23] However, with the passage of time, incorporation of the function of these cells into the "sense" of cutaneous immunology has not occurred.

Along the same lines, it has recently been discovered that a particular subpopulation of NK T cells (cells with Tcr that almost always contain $V_\alpha 14$) recognizes a glycolipid on CD1 molecules on APC.[24,25] Unexpectedly, recognition of CD1 by NK T cells has been found to be essential when immune privilege is offered to antigens placed in the anterior chamber of the eye. The possibility exists that CD1 molecules on cutaneous APC may signal an innate/adaptive immune response that regulates and inhibits cutaneous immunity. Thus, there may very well be a "yang" for the "yin" of the danger hypotheses, i.e., cells of *the innate immune system*, through recognition of xenobiotics expressed via CD1, *may inhibit, rather than promote*, the ability of the adaptive immune system to detect and respond to cutaneous antigens via contact hypersensitivity. Much more needs to be learned about the role of CD1 and other so-called class Ib molecules in the process by which xenobiotics placed on the skin become (or not) immunogenic haptens.

D. SIMILARITIES AND DIFFERENCES AMONG UNIVERSAL AND NONUNIVERSAL SENSITIZERS

Strong haptens, such as DNCB, TNCB, urushiol, nickel, etc., have been widely studied for their chemical properties and for their biochemical interactions with cells and molecules of the skin. Certain patterns of biochemical reactivity have emerged from these studies, and we think we know the nature of the immunogenicity of these haptens at the molecular level. This knowledge has been gained, in part, because these haptens are universal sensitizers, i.e., when applied epicutaneously in sufficient dosage, virtually everyone becomes contact sensitized. Although much remains to be learned about these types of haptens, it is not completely clear that the rules that have emerged (or that will emerge) from their study can be applied to nonuniversal sensitizers, i.e., molecules that, irrespective of dosage, are only capable of sensitizing a portion (often minor) of the population. In fact, devising experimental animal models for molecules (such as drugs) that sensitize only some individuals of a species has proven to be extremely difficult — some would say, as of yet, "impossible." We need to develop novel strategies to gather information about certain properties of nonuniversal sensitizers: their capacity to act as irritants; their capacity to act as toxins; and their capacity to serve as antigenic moieties that can be recognized by T cells.

E. GENETIC POLYMORPHISMS AND THEIR INFLUENCE ON CONTACT HYPERSENSITIVITY AND ALLERGIC CONTACT DERMATITIS

We are only beginning to appreciate the importance in cutaneous immunology of subtle genetic diversities, known as polymorphisms, among individual human beings. Mention was made above of two types of polymorphisms that have already been implicated in determining whether and what type of immune response will be initiated by epicutaneous application of a xenobiotic. At the moment we have no idea to what extent the nonuniversality of certain contact sensitizers depends upon genetic differences among individuals in a species. The polymorphism of the P450 enzyme described above makes this point dramatically.[7]

A list of staggering length can be generated of gene loci for which potential polymorphisms exist that are relevant to CH and ACD: loci determining metabolic pathways of detoxification, pathways to apoptosis, production of individual cytokines and chemokine, and expression of receptors for individual cytokines, chemokines, and neuropeptides. Evidence defining polymorphisms at loci encoding various cytokines is already present; it is known that there is significant individual variation (genetically determined) in the amount of IFN-γ made during antigenic challenge.[26–28] It may turn out that the degree of heterogeneity among human beings at gene loci pertinent to CH and ACD is enormous, thereby lessening optimism that "silver bullet"-type cures or treatments are even possible.

F. Definition of the Important Details of the Processes of Hapten Sensitization and Expression

The pathway that leads from epicutaneous application of hapten to activation of naive hapten-specific T cells in the draining lymph node has been carefully studied. But by no means is each step in the pathway known, nor is it always clear how one step leads to the next. In many ways, our current knowledge of the sensitization process resembles a map of Europe in which all of the capitol cities are identified, but no motorways are depicted. While the direction one would have to take to get by car from London to Rome is apparent from the map, and one could even identify the cities through which the journey would pass, in the absence of the details and locations of highways, bridges, tunnels, etc., the car's driver would be unable to reach Paris, much less pass the Alps and enter Tuscany. It is this level of detail that is still missing from our "road map" of the induction of CH. Until this "map" is complete, it will be impossible to either reach "Rome," or avoid it if trouble awaits there.

We know even less about the details of elicitation of CH. The recent contribution from Grabbe and Schwartz[12] has considerably advanced our understanding of CH expression, by emphasizing the importance of "irritant" properties of haptens. In a very real sense, this information supports the view that we need to learn much more about the role that innate immunity plays — not only in induction, but also in expression of CH.

Finally, very little is known about the process by which a simple contact hypersensitivity reaction degenerates into allergic contact dermatitis. In general, it has been difficult to generate animal models of chronic immunologic diseases, irrespective of tissue or organ of interest. Research in ACD suffers from the lack of a suitable animal model of chronicity, because only in a chronic model would it be possible to dissect out the factors responsible for turning a self-limited immune response into a self-sustaining one.

V. WHAT WOULD WE REALLY LIKE TO KNOW NEXT?

Because so much remains to be learned about CH and ACD, it is difficult to cull out a few and elevate them to prominence by highlighting them. Yet, creating such a list may help to clarify approaches to future experiments. My list of answer to questions I think would be extremely important follows.

A. Considering the Universe of Molecules in Our Environment, Can We Predict Which Molecules Are Likely to Act as Sensitizing Haptens, Which Are Merely Irritants, and Which Have No Pathologic Potential?

There are many approaches to be taken to answering this question. On the one hand, careful analysis of the chemical properties and biochemical interactions of known haptens and irritants must continue, in the hope that rules will emerge that can allow predictions to be made about new and novel molecules of interest. On the other hand, it is important to continue the development of in vivo and (more pertinent) in vitro assays that distinguish between irritants and haptens. Investigators need to go beyond multicellular responses to chemical irritants and haptens in order to analyze effects within individual cells. A promising approach of this type was recently reported by Kuhn et al.,[29] who demonstrated that contact sensitizers (but not irritants) have the interesting effect of promoting tyrosine phosphorylation within MHC class II positive antigen-presenting cells. While the nature of the phosphorylated proteins remains to be determined, this result indicates that intracellular consequences of exposure of cells to haptens is likely to include up- and downregulation of signaling pathways important in cell function — in this case, among antigen presenting cells.

The generation of in vitro models to assess and distinguish contact sensitizers from irritants at the immune cell level is a very worthy goal. D. Schmitt and colleagues claim to have developed a culture system that enables dendritic cells prepared from peripheral blood to be differentiated in vitro into potent APCs.[30] They then demonstrate that these cells, when interacted with haptens, can activate presumptive hapten-specific T cells, a response that can be quantified in vitro. Whether this approach can be used to distinguish haptens from irritants, or to discriminate weak from strong sensitizers is still an open question.

B. CONSIDERING THAT POTENT HAPTENS POSSESS IRRITANT PROPERTIES, WHAT FACTORS CAN TIP THE BALANCE IN ANY GIVEN INDIVIDUAL, THEREBY DETERMINING WHETHER THE RESULT OF EXPOSURE IS IRRITATION ALONE, CONTACT HYPERSENSITIVITY, OR EVEN CHRONIC ALLERGIC CONTACT DERMATITIS?

The irritant response that is evoked in skin is multifactorial in origin, but especially reliant upon changes in the dermal microvasculature and the recruitment of inflammatory cells from the blood. We would like to know which features of the irritant response are the stepping stones to contact sensitization so that we can work to reduce or eliminate these particular dimensions of the irritant response. Recent attention has been called to quick response elements in the skin, such as mast cells and cutaneous nerves. Undoubtedly, there must be host response genes — perhaps expressed in particular cutaneous cell types (nerves, mast cells, endothelium) — that lead to strong irritant responses in some individuals but not in others. If we knew the identity of these genes and the relationship of the gene product to the irritant reaction, it might be possible to predict which individuals are likely to make an irritant response to a chemical that promotes the eventual emergence of contact hypersensitivity.

C. IF A MOLECULE IS KNOWN TO HAVE CONTACT SENSITIZING CAPACITY, HOW CAN AN IMMUNE RESPONSE TO THAT MOLECULE BE PREVENTED LOCALLY OR SYSTEMICALLY?

Now that it appears that the CH response is dominated by CD8+ T cells, we need to discover whether there might be local maneuvers — within the exposed skin itself — that could be used to circumvent this type of sensitization. Perhaps what has been learned about the ability of acute, low dose ultraviolet B radiation to impair the induction of contact hypersensitivity to universal sensitizers (such as DNCB, TNCB, etc.) can be applied to prevent sensitization by a novel chemical placed on the skin. Some investigators believe that UVR deviates the conventional hapten-specific immune response toward the Th2 direction which is supposed to inhibit, rather than promote, contact hypersensitivity. Another perspective is that UVR damages cutaneous APCs and for a transient interval of time robs the skin of its capacity to promote CH when hapten is applied locally.

D. ARE THERE MANEUVERS OR STRATEGIES THAT CAN PREVENT SYSTEMIC IMMUNITY FROM EMERGING ONCE A HAPTEN HAS BEEN PAINTED EPICUTANEOUSLY?

The literature of immunologic tolerance is rich in models that inhibit immunity, ranging from neonatal exposure to antigens to the tolerance-promoting capacities of certain immunosuppressive drugs. Lessons from the study of cutaneous immunity and tolerance may be helpful in this regard. The systemic immune deficiencies created by exposure to ultraviolet B radiation suggest that mechanisms exist that can control and/or curtail immunity to cutaneous antigens — mechanisms that arise from the effects of UVR on skin itself.

E. MIGHT IT BE POSSIBLE TO PREVENT THE LOCAL CUTANEOUS EXPRESSION OF CONTACT HYPERSENSITIVITY ONCE IT HAS ALREADY BEEN ESTABLISHED SYSTEMICALLY?

It is an immunologic axiom that inhibiting the expression of immunity is fundamentally more difficult than inhibiting its induction. Contact hypersensitivity is no exception to this rule. There is no evidence to suggest that UVR, in either its acute, low dose form or in the high dose form, can suppress preexistent immunity at a systemic level. However, there is some evidence that skin that has been exposed to UVR may display an immune deficit to immune expression for a short interval of time.[31,32] But the evidence in this regard is controversial and mixed.

There are, however, other strategies for suppressing preexisting immunity. For example, oral tolerance, which is achieved by feeding antigens by mouth, inhibits both the induction and the expression of immunity.[33,34] Feeding of an antigen to an individual with preexisting immunity has been found to suppress expression of immunity to that antigen. It remains to be seen whether feeding haptens can suppress presensitization of the contact hypersensitivity type. Another example is anterior chamber-associated immune deviation. In this model system, which is related to the immune privileged nature of the anterior chamber of the eye, injection of hapten-bearing lymphoid cells into the anterior chamber suppresses the induction of contact hypersensitivity.[35] There is good evidence that efferent T suppressor cells are generated in ACAID, and these cells effectively limit the expression of delayed hypersensitivity as well as contact hypersensitivity.

VI. CONCLUSION

Contact hypersensitivity is a complex immune response. As research probes deeper into the cellular and molecular mechanisms that operate in contact hypersensitivity, we seem to be straying further and further from a simplistic explanation. Only a decade ago, we thought that the fundamental elements of contact hypersensitivity induction — hapten, cutaneous antigen-presenting cells, hapten-specific T cells — had been identified, and that manipulation of the response was within our grasp. Now, as we enter the year 2000, we are not at all sure what the *essential* characteristics of a hapten are (in a predictive sense), nor do we know how haptens differ from irritants. We are confronted with more cutaneous APCs than we thought necessary, and we are unsure how each participates. We cannot even be sure of the precise functional phenotype of the hapten-specific T cells that are responsible for effecting contact hypersensitivity. Moreover, we must now (somehow) incorporate dermal mast cells, cutaneous nerves, vascular endothelial cells, and cells of the innate immune system into an overall synthesis. To top it off, we are beginning to understand that genetic differences among human beings influence whether contact hypersensitivity to a given hapten will emerge, whether it will be intense and/or long-lasting, and whether the response will degenerate into a chronic inflammatory skin disease.

In the setting, the prospects are bleak for creation of simple strategies to either prevent sensitization, to promote tolerance, or to suppress preexisting immunity to epicutaneously applied haptens. Immune responses to haptens may be as complex as immune responses to neoantigens expressed by malignant tumor cells or to transplantation antigens encoded by major and minor histocompatibility gene. If that is the case, managing immune responses to individual haptens may require tailored rather than stereotypic strategies of great diversity.

REFERENCES

1. Gocinski BL and Tigelaar RE. Roles of CD4+ and CD8+ T cells in murine contact sensitivity revealed by in vivo monoclonal antibody depletion. *J. Immunol.* 1990, 144: 4121–4128.
2. Bour H, Peyron E, Gaucherand M, Garrigue JL, Desvignes C, Kaiserlian D, Revillard JP, and Nicolas JF. Major histocompatibility complex class I-restricted CD8+ T cells and class II-restricted CD4+ T cells, respectively, mediate and regulate contact sensitivity to dinitrofluorobenzene. *Eur. J. Immunol.* 1995, 25: 3006–3010.
3. Kohler J, Martin S, Pflugfelder U, Ruh H, Vollmer J, and Weltzien HU. Cross-reactive trinitrophenylated peptides as antigens for class II major histocompatibility complex-restricted T cells and inducers of contact sensitivity in mice. Limited T cell receptor repertoire. *Eur. J. Immunol.* 1995, 25: 92–101.
4. Cavani A, Hackett CJ, Wilson KJ, Rothbard JB, and Katz SI. Characterization of epitopes recognized by hapten-specific CD4+ T cells. *J. Immunol.* 1995, 154: 1232–1238.
5. Gelber C, Gemmell L, McAteer D, et al. Down-regulation of poison ivy/oak-induced contact sensitivity by treatment with a class II MHC binding peptide:hapten conjugate. *J. Immunol.* 1997, 158: 2425–2434.
6. Niizeki H, Kurimoto I, and Streilein JW. A substance p agonist acts as an adjuvant to promote hapten-specific skin immunity. *J. Invest. Dermatol.* 1999, 112: 437–442.
7. Anderson C, Hehr A, Robbins R, Hasan R, Athar M, Mukhtar H, and Elmets CA. Metabolic requirements for induction of contact hypersensitivity to immunotoxic polyaromatic hydrocarbons. *J. Immunol.* 1995, 155(7): 3530–3537.
8. Streilein JW and Bergstresser PR. Genetic basis of ultraviolet-B effects on contact hypersensitivity. *Immunogenetics* 1988, 27: 252.
9. Vincek V, Kurimoto I, Medema J-P, Prieto E, and Streilein JW. TNFα polymorphism correlates with deleterious effects of ultraviolet B light on cutaneous immunity. *Cancer Res.* 1993, 53: 728–732..
10. Kurimoto I and Streilein JW. Characterization of the immunogenetic basis of ultraviolet-B light effects on contact hypersensitivity induction. *Immunology* 1994, 81: 352–358.
11. Grabbe S, Steinert M, Mahnke K, Schwarz A, Luger TA, and Schwarz T. Dissection of antigenic and irritative effects of epicutaneously applied haptens in mice. Evidence that not the antigenic component but nonspecific proinflammatory effects of haptens determine the concentration-dependent elicitation of allergic contact dermatitis. *J. Clin. Invest.* 1996, 98: 1158–1164.
12. Grabbe S and Schwarz T. Immunoregulatory mechanisms involved in elicitation of allergic contact hypersensitivity. *Immunol. Today* 1998, 19: 37–44.
13. Watschinger B, Gallon L, Carpenter CB, and Sayegh MH. Mechanisms of allo-recognition. Recognition by in vivo-primed T cells of specific major histocompatibility complex polymorphisms presented as peptides by responder antigen-presenting cells. *Transplantation* 1994, 57(4): 572–576.
14. Shearer GM, Rehn TG, and Garbarino CA. Cell-mediated lympholysis of trinitrophenyl-modified autologous lymphocytes. *J. Exp. Med.* 1975, 141: 1348–1357.
15. Friedman SM, Kuhns J, Irigoyen O, and Chess L. The induction of TNP-altered, self-reactive human cytotoxic T cells by soluble factors: the role of Ia antigens. *J. Immunol.* 1979, 122: 1302–1311.
16. Carroll MC and Prodeus AP. Linkages of innate and adaptive immunity. *Curr. Opin. Immunol.* 1998, 1: 36–40.
17. Matzinger P. Tolerance, danger, and the extended family. *Annu. Rev. Immunol.* 1994, 12: 991–1045.
18. Griem P, Wulferink M, Sachs B, Gonzalez JB, and Gleichman E. Allergic and autoimmune reactions to xenobiotics: how do they arise? *Immunol. Today,* 1998, 19(3): 133–141.
19. Zeng Z, Castano AR, Segelke BW, Stura EA, Peterson PA, and Wilson IA. Crystal structure of mouse CD1: an MHC-like fold with a large hydrophobic binding groove. *Science* 1997, 277(5324): 339–345.
20. Beckman EM, Porcelli SA, Morita CT, Behar SM, Furlong ST, Brenner MB. Recognition of a lipid antigen by CD1-restricted alpha beta+ T. *Nature* 1994, 372 (6507): 691–694.

21. Sugita M, Moody DB, Jackman RM, Grant EP, Rosat JP, Behar SM, Peters PJ, Porcelli SA, and Brenner MB. CD1 — a new paradigm for antigen presentation and T cell activation. *Clin. Immunol. Immunopathol.* 1998, 87: 8–14.

22. Bergstresser PR, Tigelaar RE, Dees JH, and Streilein JW. Thy-1 antigen-bearing dendritic cells populate murine epidermis. *J. Invest. Dermatol.* 1983, 81(3): 286–268.

23. Tschachler E, Schuler G, Hutterer J, Leibl H, Wolff K, and Stingl G. Expression of Thy-1 antigen by murine epidermal cells. *J. Invest. Dermatol.* 1983, 81(3): 282–285.

24. Burdin N, Brossay L, Koezuka Y, Smiley ST, Grushy MJ, Gui M, Taniguchi M, Hayakawa K, and Kronenberg M. Selective ability of mouse CD1 to present glycolipids: alpha-galactosylceramide specifically stimulates V alpha 14+ NK T lymphocytes. *J. Immunol.* 1998, 161(7): 3271–3281.

25. Kawano T, Cui J, Koezuka Y, Toura I, Kaneko Y, Motoki K, Ueno H, Nakagawa R, Sato H, Kondo E, Koseki H, and Taniguchi M. CD1d-restricted and TCR-mediated activation of Valpha14 NKT cells by glycosylceramides. *Science* 1997, 278(5343): 1626–1629..

26. Cork MJ, Crane AM, and Duff GW. Genetic control of cytokines. Cytokine gene polymorphisms in alopecia areata. *Dermatol. Clin.* 1996, (4): 671–678.

27. Turner D, Grant SC, Yonan N, Sheldon S, Dyer PA, Sinnott PJ, and Hutchinson IV. Cytokine gene polymorphism and heart transplant rejection. *Transplantation* 1997, 64(5): 776–779.

28. Hutchinson IV, and Pravica V, Perrey C, and Sinnott P. Cytokine gene polymorphisms and relevance to forms of rejection. *Transplant. Proc.* 1999, 31(1–2): 734–736.

29. Kuhn U, Brand P, Willemsen J, Jonuleit H, Enk AH, Brandwijk-Petershans R, Saloga J, Knop J, and Becker D. Induction of tyrosine phosphorylation in human MHC class II-positive antigen-presenting cells by stimulation with contact sensitizers. *J. Immunol.* 1998, 160(2): 667–673.

30. Rougier N, Redziniak G, Schmitt D, Vincent C. Evaluation of the capacity of dendritic cells derived from cord blood CD34+ precursors to present haptens to unsensitized autologous T cells in vitro. *J Invest Dermatol.* 1998, 110(4): 348–352.

31. Kripke ML. Immunological unresponsiveness induced by ultraviolet radiation. *Immunol. Rev.* 1984, 80: 87–102.

32. Tie C, Golomb C, Taylor JR, and Streilein JW. Suppressive and enhancing effects of ultraviolet B radiation on expression of contact hypersensitivity in man. *J. Invest. Dermatol.* 1995, 104(1): 18–22..

33. Garcia G and Weiner HL. Manipulation of Th responses by oral tolerance. *Curr. Top. Microbiol. Immunol.* 1999, 238: 123–145.

34. Friedman A, al-Sabbagh A, Santos LM, Fishman-Lobell J, Polanski M, Das MP, Khoury SJ, and Weiner HL. Oral tolerance: a biologically relevant pathway to generate peripheral tolerance against external and self antigens. *Chem. Immunol.* 1994, 58: 259–290.

35. Waldrep JC and Kaplan HJ. Anterior chamber associated immune deviation induced by TNP-spleno-cytes (TNP-ACAID). I. Systemic tolerance mediated by suppressor T-cells. *Invest. Opthalmol. Vis. Sci.* 1983, 8: 1086–1092.

Index

A